Hearing Science

Hearing Science

Diana C. Emanuel, PhD, CCC-A
Professor and Audiology Graduate Program Director
Audiology, Speech–Language Pathology, and Deaf Studies
Towson University
Towson, Maryland

Tomasz Letowski PhD, ScD
Senior Research Scientist
Human Factors and Engineering Directorate
U.S. Army Research Laboratory
United States Army
Aberdeen Proving Ground, Maryland

Wolters Kluwer Health | Lippincott Williams & Wilkins
Philadelphia • Baltimore • New York • London
Buenos Aires • Hong Kong • Sydney • Tokyo

Acquisitions Editor: Peter Sabatini
Managing Editor: Andrea Klingler
Marketing Manager: Alison Noplock
Production Editor: Eve Malakoff-Klein
Designer: Doug Smock
Compositor: International Typesetting and Composition
Printer: Data Reproductions Corporation

351 West Camden Street
Baltimore, MD 21201

530 Walnut Street
Philadelphia, PA 19106

Printed in the United States

9 8 7 6 5 4 3 2 1

Library of Congress Cataloging-in-Publication Data

Emanuel, Diana C.
Hearing science / Diana C. Emanuel, Tomasz Letowski.—1st ed.
p. ; cm.
Includes bibliographical references and index.
ISBN-13: 978-0-7817-8047-6
ISBN-10: 0-7817-8047-0
1. Hearing. 2. Hearing disorders.
[DNLM: 1. Hearing. 2. Hearing Disorders. WV 270 E52h 2009] I. Letowski, Tomasz. II. Title.
QP461.E46 2009
612.8'95—dc22

2007025944

DISCLAIMER

Care has been taken to confirm the accuracy of the information present and to describe generally accepted practices. However, the authors, editors, and publisher are not responsible for errors or omissions or for any consequences from application of the information in this book and make no warranty, expressed or implied, with respect to the currency, completeness, or accuracy of the contents of the publication. Application of this information in a particular situation remains the professional responsibility of the practitioner; the clinical treatments described and recommended may not be considered absolute and universal recommendations.

The authors, editors, and publisher have exerted every effort to ensure that drug selection and dosage set forth in this text are in accordance with the current recommendations and practice at the time of publication. However, in view of ongoing research, changes in government regulations, and the constant flow of information relating to drug therapy and drug reactions, the reader is urged to check the package insert for each drug for any change in indications and dosage and for added warnings and precautions. This is particularly important when the recommended agent is a new or infrequently employed drug.

Some drugs and medical devices presented in this publication have Food and Drug Administration (FDA) clearance for limited use in restricted research settings. It is the responsibility of the health care provider to ascertain the FDA status of each drug or device planned for use in their clinical practice.

To purchase additional copies of this book, call our customer service department at **(800) 638-3030** or fax orders to **(301) 223-2320.** International customers should call **(301) 223-2300.**

Visit Lippincott Williams & Wilkins on the Internet: http://www.lww.com. Lippincott Williams & Wilkins customer service representatives are available from 8:30 am to 6:00 pm, EST.

With love and appreciation to my husband, Peter; my daughter, Isabel; my son, Devon Benjamin; my parents, Jeremy and Rosalind Wright; and my hearing science teachers, Dr. Barbara Laufer, Dr. Tom Frank, and Dr. Tomasz Letowski.
DCE

To my parents, Prakseda and Henryk; my wife, Anna; and my sons, Szymon and Jan, who all in various ways helped make this book a reality.
TRL

Preface

Hearing science encompasses all physiologic, physical, psychological, and technical phenomena related to normal aspects of sound perception, including the creation and transmission of auditory signals. It is a multidisciplinary field formed by the combination of many different topic areas. To study hearing science is to learn various aspects of mathematics, physics, biology, psychology, and engineering without becoming a mathematician, physicist, biologist, psychologist, or engineer. In a hearing science course, topics from these disciplines are generally structured into three main subject areas: *anatomy and physiology* of the ear, physical *acoustics* (the study of the physical properties of sound), and *psychoacoustics* (the study of human response to sound), with some audio signal transmission, measurement, and reproduction issues covered at the end of the course. Hearing science, however, is more than just the combination of these topics areas. Although it requires a foundation in many areas of scientific knowledge, hearing science is a unique science focused on human interactions in the world of sound. At the heart of the discipline is an understanding that the ability to hear connects us with the natural world and, most importantly, with our fellow human beings. The vast majority of people communicate via spoken language and music. To understand this communication at its basic level, one must begin with a study of how sound is created, how it travels from the sound source to the ear, how it travels through the auditory (hearing) system from the external part of the ear that we can see all the way to the brain, and how the sound is perceived by the listener once it reaches the brain. Sounds are received, interpreted, evaluated as esthetically pleasing or unpleasant, and used as a means of expression for our thoughts and feelings. Last but not least, sounds have a profound effect on our behavior, health, and ability to function as a community.

The term *sound* can be described in two different ways. An *acoustician*, someone who studies the physical properties of sound, would define sound as a mechanical disturbance propagating through the environment. A *psychoacoustician*, someone who studies human response to sound, would define sound as our awareness of a stimulus received by the auditory system. These two definitions are fundamentally different; building a bridge between them is the main challenge of hearing science. Acoustics defines sound based on a physical phenomenon that exists in nature without the need for our awareness of it (i.e., without the need for a listener). Psychoacoustics defines sound based on the perception of sound by a listener.

Students of hearing science come from varied backgrounds. Some students are returning adults with math and science classes taken many years before the study of hearing science. Some students have a fear of mathematics and others have always identified themselves as "weak in math" due to difficulties in early mathematics courses. Some students found hearing science through disciplines such as psychology and speech-language pathology, where the emphasis was on human interaction and not on mathematics and physics. Others simply have not reviewed the basic foundation skills since they prepared for the SAT examination. It is possible for hearing science students to seek out algebra, geometry, trigonometry, and physics textbooks to prepare for hearing science, but this is an extraordinarily time-consuming task with an overwhelming amount of reading, most of which is not immediately necessary for the study of hearing science. This textbook is designed to provide a guide through the fascinating subject of hearing science, with an emphasis on problem solving as a means to provide feedback to the reader regarding his or her understanding of the material each step of the way.

Organization

The book is divided into four parts: Foundation Skills, Acoustics, Hearing, and Audio Systems. Part I, Foundation Skills (with contributions from Szymon Letowski), reviews a limited number of concepts in mathematics and physics that are needed to study the other topic areas in the text. This portion of the book was written in response to years of requests from hearing science students for a textbook that reviews basic problem-solving skills necessary for hearing and speech science, before the actual hearing science content is taught. Students who approach chapters labeled "mathematics" and "physics" with a certain amount of fear should find these chapters written at a level that is helpful rather than terrifying. After the explanation of each concept, practice problems are provided to allow students to apply the concepts to problem solving and check their level of understanding. The companion student website provides step-by-step solutions to the practice problems and supplemental material to enhance learning. Readers with a strong mathematics and physics background should be able to skip Chapters 1 and 2 or to select specific sections to review based on their knowledge base. Likewise, professors can tailor reading assignments within these two chapters to the level of mathematics used in their specific course. The companion website also includes some further elaboration on selected topics included in the written text for those readers who are interested in expanding their knowledge slightly beyond the material offered by the text.

Part II, Acoustics, provides the bulk of material taught in many hearing science courses. The chapters begin with a simple review of mechanical vibration using straightforward models (pendulum, mass and spring) to study how things move. The concepts become progressively more complex as the topics of complex vibrating systems, the nature of sound waves, sound propagation, and the decibel are covered in detail. The more advanced concept of impedance, which is usually explained at the end of a hearing science course, is integrated into the book in four places: first, as it relates to mechanic systems; second, as it relates to acoustic systems; third, as it relates to the physiology of the ear; and fourth, as it is used in audio systems. The concept of the decibel, covered in Chapter 7 (written with Szymon Letowski), requires quite a lot of problem solving to truly understand its range of applications; however, it should be a very approachable topic for students who have reviewed the mathematics chapter. It begins with the concept of the decibel and takes students step by step through decibel problem solving, using the same format as that in the mathematics chapter.

Part III, Hearing, covers the anatomy and physiology of the outer, middle, and inner ears and the central auditory nervous system; the conduction of sound via bone conduction; and psychoacoustics. Concepts from the acoustic section of the book are re-emphasized as they apply to the auditory system throughout this section of the textbook. Chapter 10 (written with Laurie Williams-Hogarth) discusses the central auditory nervous system and provides an overview not only of the central auditory nevous system, but also of the important parts of the overall central nervous system, so students are not just studying the isolated pathway of the auditory nervous system in a vacuum. Chapter 12, the final chapter of this section, focuses on psychoacoustics, the study of human response to sound. The chapter covers responses of the auditory system to a number of physical dimensions and various psychological phenomena, including spatial perception of sound.

Part IV, Audio Systems, covers more technical topics related to hearing science, divided into three chapters: Electricity and Electric Circuits (Chapter 13, written with Stephen Pallett), Audio Signals and Devices (Chapter 14), and Digital Signal Processing (Chapter 15). For students who have always wanted to know more about how sound is processed in audio systems, computers, CD players, hearing aids, and so forth, these chapters provide an introduction to basic electronics and the way sound is transferred back and forth between its acoustic form and electric (audio) form.

This book begins at an easy level and gradually increases in difficulty with each chapter. Each chapter expands and integrates information from the preceding chapters and refers back to them when needed. The bulk of the text is written at an intermediate difficulty level, although some more difficult topics should probably be read more than once. For example, topics such as impedance are quite challenging to grasp the first time they are presented; however, this information is critical to the understanding of hearing science.

Features

Each chapter begins with a list of **Objectives** that provide a highlight of the main ideas presented in the chapter. A list of **Key Terms** is also included. These terms are bolded within the text. Because multiple terms are used by people working in different areas to describe the same concept, we have tried to include the most common of these terms to make an easy transition between this book and others. In some cases, multiple spellings are acceptable for various terms (e.g., sound field vs. soundfield and ear muff vs. earmuff). We have selected what we have found to be the most common spelling, although instructors may wish to point out alternate spellings as they work through the material. **Examples** show the reader how to work through problems related to each major concept, and then **Practice Problems** at the end of each main section allow students to try to apply the concepts themselves. A **Summary** and a list of **Key Points** end each chapter and provide a review of the main concepts.

Links are included online to provide help in understanding basic concepts, to provide more information on a topic, or to help students work through the text's practice problems step by step. Links are called out in the text with an icon ( ). Four chapters also include online **Audio Clips** illustrating examples of sounds, which are called out in the text with an icon ( ). Four of these chapters are duplicated online in text format, so students can access the audio clips while reading the chapter. The website also includes a **Quiz** for each chapter and **Labeling Exercises** of anatomic illustrations to give students extra practice. In addition, instructors have online access to video clips of possible classroom demonstrations, homework suggestions for each chapter, the answers to the online quizzes, a Test Bank, PowerPoint lecture outlines, and an Image Bank. It was our intention to create a package that may be appealing to all students regardless of their initial level of knowledge and to all hearing science instructors regardless of the specific focus of their hearing science course.

Many scientific books, textbooks, and brochures are available in bookstores and libraries that cover sound, acoustics, and auditory perception. None of these books, however, covers with uniform stress all the topic areas of hearing science with a focus on teaching the phenomena rather than just presenting information. Students have varying abilities and different strengths and weaknesses, and it is crucial that all these different abilities are addressed by a single textbook. Our intention was to write a book with a focus on the systematic explanation of both fundamental and advanced concepts, thereby providing a comprehensive look at the many different areas that contribute to a good understanding of hearing science.

Diana C. Emanuel
Tomasz Letowski

Acknowledgements

Writing a book is an adventure. To begin with, it is a toy and an amusement; then it becomes a mistress, and then it becomes a master, and then a tyrant. The last phase is that just as you are about to be reconciled to your servitude, you kill the monster, and fling him out to the public.

—Winston Churchill

It cannot be said any better. Writing this book was an arduous journey, sometimes joyful and sometimes torturous, but it would never have been completed without the support of many people. First and foremost, we are very thankful to our contributing authors Szymon Letowski, Dr. Laurie Williams-Hogarth, and Dr. Stephen Pallett for their contributions, discussions, and steadfast support that they gave to the project. We would like to acknowledge the critical review and supportive comments of our colleagues who conducted the formal review of the manuscript. We are also very thankful to our colleagues Dr. Dana Boatman, Dr. Margaret Jastreboff, Dr. Powell Jastreboff, Dr. Peggy Korczak, Dr. Alex Storrs, and Mr. Pete Liiva, who provided advice and informally reviewed pieces of the book along the way. We both take full responsibility for all the errors and mistakes that may be still left in the book, but their number would be much higher without the help of doctoral students Harmony Evans, Megan Glascock, Rebecca Book, and Mary Carson, who spent many hours on various mundane tasks with us and provided priceless feedback regarding the clarity and integrity of the text.

Contributors

Szymon Letowski, BS
Knowledge Engineer
Evidence Based Research, Inc.
Vienna, Virginia

Stephen Pallett, AuD
Clinical Faculty
Department of Audiology, Speech-Language Pathology, and Deaf Studies
Towson University
Towson, Maryland

Laurie Williams-Hogarth, PhD
Senior Lecturer
Biological Sciences
Towson University
Towson, Maryland

Reviewers

Connie Barker, PhD
Department of Communication Disorders and Deaf Education
Lamar University Speech and Hearing Clinic
Beaumont, Texas

Deborah Culbertson, PhD, Audiology
Clinical Associate Professor
Communication Sciences and Disorders
East Carolina University
Greenville, North Carolina

Jackie M. Davie, PhD
Assistant Professor
Department of Audiology and Speech Pathology
Bloomsburg University
Bloomsburg, PA

Tom Frank, PhD
Professor of Audiology
Communication Disorders
The Pennsylvania State University
University Park, PA

Paula P. Henry, PhD
Research Audiologist
Army Research Laboratory
Aberdeen Proving Ground, MD

James Lynn, PhD
Dean
College of Fine and Applied Arts
The University of Akron
Akron, Ohio

Robert Oyler, PhD
Auditory Habilitation Specialist
Chattering Children McLean, VA

John P. Preece, PhD
Professor of Communication Sciences
Hunter College
and
Professor of Audiology
The Graduate Center—City University of New York
New York, New York

Tracie Rice, AuD
Visiting Assistant Professor
Human Services
Western Carolina University
Cullowhee, North Carolina

Barbara Snelling, MBA, AuD
Communication Sciences and Disorders
University of Houston
Houston, Texas

Carmen Taylor, PhD
Associate Professor
Communicative Disorders
The University of Alabama
Tuscaloosa, Alabama

Contents

PART I

Foundation Skills

Chapter Outline

CHAPTER 1

Mathematics

Diana C. Emanuel, Tomasz Letowski, and Szymon T. Letowski

Objectives

- To review basic algebra including order of operations and solving for *x*
- To review basic geometry including angles and the Pythagorean Theorem
- To review basic trigonometry including sine, cosine, and tangent functions
- To provide students with opportunities to practice basic algebra, geometry, and trigonometry prior to their application in hearing science
- To review polar and Cartesian coordinate systems and the method for converting between these two systems

Key Terms

Adjacent side
Algebra
Angle
Arithmetic
Azimuth
Base
Calculus
Cartesian coordinates (rectangular coordinates)
Circumference
Constant
Coordinates
Cylindrical coordinates
Diameter
Equation
Function
Geometry
Hypotenuse
Integer
Logarithm (exponent, power)
Opposite side
Order of operations
Origin
Orthogonal
Phase angle
Pythagorean Theorem
Polar coordinate system
Radian
Radius
Right triangle
Scientific notation
Simplification
Slope
Solving for *x*
Steps to solving equations
Substitution
Symbol
Trigonometry
Variable
y-intercept

Students entering hearing science class have a variety of experiences with mathematics. This chapter offers a tutorial for students with weak to moderate math skills, a review of concepts for students with good but "rusty" math skills, and a teaching guide for students with excellent math skills who wish to assist other students. This chapter will review the fundamental aspects of four areas of mathematics: arithmetic (the study of numbers), algebra (the study of relationships between numbers and the use of variables in equation solving), geometry (the study of points, lines, angles, surfaces, and shapes), and trigonometry (the study of triangles). Since each of these topics can easily serve as the subject for an entire textbook, this chapter is not intended as a comprehensive treatment of the material; rather, it presents only those key aspects of each topic that are needed to begin the study of hearing science. You will need a scientific calculator to do the problems in this chapter. A scientific calculator contains logarithm keys (log, 10^x) and trigonometry keys (sin, cos, tan). The calculator does not have to be an expensive "bells and whistles" calculator with graphing functions. An inexpensive scientific calculator is fine and can be purchased online, in your college bookstore, or in just about any store that sells school supplies.

Box 1.1 Steps to Solving Equations

Substitute

Substitute real numbers for variables when possible. A **variable** is a letter or symbol representing an unknown number.

Simplify

Simplify both sides of the equation using the Order of Operations (PEMDAS). All operations within the same step are done from left to right:

- Parentheses
- Exponentiation
- Multiplication and division
- Addition and subtraction

Solve for *x*

Solve for *x* (or any other variable) by isolating *x*. In other words, *x* should be by itself on one side of the equation. To do this, use the **reverse of the Order of Operations** to remove unwanted information from the variable side of the equation. Instead of PEMDAS you would use SADMEP.

- Subtraction and addition
- Division and multiplication
- Exponentiation
- Parentheses

ARITHMETIC AND ALGEBRA

The mathematical concepts and problems presented in this book begin at a basic level and increase gradually in difficulty. First, a solid grasp of basic arithmetic concepts including whole numbers (cardinal numbers), positive and negative numbers, and rational numbers (fractions) is needed. These concepts are familiar to most students and are provided online for students who need a review. **Link 1-1 and 1-2**

Second, a clear understanding of the principle of the Order of Operations is required to be able to apply it effectively to any type of problem. These two concepts form the basis for the process of solving equations, which in turn is the foundation for all problem solving. An **equation** is a statement asserting the equality of two quantities. Every equation is made up of two strings of numbers and/or symbols that are connected by an equals ("=") sign. Equations can be simple, like $x = 4$, or complex, like $7x^3 = [(x + 3)^2 - 7](x^2 - 1)$. They may include unknown **variables** (e.g., x), **constants** (numbers), and **symbols** for mathematical operations (e.g., +).

Steps to Solving Equations

To solve an equation means to rewrite it so that one side of the equation ends up being just the unknown variable and the other side being a number, as in $x = 4$. This process involves the following three steps: substitution, simplification, and solving for *x*. These steps are highlighted in Box 1.1.

Substitution and Simplification

The first step in solving an equation is substitution. **Substitution** is the act of replacing something with something else. In mathematics, this means putting a known value or another equation in the place of an unknown variable. For example, if you need to solve the equation $x = 4 + b$ and you know that $b = 5$, you would substitute 5 for *b* in the equation and quickly find that $x = 9$.

The second step in equation solving is simplification. Fundamental to solving any equation is the process of **simplification**, which is the step-by-step process for making an equation progressively simpler. This process is described by a sequence known as the **Order of Operations.** The Order of Operations tells us which mathematical operations in an equation to do first. An equation is considered simplified when all the operations in it have been applied. The Order of Operations is listed below.

Order of Operations

1. Operations within parentheses
2. Exponential (logarithmic) operations
3. Multiplication or division
4. Addition or subtraction

Box 1.2 PEMDAS

The Order of Operations is often remembered using the sentence "Please Excuse My Dear Aunt Sally" or the acronym PEMDAS for Parentheses, Exponents, Multiplication, Division, Addition, and Subtraction.

Example 1.1

Consider the equation $x = 45 + 7 \times (45 + 2) + 10^2$. This equation involves parentheses, an exponent, multiplication, and addition. It cannot be solved by beginning with the first 45 and proceeding from left to right. It must be solved in the specific order dictated by the Order of Operations.

First, consider operations within parentheses:

$$x = 45 + 7 \times \underline{(45 + 2)} + 10^2$$

Second, consider exponents:

$$x = 45 + 7 \times 47 + \underline{10^2}$$

Third, multiplication:

$$x = 45 + \underline{7 \times 47} + 100$$

Fourth, addition:

$$x = \underline{45 + 329 + 100}$$

$$x = 474$$

Answer: $x = 474$

If you need to practice solving problems to master the Order of Operations, complete the practice problems that follow. If your answers do not agree with the answers provided, step-by-step solutions are provided online.

PRACTICE PROBLEM: SIMPLIFICATION

Solve for *x:*

1. $x = 8 \times 16 + 4$
2. $x = 68 + 8 \times (32 + 1) + 10(5)$
3. $x = 45 \times 16 + \frac{21}{3} + 1$
4. $x = (34 + 23 \times 7) - 18(4) + \frac{4}{2}$

Answers (If you need help with these problems, consult the website.) **Link 1-3**

1. $x = 132$
2. $x = 382$
3. $x = 728$
4. $x = 125$

Solving for x

The third step in equation solving is called **solving for x.** *X* is actually a generic term for any variable that is unknown, so in some cases instead of *x* you may see another letter or symbol such as f, I, θ, λ, and so forth. In Example 1.1, *x* was alone on one side of the equation. For most problems, this will not be the way the equation will initially appear. Thus, before the equation can be solved, it must first be manipulated to isolate the *x* on one side. In the process of doing this, you should follow the **Steps to Solving Equations** regardless of the complexity of the equation.

Example 1.2

$x + 2 = 14$ Solve for *x*

To isolate *x* on one side of the equation, simply subtract 2 from both sides.

$$x + 2 \underline{- 2} = 14 \underline{- 2}$$

$$x = 12$$

To check your work, you can substitute the answer you found into the original equation and make sure both sides of the equation are equal, as shown below. Although this is an easy example, you may find this process of working backwards a useful way to check your work for more complex problems. The original equation was:

$$x + 2 = 14$$

Substitute the answer you found (12) for the variable *x*.

$$12 + 2 = 14$$

$$14 = 14$$

Since both sides are equal, you have confirmed that the answer you found, $x = 12$, was correct.

Most students are comfortable solving problems involving only addition and subtraction, so we will begin our review with multiplication and division. If you need further help with beginning equation solving and practice with addition and subtraction, see the website. **Link 1-4**

In the following few sections, we will introduce the mathematical operations in reverse order to the Order of Operations, beginning with the easier topics of multiplication and division and working our way to the more complex topic of exponents/logarithms.

Multiplication and Division

The operations of multiplication and division can be expressed in a number of ways. These are presented below and you should be familiar with all of them. Do not confuse × (meaning multiplication) with the variable *x*, which is written as an italicized letter.

Multiplication	Division
$4 \cdot 3 = 12$	$12 \div 3 = 4$
$4 \times 3 = 12$	$12/3 = 4$
$4(3) = 12$	$\frac{12}{3} = 4$
$4y = 12$, where $y = 3$	

The next two examples demonstrate the use of the steps to solving equations for problems involving multiplication, division, addition, and subtraction. Review these examples and complete the problems provided at the end of the section.

Example 1.3

$$x \times 13 = 4(y) + 5r$$

Solve for x where $y = 10$ and $r = 17$

First, substitute the values of all known variables. Recall that $4(y)$ and $5r$ both express multiplication (i.e., 4 multiplied by y and 5 multiplied by r). We know that $y = 10$ and $r = 17$, so after substituting the equation looks like:

$$x \times 13 = 4 \times 10 + 5 \times 17$$

Simplify. Remember to follow the Order of Operations (PEMDAS). First, do the multiplication and then the addition.

$$x \times 13 = \underline{4 \times 10} + \underline{5 \times 17}$$

$$x \times 13 = \underline{40 + 85}$$

$$x \times 13 = 125$$

Solve for x. The left side contains $x \times 13$, so we need to remove the 13. Divide both sides of the equation by 13.

$$\frac{\{x \times 13\}}{13} = \frac{\{125\}}{13}$$

Based on the Fundamental Rule of Fractions (see **Link 1-2**), 13 can be removed (cancelled) from the numerator and denominator of the left fraction.

$$\frac{x \times 13}{13} = \frac{125}{13}$$

$$x = \frac{125}{13}$$

$$x = 9.6153846154$$

Answer: 9.62

Notice that the answer to Example 1.3 was rounded, so instead of reporting the answer as 9.6153846154 with as many digits as your calculator can display, the answer was rounded to 9.62. The number of decimal places you choose to report will affect the precision (accuracy) of your answer. For example, using four decimal places is more precise than using only one. In this book, we will generally round the *final* answer to two decimal places, but keep a larger number of decimal places during the problem-solving stages to decrease the probability of rounding error and to more closely approximate the numbers you will see on your calculator as you work through the problems. If you are not familiar with the rules of rounding, rounding error, or estimation, see the website. **Link 1-5**

In hearing science, numbers that are in fraction form (such as $p = 1/500$) are usually converted into their decimal equivalent (i.e., $p = 1/500 = 0.002$) before the values are substituted into the equation. This avoids having to perform operations on fractions, which often necessitates the calculation of a common denominator. In some cases, however, it is necessary to manipulate fractions, as seen in the next example.

Example 1.4

$$p \times \lambda = d \times s/f - 3$$

Solve for f where $p = 0.001$,
$\lambda = 27440$, $s = 343$, and $d = 80$

First, substitute the values of all known variables. Here p, λ, s, and d are known.

$$0.001 \times 27440 = 80 \times \frac{343}{f} - 3$$

Next, simplify the equation. Remember to follow the Order of Operations (PEMDAS). First, complete the multiplication on the left side of the equation.

$$27.44 = 80 \times \frac{343}{f} - 3$$

Next, complete the multiplication on the right side of the equation. Multiplication and division are on the same order of operations, which is why 80 and 343 can be multiplied even though 343 is divided by f.

$$27.44 = \frac{27440}{f} - 3$$

Solve for f using the reverse Order of Operations (SADMEP). First, add 3 to both sides.

$$\{27.44\} + 3 = \left\{\frac{27440}{f} - 3\right\} + 3$$

$$30.44 = \frac{27440}{f}$$

Next, use cross-multiplication. If you are not familiar with cross-multiplication, see the website. **Link 1-6**

$$\frac{30.44}{1} = \frac{27440}{f}$$

$$30.44 \times f = 27440 \times 1$$

Solve for f by dividing each side of the equation by 30.44.

$$\frac{30.44 \times f}{30.44} = \frac{27440}{30.44}$$

The removal of 30.44 from both the numerator and denominator of the left side of the equation is based on the Fundamental Rule of Fractions.

$$f = \frac{27440}{30.44}$$

$$f = 901.445$$

Answer: 901.45

PRACTICE PROBLEMS: MULTIPLICATION AND DIVISION

Solve for the unknown variable.

1. $x = 1/y$ Solve for x where $y = 4/3$
2. $8 \div \frac{1}{3} = 3 - x$ Solve for x
3. $\frac{1}{x} = 0.125$ Solve for x
4. $\frac{32}{4x} = 100$ Solve for x
5. $\frac{3x}{47} = 64$ Solve for x
6. $\lambda = \frac{s}{f}$ Solve for f where $\lambda = 1.2$ and $s = 343$
7. $\frac{y}{7} = 3$ Solve for y
8. $p = \frac{1}{f}$ Solve for f where $p = 0.002$
9. $\frac{42}{x} + 7 - 4 + C = 5$ Solve for x where $C = 3$
10. $p - y = d \times \frac{f}{t} + q$ Solve for q where $y = -3$, $d = 5.7, f = -2, p = 7,$ and $t = 1/3$.
11. $\frac{42}{x} + 7 - 4 + C \times D = 5$ Solve for x where $C = 43$

Answers (If you need help with these problems, consult the website.) **Link 1-7**

1. $x = \frac{3}{4}$ or $x = 0.75$
2. $x = -21$
3. $x = 8$
4. $x = \frac{2}{25}$ or $x = 0.08$
5. $x = \frac{3008}{3}$ or $x = 1002.67$
6. $f = 285.83$
7. $y = 21$
8. $f = 500$
9. $x = -42$
10. $q = 44.2$
11. $x = \frac{42}{2 - 43D}$

Box 1.3 Ready for More?

If you are doing well, congratulations: You have most of the basic skills you need at this point to move on to more advanced problem solving. If you are struggling, go back and review the previous sections before proceeding or ask your professor for a recommendation for a basic algebra textbook.

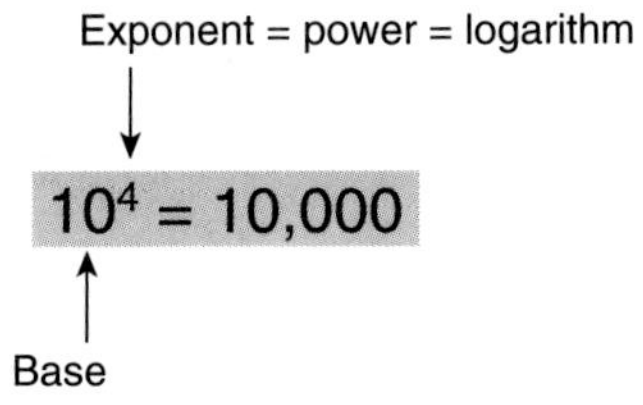

Figure 1.1. The base 10 raised to the fourth power is equal to 10,000. A power is also called an exponent or a logarithm (log).

Exponents

An **exponent** represents the number of times a **base** number is multiplied by itself. In Figure 1.1, the base is 10 and the exponent is 4. Both the base and the exponent can be any number. If the exponent is positive (greater than 0), we multiply the base by itself that many times. In Figure 1.1, the base 10 is multiplied four times. In other words: $10^4 = 10 \times 10 \times 10 \times 10 = 10{,}000$. When a base number has an exponent, we say that the number is **raised to a power.** In Figure 1.1, the mathematical expression would be read: "ten raised to the fourth power" or "ten to the fourth power" or just "ten to the fourth." If the exponent is 2, then we just say "squared," so if the base is 5 and the exponent is 2, we say "five squared" rather than "five to the second." Table 1.1 lists some powers of 5 and their equivalents written without an exponent.

If the exponent is equal to 0, then the result is *always* 1: for example, $10^0 = 1$, $7^0 = 1$, and $(0.2)^0 = 1$. If the exponent is negative (less than 0), we first calculate the product as if the exponent were positive, and then we divide 1 by that product. So, to find 10^{-3}, we start by calculating $10^3 = 10 \times 10 \times 10 = 1000$, and then we divide $1/1000 = 0.001$. Thus, $10^{-3} = 0.001$.

Table 1.1. Some Powers of 5

5^{-4}	5^{-3}	5^{-2}	5^{-1}	5^0	5^1	5^2	5^3	5^4
$\frac{1}{5^4} =$	$\frac{1}{5^3} =$	$\frac{1}{5^2} =$	$\frac{1}{5^1} =$					
$\frac{1}{625} =$	$\frac{1}{125} =$	$\frac{1}{25} =$	$\frac{1}{5} =$					
0.0016	0.008	0.04	0.2	1	5	25	125	625

An **integer** is a positive or negative whole number or zero (i.e., −1, 0, 1, 2); in other words, an integer is a number without decimals. When a base is raised to an integer power, it is quite easy to calculate. It is especially easy (and very important) to be able to quickly calculate the powers of 10. Looking at the sequence of powers below, it should be no problem to discern a clear and predictable pattern.

$10^0 = 1$ (exponent = 0, no zeros in result)
$10^1 = 10$ (exponent = 1, 1 zero in result)
$10^2 = 10 \times 10 = 100$ (exponent = 2, 2 zeros in result)
$10^3 = 10 \times 10 \times 10 = 1000$
$10^4 = 10 \times 10 \times 10 \times 10 = 10{,}000$

If the exponent is a negative whole number, a predictable pattern is likewise seen.

$10^{-1} = 0.1$ (exponent = −1, one decimal place in result)
$10^{-2} = 0.01$ (exponent = −2, two decimal places in result)
$10^{-3} = 0.001$ (exponent = −3, three decimal places in result)
$10^{-4} = 0.0001$ (exponent = −4, four decimal places in result)

Box 1.4 Base 10 Raised to a Whole Number

When base 10 is raised to a power that is a positive whole number, the exponent is equal to the number of zeros following the number 1. In other words, 0^x = 1 followed by *x* zeros.

When 10 is raised to a power that is a negative whole number, the exponent is equal to the number of decimal places to the right of the decimal point.

Any base may also be raised to a power that is not an integer, such as:

$2^{1.5} = 2.83$
$(7.25)^{0.67} = 3.77$
$10^{-3.5} = 0.000316228$

As you can imagine, such calculations cannot be done without a calculator, even if the base is 10. If you're not sure how to perform exponential calculations on your calculator, consult your user's guide, but most calculators follow the steps shown in these examples.

Box 1.5 Calculator Tip

Calculators capable of performing these calculations will have a [x^y], [y^x], or [^] button. Some more advanced calculators may have different steps for solving these problems.

Example 1.5

$2^{1.5} = x$ Solve for x

Calculator solution

2 [y^x] 1.5 [=]

or

2 [x^y] 1.5 [=]

or

2 [^] 1.5 [=]

Answer: 2.83

Example 1.6

$10^{-3.5} = x$ Solve for x

This problem involves entering a negative exponent. Although some calculators allow for direct entry of −3.5 using the (−) key, many require you to enter the number first and then the sign using the [±] button. Check your calculator's user's manual for instructions if one of these steps does not yield the correct answer.

Calculator steps:

10 [y^x] 3.5 [+/−] [=]

or

10 [x^y] 3.5 [+/−] [=]

or

10 [^] 3.5 [+/−] [=]

Answer: 0.00032

The answer to this problem may appear in scientific notation on your calculator. If so, the answer will probably look like one of these:

3.16 E −4
3.16×10^{-4}
3.16 ^ 10^{-4}

Some calculators may indicate scientific notation in other ways. Scientific notation is discussed at the end of this chapter.

Since the number 10 is used as the base in scientific notation ($3.16 \times \mathbf{10}^{-4}$), some calculators have a separate button for calculating powers of 10. The button looks like this: [10^x]. If your calculator has this button, you could have used it instead:

$10^{-3.5}$ = 3.5 [+/−] [10^x] [=] 0.0003162277

Try the practice problems until you feel comfortable with the specific steps required by your calculator. Be sure to use a calculator you are familiar with during hearing science examinations.

PRACTICE PROBLEMS: EXPONENTS

1. $10^{1/2} =$
2. $2^6 =$
3. $10^{-4} =$
4. $10^{2.3} =$
5. $6^{3.8} =$
6. $10^{-0.75} =$
7. $10^0 =$
8. $10^{-0.007} =$

Answers (If you need help with these problems, consult the website.) **Link 1-8**

1. 3.16
2. 64
3. 0.0001
4. 199.53
5. 905.68
6. 0.18
7. 1
8. 0.98

Box 1.6 Ready for More?

Keep in mind that no matter how complex the next few sections appear, all of the problems are based on a pyramid of learning. You now have a solid foundation; just stack the new blocks (new material) on top of these bottom building blocks. If you are struggling, go back and review the previous sections before proceeding or ask your professor for a recommendation for a basic algebra textbook.

Logarithms (Logs)

A **logarithm** is an exponent. If we consider the base and exponent shown in Figure 1.1, notice you can use the term exponent or logarithm (log) to describe the same thing. Solving a logarithm problem simply means finding an unknown exponent, as in solving for x in the equation $10^x = 10{,}000$. Since it is the exponent that is unknown in this equation, logarithm problems use a specific notation.

$$\text{Log}_{10}10{,}000 = 4$$

$$10^4 = 10{,}000$$

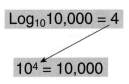

Figure 1.2. The log, base 10, of 10,000 is four. This is a common format for expressing log equations. The translation between this notation and Figure 1.1 is indicated.

Figure 1.2 illustrates a common way of presenting logarithm problems in hearing science. Notice that only the format has changed; compared with the information provided in Figure 1.1, all of the information is still the same. This equation is read: "The log, base 10, of 10,000 is 4." Some additional examples are shown here:

$\text{Log}_2\ 16 = x$	Here $x = 4$ and it is the same as writing $2^4 = 16$.
$\log_5 25 = x$	Here $x = 2$ and it is the same as writing $5^2 = 25$.
$\log_7 343 = x$	Here $x = 3$ and it is the same as writing $7^3 = 343$.
$\log_{10} 0.0003 = x$	Here $x = -3.5$ and it is the same as writing $10^{-3.5} = 0.0003$.

Now, although, as you saw above, the base in a logarithm problem can be any number, it is usually restricted to 10 for most hearing science purposes; therefore, all the logarithm problems you will encounter in this text will have 10 as their base. Note that for simplicity, $\log_{10}$ is often simply written as log; that is, "$\log_{10} 4$" is the same as "log 4" in most applications.

Example 1.7

$\log 6.85 = x$ Solve for x

To calculate the log, enter 6.85 into the calculator and press the [log] button. The number 0.8356905715 should appear on your calculator. Some calculators require the reverse order of entry: first press [log] and then enter 6.85. If neither of these steps results in the right number, consult your calculator's user's manual.

Answer: 0.84

Remember that the number we found, 0.84, is the log (exponent) to which we need to raise 10 to end up with 6.85 as our result:

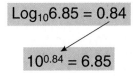

$$\text{Log}_{10}6.85 = 0.84$$

$$10^{0.84} = 6.85$$

Example 1.8

In some cases, a problem to be solved will involve the following notation:

$$10^x = 2500 \text{ Solve for } x$$

In this situation, just like Example 1.7, you are trying to determine the log. The problem can be rewritten in the same format as the previous example.

$$\log_{10} 2500 = x \text{ Solve for } x$$

To calculate the log, enter 2500 into the calculator and press [log]. The number 3.397940009 should appear on your calculator. Again, some calculators require reverse order of entry: first press [log] and then enter 2500. If neither of these steps results in the right number, consult your calculator's user's manual.

Answer: $\log_{10} 2500 = 3.397940009 = 3.40$

In other words, $10^{3.40} = 2500$

PRACTICE PROBLEMS: LOGARITHMS

Solve for *x*.

1. $\log_{10} 1000 = x$
2. $\log_{10} 3400 = x$
3. $10^x = 3000$
4. $10^x = 0.0089$
5. $10^x = 0.324$
6. $\log_{10} 0.57 = x$
7. $\log_{10} 5.4 = x$
8. $\log_{10} 2.98 = x$
9. $\log_{10} 2 = x$
10. $\log_{10} 300 = x$

Answers (If you need help with these problems, consult the website.) **Link 1-9**

1. 3
2. 3.53
3. 3.48
4. −2.05
5. −0.49
6. −0.24
7. 0.73
8. 0.47
9. 0.30
10. 2.48

Box 1.7 Calculator Tip

To solve log problems ($\log_{10} A = x$), enter *A* into the calculator and press [log].

Antilogs

The opposite of a log is an antilog. You have already solved antilog problems, probably without even realizing it. In the section on exponents, all of the practice problems were solved for the antilog. The antilog is identified in the familiar equation from the last two sections.

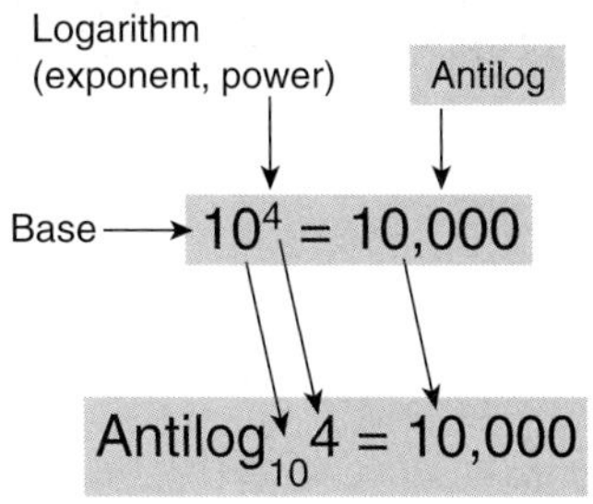

Figure 1.3. The antilog, to the base 10, of four is 10,000.

As we saw in the logarithm problems, a common format is used for antilog problems. The conversion to the new format is also provided in Figure 1.3. This alternate format is read as follows: "The antilog, to the base 10, of 4 is 10,000."

Box 1.8 Calculator Steps for Solving Antilog Problems

To solve antilog problems in this format: $\text{antilog}_{10} A = x$, try one of these steps:

A [10^x]	*A* [2nd] [log]	*A* [shift] [log]
10 [y^x] *A* [=]	10 [x^y] *A* [=]	10 [^] A [=] 10 [^] A [enter]

PRACTICE PROBLEMS: SOLVING PROBLEMS WITH ANTILOGS

Solve for *x*.

1. $\text{antilog}_{10} 4 = x$
2. $\text{antilog}_{10} 2 = x$
3. $\text{antilog}_{10} 0.6 = x$
4. $\text{antilog}_{10} 0.0845 = x$
5. $10^{4.2} = x$
6. $10^{9.5} = x$
7. $10^{-6.0} = x$

Answers (If you need help with these problems, consult the website.) **Link 1-10**

1. 10,000
2. 100
3. 3.98
4. 1.21
5. 15848.93 or 1.58×10^4
6. 3162277660 or 3.16×10^9
7. 0.000001 or 1.0×10^{-6}

Complex Problems

Now that logarithms have been reviewed, problems involving any combination of operations can be solved. Review the example and complete the practice problems. If you do not arrive at the same answers as the answer key, follow the step-by-step solutions provided online.

Example 1.9

$20^2 + 10 \times y + \log\left(\frac{x}{200}\right) = \frac{37008}{z}$ Solve for x where $y = 10.7$ and $z = 72$

Substitute known variables. Here, y and z are known.

$$20^2 + 10 \times 10.7 + \log\left(\frac{x}{200}\right) = \frac{37008}{72}$$

Simplify, following the Order of Operations. First, consider parentheses. The operation within the parentheses, $\left(\frac{x}{200}\right)$, cannot be performed because it contains an unknown variable. Next, consider any exponents and logs. Here 20^2 can be calculated, but the logarithm cannot be calculated because of the unknown variable x.

$$400 + 10 \times 10.7 + \log\left(\frac{x}{200}\right) = \frac{37008}{72}$$

Next, perform the multiplication and division.

$$400 + 107 + \log\left(\frac{x}{200}\right) = 514$$

Next, perform the addition.

$$507 + \log\left(\frac{x}{200}\right) = 514$$

Solve for x by following the Order of Operations in reverse order. First, remove 507 by subtracting it from both sides.

$$\left\{507 + \log\left(\frac{x}{200}\right)\right\} \mathbf{- 507} = \{514\} \mathbf{- 507}$$

$$\log\left(\frac{x}{200}\right) = 7$$

Next, find the antilog of both sides. Keep in mind that log is short for $\log_{10}$ and the antilog is simply base 10 raised to the specified power. The antilog and log steps cancel each other.

$$\textbf{antilog}\left\{\log\left(\frac{x}{200}\right)\right\} = \textbf{antilog}\{7\}$$

$$\frac{x}{200} = 10^7$$

To isolate x on one side, multiply both sides by 200.

$$\left\{\frac{x}{200}\right\} \mathbf{\times 200} = \{10^7\} \mathbf{\times 200}$$

$$x = 10^7 \times 200$$

Now we need to simplify again, this time by just multiplying.

$$x = 10000000 \times 200$$

$$x = 2000000000$$

Answer: 2000000000

PRACTICE PROBLEMS: COMPLEX PROBLEMS

1. $33 + 9(y - 7) + 3y = x$ Solve for x where $y = 11$
2. $\frac{13}{2} - 9(4y + 1) = x$ Solve for x where $y = 7$
3. $\frac{-7y(14 - y - 2)}{y - 2} = x$ Solve for x where $y = 5$
4. $\frac{-8y^2(y + 2)^2}{y^2 - 1} = x$ Solve for x where $y = 3$
5. $x = 20 + 20 \times \log_{10}\left(\frac{y}{20}\right)$ Solve for x where $y = 40$
6. $x = 6 - 4 + \frac{3}{f} - 10 \times \log_{10}\left(\frac{y + 64}{20}\right)$ Solve for x where $f = 2$ and $y = 39$
7. $x = 59 - 4 + 6y - 20 \times 10^{(52/13)}$ Solve for x where $y = 1.3$
8. $y = 64 + 20 \times \log_{10}\left(\frac{x}{20}\right)$ Solve for x where $y = 7.0$
9. $y = 78 + 10 \times \log_{10}\left(\frac{x}{10^2}\right)$ Solve for x where $y = 20$

Answers (If you need help with these problems, consult the website.) **Link 1-11**

1. 102
2. −254.5
3. −81.67
4. −225
5. 26.02
6. −3.62
7. −199937.2 (or -2.0×10^5)
8. 0.03
9. 0.00016

SCIENTIFIC NOTATION

Scientific notation, also called exponential notation or power-of-10 notation, is a way of representing very large or very small numbers in a condensed form. A number is expressed in scientific notation when it is in the form $a \times 10^n$, where a is a number greater than or equal to 1 but smaller than 10 and n is an exponent. This notation is used to write down numbers without trailing, or leading, **zeros.** This is useful when working with numbers like 385,000,000,000 or 0.00000000127.

To convert a number into scientific notation, follow the steps outlined in Box 1.9.

Box 1.9 Converting From Standard to Scientific Notation

1. Take the first nonzero digit and place a decimal point after it.
2. Write the remaining nonzero digits after the decimal point.
3. Add the phrase "$\times$ 10."
4. Count the number of decimal places you moved the decimal point.
5. Attach this number as an exponent to the 10 from Step 3. If the original number was less than one, make the exponent negative.

Example 1.10

Convert the numbers 385,000,000,000 and 0.00000000127 from standard to scientific notation. Follow the steps in Table 1.2.

Answer: 3.85×10^{11} and 1.27×10^{-9}

Some calculators may automatically display numbers in scientific notation. Note that numbers in scientific notation may appear in one of several different ways.

Example 1.11

Use a calculator to multiply 385,000 $\times$ 1,000,000

Answer: 3.85×10^{11}

The calculator display may look like one of the following:

3.85×10^{11}

3.85 E 11

3.85^{11}

3.85 ^ 11

Be careful not to misinterpret the last three entries. These are all ways of showing 3.85×10^{11} on a calculator or computer display. They do NOT indicate 3.85 to the 11th power ($\neq 3.85^{11}$).

To convert from scientific to standard notation, simply move the decimal place the number of spaces indicated by the exponent. For a positive exponent, move the decimal point to the right; for a negative exponent, move the decimal point to the left.

Example 1.12

Convert from scientific notation to standard notation.

3.21×10^{-4}

The exponent is negative, so move the decimal four places to the left.

.0003.21 ←

Answer: 0.00032

Example 1.13

Convert from scientific notation to standard notation.

3.21×10^{4}

The exponent is positive, so move the decimal four places to the right.

3.2100. →

Answer: 32,100

Remember that if the exponent in scientific notation is negative, the number is small (less than 1), and if the exponent is positive, the number is large (greater than 1).

▸ Table 1.2. Converting Between Standard and Scientific Notation

		Two Examples	
	Conversion Steps:	**385,000,000,000.**	**0.00000000127**
Standard notation	1. Place the decimal after the first nonzero digit.	3. ←	1. →
	2. Place the rest of the nonzero digits after the decimal.	3.85	1.27
	3. Include the phrase "$\times$ 10"	3.85×10	1.27×10
	4. Count the number of places you moved the decimal.	3.85,000,000,000. 11 spaces	0.000000001.27 9 spaces
	5. Use this number as an exponent for the 10. If the original number is less than one, make the exponent negative.	385,000,000,000 >1 Exponent = 11	0.00000000127 <1 Exponent = -9
Scientific notation	6. Place the exponent.	3.85×10^{11}	1.27×10^{-9}

PRACTICE PROBLEMS: SCIENTIFIC NOTATION

Convert from standard to scientific notation for problems 1 to 6 and from scientific to standard notation for problems 7 to 10.

1. 373,000,000,000,000
2. 0.0000053
3. 452,000,100,000
4. 0.0000000000008
5. 486.209000
6. 43.76
7. 4.28×10^2
8. 6.79×10^{-3}
9. 1.0×10^1
10. 6.43×10^{-8}

Answers (If you need help with these problems, consult the website.) **Link 1-12**

1. 3.73×10^{14}
2. 5.3×10^{-6}
3. 4.520001×10^{11} or (rounded) 4.52×10^{11}
4. 8.0×10^{-13}
5. 4.86209×10^2 or (rounded) 4.86×10^2
6. 4.376×10^1 or (rounded) 4.38×10^1
7. 428
8. 0.00679
9. 10
10. 0.0000000643

Dividing Numbers in Scientific Notation

Dividing numbers in scientific notation can be problematic when using a calculator unless the appropriate steps are taken. Entering the division problem into a standard calculator straight from beginning to end will not give the right answer.

Example 1.14

$$\frac{3.48 \times 10^{11}}{7.29 \times 10^{12}} = x$$

If you enter this equation into a standard calculator from left to right and top to bottom as follows,

$$3.48 \times 10^{11} \div 7.29 \times 10^{12} =$$

you actually end up entering the following, different, equation:

$$☹ \frac{3.48 \times 10^{11}}{7.29} \times 10^{12} = x ☹$$

The mistake here is that 10^{12} was moved out of the denominator. This occurred because of the Order of Operations. Since multiplication and division are on the same level, the calculator immediately divides by 7.29, without waiting for the entire denominator in scientific notation to be entered.

Example 1.14 can be solved easily with a calculator using one of three following methods.

1. Use parentheses (available on some calculators) to group the denominator.

$$\frac{3.48 \times 10^{11}}{(7.29 \times 10^{12})} =$$

2. Use the memory button on the calculator. Calculate the denominator first, 7.29×10^{12}, and store the result in memory. Clear the display. Then calculate 3.48×10^{11} and divide the result by the number in memory. If you want to use this method, make sure you are familiar with using your calculator's memory feature.
3. Split the fraction. Since multiplication and division are on the same level in the Order of Operations, a fraction of the type $\frac{a \times b}{c \times d}$ can be split into $\frac{a}{b} \times \frac{b}{d}$. Note that each numerator term becomes its own numerator and each denominator term its own denominator. This is actually the easiest and most straightforward method for dividing numbers in scientific notation. Moreover, splitting the fraction is a useful tool for problem solving in hearing science.

$$\frac{3.48 \times 10^{11}}{7.29 \times 10^{12}} = \frac{3.48}{7.29} \times \frac{10^{11}}{10^{12}}$$

From here, do each division problem separately. The second division problem is in fact extremely simple. To divide one power of a number by another power with the same base, just subtract the exponent in the denominator from the exponent in the numerator. This will probably be clearer written as a mathematical formula:

$$\frac{x^A}{x^B} = x^{A-B} \quad \textbf{(1.1)}$$

Thus, $\frac{10^{11}}{10^{12}} = 10^{11-12} = 10^{-1}$, and so

$$\frac{3.48 \times 10^{11}}{7.29 \times 10^{12}} =$$

$$\frac{3.48}{7.29} \times \frac{10^{11}}{10^{12}} =$$

$$0.4773662551 \times 10^{-1} =$$

$$0.4773662551 \times 0.1 =$$

$$0.04773662551$$

Answer: 0.048

Sometimes splitting the fraction can create an answer that looks similar to scientific notation; that is, it has a number and then "$\times 10^n$" but it is not in scientific notation because either the first part of the notation is zero, such as in the expression:

$$0.4773662551 \times 10^{-1}$$

or more than one digit is to the left of the decimal place, for example:

$$24.354 \times 10^{14}$$

To convert these numbers into scientific notation involves two steps.

1. Alter the first part of the number in scientific notation so there is one nonzero integer to the left of the decimal place.
2. Because the first portion of the notation has been altered, the second step is to adjust the power of 10 to account for this change. If the decimal is moved to the right in the first step, this makes the first part of the expression larger, so the second part, the power of 10, must become smaller. If, on the other hand, the decimal is moved to the left, this makes the first part smaller, so the power of 10 must become larger. For each shift of one decimal place, the exponent of the 10 should either be increased or decreased by one. Clearly, if the power of 10 is to become smaller, the exponent needs to decrease, and if the power of 10 is to become larger, the exponent needs to increase.

Example 1.15

Convert $0.4773662551 \times 10^{-1}$ into scientific notation.

First, shift the decimal to the right in the first part of the expression, which becomes

$$4.773662551$$

Since this part of the expression became larger, the second part must become smaller, so subtract 1 from the power of 10. So 10^{-1} changes to 10^{-2}.

Answer: 4.77×10^{-2}

Example 1.16

Convert 24.354×10^{14} into scientific notation.

First, shift the decimal to the left in the first part of the expression, which becomes

$$2.4354$$

Since this part of the expression became smaller, the second part must become larger, so add 1 to the power of 10. So 10^{14} changes to 10^{15}.

Answer: 2.44×10^{15}

PRACTICE PROBLEMS: DIVIDING NUMBERS IN SCIENTIFIC NOTATION

Solve for x. Answer problems 1 to 4 in standard notation and problems 5 to 7 in scientific notation.

1. $x = \dfrac{2.8 \times 10^{-10}}{3.7 \times 10^{-12}}$
2. $x = \dfrac{2.8 \times 10^{-12}}{3.7 \times 10^{-12}}$
3. $x = \dfrac{8.76 \times 10^{2}}{3.45 \times 10^{4}}$
4. $x = \dfrac{7.77 \times 10^{1}}{4.82 \times 10^{1}}$
5. $x = \dfrac{1.0 \times 10^{0}}{2.0 \times 10^{1}}$
6. $x = \log\left(\dfrac{5 \times 10^{2}}{2 \times 10^{1}}\right)$
7. $x = 10 + 10 \times \log\left(\dfrac{3 \times 10^{-12}}{10^{-12}}\right)$

Answers (If you need help with these problems, consult the website.) **Link 1-13**

1. 75.68
2. 0.76
3. 0.025
4. 1.61
5. 5.0×10^{-2}
6. 1.40×10^{0}
7. 1.48×10^{1}

Multiplying Numbers in Scientific Notation

Multiplication with scientific notation is much easier than division. Example 1.17 can be entered directly into a calculator. The calculator automatically calculates the exponents first and proceeds from left to right with the multiplication.

Example 1.17

$$\{5.92 \times 10^{-3}\} \times \{4.83 \times 10^{-7}\} =$$

This problem can be entered directly into a calculator from left to right. One set of calculator steps is provided here. You should know from previous sections in this chapter how to alter these steps based on the calculator you are using. If your calculator creates an open parenthesis "(" for exponents, keep in mind that you will need to close the parenthesis by entering a ")" before entering the next multiplication problem.

5.92 [×] 10 [y^x] 3 [+/−] [×] 4.83 [×] 10 [y^x] 7 [+/−] =

Answer: 2.86×10^{-9}

In some cases, it may be easier to apply the following formula for use in equation solving:

$$x^A \times x^B = x^{A+B} \quad (1.2)$$

Thus, a problem such as $10^{-3} \times 10^{-7}$ becomes $10^{(-3)+(-7)} = 10^{-10}$.

PRACTICE PROBLEMS: MULTIPLICATION IN SCIENTIFIC NOTATION

1. $(3.12 \times 10^{-1}) \times (5.37 \times 10^{7})$
2. $(7.39 \times 10^{3}) \times (4.83 \times 10^{4})$

Answers (If you need help with these problems, consult the website.) **Link 1-14**

1. 16754400 (standard) or 1.68×10^{7} (scientific)
2. 356937000 (standard) or 3.57×10^{8} (scientific)

GEOMETRY

Geometry is the branch of mathematics concerned with the study of points, lines, angles, surfaces, and shapes and the relationships among them. The two basic fields of geometry are plane geometry and solid geometry. Plane geometry is concerned with lines, squares, circles, polygons, etc., that can be drawn on a two-dimensional plane. Solid geometry deals with three-dimensional figures and surfaces such as cubes, spheres, and cylinders.

A basic understanding of both plane geometry and solid geometry is necessary for hearing science to understand the way sound waves travel and how sound waves are affected by surfaces and objects in the environment. This chapter assumes that the reader is familiar with basic geometry terms including point, line, horizontal line, vertical line, perpendicular, parallel, and vertex. If these terms are unfamiliar, see the website. **Link 1-15**

Line and Angle

In the study of geometry, considerable time is spent on proving the properties of various geometric relationships involving lines and angles. This text will not focus on proofs, but will review the concepts needed for the study of sound. First, it is important to recall the classification of angles and some key relationships between lines and angles (Fig. 1.4). An **angle** is the space between two lines or planes that intersect or the inclination of one line compared to another. Note that a right angle is drawn with a square in the angle. Examine the intersecting lines shown on the bottom of Figure 1.4. Notice line AB is intersected by line EF at point C. The angles created above line AB are ∠ACE and ∠BCE. If we add ∠ACE and ∠BCE together, the result is ∠ACB, which we know is a straight angle (180°). So, the sum of ∠ACE and ∠BCE will be equal to 180°. Furthermore, we know several things about the angles below line AB, including the fact that ∠ACE = ∠BCF, ∠BCE = ∠ACF, and the sum of BCF and FCA is 180°.

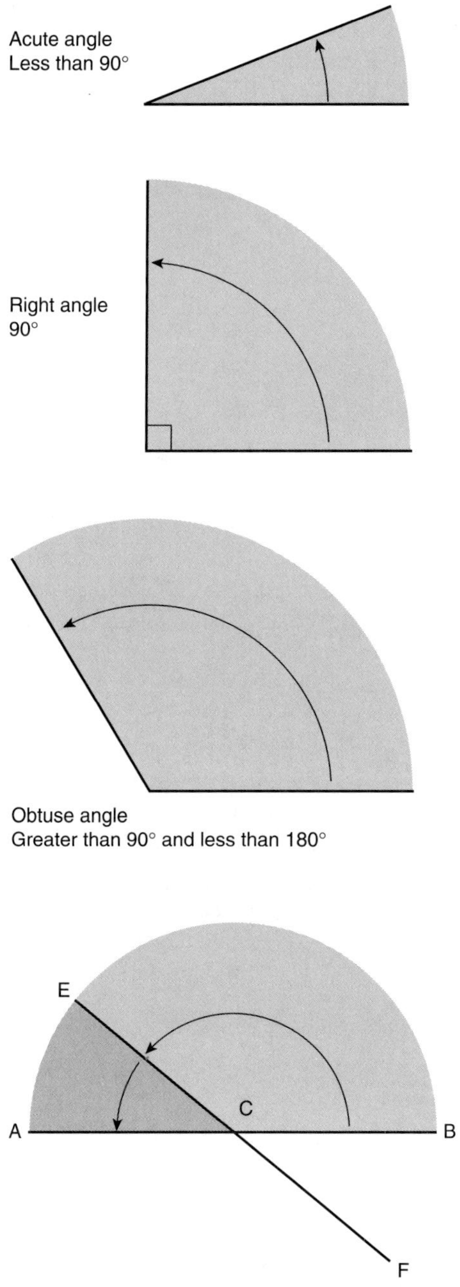

Figure 1.4. Examples of angles and relationships among angles created by the intersection of two straight lines.

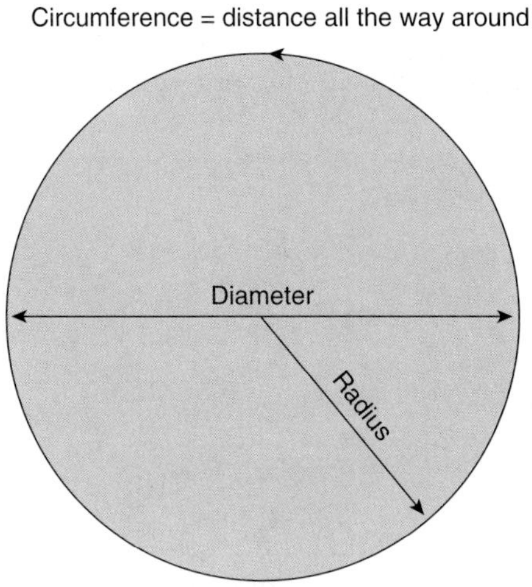

Figure 1.5. Aspects of a circle.

Circle

A circle is a curved line drawn such that every point on it is the same distance away from a given center point (Fig. 1.5). The **circumference (*l*)**, also called the perimeter, of a circle is the entire curved line all the way around the circle. The same term is also used to describe the whole distance around the circle. The **radius (*r*)** is a line drawn from the central point of the circle to any point on the circle. The relationship between the radius and the length of the circumference (*l*) is given in Equation 1.3.

$$l = 2\pi r, \text{ where } \pi \approx 3.14 \tag{1.3}$$

A straight line between two points on a circle that passes through the center of the circle is called the **diameter (*d*).** The diameter is equal to two times the radius of the circle.

Imagine a radius (indicated by the arrow in Fig. 1.6, *top*) traveling counterclockwise around a circle (like the

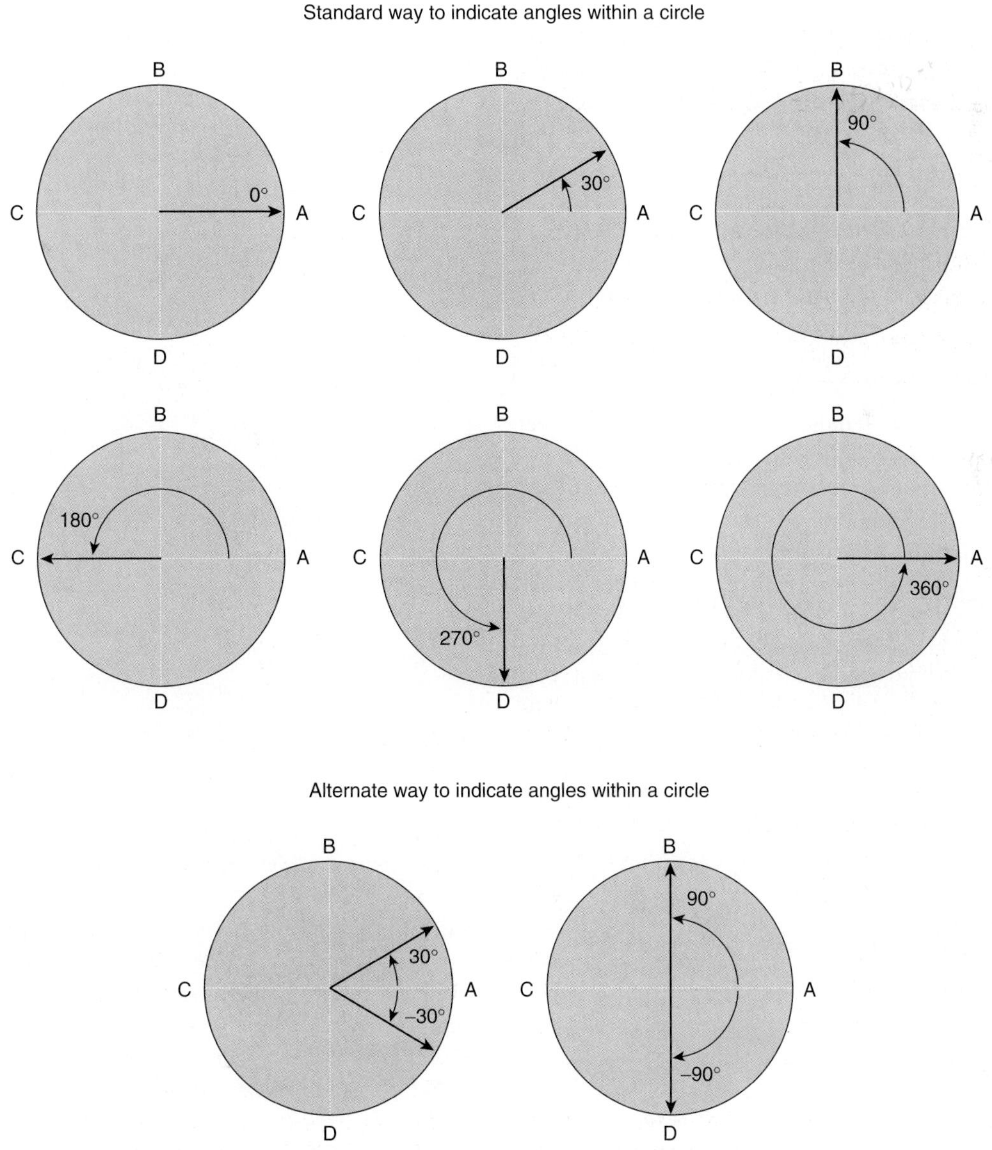

Figure 1.6. Angles within a circle as they are generally denoted (*top*) and an alternate way to indicate angles within a circle that is sometimes used in hearing science (*bottom*).

long arm of a clock traveling backwards) beginning at point A. When the radius has rotated from its initial position to a new position, it is said that it has moved by a certain angle (written θ and pronounced "theta"). Angles are measured in degrees (°) and one full rotation of the radius corresponds to 360°. This number was probably adopted by analogy to ≈ 360 days in a year and because it is easily divisible into smaller pieces. One degree can be further divided into 60 (angular) minutes (‘), and one minute into 60 (angular) seconds ("). Sometimes the names arcminute and arcsecond are also used.

When the radius in Figure 1.6 has rotated one third of the way between points A and B, the angle between the radius and its start position is 30°. This angle changes as the radius travels around the circle and will vary from 0° to 360° as the radius completes its rotation around the circle. When the radius reaches point B, the angle will have become 90°. At point C the angle will be 180°, and at D it will be 270°. When the radius returns to its starting position, it will have swept through the whole circle, and the angle can be considered to be 360°. Because the radius is exactly where it started from, the angle can likewise be considered to be 0°.

In some hearing science applications, the angle of rotation around a circle is not based on a 0° to 360° range. In these situations, the circle is divided into two halves, each containing 180°. Angles in the lower half of the circle are assigned values from 0° to −180° starting from point A and moving in a clockwise manner to point C. Angles in the upper half keep their standard values. This alternate description of the angles in a circle is shown in Figure 1.6.

The convention of assigning the label "0°" to the direction indicated by point A on the circle is just a convention. In some cases it is convenient to assign the label "0°" to another direction, including the direction we are facing or the north direction. As long as the direction indicating "0°" is clearly labeled, it can be represented by any point on the circle. Angles described to the left of "0°" should be labeled as positive (+) and angles to the right of "0°" direction should be labeled as negative (−), although in some books the convention of negative to the left is used, which can be confusing. Since the full circle has 360°, the same point on the circle can be reached by traveling 270° or −90°.

The degree is not the only measure used to describe angles. The other less common but very important scientific unit for measuring angles is the radian (rad). One **radian** is an angle of a circle that is subtended by an arc (segment of a circle) equal in length to the radius of the circle. The concept of the radian began around the year 1714, with the name *radian* applied in 1873 (Cajori, 1919; O'Connor & Robertson, 2005). Since the circumference of a circle is equal to $2\pi r$, the whole circle has 2π radians. In other words, the circle encompasses an angle of 360° or 2π radians; therefore:

$$1 \text{ rad} = \frac{360^\circ}{2\pi} \approx 57.3^\circ$$

and

$$1^\circ = \frac{2\pi}{360^\circ} \approx 0.0175 \text{ rad}$$

The exact value of 1 rad expressed in degrees, minutes, and seconds is 57°17'44.6".

To convert from degrees to radians, use this equation:

$$x\ (\text{rad}) = y\ (^\circ) \times \frac{\pi}{180^\circ} \tag{1.4}$$

To convert from radians to degrees, use this equation:

$$x\ (^\circ) = y\ (\text{rad}) \times \frac{180^\circ}{\pi} \tag{1.5}$$

PRACTICE PROBLEMS: CIRCLE

Estimate the angle or use a protractor to measure the angle on each circle. If you need help with problems 4 to 7, consult the website. Link 1-16

1.

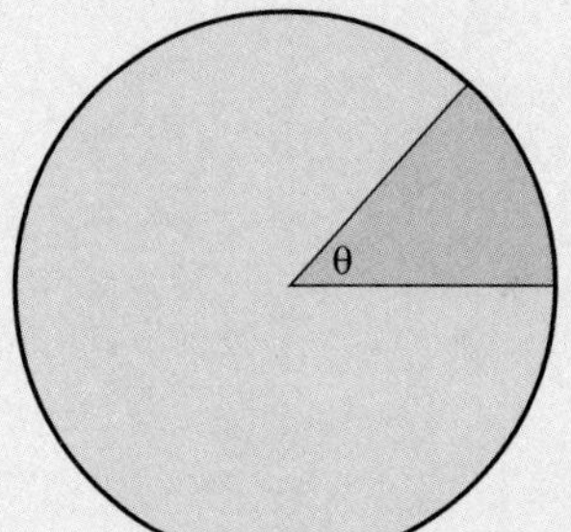

2.

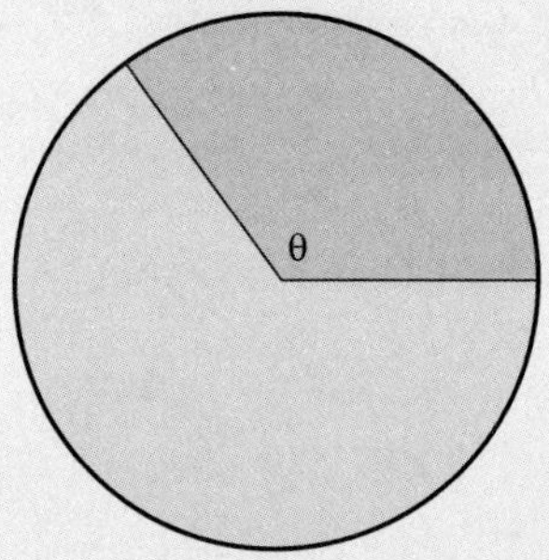

3.

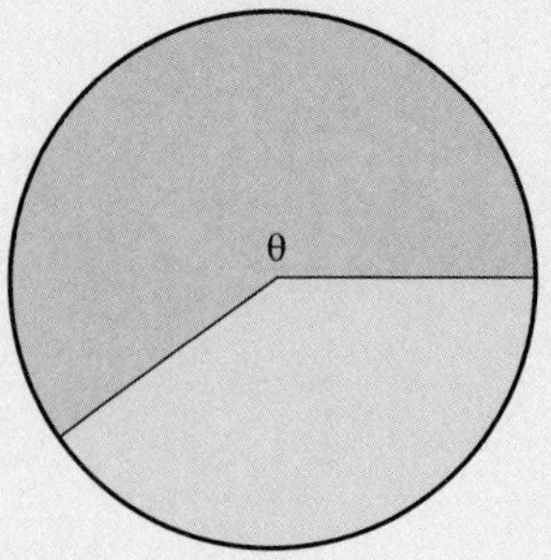

4. Convert 56° into radians.
5. Convert 225° into radians.

6. Convert 0.67 radians into degrees.
7. Convert 1.34 radians into degrees.

Answers

1. Approximately 50° (measured angle = 48°)
2. Approximately 130° (measured angle = 127°)
3. Approximately 225° (measured angle = 216°)
4. 0.98 radians
5. 3.93 radians
6. 38.39°
7. 76.78°

TRIGONOMETRY

Trigonometry is the branch of mathematics concerned with the study of triangles. It builds upon basic concepts of geometry and applies them to a triangle. An understanding of trigonometry is critical to the understanding of most of the mathematical and physical concepts that are explored in acoustics and hearing science.

A triangle is any three-sided geometric figure. A basic fact about triangles is that the sum of the angles in any triangle will always be equal to 180°. Certain types of triangles are more important than others and for that reason they have been given their own names. Examples of these specific types of triangles are shown in Figure 1.7.

The **right triangle,** which is a triangle containing a 90° angle, is of special interest in the study of trigonometry. Each of the three sides of a right triangle has its own name. The longest side of the right triangle is called the **hypotenuse.** The side of the triangle that is adjacent to the hypotenuse and forms the angle θ (theta) with the hypotenuse is called the **adjacent side.** The third side, opposite to the angle θ, is called the **opposite side.** The relationships between the lengths of the hypotenuse, adjacent side, and opposite side in a right triangle and the degree of the angle θ are of great interest in trigonometry.

Pythagorean Theorem

The **Pythagorean Theorem** (named after Pythagoras of Samos; 540–480 BC) states that the sum of the squares of the two shorter sides of a right triangle is equal to the square of the longest side (the hypotenuse). In other words, looking at the triangle in Figure 1.8, the lengths of the sides, a, b, and c, are related such that:

$$a^2 = b^2 + c^2 \quad (1.6)$$

If we know the length of b and c and wish to find the length of a, we can rewrite Equation 1.6 as:

$$a = \sqrt{b^2 + c^2} \quad (1.7)$$

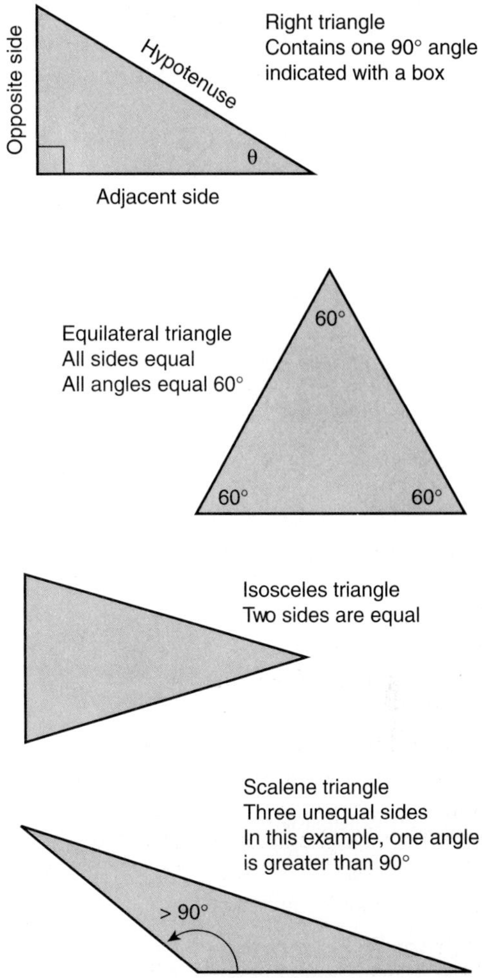

Figure 1.7. Several types of triangles, including a right triangle, with the angle θ and the adjacent side, opposite side, and hypotenuse labeled.

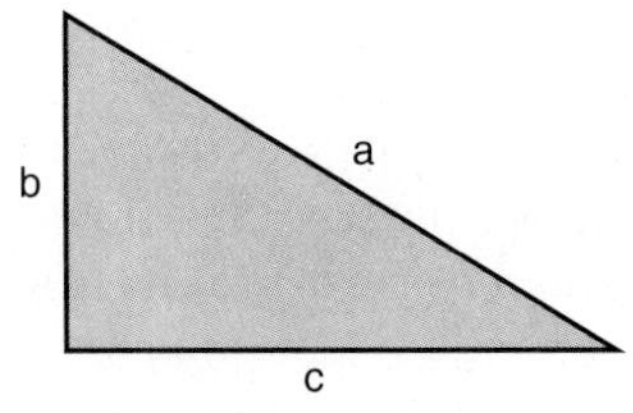

Figure 1.8. With the sides of the right triangle labeled such that a is the hypotenuse and b and c are the other sides, the relationship between the length of the sides can be explained with the Pythagorean Theorem.

Example 1.18

If the two shorter sides of a triangle are 5.4 cm and 6.3 cm, what is the length of the hypotenuse?

First, select Equation 1.7.

$$a = \sqrt{b^2 + c^2}$$

Next, substitute known variables.

$$a = \sqrt{5.4^2 + 6.3^2}$$

(continued)

Solve for a.

$$a = \sqrt{29.16 + 39.69}$$

$$a = \sqrt{68.85}$$

$$a = 8.2975900115$$

Answer: The hypotenuse is 8.30 cm long.

PRACTICE PROBLEMS: PYTHAGOREAN THEOREM

1. If side $b = 12$ cm and side $c = 14$ cm, what is the length of side a?
2. If side $b = 13.2$ m and side $c = 8.3$ m, what is the length of side a?
3. If side $b = 0.2$ km and side $c = 0.8$ km, what is the length of side a?

Answers (If you need help with these problems, consult the website.) **Link 1-17**

1. The length of side a is 18.44 cm.
2. The length of side a is 15.59 m.
3. The length of side a is 0.82 km.

Trigonometric Functions

Trigonometric functions are functions of an angle that are expressed as the ratio of two of the sides of a right triangle that contains that angle. In other words, these functions result when you divide the length of any one side of the right triangle by the length of another side. Trigonometric functions include sine, cosine, tangent, secant, cosecant, and cotangent functions. For example, the sine of the angle θ is the length of the opposite side divided by the length of the hypotenuse. Formulas for the three main properties (functions)—the sine, cosine, and tangent of an angle θ—are given below.

$$\sin \theta = \frac{\textit{opposite}}{\textit{hypotenuse}}$$

$$\cos \theta = \frac{\textit{adjacent}}{\textit{hypotenuse}}$$

$$\tan \theta = \frac{\textit{opposite}}{\textit{adjacent}}$$

Box 1.10 Helpful Hint

One way to remember these equations is "Ollie had a heap of apples" for o/h (sine), a/h (cosine), and o/a (tangent).

In addition, three other functions are the inverse of the above functions:

$$\text{cosecant } \theta = \frac{\textit{hypotenuse}}{\textit{opposite}} = \frac{1}{\sin \theta}$$

$$\text{secant } \theta = \frac{\textit{hypotenuse}}{\textit{adjacent}} = \frac{1}{\cos \theta}$$

$$\text{cotan } \theta = \frac{\textit{adjacent}}{\textit{opposite}} = \frac{1}{\tan \theta}$$

Trigonometric functions can also be applied to triangles that are not right triangles using the Sine Law and the Cosine Law; see the website if you are interested in this topic. **Link 1-18**

Example 1.19

Calculate the sine of the angle θ shown here:

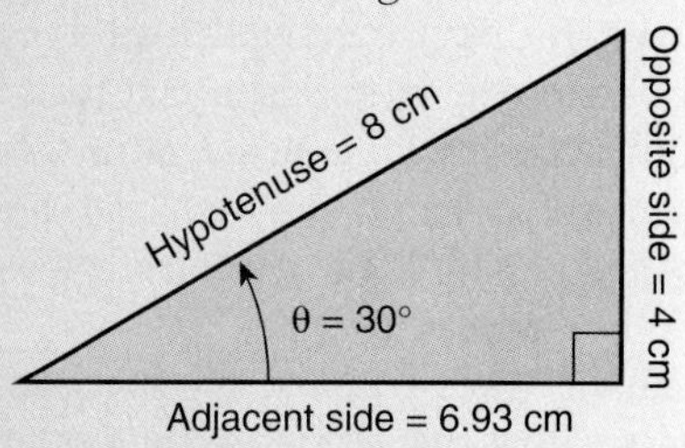

First, select the appropriate equation, the equation for the sine.

$$\sin \theta = \frac{\textit{opposite}}{\textit{hypotenuse}}$$

Substitute known variables and solve.

$$\sin \theta = \frac{4 \textit{ cm}}{8 \textit{ cm}}$$

$$\sin \theta = 0.5$$

Answer: The sine of the angle θ is 0.5.

In Example 1.19, the value of the angle θ was shown in the figure provided in the problem; therefore, a simpler way of determining the sine of θ would have been to use the sine function on a calculator. The sine of any angle can be computed on a calculator by entering the angle and then pressing the [sin] button, that is, 30 [sin] for the example. Consult your calculator's user's manual if this does not produce the correct answer. Similarly, the cosine and tangent of an angle can be calculated using the [cos] and [tan] buttons on a scientific calculator.

In addition to finding the sine, cosine, and tangent if the angle θ is known, sine, cosine, and tangent operations can also be performed in reverse to find the angle θ. In other words, instead of entering the angle and finding the sine, cosine, or tangent, we can use the inverse sine (arcsine or $\sin^{-1}$), inverse cosine ($\cos^{-1}$), or inverse tangent ($\tan^{-1}$) functions to find the angle θ. To find the inverse sine, enter the sine of the angle and then press the [$\sin^{-1}$] button on your calculator. For calculators without a [$\sin^{-1}$] button, you may need to use an [inv] (inverse) or [2nd] (2nd function) button and then the [sin] button. If none of these steps works with your calculator, consult the user's manual to determine how to find the right steps.

Example 1.20

If $\sin \theta = 0.25$, what is the value of θ?

Use a scientific calculator to enter 0.25 and then find $\sin^{-1}$ (inverse sine function) using the appropriate button(s), either [$\sin^{-1}$], [inv][sin], [2nd][sin], or [shift][sin].

Answer: $\theta = 14.47751219° = 14.48°$

PRACTICE PROBLEMS: SINE, COSINE, AND TANGENT

1. Calculate the sine of the angle θ given the following dimensions:

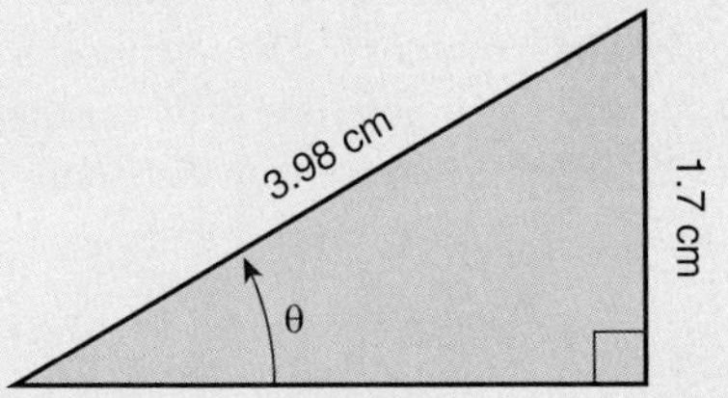

2. Calculate the sine of the angle θ when the hypotenuse = 7 cm, adjacent side = 6.4 cm, and opposite side = 2.8 cm.
3. Calculate the cosine of the angle θ when the hypotenuse = 9 km, adjacent side = 8.48 km, and opposite side = 3 km.
4. Calculate the tangent of the angle θ when the hypotenuse = 2.8 m, adjacent side = 2 m, and opposite side = 2 m.
5. Calculate the cotangent of the angle θ when the hypotenuse = 2.8 m, adjacent side = 2 m, and opposite side = 2 m.
6. Calculate the sine of the angle $\theta = 60°$.
7. Calculate the sine of the angle $\theta = 55°$.
8. Calculate the cosine of the angle $\theta = 45°$.
9. Calculate the tangent of the angle $\theta = 23°$.
10. Find the angle θ when $\sin \theta = 0.866$.
11. Find the angle θ when $\cos \theta = 0.707$.
12. Find the angle when $\tan \theta = 0.819$.

Answers (If you need help with these problems, consult the website.) **Link 1-19**

1. 0.43
2. 0.4
3. 0.94
4. 1
5. 1
6. 0.87
7. 0.82
8. 0.71
9. 0.42
10. 60°
11. 45.01°
12. 39.32°

COORDINATE SYSTEMS

When points (or sets of points such as lines) need to be referred to or identified in space, they must be referenced to a system of coordinates. **Coordinates** are distances or angles that uniquely identify the position of specific points in space in reference to a certain central point called the **origin.** Two basic systems of coordinates used in mathematics are the Cartesian coordinate system and the polar coordinate system. René Descartes (1596−1650), known also under the name Cartesius, introduced the Cartesian coordinate system based on the **orthogonal** (right angle) coordinates x and y for a plane or x, y, and z for three-dimensional space. These two- and three-dimensional systems are referred to as Cartesian systems. Similar systems based on angles from baselines are referred to as polar systems.

Cartesian Coordinates

Cartesian coordinates, also called **rectangular coordinates,** describe a system for locating points on a plane (flat surface) or in three-dimensional space (Fig. 1.9). The Cartesian coordinates of a plane consist of two perpendicular axes (called x and y)* that cross at a central point called the origin. Similarly, the Cartesian coordinates of three-dimensional space consist of three perpendicular (orthogonal) axes x, y, and z crossing at the origin. This space is called Euclidean space after the Greek mathematician Euclid (365−275 BC) and it is the foundation of Euclidean geometry. The axes are customarily drawn according to the east/west (x), north/south (y), and front/back (z) directions from the origin. Each point in space is uniquely specified by two (x, y) or three (x, y, z) numbers representing

*The x (horizontal) axis is sometimes called the abscissa and the y (vertical axis) is sometimes called the ordinate.

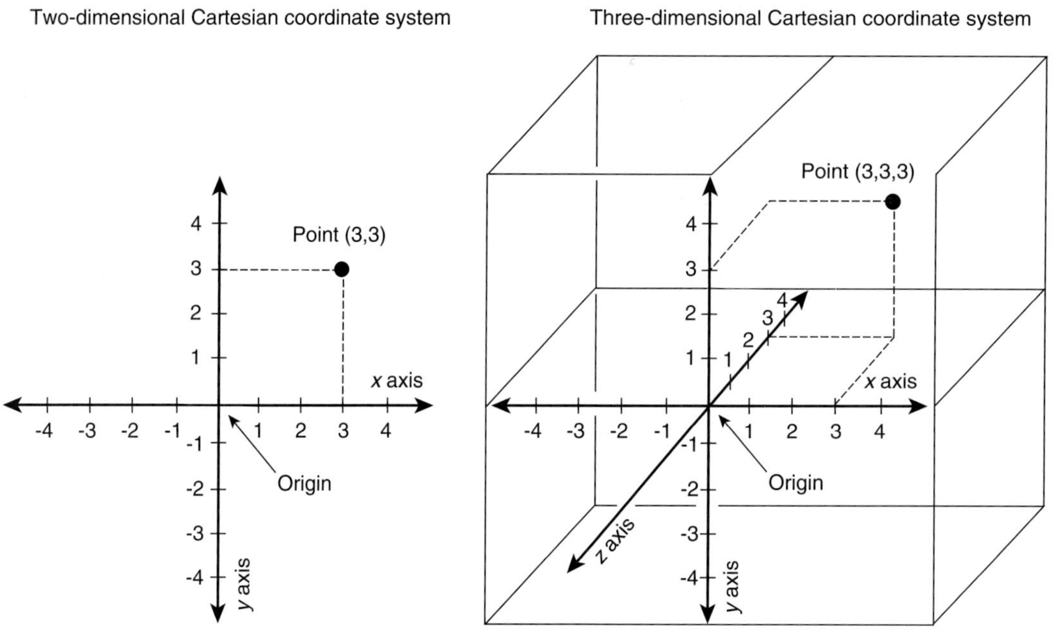

Figure 1.9. Two- (x, y) and three-dimensional (x, y, z) Cartesian coordinates.

the distance of the point from the origin along each of the axes. An example of a point defined on a plane and in three-dimensional space using Cartesian coordinates is shown in Figure 1.9. The points shown are (3, 3) for the plane and (3, 3, 3) in three-dimensional space. The origin of the coordinate system is assigned the value (0, 0) in two dimensions and (0, 0, 0) in three dimensions. On a plane, if points are plotted on an $x-y$ graph, the distance between any two points can be determined easily using the Pythagorean Theorem.

Example 1.21

What is the distance between two points, where point A is located at (2, 2) and point B is located at (4, 4)?

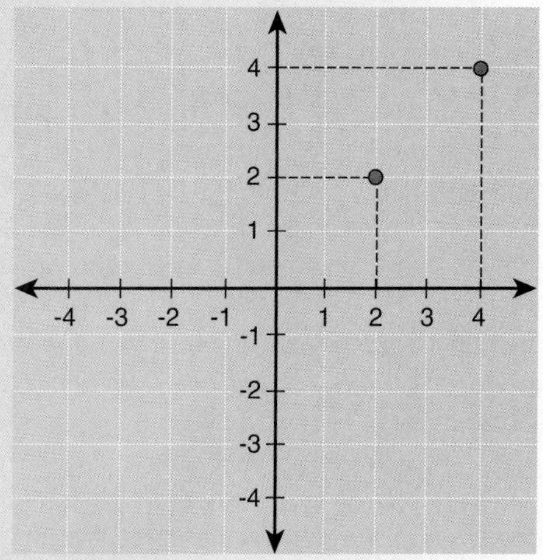

Since point A is located at (2, 2) and point B is located at (4, 4), the distance between the points along the x axis is $4 - 2 = 2$ and the distance between the two points along the y axis is $4 - 2 = 2$. If we draw a right triangle with the line AB as the hypotenuse, the distance along the x axis is equal to the length of one side of the triangle and the distance along the y axis is equal to the length of another side of the triangle. The length of the hypotenuse of the triangle is missing; therefore, the distance between the two points can be found using the Pythagorean Theorem.

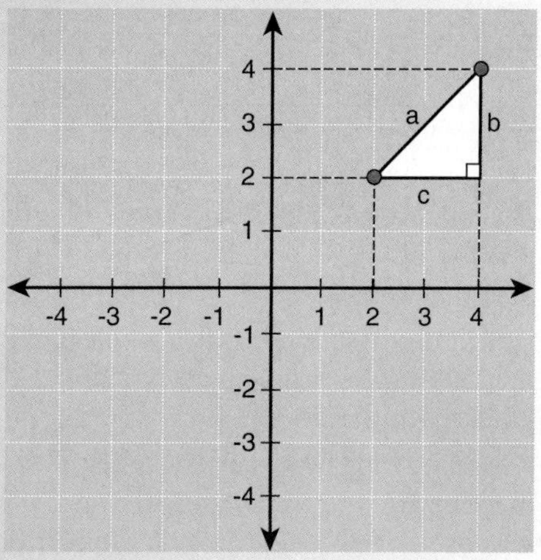

Applying the Pythagorean Theorem to this problem is as follows:

$$a = \sqrt{c^2 + b^2}$$

$$a = \sqrt{2^2 + 2^2}$$

$$a = \sqrt{4 + 4}$$

$$a = \sqrt{8}$$

$$a = 2.828427125$$

$$a = 2.83$$

Answer: The distance between point A and point B is 2.83 (units unspecified).

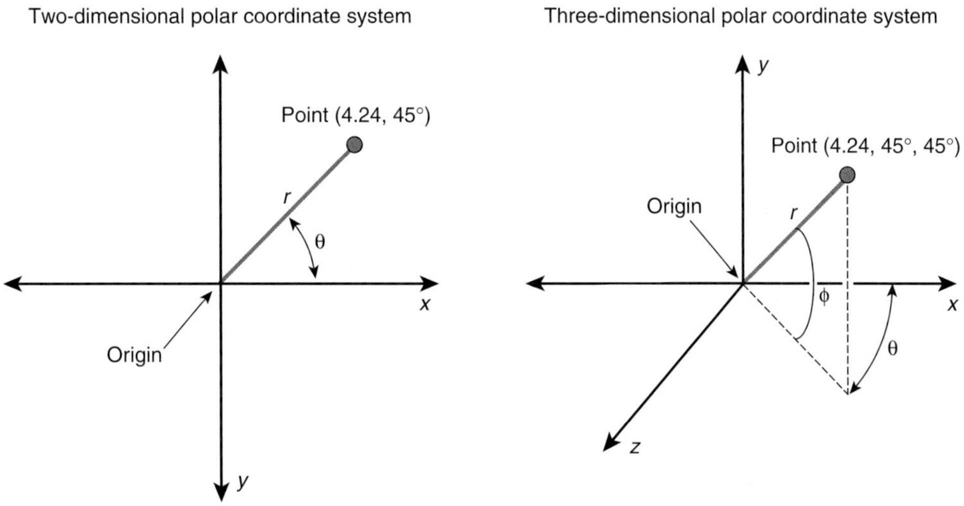

Figure 1.10. Two- (r, θ) and three-dimensional (r, θ, φ) polar coordinates.

> **PRACTICE PROBLEMS: CARTESIAN COORDINATES**
>
> 1. If two points are located at positions (2.4, 4.5) and (5.1, 4.0), what is the distance between the two points?
> 2. If two points are located at positions (0.9, −3) and (−2, 5), what is the distance between the two points?
>
> **Answers** (If you need help with these problems, consult the website.) **Link 1-20**
>
> 1. The distance between the two points is 2.75 (units unspecified).
> 2. The distance between the two points is 8.51 (units unspecified).

Polar Coordinates

The **polar coordinate system** is a coordinate system in which each point in space is uniquely specified by two or three numbers: (r, θ) for two-dimensional space and (r, θ, φ) for three-dimensional space (Fig. 1.10). The distance between the point of interest and the origin is indicated by the letter r. The angle between the x axis and the line connecting the point of interest with the origin is indicated with the symbol θ (theta) and it is called the **phase angle.** In three-dimensional space, the angle θ represents the direction in the horizontal plane (also called the azimuth) and the angle φ represents the direction in the vertical plane (also called the polar angle or elevation).* The origin of the coordinate system is assigned the value (0, 0) in two-dimensional space and (0, 0, 0) in three-dimensional space.

Graphically, the polar plot looks similar to the Cartesian coordinate plot. In some instances, the Cartesian coordinate system will be preferable for graphing and in other instances the polar coordinate system will be easier. In solving hearing science problems, you may need to use both. In some cases, you may need to convert between Cartesian and polar coordinates. To convert from polar to Cartesian coordinates, use Equations 1.8 and 1.9:

$$x = r \cos \theta \tag{1.8}$$

$$y = r \sin \theta \tag{1.9}$$

Example 1.22

Translate the polar coordinates (10, 45°) into Cartesian coordinates.

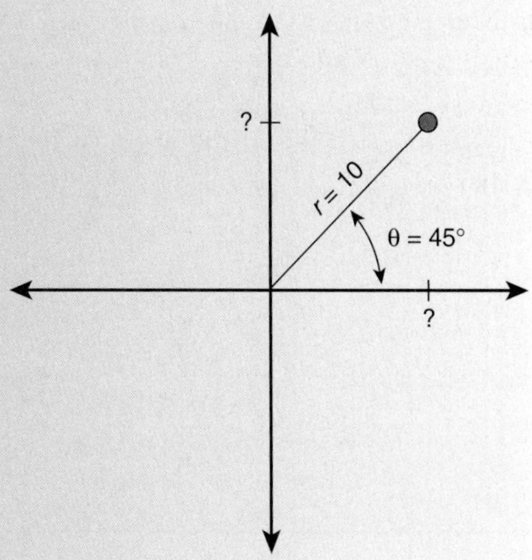

*Physicists, engineers, and *non-American* mathematicians interchange the symbols φ and θ, using φ to denote the azimuth and θ the elevation. In some cases, the z Cartesian coordinate rather than the φ coordinate may be added to polar coordinates in the x–y plane. These hybrid Cartesian–polar coordinates are called **cylindrical coordinates** and are occasionally used to describe some sound phenomena in three-dimensional space.

First, to calculate the x coordinate, select Equation 1.8.

$$x = r \cos \theta$$

Next, substitute known variables. Here r is known (it is 10) and θ is known (it is 45°).

$$x = 10 \times \cos 45$$

Perform the cosine operation first. Enter 45 into your calculator. Press the cos button. You should get the number 0.7071067812. (Note: If you did not get this number, your calculator may be reporting the answer in radians instead of degrees.)

Multiply this number by 10 and round.

$$x = 10 \times 0.7071067812$$

$$x = 7.071067812$$

$$x = 7.07$$

Next, calculate the y coordinate. Use Equation 1.9 from the previous section.

$$y = r \sin \theta$$

Substitute known variables.

$$y = 10 \sin 45$$

$$y = 10 \times 0.7071067812$$

$$y = 7.071067812$$

$$y = 7.07$$

Answer: The Cartesian coordinates are (7.07, 7.07).

Notice in this figure how the polar coordinates are related to the Cartesian coordinates. The Cartesian coordinates specify the relationship of the point to the x and y axes, and the polar coordinates specify the distance from the origin and the angle in relationship to the x axis.

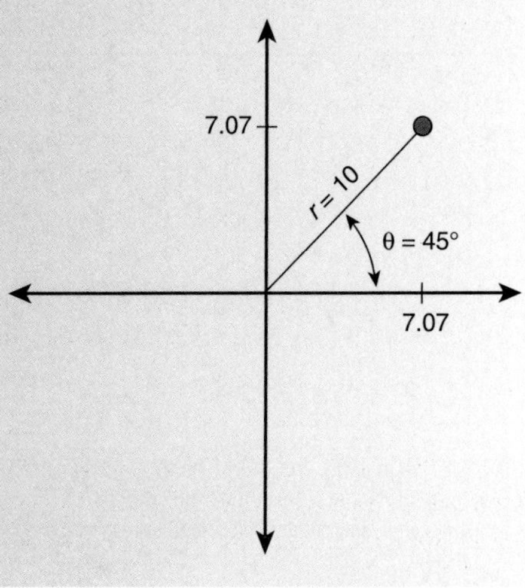

If Cartesian coordinates are given and they must be translated into polar coordinates, use these formulas.

$$r = \sqrt{x^2 + y^2} \quad \textbf{(1.10)}$$

$$\theta = \tan^{-1}\left(\frac{y}{x}\right) \quad \textbf{(1.11)}$$

In Equation 1.11, if $x < 0$, you must add 180° to get the correct answer. Notice the expression $\tan^{-1}$ in Equation 1.11. Recall from the sine, cosine, and tangent section of this chapter that this is just one of the ways to label the inverse tangent, also known as the arctangent. To perform this operation, press the $\tan^{-1}$ button (or the inv or 2nd buttons and then the tan). If none of these steps works with your calculator, consult the user's manual to determine how to find the right steps.

Example 1.23

If the Cartesian coordinates are (2.4, 5.1), what are the polar coordinates?

First, select the appropriate equations. Calculate r first using Equation 1.10.

$$r = \sqrt{x^2 + y^2}$$

Substitute known variables. We know that $x = 2.4$ and $y = 5.1$.

$$r = \sqrt{2.4^2 + 5.1^2}$$

$$r = \sqrt{5.76 + 26.01}$$

$$r = \sqrt{31.77}$$

$$r = 5.636488268 = 5.64$$

Next, select Equation 1.11 to calculate θ.

$$\theta = \tan^{-1}\left(\frac{y}{x}\right)$$

Substitute known variables. We know that $x = 2.4$ and $y = 5.1$

$$\theta = \tan^{-1}\left(\frac{5.1}{2.4}\right)$$

$$\theta = \tan^{-1}(2.125)$$

Take the inverse tangent of 2.125.

$$\theta = 64.79887635$$

$$\theta = 64.80°$$

Answer: The polar coordinates are (5.64, 64.80).

Graphically, this point looks like this:

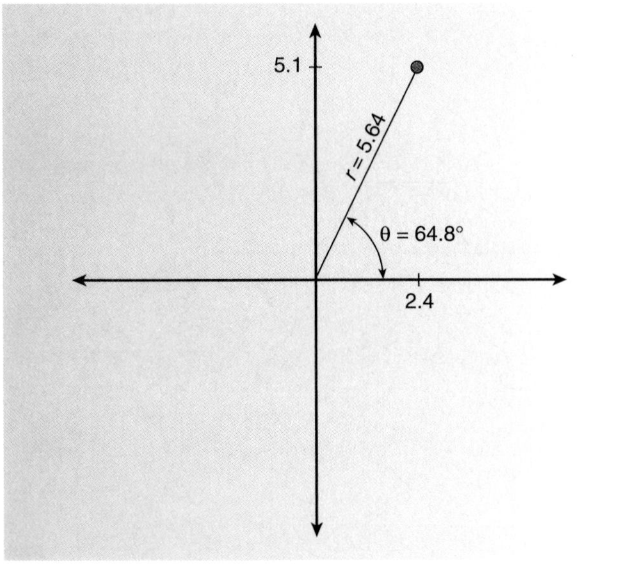

PRACTICE PROBLEMS: POLAR COORDINATES

1. Convert Cartesian coordinates (17, −4) to polar coordinates.
2. Convert Cartesian coordinates (3.2, 1.5) to polar coordinates.
3. Convert polar coordinates (4.2, 23°) to Cartesian coordinates.
4. Convert polar coordinates (1.3, 2°) to Cartesian coordinates.

Answers (If you need help with these problems, consult the website.) **Link 1-21**

1. The polar coordinates are (17.46, −13.24°).
2. The polar coordinates are (3.53, 25.11°).
3. The Cartesian coordinates are (3.87, 1.64).
4. The Cartesian coordinates are (1.30, 0.05).

Functions

Cartesian and polar coordinates are seldom used to describe one fixed point in space. Much more frequently these coordinates are used to describe a series of points that form a line. The relationship between the coordinates that form a line is called a function. In general, a **function** is an equation that shows the relationship between two sets of numbers. The function describes the specific value of the coordinate along one axis when the other coordinate is known. For example, let us consider the following equation.

$$y = 2x + 3 \qquad \textbf{(1.12)}$$

If you replace the variable x in the equation with 0 and then simplify, you will find that $y = 3$. If $x = 1$, then $y = 5$. For any other value of x, there will be a specific value of y. We can graph such a function and analyze graphically the behavior of one variable (y) when the other variable (x) varies.

Functions are usually denoted by letters such as f, g, F, and G. For example, a function can be generally written like this:

$$y = f(x) = 2x + 3 \qquad \textbf{(1.13)}$$

The symbol $f(x)$ is read "f of x" and indicates that the value of variable y depends on the value of variable x. The expression $f(x)$ is typically used when we know that y depends on x but we either do not know the specific relationship or we are not concerned with the specific relationship. For example, if we know that distance traveled (d) depends on the speed of a car (v) and duration of driving (t) but we do not know how, we can write this relationship as function $d = f(v, t)$. If we know that distance is a product of speed and time, we can write this function explicitly as $d = v \times t$.

Graphing Functions

As you know, a function is a formula expressing the relationship between two sets of numbers. A function can be illustrated using a Cartesian coordinate system. An example of a simple two-dimensional function, $x = y^2$, is shown in Figure 1.11. Recall that for every value of x, the value of y can be determined. For example, when $y = 1$, $x = 1^2 = 1$ and so forth. Several individual plotted points are shown in Figure 1.11A and, when an infinite number of points are plotted for this function, the function looks like Figure 1.11B.

When a straight line is plotted, its function has a characteristic form such that $y = mx + b$, where m is the slope of the line and b is the y-intercept. The **y-intercept** is the value of y where the line passes through the y axis. The **slope** of the line is the line's slant (inclined, declined). This can be calculated by finding the coordinates of any two points on the line and finding the difference between the y coordinates over the difference between the x coordinates; in other words, the slope $= \frac{\Delta y}{\Delta x} = \frac{y_2 - y_1}{x_2 - x_1}$. Note here that the symbol Δ (delta) means a change or difference.

To learn more about graphing mathematical functions, it will be necessary to study calculus. **Calculus** is the branch of mathematics that deals with the limits and slopes of functions as well as the areas under the functions of one or more variables.

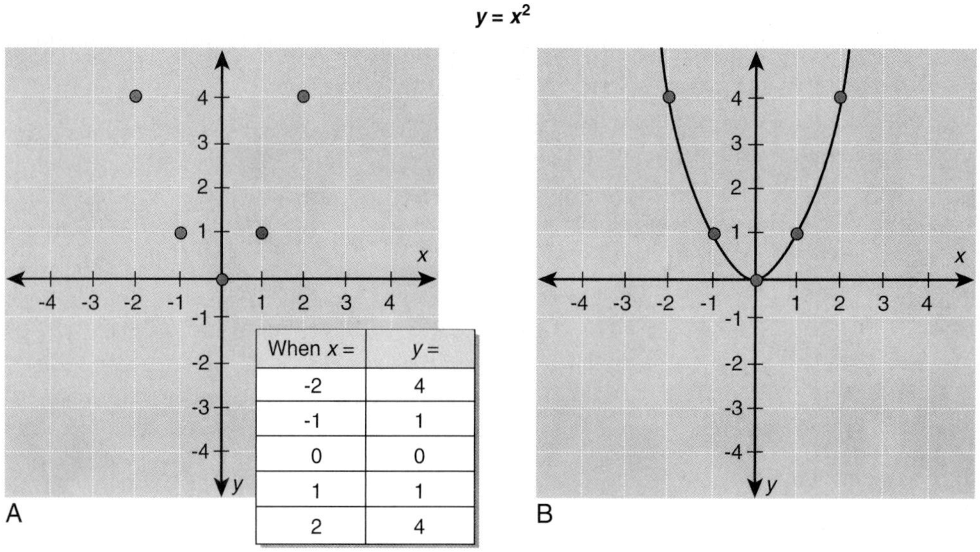

When $x =$	$y =$
-2	4
-1	1
0	0
1	1
2	4

Figure 1.11. Several plotted points (*left*) and many plotted points (*right*) for the function $x = y^2$.

Example 1.24

Find the function of the line shown on this plot:

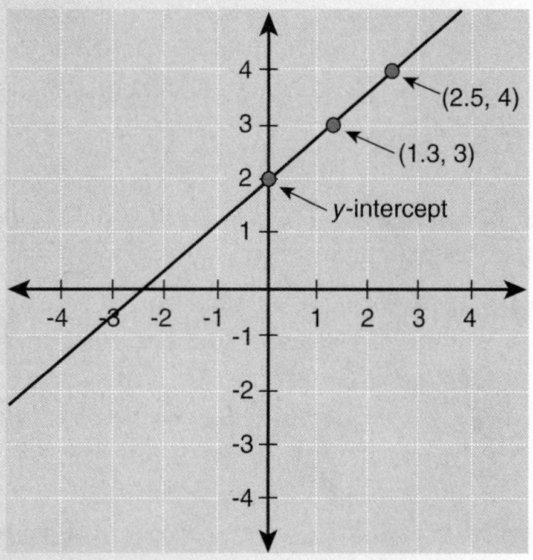

The line passes through the y axis at (0, 2). Therefore, the y-intercept is 2. The slope can be determined by finding two points along the line and determining their coordinates. Two points are shown, (1.3, 3) and (2.5, 4). The slope is calculated as follows.

$$slope = \frac{\Delta y}{\Delta x} = \frac{y_2 - y_1}{x_2 - x_1} = \frac{4 - 3}{2.5 - 1.3} = \frac{1}{1.2} = 0.83$$

With the value of the slope, 0.83, and the value of the y-intercept, 2, the function can be written.

$$y = mx + b$$

$$y = 0.83x + 2$$

To test out the function, calculate the value of y given any value of x and see if it falls on the line. If $x = 2$, $y = (0.83 \times 2) + 2 = 3.66$. Does (2, 3.66) fall on the line? Yes.

Summary

This chapter reviews the basic mathematics necessary for the study of hearing science including the relationships between numbers and the use of variables in equation solving (algebra); the study of points, lines, and angles (geometry); and the study of triangles and the sine, cosine, and tangent functions (trigonometry).

An equation may include unknown variables, constants (numbers), and symbols for mathematical operations. Fundamental to solving equations is the step-by-step process for making equations progressively simpler. This process involves following a sequence of steps known as the Order of Operations, which includes (in this order) parentheses, exponents (logs), multiplication, division, addition, and subtraction. Very large and very small numbers are usually expressed using scientific notation ($a \times 10^n$).

The right triangle is of special interest in the study of geometry and trigonometry. Each of the three sides of a right triangle has its own name. The longest side is called the hypotenuse, the side forming the angle θ with the hypotenuse is called the adjacent side, and the third side, opposite the angle θ, is called the opposite side. The Pythagorean Theorem states that the sum of the squares of the adjacent and opposite sides of a right triangle is equal to the square of the hypotenuse. The result of dividing the length of any one of the sides by the length of another is a function of the angle θ (such as the sine, cosine, and tangent of θ).

When points need to be identified in a two-dimensional plane or three-dimensional space, they must be referenced to a system of coordinates. Coordinates are distances or angles that uniquely identify the position of specific points in space in reference to a certain central point called the origin. Two basic systems of coordinates used in mathematics are the Cartesian coordinate system and the polar coordinate system.

Key Points

- Fundamental to solving any equation is the process of simplification. This process is described by a sequence known as the Order of Operations including (1) operations within parentheses, (2) exponential (logarithmic) operations, (3) multiplication and division, and (4) addition and subtraction.
- A logarithm is another way of looking at an exponent (or power). The opposite of a log is an antilog. In the equation $y = 10^x$, x is the log and y is the antilog.
- Scientific notation is a way of representing very large or very small numbers in a condensed form. A number is expressed in scientific notation when it is in the form $a \times 10^n$, where a is a number equal to or greater than 1 but smaller than 10 and n is an exponent.
- The Pythagorean Theorem states that the sum of the squares of the two shorter sides of a right triangle is equal to the square of the longest side called the hypotenuse. To find the length of the hypotenuse, use the formula $a = \sqrt{b^2 + c^2}$.
- Important characteristics of the circle include the circumference (the line, or distance of the line, all the way around the circle), the radius (the line, or distance of the line, drawn from the central point of the circle to any point on the circle), the diameter (two times the radius of the circle), and the angles within the circle, which vary from 0° to 360°.
- The result of dividing the length of any one of the sides of a right triangle (hypotenuse, adjacent side, and opposite side) by the length of another results in a function of the angle θ. These functions include the $\sin\theta$ = opposite/hypotenuse, $\cos\theta$ = adjacent/hypotenuse, and $\tan\theta$ = opposite/adjacent.
- Coordinates are distances or angles that uniquely identify the position of specific points in space in reference to a certain central point called the origin. Cartesian coordinates (rectangular coordinates) locate a point on a plane or three-dimensional space in the format (x, y) and (x, y, z). Polar coordinates locate a point on a plane or three-dimensional space using a radius (r) and one angle (two-dimensional space/plane) or two angles (three-dimensional space).
- A function is an equation that shows the relationship between two sets of numbers.

CHAPTER 2

Physics

Szymon T. Letowski, Tomasz Letowski, and Diana C. Emanuel

Chapter Outline

Learning Objectives

- To review basic physics concepts including fundamental physical characteristics such as magnitudes and units, force, work, power, and energy
- To review the concept of scalar and vector quantities, including vector addition
- To review the two fundamental areas of physics: kinematics, the study of motion, and dynamics, the study of the effects of force on the state of an object
- To demonstrate problem solving involving basic physical concepts
- To review the international system of units, including conversion between metric units

Key Terms

Acceleration (*a*)
Area (*A*)
CGS System
Density (*ρ*)
Displacement (*d*)
Distance (*d*)
Dynamics
Elasticity
Energy (*E*)
Force (*F*)
Gravity (*g*)
Inertia
Instantaneous acceleration
Instantaneous velocity
International System of Units (SI)
Joule (J)
Kinematics
Kinetic energy (E_k)
Law of Conservation of Energy
Law of Conservation of Momentum
Law of Universal Gravitation
Magnitude
Mass (*m*)
Momentum
MKS System
Newton (*N*)
Newton's First Law of Motion
Newton's Second Law of Motion
Newton's Third Law of Motion
Potential energy (E_p)
Power (*P*)
Scalar
Unit
Vector
Vector addition
Velocity (*v*)
Volume (*V*)
Watt (*W*)
Weight
Work (*W*)

Physics is the science of matter and energy and the interactions between them. Since energy exists in a variety of different forms, physics as a discipline is divided into numerous energy-specific fields such as acoustics, optics, mechanics, thermodynamics, electromagnetism, and atomic physics. Physics also plays an integral part in many other sciences like music, electronics, and hearing science. The methods of physics involve observing and measuring objective characteristics (properties) of objects and the space surrounding them. These characteristics include length, volume, mass, density, electrical charge, and many others. This chapter will review some of the basic physical characteristics essential to the study of hearing science.

BASIC PHYSICAL MAGNITUDES AND UNITS

If we want to study an object or a space, we must first measure one or more of its physical characteristics. Each and every physical measurement consists of two elements: a number, called a magnitude (value), and a unit of measurement. The **magnitude** indicates the quantity (or extent) of a property of the object. The **unit** of measurement is a quantity accepted as a standard of measurement against which other measured quantities are compared. When reporting a physical measurement, it is essential to include both of these pieces of information. A magnitude by itself is meaningless. Imagine if you asked someone how much water he or she drank yesterday, and he or she answered, "Two." You wouldn't have gained any information, and you would have to follow up with, "Two what?" The person may have drunk a lot of water (2 gallons) or not much at all (2 fluid ounces). To be useful, every measurement requires the presence of a unit. In the water example above, gallon and fluid ounce are units of volume. Note that for each physical characteristic, a number of units can be used. Other units used in reporting volume are pint, milliliter, and liter. Milliliter and liter are units in the International System of Units (SI), which is the preferred system for reporting physical measurements in science. This system will be described at the end of this chapter. First, though, we will review some of the basic physical characteristics applicable to hearing science. This review will begin with a description of physical magnitudes and units and then focus on two fundamental fields of physics: **kinematics**, the study of motion, and **dynamics**, the study of energy.

Distance, Area, and Volume

The **distance** (d) between two points is the length of the shortest line connecting them. Distance is reported in units of length such as meter (m), kilometer (km), mile (mi), or yard (yd). In the SI system, the basic unit of length (and distance) is the meter, which is equal to the distance light travels in 1/299,792,458 of a second. Common units of measurement are included in Table 2.1. If you would like to learn about the history of the metric system, consult the website. **Link 2-1**

It is important to realize that in the case of a curved surface, such as a sphere, the shortest path between two points is the straight line connecting the points through the inside of the sphere. This may not always be a practical path, however. In many situations, such as when traveling between two points on the surface of a planet, the shortest path between two points must follow the curved surface and will differ from the straight line between them. For example, on a sphere, the path will make an arc.

Area (A) is the amount of space occupied by a surface. It is a two-dimensional measure, reported in square units of length such as square meters (m^2) or square centimeters (cm^2). Figure 2.1 includes formulas for calculating the area of many common surfaces.

Volume (V) is the amount of space occupied by a substance or an object. It is a three-dimensional measure and it is commonly reported in cubic units of length, such as cubic centimeters (cc or cm^3) or cubic meters (m^3), or in units of fluid volume, such as liters. A liter is the volume occupied by 1 kg of water at a temperature of 4°C and at an atmospheric pressure of 1 atmosphere. It is practically identical to the cubic decimeter (dcm^3) (1 liter = 1.000028 dcm^3). The base unit of measurement for volume is the cubic meter (m^3).

The formulas for calculating volume depend on the shape of the object. Figure 2.1 shows the formulas for the volume of many common shapes.

PRACTICE PROBLEMS: AREA AND VOLUME

1. Calculate the area of a circle with a radius of 3 cm.
2. Calculate the volume of a cylinder with a radius of 6 m and a height of 10 m.
3. Calculate the area of a triangle with a base length of 5.6 m and a height of 7 m.
4. Calculate the volume of a sphere with a radius of 0.5 m.
5. Calculate the total surface area of the cylinder in Problem 2. (Note: For this problem you must calculate the circumference of a circle to determine the area of the sides of the cylinder. The formula for the circumference of a circle is $l = 2\pi r$.)
6. Calculate the difference between the area of a square with a side of 4 cm and the circle inscribed in the square shown below.

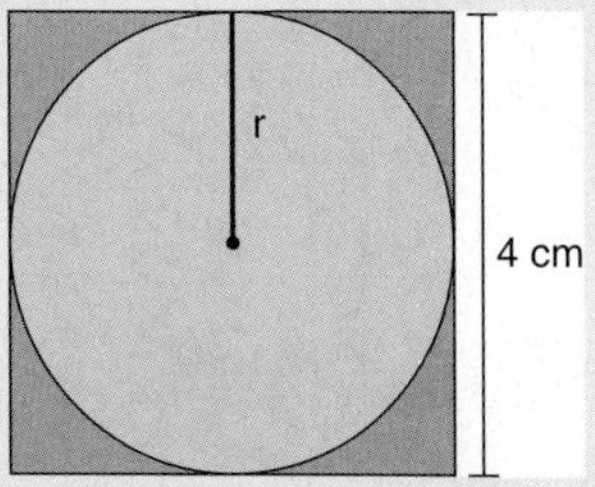

Answers (If you need help with these problems, consult the website.) **Link 2-2**

1. 28.27 cm^2
2. 1130.97 m^3
3. 19.6 m^2
4. 0.52 m^3
5. 603.07 m^2
6. The area of the square is larger than the area of the circle by 3.44 cm^2.

Table 2.1. Basic Units of Measurement in the SI System

Parameter	Unit	Symbol	Formal Definition	Formulas and Comments
Distance (*d*)	meter	m	The meter is the length of path traveled by light in vacuum in 1/299792458 of a second.	
Mass (*m*)	kilogram	kg	The kilogram is the mass of an international standard in the form of a platinum-iridium cylinder kept by the International Bureau of Weights and Measures at Sevres in France.	The kilogram is the only SI unit defined with a prefix (*kilo*), whereas the basic unit of the decimal system is the gram; 1 kg = 1000 grams. It is also the only SI unit defined as a material object.
Time (*t*)	second	s	The second is equal to the duration of 9192631770 periods of the radiation corresponding to the transition between two hyperfine levels of the ground state of the caesium-133 atom.	The second is a metric unit since its smaller units are products of the division by 10 (e.g., millisecond, microsecond).
Temperature (*T*)	kelvin	K	The kelvin is 1/273.16 of the thermodynamic temperature of the triple point of water. The zero point of the Kelvin scale is equivalent to –273.16°C on the Celsius scale. This zero point is considered the lowest possible temperature of anything in the universe.	The former name of this unit—*degree Kelvin* (°K)—was changed to *kelvin* (K) by international agreement in 1967.
Light intensity (*L*)	candela	cd	The candela is the luminous intensity in a given direction of a source that emits monochromatic radiation of a frequency 540×10^{12} Hz and has a radiant intensity in that direction of 1/683 watt per steradian.	
Electric current (*I*)	ampere	A	The ampere is the amount of constant current flowing in two straight parallel conductors of infinite length and negligible cross section separated by a distance of 1 meter in vacuum that produces the force between these conductors equal to 2×10^{-7} newton per meter of length.	One ampere is equal to the amount of electricity contained in 6.24×10^{18} (6.24 quintillion) electrons passing through a point of observation in 1 second. One ampere represents the change in electrical charge with a rate of 1 coulomb per 1 second.
Amount (*a*)	mole	mole	The mole is the amount of substance that contains as many elementary entities as there are atoms in 0.012 kilograms of carbon-12. This number of entities is equal to 6.02×10^{23} (Avogadro's number). The elementary entities may be atoms, molecules, ions, electrons, etc., and must be specified. Note: In this definition, it is understood that the carbon-12 atoms are unbound, at rest, and in their ground state.	
Frequency (*f*)	hertz	Hz	The hertz is equal to a frequency of one cycle per second.	1 Hz = 1 s^{-1}

(continued)

▶ **Table 2.1.** Basic Units of Measurement in the SI System (*Continued*)

Parameter	Unit	Symbol	Formal Definition	Formulas and Comments
Force (*F*)	newton	N (kg × m/s^2)	The newton is the force required to give a mass of 1 kilogram an acceleration of 1 m/s^2.	1 dyne = 1 g cm/s^2 = 10^{-5} N 1 kG = 9.81 N
Stiffness (*K*)	N/m	N/m*		The inverse (opposite) of stiffness is compliance (C) (m/N).
Pressure (*p*)	pascal	Pa (N/m^2)	The pascal is the pressure produced by a force of 1 newton acting on an area of 1 m^2.	1 μbar = 1 dyne/cm^2 1 μbar = 0.1 N/m^2 = 0.1 Pa
Energy, work (*E*)	joule	J (N × m)	The joule is the unit of work and energy equal to the work done when the point of application of a force of 1 newton moves a distance of 1 meter in the direction of the force.	The calorie (cal) is the quantity of heat required to raise the temperature of 1 gram of water by 1°C (1K). 1 cal = 4.1868 J = 41868 × 10^3 erg 1 erg = 1 dyne cm = 10^{-7} J
Power (*P*)	watt	W (J/s)	The watt is a power of 1 joule per second.	
Voltage (*V*)	volt	V (W/A)	The volt is the difference of potential between two points on a conductor carrying a constant current of 1 ampere when the power dissipated between the points is 1 watt.	
Electric charge (*C*)	coulomb	C (A × s)	The coulomb is the electric charge transferred by a current of 1 ampere in 1 second.	
Resistance (*R*)	ohm	Ω (V/A)	The ohm is the resistance between two points on a conductor when a constant potential difference of 1 volt applied between these points produces a current of 1 ampere.	The inverse (opposite) of resistance is admittance (*G*) (A/V).
Acoustic resistance	rayl	Ω (kg/m^{2}s)	The rayl is the opposition of acoustic matter when the acoustic pressure of 1 pascal produces a particle velocity of 1 meter per second (Pa × s/m = kg/m^{2}s).	The rayl is also called the acoustic ohm. Confusingly, the same name, rayl, is used for MKS and CGS units. Therefore, the CGS rayl equals 10 MKS rayls.
Magnetic flux	weber	Wb (V × s)	The weber is the magnetic flux that when uniformly reduced to zero in the span of 1 second produces in a one-turn coil an electromagnetic force equal to 1 volt.	
Magnetic flux density	tesla	T (Wb/m^2)	The tesla is the magnetic flux density equal to 1 weber of magnetic flux over 1 m^2.	1 T = 10^4 gauss
Inductance (*L*)	henry	H (Wb/A)	The henry is the inductance of a closed circuit in which an electromagnetic force of 1 volt is produced when the electric current in the circuit varies uniformly at a rate of 1 ampere per second.	
Capacitance (*C*)	farad	F (C/V)	The farad is the capacitance of a capacitor that when charged with 1 coulomb has a potential difference of 1 volt between its plates.	

**There are two forms of stiffness, axial stiffness measured in N/m and bulk stiffness measured in N/m^2.*

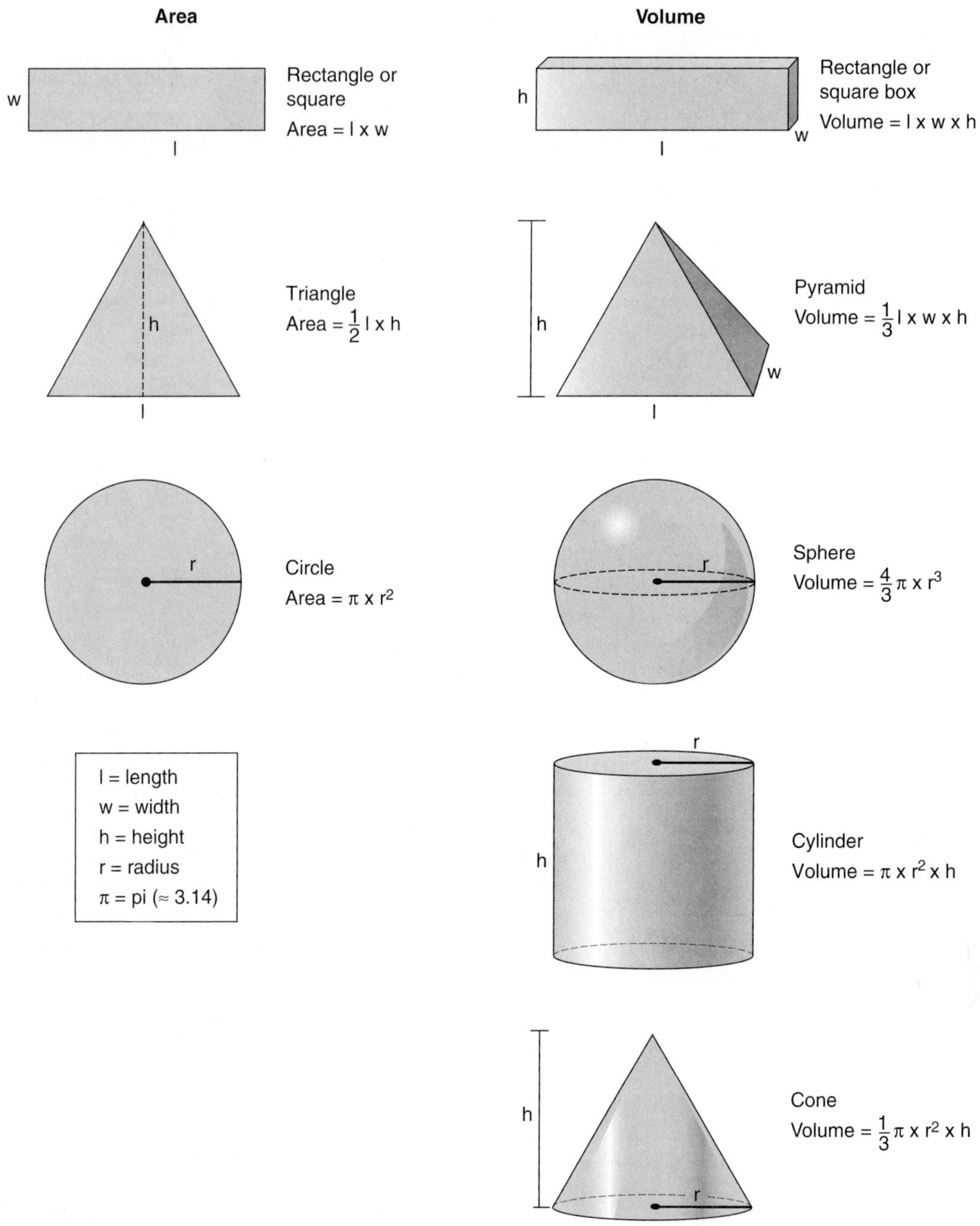

Figure 2.1. The area and volume formulas for several common shapes.

Mass, Density, and Elasticity

Mass (m) is the amount of matter that is present in a substance. Mass is commonly reported in kilograms for larger masses and in grams for smaller ones. It is tempting to think of mass as the same thing as weight, but the two are quite different. Weight is mass affected by the force of **gravity**, which will be discussed later. On grocery store items, various amounts of mass are reported in units of mass such as pounds, ounces, kilograms, or grams but they are listed as the "weight" of the item. The direct translation between weight and mass in this application is faulty. "Net weight" should actually be reported in a force unit, such as newtons.

Density (ρ) is the amount of matter in a given unit of volume. If the mass (m) and volume (V) of a substance are known, the density of a solid or a liquid can be easily calculated with the following formula:

$$density(\rho) = \frac{mass}{volume} = \frac{m}{V} \quad \textbf{(2.1)}$$

Example 2.1

If a substance has a mass of 5 kg and a volume of 25 cubic centimeters, what is its density?

$$\rho = \frac{m}{V}$$

$$\rho = \frac{5\ \text{kg}}{25\ \text{cm}^3}$$

$$\rho = 0.2\ \frac{\text{kg}}{\text{cm}^3}$$

Answer: The density is 0.2 kg/cm^3

Notice in Example 2.1 that the unit for density includes both a mass unit, kilograms in this example, and a volume unit, cubic centimeters in this example. Other mass units (e.g., gram) and volume units (e.g., liter) can also be used. The density of a substance can change in response to changes in temperature or pressure. For example, increasing the temperature of water to past its boiling point will turn the water into steam and drastically change its density. Similarly, decreasing the temperature of water to below its freezing point will turn the water into ice, again affecting its density. Pressurized air, such as the air pumped into a tire or a scuba tank, has a much greater density than the air around us. Although most liquids and solids are virtually incompressible, gases, such as air, can be compressed easily.

A physical characteristic related to compression is elasticity. **Elasticity** is the property of matter that allows matter to recover its form (size and shape) after it has been distorted (expanded or compressed). Rubber, for example, is a highly elastic material. Think of a rubber band. If you stretch it and let it go, it will immediately return to its original size and shape. Air is another highly elastic material. If a tire filled with compressed air pops, the air inside will quickly escape and return to the density of the surrounding air. Elasticity is thus a property that preserves the original shape or density of the matter and when disturbed may become a source of motion.

KINEMATICS

Kinematics is the branch of physics that describes the motion of objects in space without considering the cause of the motion. The motion can be linear (in a straight line), can be curvilinear (in a curved line), or can follow any other path. The focus of kinematics is the relationship among displacement (d), velocity (v), acceleration (a), and time (t). The first three variables are vectors, while the fourth one is a scalar.

Scalars and Vectors

The physical properties described so far (e.g., distance, mass, volume, and density) are characterized by a magnitude together with a unit of measurement. Physical characteristics

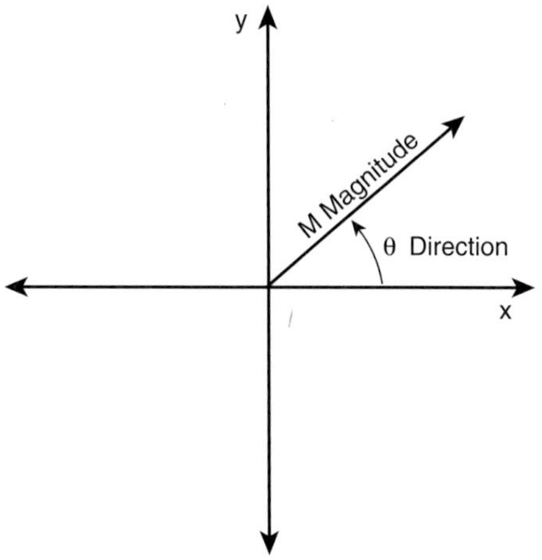

Figure 2.2. The magnitude and direction of a vector.

for which it is sufficient to provide only a magnitude and a unit are called **scalar** quantities or scalars. Other examples of scalars are speed, temperature, and pressure.

Sometimes a physical characteristic concerns motion or potential motion, and so a measurement of this characteristic also requires a statement of direction. Physical characteristics that are described by a magnitude, a unit, and a direction are called **vector** quantities or vectors. A vector is usually represented by an arrow with its length proportional to the given magnitude and pointing in the specified direction. An example of a vector in the x–y plane is shown in Figure 2.2. Examples of vector quantities are displacement, velocity, acceleration, and force. It is important to remember the distinction between vectors and their scalar counterparts, that is, displacement (vector) versus distance (scalar) and velocity (vector) versus speed (scalar). In pairs such as this, the vector is simply the scalar together with a direction. Speed by itself does not have a direction. When you specify a direction for the speed, however, speed becomes a velocity. In other words, the magnitude of a velocity is a speed, just as the magnitude of a displacement is a distance.

Displacement, Velocity, and Acceleration

Displacement (d) is defined as a change in position. As noted in the previous section, displacement is distance together with information about the direction of change. When talking about displacement, we are only interested in the change from the original position to the final position. We are not interested in the path the object took to get there. For example, in Figure 2.3, a box is positioned in front of a person, position A, and then moved to the person's left (the reader's right) to position B. Displacement at position B is 0.6 meters to the left of the person. If the box is then moved 0.3 meters back toward the person, the total displacement from position A to position C is 0.3 meters to the person's left. The path of the box is irrelevant—the total displacement is a change in position of 0.3 meters to the person's left. Here, a simple descriptor (left) was used to provide the direction, but in science, it is common to describe the

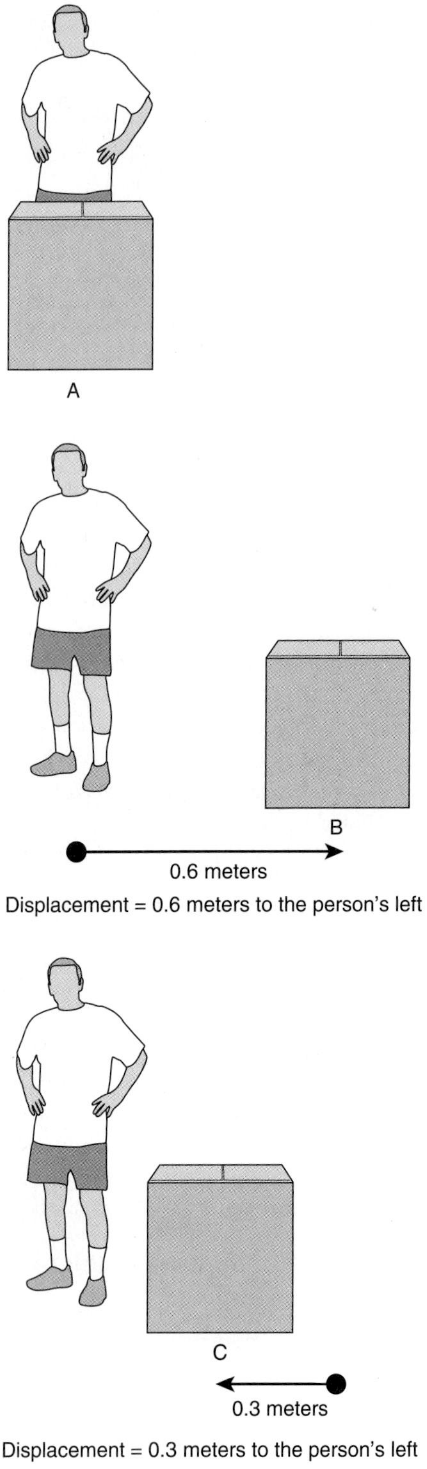

Figure 2.3. Displacement demonstrated with the movement of a box.

direction of motion as positive (+) or negative (−) or to describe it using angles.

Velocity (v) is defined as the rate of change in displacement. In science, velocity is most commonly reported in meters per second (m/s), but it can also be stated in feet per second (ft/s) or miles per hour (mph). **Average velocity** (v_{avg}) is calculated from the displacement (*d*) and the amount of time (*t*) it took for the displacement to occur. The formula for this calculation is:

$$v_{avg} = \frac{displacement}{time} = \frac{d}{t} \tag{2.2}$$

It is usually presented in a more precise fashion as follows:

$$v_{avg} = \frac{displacement}{time} = \frac{\Delta d}{\Delta t} = \frac{d_2 - d_1}{t_2 - t_1} \tag{2.3}$$

The triangle-like symbol (Δ) is actually the capital Greek letter delta, which is used in formulas to represent "difference" or "change." Other standard notation in Equation 2.3 includes *d* for displacement (position) and *t* for time. The subscripts (i.e., the 1 and 2 in d_1 and d_2) indicate either the first or second measurement. If you measure from the beginning of a motion, d_1 and t_1 are zero, so the formula simplifies to $v_{avg} = d_2 / t_2$. If the time span Δt is very short, the average velocity (v_{avg}) becomes the velocity at a given instant. This velocity is usually referred to as the **instantaneous velocity.**

In some situations, the direction of displacement is unknown or irrelevant to a discussion. In these cases, the symbol *d* in Equation 2.3 may represent the distance and contain no information about direction. In these cases, velocity (v) likewise loses its vector properties and represents speed. Remember, a velocity without a specific direction is a speed.

Example 2.2

A person has traveled 30 meters east in 6 seconds, and we want to find the person's average velocity. The calculation is as follows:

$$v_{avg} = \frac{displacement}{time}$$

$$v_{avg} = \frac{30\ m}{6\ s}$$

$$v_{avg} = 5\frac{m}{s}$$

Answer: The average velocity is 5 m/s east.

As demonstrated in Example 2.2, do not let yourself think of velocity as the same thing as speed; notice that the answer included a direction (east). Speed is a scalar quantity; velocity is a vector quantity. Velocity must be reported with both a magnitude (a speed) and a direction. Consider the following example in which average velocity and average speed are very different because the calculation of velocity must take direction into account although the calculation of speed does not.

Example 2.3

If Mary walks due east for 1 hour and travels 6 kilometers and then turns around and walks due west for 1 hour and travels 6 kilometers, her average *speed* is clearly 6 km/hr. What is her average *velocity* for the entire trip (Fig. 2.4).

$$v_{avg} = \frac{displacement}{time}$$

$$v_{avg} = \frac{0 \text{ km}}{1 \text{ hr}}$$

$$v_{avg} = 0 \text{ km/hr (east)}$$

Answer: The average velocity is 0 km/hr (east).

From Example 2.3 you have seen that Mary's average velocity is 0 km/hr (east). Remember, displacement is a change in position and, as mentioned earlier, it does not concern the path of motion. At the end of the walk, Mary is back to where she started. Since there was no change in her position at the end of the walk as compared to her position at the beginning of the walk, her displacement was zero kilometers (east). Keep in mind that we could have calculated her average velocity just for the first or second part of her walk or we could have calculated her instantaneous velocity at any time during the walk, but the point of this example was to demonstrate the difference between calculating speed and calculating velocity.

PRACTICE PROBLEMS: VELOCITY

1. John travels north for 0.5 hour and travels 2.5 kilometers. Then he travels south for 0.5 hour and travels 2.5 kilometers. What is John's average velocity over his total 1-hour walk?
2. In Problem 1, what is John's average velocity for the first $\frac{1}{2}$ hour of the walk?
3. If a car moves west for 1 hour and travels 60 kilometers and then east for half an hour and travels 30 kilometers, what is the car's average velocity for the entire $1\frac{1}{2}$-hour trip?
4. In Problem 3, what is the car's average speed?

Answers (If you need help with these problems, consult the website.) **Link 2-3**

1. John's average velocity for the 1-hour walk was 0 km/hr north.
2. John's average velocity for the first $\frac{1}{2}$ hour was 5 km/hr north.
3. The car's average velocity for the $1\frac{1}{2}$-hour trip was 20 km/hr west.
4. The car's average speed was 60 km/hr.

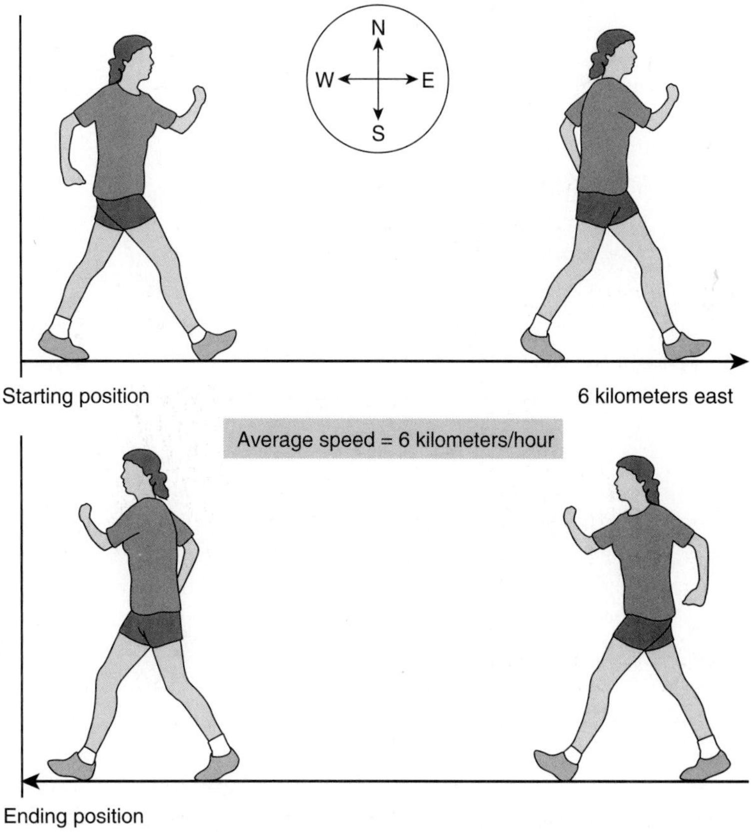

Figure 2.4. Velocity demonstrated with a walker changing direction.

Acceleration (a) is defined as the rate of change in velocity. It is usually reported in meters per second squared (m/s^2). To get a clear picture of the difference between velocity (rate of change in displacement) and acceleration (rate of change in velocity), consider this example. A car is stopped on the entrance ramp of a highway and then quickly accelerates to highway speed to join traffic. Just as the car is "taking off" from the ramp, its velocity is at its lowest (it's not going very fast), but its acceleration is at its greatest because the driver just pressed down on the accelerator to get the car from 0 to 55 mph as quickly as possible. Once the car reaches highway speed, its velocity is at its greatest, but since its velocity is no longer changing, its acceleration is now at its lowest (i.e., zero).

Box 2.1 Understanding Why the Unit for Acceleration is m/s²

Acceleration is equal to velocity over time. The unit for velocity is m/s and the unit for time is s. Thus, if we solve an acceleration problem in which the velocity is 15 m/s and the time is 10 s, the acceleration is 1.5, and the units end up as m/s/s as shown here.

$$accelearation = \frac{velocity(m/s)}{time(s)} = \frac{15\frac{m}{s}}{10\ s} = 1.5\frac{\frac{m}{s}}{s}$$

However, the unit for acceleration is reported in m/s^2. How can m/s/s be reported as m/s^2? These two units are equal mathematically. You may need to review the mathematics chapter to understand this concept, but consider this:

In the unit m/s/s, the top portion of the unit m/s is divided by seconds. Dividing by any quantity is the same as multiplying by its inverse. The inverse of s is 1/s. Thus, the following conversions can be made:

$$\frac{\frac{m}{s}}{s} = \frac{m}{s} \div s = \frac{m}{s} \times \frac{1}{s} = \frac{m}{s \times s} = \frac{m}{s^2}$$

Thus, m/s/s can be rewritten m/s^2.

Average acceleration can be determined by measuring the velocity of a moving object at two points in time. The initial velocity (v_1) is subtracted from the final velocity (v_2) and the time of the first measurement (t_1) is subtracted from the time of the second measurement (t_2). The difference in the velocity (Δv) is then divided by the difference in time (Δt). Written mathematically:

$$a_{avg} = \frac{velocity}{time} = \frac{\Delta v}{\Delta t} = \frac{v_2 - v_1}{t_2 - t_1} \qquad (2.4)$$

Just as for velocity, if Δt is very small, we can calculate **instantaneous acceleration.**

Acceleration, like displacement and velocity, is a vector quantity. The direction of acceleration, however, is influenced by the direction of motion *and* by whether the object is accelerating (speeding up) or decelerating (slowing down). A negative acceleration indicates that the object is either accelerating in the negative direction or decelerating in the positive direction. If we consider the magnitude of acceleration on its own, it becomes a scalar. Unlike displacement and velocity, acceleration without direction does not have its own special name, which can be confusing at times.

One useful number to remember regarding acceleration is $9.8\ m/s^2$. This is the acceleration due to the force of gravity on Earth. All falling objects on Earth accelerate steadily at this rate. This is true regardless of the mass of the object, although an object such as a feather will fall slower than a lead ball because of the effect of air resistance against the feather. If both objects were dropped in a vacuum (space with no air), they would fall at the same rate. If you are interested in the mathematical relationship between displacement, velocity, and acceleration of an object moving with a constant acceleration, consult the website. **Link 2-4**

Example 2.4

While watching a car accelerate down a straight road, you take two velocity measurements, the first at 2 seconds into the acceleration and the second at 4 seconds into the acceleration. If the velocity at 2 seconds was 2 m/s and the velocity at 4 seconds was 20 m/s, what was the car's average acceleration?

First, select the appropriate equation to determine the acceleration.

$$a_{avg} = \frac{velocity}{time} = \frac{\Delta v}{\Delta t} = \frac{v_2 - v_1}{t_2 - t_1}$$

Second, substitute known variables. We know the times of the two measurements, 2 seconds and 4 seconds into the acceleration, and we know the velocities at those times, 2 m/s and 20 m/s.

$$a_{avg} = \frac{20\frac{m}{s} - 2\frac{m}{s}}{4\ s - 2\ s}$$

$$a_{avg} = \frac{18\frac{m}{s}}{2\ s}$$

$$a_{avg} = 9\frac{m}{s^2}$$

Answer: The car's acceleration was $9\ m/s^2$.

PRACTICE PROBLEMS: ACCELERATION

1. While watching a car accelerate down a road, you take two velocity measurements, the first at 1 second into the acceleration and the second at 3 seconds into the acceleration. If the velocity at 1 second was 3 m/s and the velocity at 3 seconds was 17 m/s, what was the car's average acceleration?
2. While watching a marble accelerate down an incline, you take two velocity measurements, the first at 1 second into the acceleration and the second at 3 seconds into the acceleration. If the velocity at 1 second was 0.5 m/s and the velocity at 3 seconds was 0.7 m/s, what was the marble's average acceleration?
3. If an object is free falling, with minimal friction, what is its acceleration?
4. If the velocity of a falling object increases by 9.8 m/s in 2 seconds, what is the object's average acceleration?

Answers (If you need help with these problems, consult the website.) **Link 2-5**

1. The car's acceleration was 7 m/s^2.
2. The marble's average acceleration was 0.1 m/s^2.
3. Acceleration due to gravity is 9.8 m/s^2.
4. The acceleration is 4.9 m/s^2.

Vector Addition

Numbers (scalars) can be added, subtracted, multiplied, divided, and so forth. Similar operations can be performed on vectors. For the purposes of this text, only the addition of vectors will be considered.

Frequently two or more vectors must be added together to find a combined vector, for example, if we want to find the total displacement of an object that first moves in one direction and then later in a second direction. Since vector quantities consist of both a magnitude and a direction, the problem cannot be solved by simply adding together the magnitudes of the individual vectors. We must consider the magnitudes relative to the directions. This is done using vector addition.

Vector addition is the method for adding two vectors together taking both their individual magnitudes and their individual directions into account. It is not a difficult concept, but if you do not feel comfortable with Cartesian and polar coordinates or the Pythagorean Theorem, it might be worthwhile to go back and review those sections from Chapter 1 before continuing here.

Example 2.5

Imagine you are the pilot of a small airplane traveling at 300 mph due east. A wind from the southwest is pushing the airplane at 25 mph in a northeast direction. What is the velocity of the airplane relative to the ground?

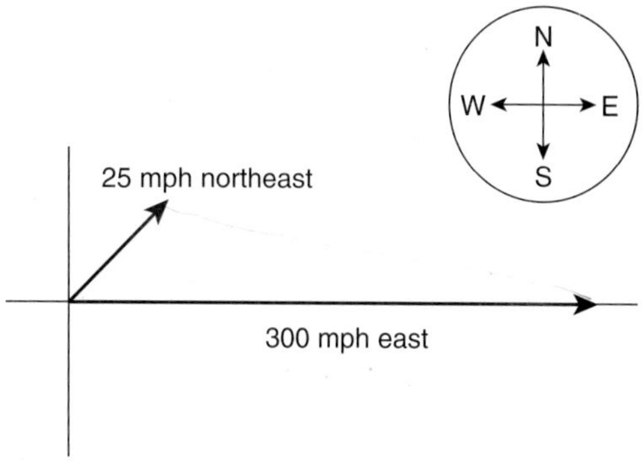

Figure 2.5. Two velocity vectors.

To answer this problem, we must consider both things influencing the overall velocity of the airplane, the airplane's own velocity (300 mph east) and the wind velocity (25 mph northeast). If you ignore the effect of the wind and try to predict the location of the plane, your prediction will be miles away from the actual location.

First, we note that the two velocity vectors can be plotted on a graph, shown in Figure 2.5.

Notice in Figure 2.5 the two arrows representing the two vectors. The direction is clearly indicated by the way the arrows are pointing. The magnitudes of the vectors are clearly visible; the 300 mph east vector is much longer than the 25 mph northeast vector.

The main idea behind vector addition is that the two vectors acting simultaneously can be considered to act sequentially (one after the other) for problem solving. This allows us to plot the second vector starting from the tail (arrowhead end) of the first vector. A third vector can be drawn from the head (start) of the first vector to the tail of the second. This third vector is called the resultant vector and represents the sum of the first two vectors. Once we determine the magnitude and direction of the resultant vector, shown in Figure 2.6, we have added the first and second vectors.

Determining the magnitude and direction of the resultant vector requires a few steps. Since the direction of the first vector is due east, it aligns with the x axis on a standard x–y plot and determining the Cartesian (x, y) coordinates of its tail is very easy (Fig. 2.7). Its magnitude is 300 mph, so it ends at 300 on the x axis, and since it is pointing due east, its coordinate on the y axis is zero. Thus, the Cartesian coordinates of its tail are (300, 0).

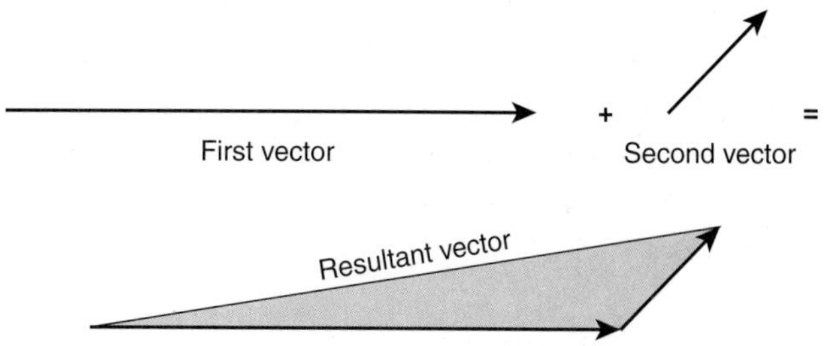

Figure 2.6. The resultant vector created by the addition of two vectors.

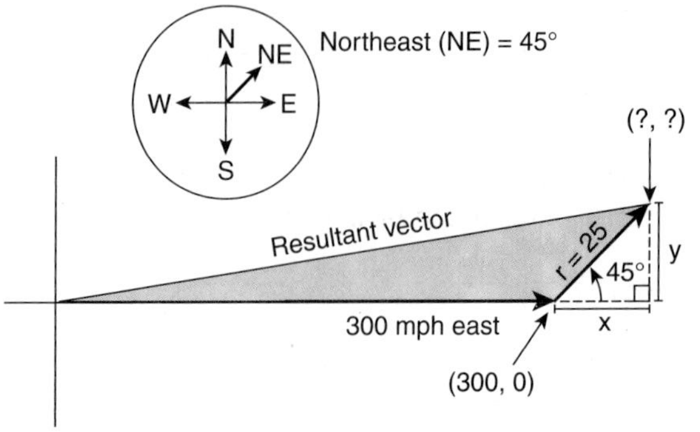

Figure 2.7. A velocity of 300 mph east yields the Cartesian coordinates of (300, 0). The polar coordinates of the second vector (25, 45°) are used to calculate the Cartesian coordinates of the second vector.

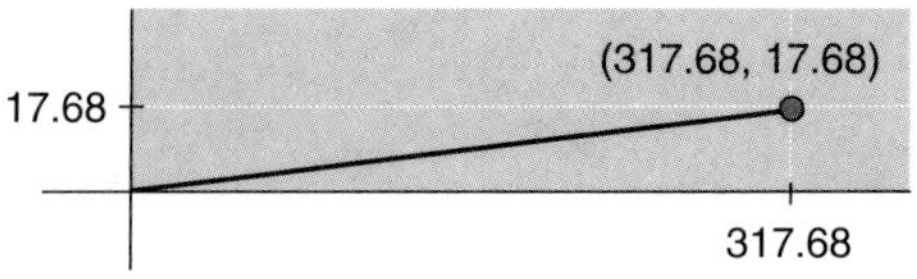

Figure 2.8. Cartesian coordinates determined for the tail of the resultant vector.

Now what about the second vector? Since the first vector points east and the second vector points northeast, the angle between the two vectors is 45° (Fig. 2.7). Since we know the length (magnitude) of the second vector (given in the problem as 25 mph) and the angle between the first vector and the second vector (45°), this means we know the polar coordinates of the second vector (25 mph, 45°). Since we know the Cartesian coordinates of the first vector and the polar coordinates of the second vector, we can use this information to find the magnitude and direction of the resultant vector by following these steps:

1. Convert the polar coordinates of the second vector to Cartesian coordinates.
2. Add the Cartesian coordinates from the two vectors to determine the Cartesian coordinates of the resultant vector.
3. Convert the Cartesian coordinates of the resultant vector to polar coordinates to solve the problem.

To solve this problem, begin with step 1. Recall from Chapter 1 the necessary equations for converting from polar to Cartesian coordinates:

$$x = r\cos\theta \qquad (2.5)$$

$$y = r\sin\theta \qquad (2.6)$$

If we consider the second vector as the hypotenuse of a right triangle, as shown in Figure 2.7, x is the length of the base of the triangle and y its height. Inserting the length of the vector (25) and the angle (45°) into the above equations, we find:

$$x = r\cos\theta$$
$$x = 25 \times (\cos 45°)$$
$$x = 17.68$$

Thus, the x coordinate for the second vector is 17.68.

$$y = r\sin\theta$$
$$y = 25 \times (\sin 45°)$$
$$y = 17.68$$

Thus, the y coordinate for the second vector is 17.68.

Next, proceed to step 2. To determine the Cartesian coordinates of the tail of the resultant vector, add the x and y values from the second vector to the x and y coordinates, respectively, of the first vector (Fig. 2.8).

$$x = 300 + 17.68 = 317.68$$
$$y = 0 + 17.68 = 17.68$$

Next, proceed to step 3. To arrive at the overall velocity, that is, speed and direction, of the plane, the Cartesian (x, y) coordinates of the resultant vector must now be converted back into polar coordinates. The appropriate formulas discussed in Chapter 1 are:

$$r = \sqrt{x^2 + y^2} \qquad (2.7)$$

$$\theta = tan^{-1}\left(\frac{y}{x}\right) \qquad (2.8)$$

Substitute the Cartesian coordinates of the resultant vector into the above formulas:

$$r = \sqrt{317.68^2 + 17.68^2} = 319.17$$

$$\theta = tan^{-1}\left(\frac{17.68}{317.68}\right) = 3.19$$

Answer: The velocity of the airplane relative to the ground is 319.17 mph at 3.19°.

PRACTICE PROBLEMS: VECTOR ADDITION

1. If Mary walks 1 kilometer east then 2 kilometers northeast, what is her displacement at the end of the walk?
2. If an airplane travels at 300 mph east and the wind is blowing at 25 mph toward the southwest, what is the average velocity of the airplane relative to the ground?

Answers (If you need help with these problems, consult the website.) **Link 2-6**

1. Mary's displacement at the end of the walk is 2.79 km, 30.33°.
2. The velocity of the airplane relative to the ground is 282.87 mph at 356.42° or −3.58°.

DYNAMICS

In the kinematics portion of this chapter, we considered motion without regard for its source or cause. To cause motion or any other change in the state of an object, energy needs to be applied to the object. When energy is applied to an object, the result is a force being created that can move or alter the object. The domain of physics concerned with energy and force is called dynamics. **Dynamics** is the study of the effects of forces on the state of an object or a system of objects.

Force

Force (*F*) can be viewed as a push or a pull. More formally, force can be defined as an interaction between two objects or between an object and its environment. Force is another vector quantity; the direction of the push or pull is very important. The unit of force that is generally used in science is the **newton**. One newton is the amount of force required to accelerate a 1-kg mass at 1 m/s^2.

In Figure 2.9A, you can see a man exerting a force on an object. This may cause the object to move (depending on the mass, the force, and the friction of the surface). If a single person is not successful at moving the object and a second person pushes simultaneously, with the same force, the force is doubled. So, is the box more likely to move? It depends on the direction in which the second force is applied. Examine Figures 2.9B and 2.9C. If the second person applies a force in the same direction as the first person (Fig. 2.9B), they are working together and the box is more likely to move. If, however, the second person applies the force in the opposite direction (Fig. 2.9C), the box will not move even though the force is doubled. This is why force must be described by both magnitude and direction.

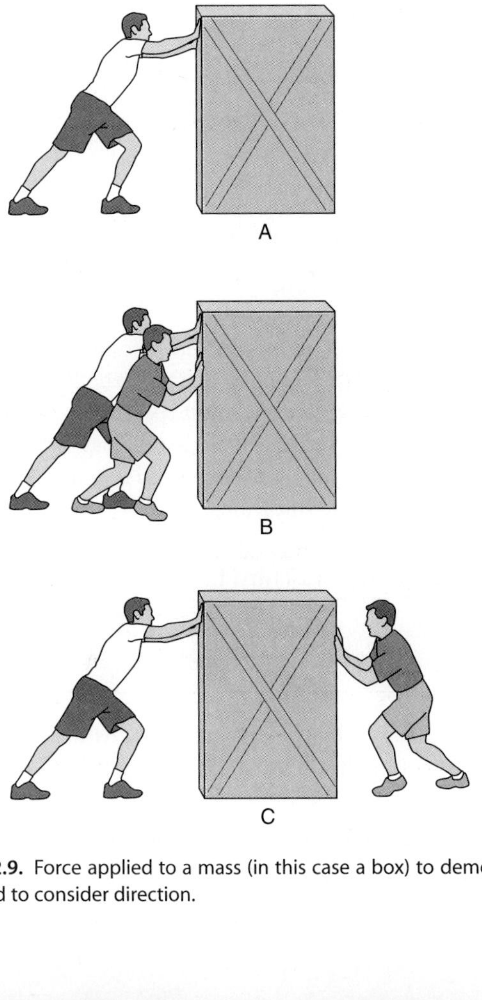

Figure 2.9. Force applied to a mass (in this case a box) to demonstrate the need to consider direction.

Newton's Laws of Motion

The basic relationships between force and motion were first formulated by Sir Isaac Newton (1642–1727) in the form of three laws of motion. They were published in 1687 and laid the foundation of classic physics. **Newton's First Law of Motion** states that an object at rest will remain at rest and an object in motion will remain in motion and move with uniform velocity unless acted upon by an external force. The First Law of Motion describes the concept of **inertia** and is based on the observation of the great Italian astronomer and mathematician Galileo Galilei (1564–1642) that a force does not need to be exerted on an object to keep it in uniform motion. This law is, therefore, also known as the Law of Inertia. Inertia is the opposition of an object to changes to its state of motion. The product of mass (*m*) and velocity (*v*) of a moving object is called **momentum** (***M***, plural: momenta) and this product remains constant if no external force acts on the mass.

Box 2.2 Newton's First Law of Motion (Law of Inertia)

An object will remain at rest or in a state of uniform motion unless there is unbalanced force acting on it.

Box 2.3 Galileo Galilei

Galileo Galilei (1564–1642) was an Italian mathematician and astronomer. His observations of the solar system via a self-made telescope supported the Copernican theory, which stated that the Earth moved around the sun. Galileo's publication of these observations was considered an insult to the Pope and he was convicted of heresy in 1633. He is described in physics texts as the "first modern physicist" because of his combination of mathematical experimentation with careful observation of the natural world (Mulligan, 1991).

Box 2.4 Sir Isaac Newton

Sir Isaac Newton (1642–1727) was a British mathematician and physicist who described the basic relationships between force and motion, which are known as Newton's Laws of Motion and the Law of Universal Gravitation. They were published by Newton in 1687 in his *Philosophiae Naturalis Principia Mathematica (Mathematical Principles of Natural Philosophy)*, the book that laid the foundations of classical physics. He was known to be rather surly and highly introspective, and often wrote down his ideas but kept them hidden for years before they were published.

Newton's Second Law of Motion describes the relationship between force, mass, and acceleration. It says that an object's acceleration is proportional to the force exerted on the object and inversely proportional to the mass of the object. This simply means that the greater the force is, the higher the acceleration, and the greater the mass is, the lower the acceleration.

Box 2.5 Newton's Second Law of Motion

An unbalanced force acting on an object will cause the object to move with an acceleration proportional to the force and inversely proportional to the mass of the object.

The mathematical expression of the Second Law of Motion is one of the most fundamental equations in all of physics: Force equals mass times acceleration.

$$F = m \times a \tag{2.9}$$

You can think of this equation in two ways: (1) as specifying the force required to cause a given acceleration or (2) as determining the acceleration a given force will cause. The Second Law of Motion is actually an extension of the First Law of Motion. Notice that if there is no force ($F = 0$), then there can be no acceleration ($a = 0$), since mass cannot be zero. Likewise, if an object is not accelerating (nor decelerating), then there can be no external force acting on it.

Example 2.6

If a mass of 6 kg is accelerated at 2 m/s^2, what is the force?

Select the appropriate equation.

$$F = m \times a$$

Substitute known variables.

$$F = 6\ \text{kg} \times 2\ \frac{\text{m}}{\text{s}^2}$$

$$F = 12\ \frac{\text{kg} \times \text{m}}{\text{s}^2}$$

Here, you need to know that 1 newton is equal to $1\frac{\text{kg} \times \text{m}}{\text{s}^2}$. Therefore, replace the unit $\frac{\text{kg} \times \text{m}}{\text{s}^2}$ with the newton (N).

$$F = 12\ \text{N}$$

Answer: The force is 12 newtons (N).

Example 2.7

If a force of 3 N is applied to a mass of 0.5 kg, what is the acceleration?

Select the appropriate equation.

$$F = m \times a$$

Substitute known variables and solve.

$$3\ \text{N} = 0.5\ \text{kg} \times a$$

$$a = \frac{3\ \text{N}}{0.5\ \text{kg}}$$

Recall from Example 2.6 that $1\ \text{N} = 1\frac{\text{kg} \times \text{m}}{\text{s}^2}$. Therefore, when an equation includes N and the units must be simplified, rewrite N as $\frac{\text{kg} \times \text{m}}{\text{s}^2}$, and simplify by canceling the kilogram unit from the numerator and denominator.

$$a = \frac{3\ \frac{\text{kg} \times \text{m}}{\text{s}^2}}{0.5\ \text{kg}}$$

Answer: The acceleration is 6 m/s^2.

PRACTICE PROBLEMS: NEWTON'S SECOND LAW OF MOTION

1. If a mass of 10 kg is accelerated at 10 m/s^2, what is the force?
2. If a force of 2 N is applied to a mass of 10 kg, what is the acceleration?
3. If a force of 100 N accelerates a mass at 20 m/s^2, what is the mass?

Answers (If you need help with these problems, consult the website.) **Link 2-7**

1. The force is 100 N.
2. The acceleration is 0.2 m/s^2.
3. The mass is 5 kg.

Newton's Third Law of Motion, also known as the Law of Action, states that for every action there is an equal and opposite reaction. This means that if object A exerts a force on object B, then object B acts with an equal force on object A. Both forces are of the same type and magnitude but they are acting in opposite directions.

Box 2.6 Newton's Third Law of Motion

Every force produces a counterforce that is equal in magnitude and opposite in direction.

Two familiar real-world events that illustrate this principle are stepping off a boat and shooting a gun. When you step off a boat onto land, the force you exert to move yourself forward also pushes the boat backwards. When you shoot a gun, the force that propels the bullet through the barrel is also what causes the gun to recoil.

Newton's three laws of motion are the main laws governing the movements and interactions of objects. Collectively, these laws represent an important physical principle called the Law of Conservation of Momentum, which is a natural extension of Newton's First Law. To understand how Newton's three laws of motion form the basis for the Law of Conservation of Momentum, consider a force (F) acting on an object with mass (m). According to Newton's Second Law, the force will accelerate the object with an acceleration (a). When the force finishes its action, then according to the first Newton's law, the object will continue to move with a uniform velocity $v = a \times t$ where t is the time interval during which the force was acting on the object. Recall that the product of mass and velocity is called momentum. Thus, an object that is not acted upon by an external force will always maintain its momentum. When two objects (or systems) moving with uniform velocities collide, however, their forces interact, resulting in changes in their velocities. Further, according to Newton's Third Law, for every action there is an equal and opposite reaction. Thus, the sum of the momenta of the two objects before the collision must be equal to the sum of the momenta after the collision; otherwise, the reaction (i.e., what happens after the collision) would not equal the action (i.e., what happened before the collision). This can be mathematically written as:

$$m_1 v_{11} + m_2 v_{21} = m_1 v_{12} + m_2 v_{22} \qquad (2.10)$$

where m_1 and m_2 are the masses of the colliding objects, v_{11} and v_{21} are the velocities of the two masses before the collision, and v_{12} and v_{22} are the velocities of the two masses after the collision. Equation 2.10 states the **Law of Conservation of Momentum,** which states that the total momentum of all the things in the universe will never change. The importance of this law as it relates to hearing science will be demonstrated in Chapter 4, where we will consider the concepts of impedance and energy transmission.

Gravity and Weight

Gravity is a universal phenomenon in which any two objects in the universe attract each other. The strength of the attraction depends on the masses of both of the objects and the distance between them: The greater the masses are, the stronger the force; the greater the distance is, the weaker the force. However, for the force to actually be noticeable, at least one of the masses must be extremely large. We notice gravity because the mass of the Earth is approximately 6,000,000,000,000,000,000,000,000 kg. This general relationship is the focus of the **Law of Universal Gravitation,** again discovered and published by Sir Isaac Newton.

Box 2.7 The Law of Universal Gravitation

Every object in the universe attracts every other object with a force directed toward its center and that is proportional to the product of their masses and inversely proportional to the square of the distance between them.

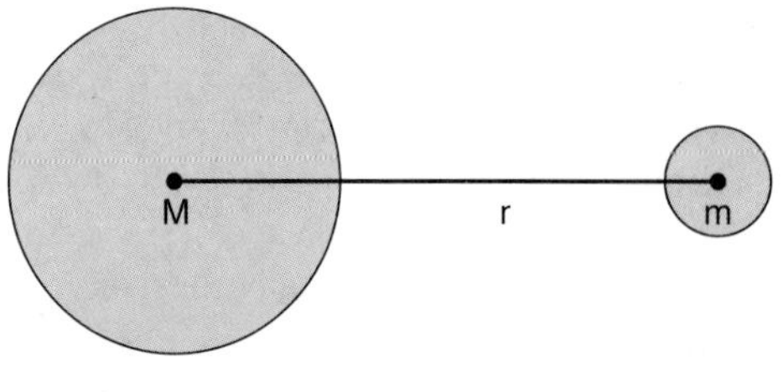

Figure 2.10 Two masses (*M* and *m*) separated by the distance (*r*).

Assuming the situation shown in Figure 2.10, the gravitational force between the two objects can be determined with the following equation:

$$F = G \times \frac{M \times m}{r^2} \qquad (2.11)$$

where G is the universal gravitational constant. To find more information about G and gravitational acceleration (g; from Equation 2.12), see the website. **Link 2-8**

Note that each object exerts the same force on the other object. The larger object attracts the smaller object and the smaller object equally attracts the larger object. The reason we see an apple fall to the ground and not the Earth being pulled toward the apple is because, as we know from the Second Law of Motion, the resulting acceleration depends on the mass of the object. Remember, the greater the mass is, the lower the acceleration. Since the mass of the Earth is so huge, its acceleration toward the apple is practically zero. The apple's mass, on the other hand, is very small compared to the Earth's, so its acceleration is quite noticeable.

The **weight** of an object is actually the force of gravity acting on the object. Note that since weight is a force, it is a vector and points toward the center of the Earth. The weight of an object on Earth can be calculated with Equation 2.12 using the acceleration due to gravity, $g = 9.8\ m/s^2$:

$$Weight = m \times g \qquad (2.12)$$

If you take an object such as a jar of pickled okra, determine its weight on Earth, and then fly to the moon and weigh it (not a NASA-worthy endeavor, perhaps), you would find the two measurements to be very different because gravity is different on the moon than on Earth. The mass of the jar, however, would be the same in both places because the amount of matter in the object does not change. Mass is easily measured on a balance scale by comparing the object of interest with another object that has a calibrated mass, as shown in Figure 2.11. In reality, we are comparing two weights, but since the force of gravity acting on both masses is the same, this measurement can be equated to comparing two masses. Weight can

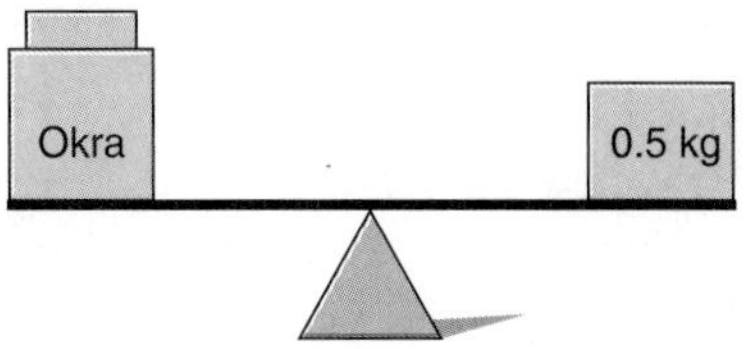

Figure 2.11. A balanced scale containing a jar on one side and a calibrated 0.5-kg mass on the other. Note that since the scale is balanced, the mass of the jar is 0.5 kg.

vary slightly based on a person's position on Earth (i.e., between the top of the tallest mountain and the bottom of the deepest cave). If you would like to know more about this topic, consult the website. **Link clip 2-9**

Work

Work (W) is the effect of force (*F*) moving an object over a distance (*d*). No matter what the force, if displacement does not occur, then no work is done on an object. For example, even if you push against a wall as hard as you can, you've done no work on the wall unless you've succeeded in pushing it a measurable distance. You may feel very tired but no work has been done on the wall. The equation used to determine the amount of work done when a force applied to an object results in movement in the direction of the force is given below:

$$W = \text{Force} \times \text{Distance} = F \times d \qquad (2.13)$$

If the force is given in newtons and the displacement is given in meters, the unit of work will be the newton meter. Since work is such a fundamental concept in physics, the newton meter has its own name, the **joule (J)**. One joule is the amount of work done when a 1-kg mass is moved 1 m.

Example 2.8

If you push the box with a force of 5 N and move it 3 m straight ahead, how much work have you done (Fig. 2.12)?

Since the direction of the force is the same as the direction of the displacement, we can use Equation 2.13. Substituting known variables, we arrive at the following answer:

$$W = F \times d$$

$$W = 5\text{ N} \times 3\text{ m}$$

$$W = 15\text{ N} \times \text{m}$$

$$W = 15\text{ J}$$

Answer: You have done 15 J of work.

If the force is acting at an angle compared to the direction of displacement, then the equation used to determine the work becomes:

$$W = F \times d \times \cos\theta \qquad (2.14)$$

Here, θ is the angle between the direction of the force and the direction of displacement.

Example 2.9

This time, a 5-N force is applied to a box by pulling it with a string at a 45° angle. Again the box is moved 3 meters along the ground. But now how much work has been done (Fig. 2.13)?

First, select the appropriate equation. Since the force was applied at an angle compared to the direction the box was moved, use Equation 2.14. All three necessary elements are known: The angle at which the force was applied is 45°, the magnitude of the force is 5 N, and the displacement is 3 m, so:

$$W = F \times d \times \cos\theta$$

$$W = 5\text{ N} \times 3\text{ m} \times \cos 45°$$

$$W = 5\text{ N} \times 3\text{ m} \times 0.71$$

$$W = 10.61\text{ J}$$

Answer: 10.61 J

PRACTICE PROBLEMS: WORK

1. If you push an object with a force of 1 N and move it 4 m (in the same direction as the push), how much work have you done?
2. If a truck pushes an object with a force of 50 N and moves it 10 m (in the same direction as the push), how much work has the truck done?
3. If a 15-N force is applied to an object at a 35° angle (compared to the direction the object moves) and the object moves 0.5 m, how much work has been done?
4. If a 100-N force is applied to an object at a 55° angle and the object moves 13 m, how much work has been done?

Answers (If you need help with these problems, consult the website.) **Link 2-10**

1. You have done 4 J of work.
2. The truck did 500 J of work.
3. 6.15 J of work was done.
4. 745.65 J of work was done.

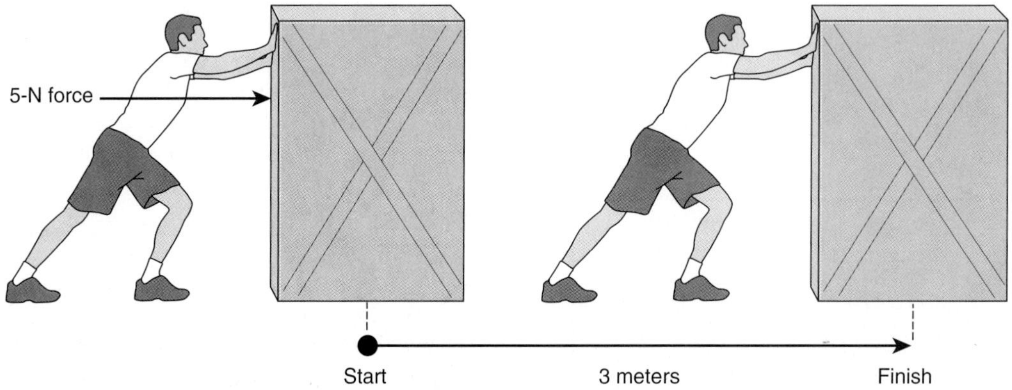

Figure 2.12. Force applied to a box causing a displacement.

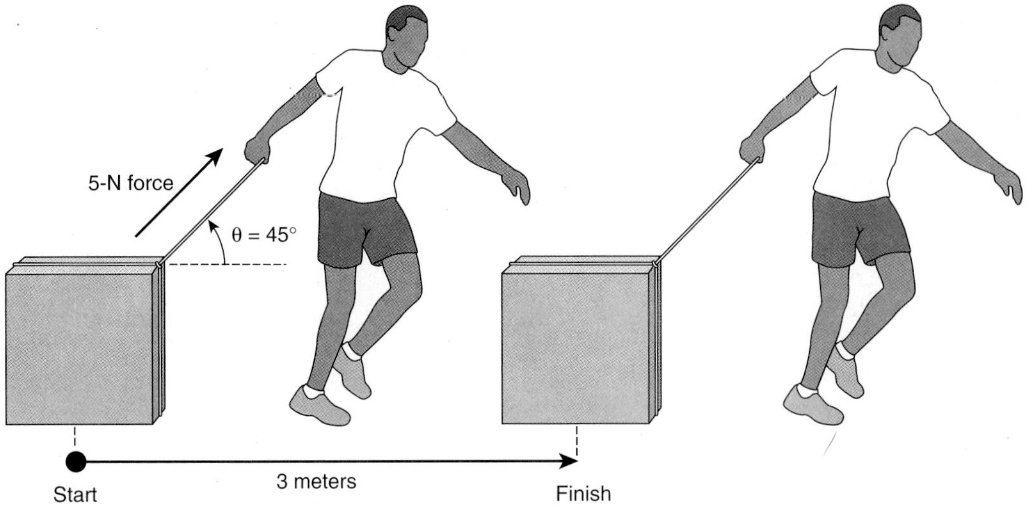

Figure 2.13. Force applied at an angle.

Energy

Energy (*E*) is defined as the ability or capacity of an object to do work. Energy is stored in an object and is gradually expended when the object does work. If we want the object to do more work, we need to provide the object with more energy. Therefore, work and energy can be treated as the same physical property seen from two different points of view. Energy is future work, whereas work is used energy. Energy has many forms including mechanical energy, electrical energy, electromagnetic energy, solar energy, and nuclear energy. However, all these different specific types of energy can be broadly classified into two categories: potential energy and kinetic energy.

Potential energy (E_p) is the energy of an object due to its position within a given physical system or environment. For example, if you hold a stone in your hand, the stone has potential energy because if you let it go it will fall to the ground. When it hits the ground, it transfers that energy into the ground. Lying on the ground, it no longer has any potential energy. So whether the stone does or doesn't have potential energy depends on its position relative to the ground. Thus, the potential energy of an object on Earth due to the force of gravity is determined by its weight and its height (h) above the ground and equals mass × gravity × height:

$$E_p = m \times g \times h \qquad (2.15)$$

The higher the object is above the surface of the Earth, the greater its potential energy. Think about the difference between dropping the same rock on somebody's foot from a height of 10 cm and from a height of 10 m. The pain the person would feel is a direct reflection of the amount of energy transferred from rock to foot, because the force (the weight of the rock) is the same regardless of the height from which it is dropped. Note that in normal speech, one might say that the rock dropped from 10 m hit the person's foot with greater force. This is an absolutely false statement within the realm of physics. It is important to be aware of this distinction between the scientific and "everyday" meanings of the word *force*. It is also important to realize that the same object taken to another planet (e.g., the moon) and held at the same distance above the surface of the planet will have a different potential energy than on Earth. This difference is due to the different masses of the planets, resulting in a different force of gravity.

Gravity is the main source of potential energy, but not the only one. Elasticity (the force of elasticity) is also a source of potential energy. Elastic materials such as extended rubber bands, stretched mechanic springs, and compressed air accumulate potential energy and can be sources of work. Elasticity is important in hearing science, because elasticity is needed for both sound generation and sound propagation. The forces of gravity and elasticity (and associated with them potential energy) are the source of vibrations and will be discussed in Chapter 3.

Kinetic energy (E_k) is the energy of motion that an object possesses due to its velocity. The dependence of kinetic energy on the velocity and mass of an object is shown in the following equation:

$$E_k = \frac{mass \times velocity^2}{2} = \frac{m \times v^2}{2} \qquad (2.16)$$

where m is the mass of a moving object and v is its velocity. The faster an object is moving, the greater its kinetic energy. (See the website for the derivation of Equation 2.16.) **Link 2-11**

One of the most important laws in physics is the **Law of Conservation of Energy,** which states that energy can change from one form to another but cannot be created or destroyed. Kinetic energy can be converted into potential energy and vice versa or transmitted from one system to another. Likewise, one specific form of energy can be transformed into another, for example, mechanical energy (motion) into thermal energy (heat). This happens, for example, when you rub your hands together to create warmth. In fact, what frequently seems like a "loss" of energy is actually energy being converted into heat. No energy is really lost or gained in the process—it has simply changed its form.

Consider again the example of the falling rock. As the rock falls, more and more of its potential energy is converted into kinetic energy; that is, its height above the ground decreases as its velocity increases. Right as it is hitting the ground, all of its potential energy has become kinetic energy, and it is this kinetic energy that is then transferred to the ground.

On the other hand, when you toss a stone straight up into the air, the transformation first goes in the opposite direction—from kinetic energy into potential energy. When you release the stone, you give it kinetic energy. While it is moving, this energy is being continually converted into potential energy; that is, its velocity decreases as its height above the ground increases. The stone continues going up until all the kinetic energy you gave it has become potential energy. At that point, because it has no more kinetic energy left, it pauses ever so briefly and then starts on its way back down because now, due to its position (height), it has potential energy.

The unit of energy is the same at the unit of work, the joule. This is because energy and work are actually two ways of looking at the same physical property. Work is the expenditure of energy. Once all of an object's energy has been spent (transferred to other objects), it can do no more work. If we say that a system has done 500 J of work, this is the same as saying that it has transferred 500 J of energy to another object. All equations, units, and various other considerations that apply to energy apply to work and vice versa.

Power

Power (*P*) is the rate at which a system is gaining or losing energy. The relationship between power and work is similar to the relationship between velocity and displacement. Velocity is the rate at which displacement occurs ($v = d/t$), whereas power is the rate at which work is done. The relationship between power (P) and work (W) or energy (E) and time (t) can be written in the following way:

$$P = \frac{W}{t} = \frac{E}{t} \qquad (2.17)$$

Thus, the power of a system that does 50 J of work in a short period of time, say 30 seconds, is greater than the power of a system that does the same amount of work (50 J) over a longer period of time, say 5 minutes. The unit of power is the **watt (W)**, which is defined as the ability of the system to do 1 joule of work in 1 second.

Example 2.10

If 100 J of work is done over 10 seconds, what is the power?

Select the appropriate equation.

$$P = \frac{W}{t}$$

Substitute known variables and solve.

$$P = \frac{100\text{ J}}{10\text{ s}}$$

$$P = 10\text{ J/s}$$
$$P = 10\text{ W}$$

Answer: The power is 10 watts.

Since power is related to work (energy) (Equation 2.17) and work is related to force (Equation 2.13), it is possible to express power as a function of force by inserting Equation 2.13 into Equation 2.17 to get:

$$P = \frac{W}{t} = \frac{F \times d}{t} = F \times \frac{d}{t} \qquad (2.18)$$

Notice that in the second part of Equation 2.18 distance (d) is divided by time (t). Since velocity (v) is equal to d/t (Equation 2.2), we can substitute velocity (v) for d/t in the above equation to arrive at a practical form of the power equation:

$$P = F \times v \qquad (2.19)$$

Equation 2.19 states that the power of any mechanical system is the product of the force acting on the system and the velocity of the system. This equation is one of the fundamental relationships describing vibrations, sound waves, and even electricity. Its practical use will be shown in future chapters that talk about force and power related to sound waves.

Please note that since Equation 2.13 is only valid when the displacement is in the same direction as that of the force being applied, Equation 2.19 may likewise only be applied if the motion is in the direction of the force. If the motion occurs at an angle to the force, Equation 2.14 must be used in the above derivation in place of Equation 2.13 and Equation 2.19 will take a different form:

$$P = F \times v \cos \theta \qquad (2.20)$$

PRACTICE PROBLEMS: ENERGY AND POWER

1. If a system produces 757 J of work over 1 hour, what is the power of the system?
2. If a system produces 0.45 J of work in 22 seconds, what is the power of the system?
3. If a system produces 27 J of work over 1 minute, what is the power of the system?
4. If a 10-N force is applied to a system and the resulting velocity is 10 m/s, what is the power consumption of the system?
5. What is the speed of a vehicle if its 60,000-W engine is producing a 10,000-N force to push it?
6. What is the energy of a 1-kg stone hitting the ground if it falls off a 19.6-m-high cliff?
7. A 0.01-kg ball is traveling with a velocity of 100 m/s. What is the energy with which it hits its target?

Answers (If you need help with these problems, consult the website.) **Link 2-12**

1. The power is 0.21 watts.
2. The power is 0.02 watts.
3. The power is 0.45 watts.

▶ **Table 2.2.** Most Common Multiplier Prefixes Used With SI Units

Prefix	Symbol	Exponent	Decimal Equivalent	Number Name	
				American	**British**
yotta	Y	10^{24}	1 000 000 000 000 000 000 000 000	septillion	quadrillion
zetta	Z	10^{21}	1 000 000 000 000 000 000 000	sextillion	—
exa	E	10^{18}	1 000 000 000 000 000 000	quintillion	trillion
peta	P	10^{15}	1 000 000 000 000 000	quadrillion	—
tera	T	10^{12}	1 000 000 000 000	trillion	billion
giga	G	10^{9}	1 000 000 000	billion	milliard
mega	M	10^{6}	1 000 000	million	million
kilo	k	10^{3}	1 000	thousand	thousand
hecto	h	10^{2}	100	hundred	hundred
deka	da	10^{1}	10	ten	ten
BASE UNIT		**10^{0}**	**1**	**one**	**one**
deci	d	10^{-1}	0.1	one tenth	one tenth
centi	c	10^{-2}	0.01	one ...	one ...
milli	m	10^{-3}	0.001	one ...	one ...
micro	μ	10^{-6}	0.000 001	one ...	one ...
nano	n	10^{-9}	0.000 000 001	one ...	one ...
pico	p	10^{-12}	0.000 000 000 001	one ...	one ...
femto	f	10^{-15}	0.000 000 000 000 001	one ...	one ...
atto	a	10^{-18}	0.000 000 000 000 000 001	one ...	one ...
zepto	z	10^{-21}	0.000 000 000 000 000 000 001	one ...	one ...
yocto	y	10^{-24}	0.000 000 000 000 000 000 000 001	one ...	one ...

Note: The term micron *is sometimes used in place of micrometer.*

4. The power is 100 watts.
5. The speed is 21.6 km/h (6 m/s).
6. The energy is 192.08 joules.
7. The energy is 50 joules.

THE INTERNATIONAL SYSTEM OF UNITS

For a measurement made by one person to be meaningful to another person, both people must agree on a unit of measurement. For a measurement to be meaningful to everyone, a globally standardized unit of measurement is required. In ancient and medieval times, each country, land, and even region might have had their own units of measurement. Moreover, such units were almost always based on parts of the human body or on common objects. This meant that they were not overly precise. For example, the Egyptian cubit was defined as the length of the arm from the elbow to the outstretched fingertips. Clearly, a lot of room for variation exists when using such a unit for measurement, as one person's arm is not necessarily the same length as another's.

In 1791, the French Academy of Scientists established the **metric system** as a global standard for physical measurement. Since then it has been adopted by every country in the world except for the United States, where the old English (Anglo-Saxon) system of units still prevails. The metric (decimal) system is based on units of distance (meter), mass (gram), and time (second) and the multiplier 10. All unit conversions in the metric system can be made by multiplying or dividing other units by a power of 10.

Selected powers of 10 from 10^{-24} to 10^{24} have been assigned unique prefixes in the metric system that can be attached to any base unit to create a larger or smaller unit. Some common examples of this are *centi*meter, *kilo*gram, and *milli*second. If you would like to know the biggest named number, see the website. **Link 2-13** Prefixes and their corresponding powers of 10 and decimal equivalents are presented in Table 2.2.Compare this system to units of length in the English system (Table 2.3).

Imagine you didn't already know how many feet are in a mile and consider how "easy" it would be to calculate the number based on the progression shown above: 8 furlongs in a mile × 40 rods in a furlong × 5.5 yards in a rod × 3 feet in a yard = 5280 feet in a mile. Not an easy calculation, is it? But as you will soon find, it is a simple to calculate how many meters are in a kilometer. There is another problem with the English system, namely, since there is no shorter unit than the inch and no longer unit than the mile, it is rather cumbersome to deal with very short or very long distances. The English system of units is not at all an appropriate system for the scientific study of the world. Thus, even in the United States, metric units are used for scientific purposes and since all other countries use the metric system, it is also required in international trade. Table 2.4 lists

▶ **Table 2.3.** Units of Length in the English System

12 inches (in)	= 1 foot (ft)
3 feet	= 1 yard (yd)
$5^1/_2$ yards	= 1 rod (rd)
40 rods	= 1 furlong (fur)
8 furlongs	= 1 mile (mi)

Note: Basic unit: 1 inch.

▸ **Table 2.4.** Conversions Between the English System, Other Nonmetric Units, and the Metric System Units

Physical Characteristic	English System or Other Nonmetric Unit	Equivalent Metric Units
Distance	1 caliper	0.254 mm
	1 inch (in)	25.4 mm
	1 foot (ft)	30.48 cm
	1 yard (yd)	01.44 cm
	1 rod	5.029 m
	1 mile	1.6 km
	1 nautical mile	1.852 km
Area	1 square inch (in^2)	6.45 cm^2
	1 square foot (ft^2)	929.0 cm^2
	1 square yard (yd^2)	0.84 m^2
	1 acre (survey)	4047.0 m^2
	1 square mile	2.59 km^2
	1 township	93.24 km^2
Volume	1 teaspoon (tsp)	5.0 cm^3
	1 tablespoon (tbs)	15.0 cm^3
	1 cubic inch (in^3)	6.387 cm^3
	1 fluid ounce (fl oz)	29.6 cm^3
	1 cup	0.2361 dcm^3
	1 pint (pt)	0.473 dcm^3
	1 quart (qt)	0.946 dcm^3
	1 gallon (gal)	3.7851 dcm^3
	1 cubic foot (ft^3)	28.3161 dcm^3
Mass	1 grain (gr)	64.8 mg
	1 carat	200.0 mg
	1 dram (dr)	1.772 g
	1 ounce (oz)	28.35 g
	1 pound (lb)	453.6 g
	1 stone	6.35 kg
	1 slug	14.59 kg
	1 short tone (st)	907 kg
	1 tone (t)	1000.0 kg
Pressure	1 mm H_2O (4°C)	98.06 Pa
	1 mm Hg (0°C) = 1 torr	133.32 Pa
	1 lb per in^2 (psi)	6.9 kPa
	1 bar	100.0 kPa
	1 atmosphere (atm)	101.3 kPa
Force, weight	1 pond (Gram-force, G)	9.81 mN
	1 kilopond (kiloGram-force, kG)	9.81 N
	1 pound of force (lbf)	4.45 N
Work, energy	1 foot-pound (ft-lb)	1.35 J
	1 calorie	4.19 J
	1 British thermal unit (BTU)	1055.0 J
Angle	1 grad	0.9°
	1 radian	57.3°
Acceleration	1 g-unit (G)	980.67 cm/s^2
Power	1 horsepower (HP)	746 W
Temperature	Celsius degree (°C)	0°C = 273.15° Kelvin (K) $[0°C] = \frac{5}{9}([0°F] - 32)$
	Fahrenheit degree (°F)	0°F = 255.38° Kelvin (K) $[0°F] = (\frac{9}{5} \times [0°C]) + 32)$

the formulas for converting most common English units into metric units. Please note that certain nonmetric units are accepted by the International System of Units because they are important to some areas of international activities and widely used. The most important of these units are listed in Table 2.5.

The original metric system proposed by the French Academy of Sciences used the centimeter, the gram, and the second as the set of basic units. This version of the metric system is known as the **CGS system.** Later the centimeter was replaced by the meter and the gram by the kilogram. This new version is known as the **MKS system.** Both the CGS and the MKS systems also include several derived units (such as the bar and the watt) that can be expressed as a combination of the three basic units. In 1954, the Tenth General Conference on Weights and Measures (CGPM) added four more basic units to the MKS system. These four additional units—the ampere, the mole, the kelvin, and the candela—expanded the scope of the original metric system into the fields of electricity, thermodynamics, and chemistry. Because of the different nature of the physical properties they measure, they cannot be reduced to (expressed by) any combination of meters, kilograms, and seconds. In 1960 the Eleventh General Conference adopted the name **International System of Units,** usually abbreviated **SI** (from the French original, **S**ystème **I**nternational d'Unités), for this collection of units. The seven SI units are currently the standard international scientific units.

Some examples of MKS and CGS units that are relevant to hearing science are listed in Table 2.6 on page 47. In this book, the SI (MKS) units will be used for most purposes. The CGS units are listed for completeness and for backward compatibility with older scientific textbooks. Please note that the units derived from names are not capitalized but that their symbols are. For example, the newton, named after Sir Isaac Newton, is abbreviated with a capital N.

Conversions Between Metric Units

Using the metric system is not difficult at all. Just remember the following basic principles:

1. The metric system is based on the number 10.
2. The relative "size" of a unit is indicated by a prefix (e.g., *centi-*, *milli-*, etc.).
3. To convert from a unit with a prefix to a base unit, multiply by the decimal equivalent. To convert from a base unit to a unit with a prefix, divide by the decimal equivalent. The following examples will step you through the process.

Box 2.8 Converting Between a Base Unit and a Unit With a Prefix

Unit with a prefix ⟶ base	MULTIPLY by decimal equivalent
Base ⟶ unit with a prefix	DIVIDE by decimal equivalent

Example 2.11

A book has a mass of 5 kg. What is its mass in grams?

Here, we are starting with a unit with a prefix (*kilo-* is the prefix) and converting to the base unit (grams). Therefore, find the appropriate decimal equivalent for *kilo* in Table 2.2 and multiply:

$$5 \text{ kg} \times 1000 \text{ g/kg} = 5000 \text{ g}$$

So the mass of the book could be reported as 5 kg or as 5000 g. Here, it makes more sense to stick with the original unit, the kilogram, since the number "5" is less cumbersome than the number "5000." In general, select the unit that minimizes the number of zeros on either side of the decimal point.

Example 2.12

A stick is 0.5 m long. What is its length in centimeters?

Here, we are starting with a base unit (meters) and converting to a unit with a prefix (*centi-* is the prefix). Therefore, find the appropriate decimal equivalent for *centi* in Table 2.2 and divide:

$$0.5 \text{ m} \div 0.01 \text{ cm/m} = 50 \text{ cm}$$

In this case, it does not matter if we use meters or centimeters to report the length of the stick, because both answers have a small number of integers. In the next example, the conversion significantly reduces the number of zeros.

Example 2.13

The period of a sound wave was found to be 0.0000003 s. How else could this time period be reported to reduce the number of zeros?

Because the time in this example (0.0000003 s) is very short, using a unit smaller than the second will eliminate most of the zeros. Consider that 0.0000003 s can also be written as 3×10^{-7} s. The prefix associated with the power of 10 closest to 10^{-7} in Table 2.2 is *micro* (10^{-6}). So we want to express 0.0000003 s in terms of microseconds (μs). Find the appropriate decimal equivalent for *micro* in Table 2.2. Since we are converting from the base unit to a unit with a prefix, divide:

$$0.0000003 \div 0.000001 \frac{\text{s}}{\mu\text{s}} = 0.3\ \mu\text{s}$$

Answer: 0.0000003 seconds = 0.3 μs

Table 2.5. Some Widely Used, Nonmetric Units That Are Accepted by the International System of Units for International Activities

Unit	Symbol	Formal Definition	Formulas and Comments
minute (time)	min		1 min = 60 s
hour (time)	h		1 h = 60 min = 3600 s
day (time)	d		1 d = 24 h = 86 400 s
degree (angle)	°		1° = (π/180) rad
minute (angle)	′		1′ = (1/60)° = (π/10 800) rad
second (angle)	″		1″ = (1/60)° = (π/648 000) rad
liter (volume)	L *or* l	The liter is the volume occupied by 1 kg of water at a temperature of 4°C and atmospheric pressure of 1 atmosphere. It is practically identical to the cubic decimeter (dcm^3) [1 liter = 1.000028 dcm^3].	1 L = 1 dm^3 = 10^{-3} m^3
bel	B	The bel is the logarithm base 10 of a ratio of two numbers.	1 B = 10 dB
nautical mile (distance)	nm		1 nautical mile = 1852 m
knot (nautical speed)	knot		1 nautical mile per hour = (1852/3600) m/s = 1.85 km/hr
acre (area)	acre		1 acre = 1 dam^2 = 100 m^2
hectare (area)	ha		1 ha = 1 hm^2 = 10^4 m^2
bar (pressure)	bar		1 bar = 100 kPa = 1000 hPa = 10^5 Pa; 1 μbar = 0.1 Pa
ångström (distance)	Å		1 Å = 0.1 nm = 10^{-10} m
barn (area)	b	Unit used in nuclear physics. A barn is approximately equal to the area of a uranium nucleus.	1 b = 100 fm^2 = 10^{-28} m^2
curie	Ci	Unit of radioactivity	1 Ci = 3.7×10^{10} decays per second
roentgen	R	Unit of exposure to gamma rays (ionizing) radiation. A lethal dose for humans is 500 R in 5 hours.	1 R = 2.58×10^{-4} coulomb/kg
gray	Gy	Physical unit of radiation dose (absorbed dose)	1 Gy = 1 J/kg (joule of energy absorbed per kilogram of tissue) 1 rad = 10^{-2} Gy
sievert	Sv	Biological unit of radiation dose (equivalent dose dependent on the type of radiation and type of exposure)	1 Sv = 1 J/kg (joule of energy absorbed per kilogram of tissue)
Electronvolt	eV	The electronvolt is the kinetic energy acquired by an electron passing through a potential difference of 1 V in vacuum. The value must be obtained by experiment, and is therefore not known exactly.	1 eV ≈ 1.60218×10^{-19} J
unified atom mass unit	u	The unified atomic mass unit (*u*) is equal to 1/12 of the mass of an unbound atom of the nuclide ^{12}C (carbon-12) at rest and in its ground state. The value must be obtained by experiment, and is therefore not known exactly. The unified atomic mass unit is also called a dalton (Da).	1 u ≈ 1.66054×10^{-27} kg

(*continued*)

▶ **Table 2.5.** Some Widely Used, Nonmetric Units That Are Accepted by the International System of Units for International Activities (*Continued*)

Unit	Symbol	Formal Definition	Formulas and Comments
astronomical unit	AU	The astronomical unit is a unit of length. Its value is formally defined in such a way that, when used to describe the motion of bodies in the solar system, the heliocentric gravitation constant is $(0.017202\,09895)^2$ $AU^3/(day)^2$. Note: The symbol AU is used in the United States and other English-speaking countries. The International Bureau of Weights and Measures, however, recommends the symbol "ua."	An astronomical unit is approximately the mean distance between the Earth and the sun. $1\ AU \approx 1.49598 \times 10^{11}$ m (about 150 million kilometers)
parsec		A unit of astronomical length based on the distance from Earth at which the stellar parallax is 1 second of arc	Equivalent to 3.262 light years

In most cases, you will be converting either to or from a base unit as shown in the previous examples. Occasions will arise, however, in which you will need to convert across the base unit, for example, from decimeters (smaller than meters) to hectometers (larger than meters). To see an example of the conversion process across the base unit (a slightly more complex process), consult the website. **Link 2-14**

If a number in scientific notation must be converted between metric units, we can manipulate the exponents instead of dividing or multiplying by the decimal equivalent. To convert from a unit with a prefix to a base unit, add the exponents. To convert from a base unit to a unit with a prefix, subtract the exponents.

Example 2.14

Convert 8.4×10^{10} meters to kilometers.

Because 8.4×10^{10} is such a large number, don't write out the number with all those zeros and then divide by the decimal equivalent—that is far too cumbersome. Instead, find the exponent column in Table 2.2 and notice that the *kilo* prefix has an exponent equivalent of 10^3. To convert from the base unit (meters) to a unit with a prefix (kilometers), subtract the exponent from the table from the exponent used in the provided magnitude.

$$8.4 \times 10^{10}\ \text{m} = 8.4 \times 10^{10-3}\ \text{km} = 8.4 \times 10^{7}\ \text{km}$$

Example 2.15

Convert 5.6×10^{12} millimeters to meters.

From Table 2.2, the *milli* prefix has an exponent equivalent of 10^{-3}. To convert from a unit with a prefix to a base unit, add the exponents.

$$5.6 \times 10^{12}\ \text{mm} = 5.6 \times 10^{12+-3}\ \text{m} = 5.6 \times 10^{9}\ \text{m}$$

PRACTICE PROBLEMS: THE METRIC SYSTEM

1. 45,000,000,000 watts = how many GW (gigawatts)?
2. 56,000 seconds = how many ms (milliseconds)?
3. 28,000,000 μs (microseconds) = how many seconds?
4. 0.0000000000475 seconds = how many ns (nanoseconds)?
5. 0.23 pascals = how many μPa (micropascals)?
6. 0.00000001 kg = how many grams?
7. Convert 3.6×10^9 meters to kilometers.
8. Convert 2.8×10^{20} millimeters to meters.

Answers (If you need help with these problems, consult the website.) **Link 2-15**

1. 45 GW
2. 56,000,000 ms
3. 28 s
4. 0.0475 ns
5. 230,000 μPa
6. 0.00001 g
7. 3.6×10^6 km
8. 2.8×10^{17} m

▶ **Table 2.6.** MKS and CGS Units of the Metric System

	Unit of Measurement	
Quantity	**MKS**	**CGS**
Distance, length	meter (m)	centimeter (cm)
Mass	kilogram (kg)	gram (g)
Time	second (s)	second (s)
Force	newton (N)	dyne (dyne)
Energy, work	joule (J)	erg (erg)
Power	watt (W)	watt (W)
Pressure	pascal (Pa)	$dyne/cm^2$

Summary

Physics is the science of matter and energy and the interactions between them. Kinematics is the branch of physics that describes the motion of objects in space without considering the cause of the motion. Dynamics is the branch of physics that describes the effects of forces on the state of an object or a system of objects. Measurements in physics require consistent use of a magnitude and a unit of measurement. Physical characteristics for which it is sufficient to provide just a magnitude and a unit are called scalar quantities or scalars. Physical characteristics that are described in addition by their direction are called vector quantities or vectors. When vectors are combined, a special procedure called vector addition must be used to take into account both direction and magnitude. In the scientific community, measurements are reported in units described by the International System of Units. Conversion between metric units is easily done by multiplying or dividing by powers of 10.

The basic relationships between force and motion were first formulated by Sir Isaac Newton. Newton's First Law of Motion (Law of Inertia) states that an object at rest will remain at rest unless acted upon by an external force and that an object in motion will neither speed up nor slow down unless acted upon by an external force. Newton's Second Law of Motion describes the relationship between force, mass, and acceleration ($F = ma$). Newton's Third Law of Motion (Law of Action) states that for every action there is an equal and opposite reaction. Newton's Law of Universal Gravitation explains that the strength of gravity (a phenomenon in which any two objects attract each other) depends on the masses of both of the objects and the distance between them.

The Law of Conservation of Energy states that energy can neither be created nor destroyed; however, energy can change form. Energy can take many forms, but all specific types of energy can be broadly classified into two categories: potential energy and kinetic energy. Potential energy is the energy of an object due to its position within a given physical system or environment. Kinetic energy is the energy of motion.

Key Points

- When reporting a physical measurement in science, it is essential to include both the magnitude and unit for scalar quantities. Scalar quantities include distance (the length of the shortest line connecting two points), area (the amount of space occupied by a surface), volume (the amount of space occupied by a substance or an object), mass (the amount of matter that is present), and density (the amount of matter in a given unit of volume).
- When vector quantities are reported, the direction must be stated. Examples of vector quantities include displacement (change in position), velocity (rate of displacement), acceleration (rate of change in velocity), and force (a push or a pull).
- Vector addition is the method for adding two vectors together taking both their individual magnitudes and their individual directions into account. It requires the use of Cartesian and polar coordinates and the Pythagorean Theorem.
- Elasticity is the property that allows matter to recover its form (size and shape) after it has been distorted (expanded or compressed).
- The basic relationships between force and motion are described by Newton's three laws of motion and the Law of Universal Gravitation.
- Weight and mass are not equivalent. The weight of an object is actually the force of gravity acting on the object.
- Work is defined as force acting over a distance and power is the rate at which work is done.
- Energy is defined as the ability or capacity of an object to do work. All forms of energy can be classified into potential energy (energy of an object due to its position) and kinetic energy (energy of motion).
- Conversion between metric units involves an understanding that (1) the metric system is based on powers of 10, (2) the relative "size" of a unit is indicated by a prefix, and (3) to convert between units you multiply (when starting from a prefix unit) or divide (when starting from a base unit) by the decimal equivalent provided in this chapter.

PART II

Acoustics

CHAPTER 3

Oscillations and Vibrations

Chapter Outline

Objectives

- To introduce the basic concept of simple harmonic motion in vibrating systems
- To use a pendulum to introduce the concepts of displacement, velocity, acceleration, frequency, period, amplitude, and phase of oscillations
- To use a mass-and-spring system to discuss vibrations and the effects of mass, stiffness, and friction on the behavior of vibrating systems
- To introduce the concepts of resonance and free and forced vibrations

Key Terms

Amplitude
Average (mean) magnitude
Closed system
Coefficient of damping
Coefficient of friction
Compliance
Critically damped system
Cycle
Damped vibration
Damping
Driving frequency
Elasticity
Equilibrium
Fall time
Forced vibration
Free vibration
Frequency
Friction
Harmonic motion
Heavily damped (overdamped) system
In-phase
Instantaneous magnitude
Minimally damped (underdamped) system
Open system
Oscillation
Out-of-phase
Peak-to-peak magnitude
Pendulum
Period
Periodic motion
Phase (phase angle, θ)
Phase difference
Phase relationship
Phase shift
Quality factor
Resonance
Resonance curve
Resonance frequency
Rise time
Root mean square (RMS) magnitude
Simple harmonic motion
Sinusoidal motion
Steady-state time
Stiffness
Temporal envelope
Unipolar (rectified) average magnitude
Vibration
Waveform
Waveform envelope

The source of sound is the back-and-forth motion of a mechanical object around its **equilibrium** (rest, neutral) position. This type of motion is called an oscillation or vibration. In general, an **oscillation** is any back-and-forth movement between two states. For example, an oscillation can be mechanical (e.g., lunar tide), psychological (e.g., hesitation between two alternatives), or electrical (e.g., alternating current). An object moving with such motion is called an **oscillator.** If the nature of the oscillation results from the presence of the force of elasticity, this oscillation is called a **vibration.** An object that vibrates is called a **vibrator.** Many textbooks and references treat the terms oscillation and vibration as synonyms since both involve a back-and-forth motion. Not all oscillations are vibrations, however, and the nature of gravitational oscillation and vibration is different. A gravitational oscillation is the back-and-forth movement of an object due to the force of gravity (e.g., the movement of a pendulum, lunar tide). Despite the different nature of both phenomena, both of them result in the same type of motion and both will be used to describe the nature of this motion. The pendulum will be used to introduce the concepts of displacement, velocity, acceleration, frequency, period, amplitude, and phase angle associated with a back-and-forth motion. The mass-and-spring system will be used to introduce the concepts of mass, stiffness, and friction and their effects on the properties of the back-and-forth motion.

THE PENDULUM

The common conceptual system used to explain the phenomenon of a back-and-forth movement is the pendulum. The **pendulum** is a bob suspended from a fixed point on a thin arm (e.g., string) that may swing freely back and forth when the pendulum is displaced from its rest position. Figure 3.1 shows a pendulum at rest and a pendulum in motion. The pendulum will not move unless it is forced out of its resting (equilibrium) position by an external force.

Once the pendulum is displaced from its resting position it will move back and forth. Why? Why doesn't it simply return to its rest position and stay there? The reason for the oscillatory swing of the pendulum is the interaction between its inertia and the restoring (counteracting) force of gravity.

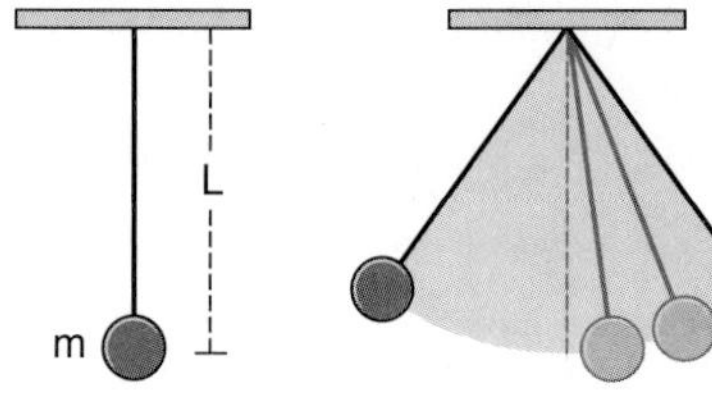

Figure 3.1. A pendulum at rest (*left*) and pendulum in motion (*right*); *m* is the mass of the bob and *L* is the length of the arm of the pendulum.

At its rest position, the pendulum is hanging straight down, toward the Earth. This is the effect of the force of gravity being counterbalanced by the force of the suspending arm. The pendulum has a certain potential energy and no kinetic energy. The potential energy depends on the pendulum mass (*m*) and its height above the Earth. An external force that swings the pendulum out of its rest position must act against the force of gravity. When an external force is applied, newly acquired potential energy creates the pulling-back effect. Thus, the force of gravity is acting as a restoring force trying to bring back the pendulum to its original rest position. Because the moving pendulum has acquired a certain amount of kinetic (motion) energy that has to be used, it does not stop when it returns to its equilibrium position. After reaching the point of equilibrium the moving pendulum starts acting against the force of gravity, gradually decreasing its speed. During this time it loses its kinetic energy and again builds up its potential energy. At a certain point, the force of gravity will exceed the force of inertia (associated with the mass of the moving pendulum) and the pendulum will begin moving again toward its rest position (equilibrium). The process of changing potential energy into kinetic energy and kinetic energy back into potential energy repeats itself over and over and keeps the pendulum moving. If no loss of energy takes place during the pendulum motion, the pendulum will continue moving back and forth until it is stopped by an external action.

Displacement of a Pendulum

Consider the pendulum swing in terms of the displacement of the pendulum arm (Fig. 3.2). Recall from Chapter 2 that displacement is a vector quantity and is described by both its magnitude and its direction. In Figure 3.2, direction is shown as positive to the right and negative to the left. Point A indicates the resting point of the pendulum (equilibrium). Point B indicates the maximum displacement in the positive direction, and point D is the maximum displacement in the negative direction. The points identified on the pendulum swing are also shown in Figure 3.2 using a simple $x-y$ plot to graphically represent the motion of the pendulum as a function of time. The x axis represents the time, and the y axis represents displacement. The positive direction is shown on the top of the y axis and the negative direction is shown on the bottom of the y axis. The plot begins at point A, when the pendulum is at its equilibrium position, which has a displacement of 0 cm. Next, point B is the maximum positive displacement of the pendulum, in this case, at 4 cm. The pendulum then swings back through equilibrium (therefore, point A is graphed again). Point D is the maximum negative displacement of the pendulum; thus, it is shown at -4 cm, indicating a 4-cm magnitude and negative direction. The pendulum then swings back through equilibrium (point A) again.

Time periods between points A–B–A–D–A in Figure 3.2 are identical, indicating that the time needed to reach maximum displacement on either side of the pendulum and the

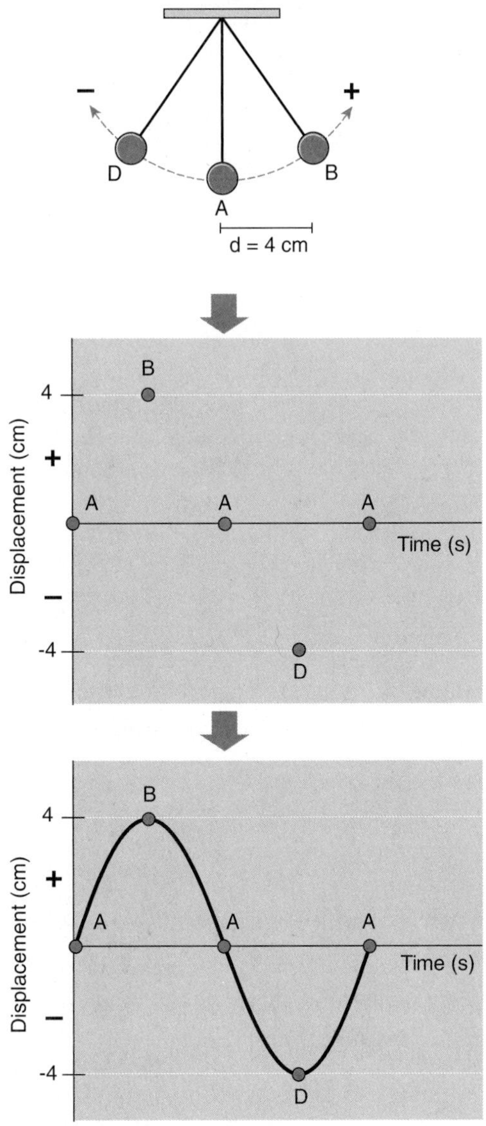

Figure 3.2. The displacement of a pendulum. Several points of displacement have been plotted.

time needed to bring the pendulum back to its neutral position are identical. However, the time needed to move the pendulum by a specific distance between these points is not always the same. The pendulum swings the fastest when it crosses its equilibrium point. At this point, the force of gravity is perpendicular to the pendulum trajectory (path) and has no effect on pendulum velocity. The pendulum swings the slowest when it reaches its maximum displacement, changes direction, and begins its backward movement toward the equilibrium position. Therefore, in the same time interval the pendulum travels much further when it is close to its equilibrium position than when it is close to its extreme displacement.

So, what does the function showing the entire pendulum displacement over time look like? Imagine the pendulum swinging from point A through points B, A, and D and then back to point A. If this function is graphed, the result is a sine function, which was introduced in Chapter 1. This concept is shown in the last illustration in Figure 3.2. The pendulum displacement changes in time as a sine function and the oscillation made by the back-and-forth motion of the pendulum is often called **sinusoidal motion.*** Mathematically, sinusoidal motion is described by Equation 3.1.

$$x = X \sin(\omega t) \tag{3.1}$$

where x is a momentary displacement of the pendulum, X is the maximum displacement of the pendulum, t is time, and ω is the angular speed, also called pulsation, which has a constant value for each specific sinusoidal motion.

Velocity of a Pendulum

The motion of the pendulum can be re-examined looking at other characteristics of the motion. Figure 3.3 illustrates the same pendulum motion described in the previous section, but this time the *velocity* of the motion is highlighted. Notice the points are now labeled A through E, which will make the discussion of velocity a little easier.

To examine the changes in the velocity of a pendulum, consider first the scalar quantity of speed. As mentioned before, the moving pendulum travels the fastest through the middle of the swing (points A, C, and E) and the slowest when it is near the edges of its swing (points B and D), where it must temporarily stop to turn around. Since the fastest point of the swing is in the middle, the greatest magnitude of the velocity is at points A, C, and E. The direction of the velocity can be determined by examining the direction in which the pendulum is traveling in Figure 3.3.

At points A and E, the pendulum is moving in the positive direction; thus, velocity is positive. At point C, the pendulum is moving in the negative direction; thus, velocity is negative. At points B and D, the magnitude is zero; therefore, the direction is not specified. With magnitude and direction identified, the velocity can be graphed on an $x-y$ plot, also shown in Figure 3.3. Notice that the graph of the velocity of the pendulum swing is similar to the graph of the displacement from Figure 3.2 except that it begins in a different place. The function describing changes in the pendulum's velocity is actually a cosine function. It has the same shape as a sine function but is shifted in time by a quarter of the time needed by the pendulum to complete one full movement back and forth.

Acceleration of a Pendulum

In addition to displacement and velocity, the acceleration of the pendulum can also be examined and graphed.

*Actually, pendulum motion only approximates simple harmonic motion because of the arc created by the swing, but it is a useful analogy to begin the study of simple harmonic motion. If the motion in just one plane (the horizontal plane) is considered, the motion can be examined as sinusoidal motion. Consult a basic physics textbook for a more complete description of the motion of the pendulum in relationship to true harmonic motion.

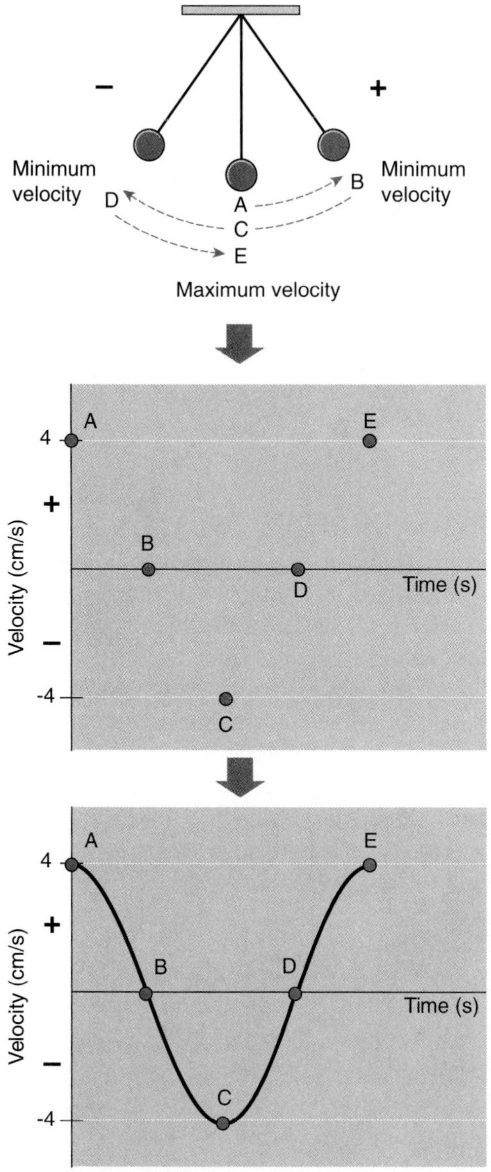

Figure 3.3. The velocity of a pendulum.

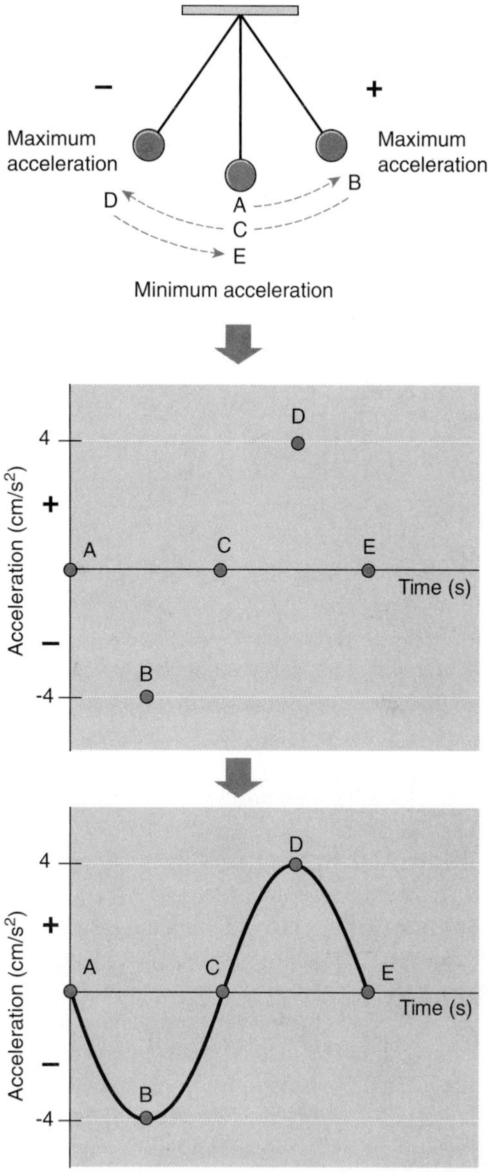

Figure 3.4. The acceleration of a pendulum.

Remember that acceleration, like velocity and displacement, is a vector quantity. First, consider the magnitude of the acceleration. Where would the magnitude of the acceleration be at its maximum? Acceleration is at its maximum magnitude at the edges of the pendulum swing as it begins to travel toward equilibrium. Remember the analogy of the accelerating car from Chapter 2. When a car is stopped and begins to accelerate into traffic, acceleration is greatest, but when the car is traveling at a high but constant velocity, the acceleration is zero. Now, look at the pendulum movement in Figure 3.4.

At the points of maximum displacement, points B and D in Figure 3.4, the pendulum arm stops briefly and then heads in the opposite direction. The point at which the magnitude of the acceleration is greatest will be from this stopped position as it begins to swing. Figure 3.4 also provides the translation of acceleration from the pendulum to the $x-y$ plot.

The direction of the acceleration is a bit more complex than it was for displacement and velocity. Acceleration is positive (+) if an object is *accelerating* from that point to the positive direction and acceleration is negative (–) if an object is *accelerating* from that point to the negative direction. However, acceleration is also positive (+) if an object is *decelerating* from that point to the negative direction and acceleration is negative (–) if an object is *decelerating* from that point to the positive direction. So the direction in an acceleration problem considers whether the object is accelerating or decelerating in addition to where it is going.

At points A, C, and E the acceleration is zero. Therefore, at these points the pendulum is traveling at a constant velocity. At points B and D, acceleration is at its maximum. Point B is negative because the pendulum is accelerating in the negative direction. Point D is positive because the pendulum is accelerating in the positive direction. All of the points between C and D are positive because the pendulum is *decelerating* in the *negative* direction (here a double negative makes a positive) and all points between A and B are negative because the pendulum is *decelerating* in the *positive* direction. Note that the acceleration function drawn in Figure 3.4 is the same familiar shape as shown before in the displacement and velocity graphs. The only difference is a different starting point. The acceleration graph is a mirror image of the displacement graph. This means that the maximum values of displacement and acceleration occur at the same time but they have different directions.

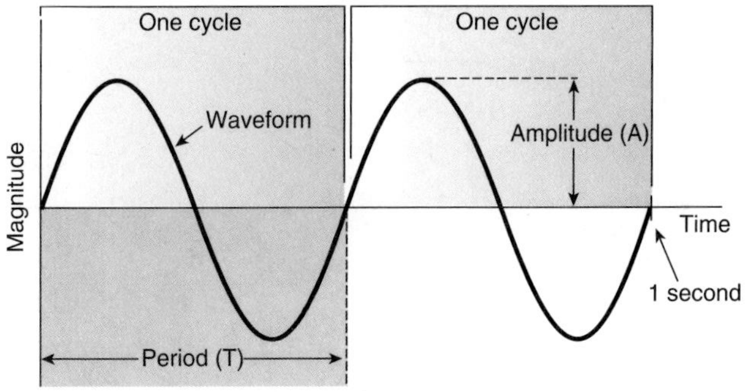

Figure 3.5. A waveform illustrating two cycles of simple harmonic motion.

SIMPLE HARMONIC MOTION

An examination of the pendulum motion described in the previous sections reveals the basic properties of a simple back-and-forth motion. First, the motion of the pendulum is periodic. **Periodic motion** is a motion that repeats itself in regular intervals until it is stopped by external action. Second, the motion is harmonic. **Harmonic motion** is a motion in which the acceleration of the object is directly proportional but opposite in direction to the displacement of the object from its equilibrium position. If a *single* object, such as a pendulum, is moving in harmonic motion, then (1) the motion has an acceleration that is directly proportional but opposite in direction to the displacement *and* (2) changes in displacement, velocity, and acceleration are sinusoidal functions of time. This motion is called **simple harmonic motion** (SHM). Simple harmonic motion is a motion described by a sinusoidal function. That is, when any characteristic of the simple harmonic motion (such as displacement, velocity, or acceleration) is graphed as a function of time, it has the shape of a sine wave. An object moving with harmonic motion is called a harmonic oscillator and an object moving with simple harmonic motion is called a simple harmonic oscillator. More complex harmonic motion takes place when the oscillating system consists of two or more objects. Such types of motion will be described in Chapter 4.

Waveform

Simple harmonic motion is fundamental to the description of vibration and, therefore, to sound. We will use this motion to define some terms that are used in the description of vibration and, later on, sound. These terms are also applicable to other, more complex back-and-forth motions, which will be described in Chapter 4. A function representing changes of any physical quantity as a function of time is called a **waveform.** A graphic representation of simple harmonic motion using a waveform is shown in Figure 3.5. The *x* axis indicates time and the *y* axis represents the magnitude of the displayed quantity, such as displacement, velocity, and acceleration, as previously discussed. From this waveform, various characteristics of the vibratory motion can be discussed such as frequency, period, phase, and amplitude.

Frequency and Period

A **cycle** is one full repetition of a periodic motion. Examples of a cycle include a rotation of the Earth around the sun (1 year), a rotation of the Earth around its own axis (1 day), and a beat in the motion of a hummingbird's wing (about 15 ms). The starting point of a cycle is arbitrary and its selection is usually determined by convenience. A cycle usually starts and ends at 0 magnitude (i.e., at equilibrium), but it can start at any magnitude. In Figure 3.5, the first cycle begins at 0 seconds and ends at 0.5 seconds. The second cycle begins at 0.5 seconds and ends at 1 second. The **frequency** (f) of a waveform is the number of cycles per second (cps).

$$\text{Frequency} = \text{Number of cycles/Time in seconds} \qquad (3.2)$$

The unit for frequency is hertz (Hz), after Heinrich Hertz, a German physicist, although you may see cycles per second (cps) in some older sources.

$$1 \text{ cycle/second} = 1 \text{ Hz}$$

If one cycle of a waveform is completed in 1 second, the frequency of the waveform is 1 cycle per second or 1 Hz; if two cycles of a waveform are completed in 1 second, the frequency is 2 Hz, and so forth. The frequency of a waveform is related to the period of the waveform. The **period** (T) is the time required for the completion of one cycle of a periodic motion. It is formally defined as the duration of one cycle of a periodic phenomenon (International Standards Organization, 2006).

$$\text{Period} = \text{Time/Number of cycles} \qquad (3.3)$$

Period can be reported in any time unit discussed in Chapter 2 such as seconds, milliseconds, and so forth. If two cycles of a waveform are completed in 1 second, the period is 0.5 s and the frequency is 2 Hz. Thus, the frequency (f) is a reciprocal (inverse) of the period (T).

$$f = \frac{1}{T} \qquad (3.4)$$

$$T = \frac{1}{f} \qquad (3.5)$$

Example 3.1

Look at the sine wave below and determine the frequency and period.

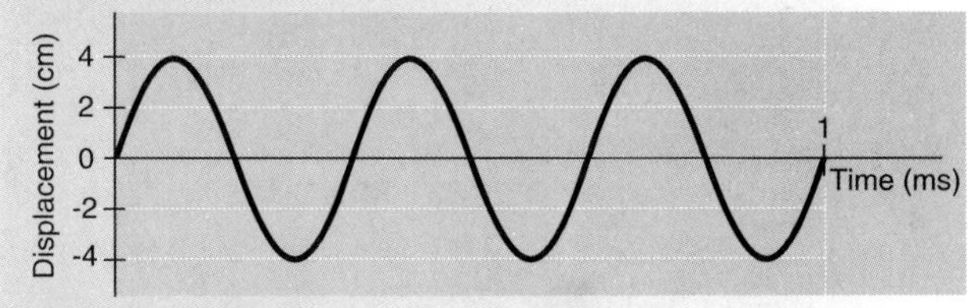

Three cycles of the waveform are displayed on the graph. Notice the x axis (time) is in milliseconds (ms) and not seconds in this example. Therefore, three cycles occurred in 1 millisecond. Although the period can be reported in any time unit, the frequency is always reported in Hz, which is cycles per *second*. So reporting this problem in cycles per millisecond would not be the conventional way to report frequency. Before solving frequency problems involving time units other than the second, use the skills from Chapter 2 to convert from milliseconds to seconds.

1 millisecond = 0.001 second

Frequency is equal to the number of cycles per second, so use Equation 3.2, substitute known variables, and solve.

Frequency = Number of cycles/Time in seconds

Frequency = 3 cycles/0.001 s

Frequency = 3000 cycles/s = 3000 Hz

Period can be determined by finding the reciprocal (inverse) of the frequency. Use Equation 3.5, substitute known variables, and solve.

$$T = \frac{1}{f}$$

$$T = \frac{1}{3000}$$

$$T = 0.00033 \text{ seconds}$$

or you can convert 0.00033 seconds to 0.33 ms

Answer: Frequency = 3000 Hz and Period = 0.33 ms

Note that the period could have been found directly from the graph (rather than using the frequency formula) by using the formula for period (Equation 3.3).

Period = Time/Number of cycles

Period = 1 ms/3 cycles

Period = 0.33 ms

(Note: Period is reported in a time unit rather than time/cycle.)

PRACTICE PROBLEMS: PERIOD AND FREQUENCY

Find the frequency and period for these three waveforms.

1.

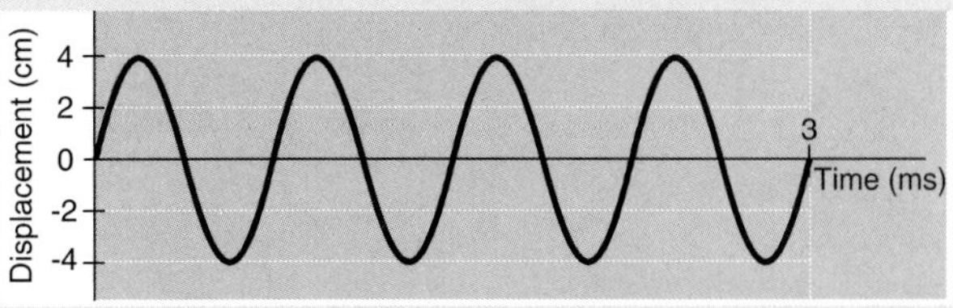

2.

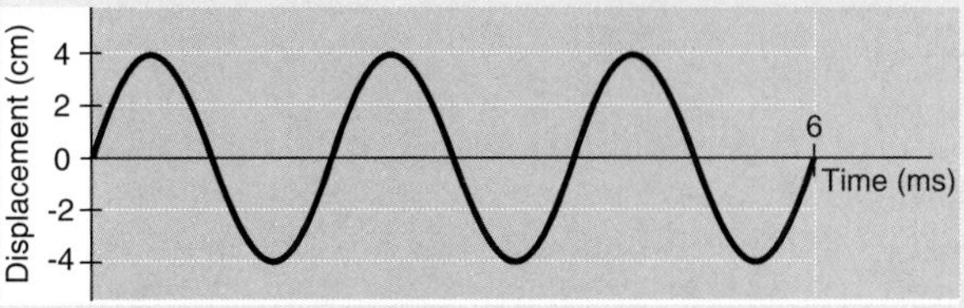

3.

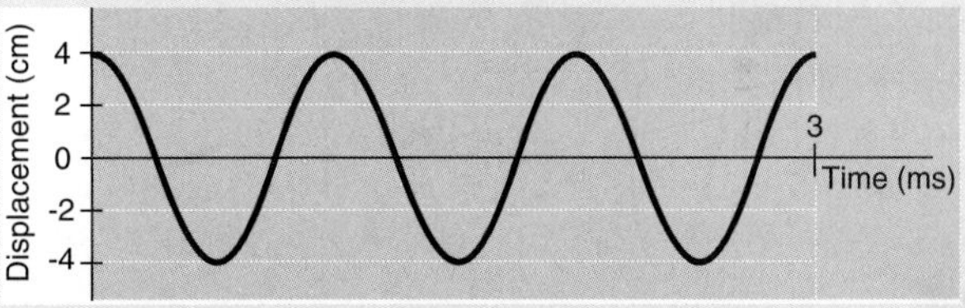

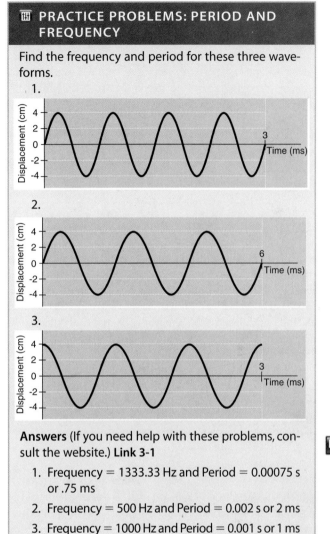

Answers (If you need help with these problems, consult the website.) **Link 3-1**

1. Frequency = 1333.33 Hz and Period = 0.00075 s or .75 ms
2. Frequency = 500 Hz and Period = 0.002 s or 2 ms
3. Frequency = 1000 Hz and Period = 0.001 s or 1 ms

Phase

The term *phase* comes from the Greek word *phasis* meaning "appearance." **Phase (phase angle, θ)** indicates a particular stage in the cycle of motion using the angles from a circle as the unit of measure (see Chapter 1 for a review of trigonometry). If the tip of a radius (r) travels around a circle and the phase angle (θ) of the circle is graphed on the x axis and sine θ is graphed on the y axis, the characteristic "sine wave" shape will appear (Fig. 3.6). One full rotation of the radius around the circle (0° to 360°) results in one complete cycle of the sine wave.

According to common convention, if the initial (rest, equilibrium) position of an object in simple harmonic motion is defined as a 0° phase, the maximum positive magnitude of the sine wave always corresponds to a phase of 90° and the maximum negative magnitude of the sine wave always corresponds to a phase of 270° (or to –90° depending on the notation). When the magnitude is zero,

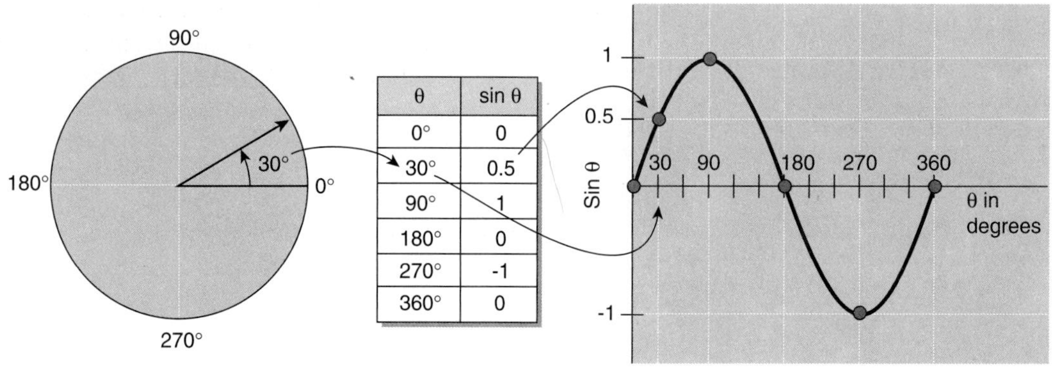

Figure 3.6. The sine wave function.

the phase angle could be 0°, 180°, or 360° depending on the direction of the vector quantity that is graphed and whether the cycle is just beginning (0°) or just ending (360°). Therefore, one cycle of a sine wave can be defined as the complete 360° rotation (change) of phase. In acoustics it is sometimes convenient to express angle in radians rather than in degrees to simplify some calculations. Recall that the circumference of a circle is equal to $2\pi r$, where r is the radius of a circle. Since an arc of one radius corresponds to one radian, the whole 360° rotation may be expressed as 2π radians. Subsequently, angular speed (used in Equation 3.1) can be expressed as:

$$\omega = \frac{2\pi}{T} = 2\pi f \qquad (3.6)$$

where T is the period of rotation and f is the frequency of the circular (harmonic) motion. Angular speed (pulsation) expressed in the above manner is one of the fundamental variables used in acoustic and engineering books.

PRACTICE PROBLEMS: PHASE

Using the sine wave below, identify the phase (in degrees) indicated by the points.

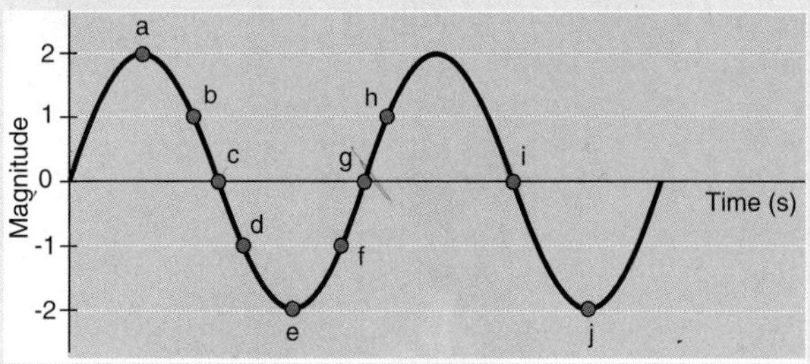

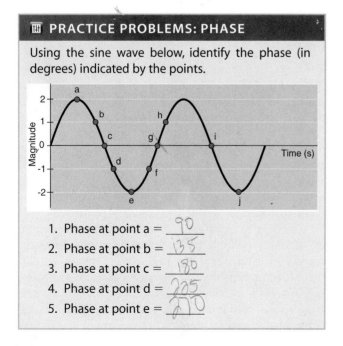

1. Phase at point a = ______
2. Phase at point b = ______
3. Phase at point c = ______
4. Phase at point d = ______
5. Phase at point e = ______
6. Phase at point f = ______
7. Phase at point g = ______
8. Phase at point h = ______
9. Phase at point i = ______
10. Phase at point j = ______

Answers (If you need help with these problems, consult the website.) **Link 3-2**

1. 90°
2. ≈135°
3. 180°
4. ≈225°
5. 270°
6. ≈315°
7. 360° or 0°
8. ≈45°
9. 180°
10. 270°

Phase Relationship

In discussing human reaction to sound, it is often necessary to compare two waveforms of the same frequency that differ in phase at the same point in time. The **phase relationship** between two waveforms is usually referred to as the phase difference or the phase shift. **Phase difference** (phase offset) is the absolute difference between the phases of two waveforms with neither of them being considered as a point of reference. The maximum possible value of phase difference is 180°. **Phase shift** is the relationship between the phase of one waveform and another where one is considered as the point of reference. The phase shift can be positive (lead) or negative (lag). The direction of the phase shift is dependent on which of the two compared waveforms is designated as the primary and which one is secondary when they are being compared. The concept of phase shift is typically used

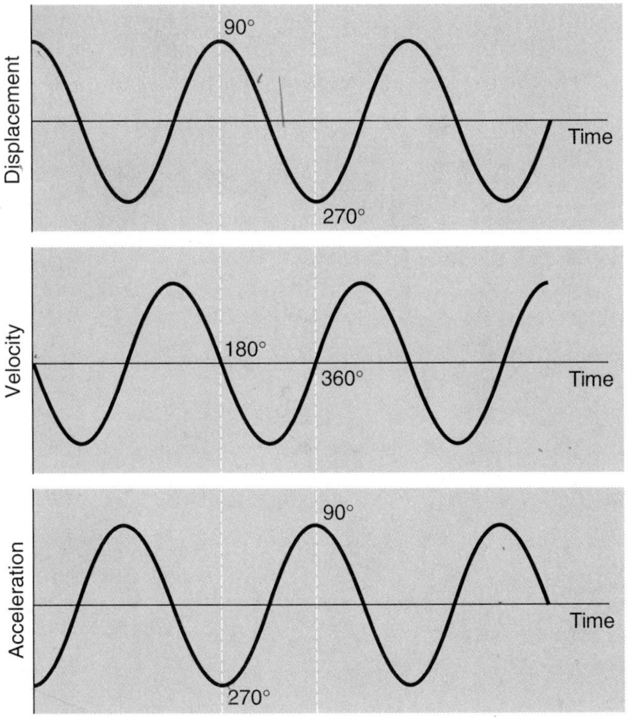

Figure 3.7. The phase relationship among displacement, velocity, and acceleration.

to describe the phase relationship between the output and input waveforms of a transmission system. Phase shift can vary from −∞ (–infinity) to +∞ (+infinity) since it can exceed one or more full 360° cycles of the waveform.

Consider, for example, the waveforms of displacement, velocity, and acceleration grouped together in Figure 3.7. The differences in phase of these three characteristics are clearly visible. The cycles begin in this figure with displacement at 90° (i.e., the pendulum or mass has been pulled to its maximum positive point to begin the motion), velocity at 180° (i.e., at minimum velocity), and acceleration at 270° (maximum acceleration in the negative direction). Since the displacement is the basic characteristic of the motion and the velocity and acceleration are dependent on the displacement, the phase of the displacement is designated as the primary waveform and used as a reference for the phase of velocity. Either displacement or velocity can be used as the reference for acceleration.

In determining the phase difference between the waveforms presented in Figure 3.7, any time point can be selected. Specifically notice the two dashed lines running parallel to the *y* axis. They indicate two arbitrary times at which phase difference can be determined. They are drawn to stress the fact that if the frequencies of the waveforms being compared are identical, the phase comparison can be made at any point in time since the same phase relationship is maintained all the time. The numbers in the graphs indicate the phase of each wave at the points where the dashed lines cross the waveforms. At the first dashed line, the phase of the displacement waveform is 90° and the phase of the velocity waveform is 180°. The phase difference between both waveforms is 90° and the phase relationship between displacement and velocity can be described as 90° out-of-phase. Similarly, the phase of the acceleration waveform at the first dashed line is 270° and the phase difference between maximum displacement and maximum acceleration is 180°. In other words, the maximum acceleration of the vibrating mass happens at the maximum displacement but it is turned in the opposite direction. If you conduct similar calculations at the second dashed line, you will arrive at the same results. This means that the difference between the phases of these three waveforms is the same regardless of which time point is selected for comparison. The phase relationship remains the same at any point of the reference wave as long as the waves have the same frequency. If you would like to calculate the phase *shift* between displacement and acceleration instead of the phase *difference* (using displacement as the reference waveform), you need to realize that for phase shift calculations you must consider the entire history of the waveforms. Examine the second dashed line in Figure 3.7. Now look at the displacement waveform. The starting phase of the displacement waveform is 90°. Then it completes one full cycle (360°) and then one additional half cycle (180°) to reach the second dashed line. The phase at this point, considering the history, is 90° + 360° + 180° = 630°. The acceleration waveform begins at a phase of 270°, and then it too completes one full cycle (360°) and one half cycle (180°) for a phase of 270° + 360° + 180° = 810°. Thus, the phase shift between the two waves is 630° – 810° = –180°. Therefore, acceleration lags behind displacement by 180°.

If the frequencies of two waveforms are different, the phase relationship between the two waveforms changes with time. For example, in Figure 3.8, the phase difference between the two waves at the first dashed line is 45° and at the second dashed line is 225°. To determine if it is possible to describe

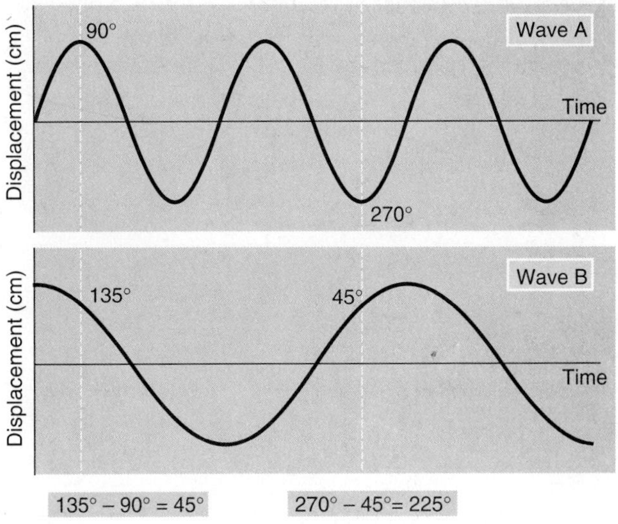

Figure 3.8. The phase relationship between two waveforms with different frequencies.

the phase relationship between two sine waves with different frequencies, it needs to be determined whether:

1. the higher frequency is an integer multiple of the lower frequency; or
2. the higher frequency is *not* an integer multiple of the lower frequency.

In the first case, for example, for the frequencies of 200 Hz and 400 Hz, the same phase relationship is repeated for every cycle of the lower frequency waveform and the phase relationship can be defined as the difference in phase between the two waves at the beginning of the cycle of the lower frequency waveform. In the second case, no fixed or periodic relationship is present between the phases of both waveforms and the concept of the phase difference does not have any practical meaning.

When two waveforms have the same frequency and the same phase, their phase relationship is described as being **in-phase.** If two waveforms have the same frequency but the phase is not the same, they are said to be **out-of-phase.** Figure 3.9 shows two waveforms that are in-phase and two waveforms that are out-of-phase. In cases where two waveforms are in a simple numerical (harmonic) relationship (e.g., 100 Hz and 200 Hz), the concept of being in-phase or out-of-phase also applies. In such cases we can say that the second waveform (200 Hz) is in-phase or out-of-phase with the first waveform (100 Hz). To report the exact phase relationship between two waveforms that are not in-phase, the phrase *out-of-phase* is preceded by the specific number of degrees (e.g., 90° out-of-phase, 180° out-of-phase, etc.). If the number of degrees is omitted, it indicates a 180° difference between the waveforms.

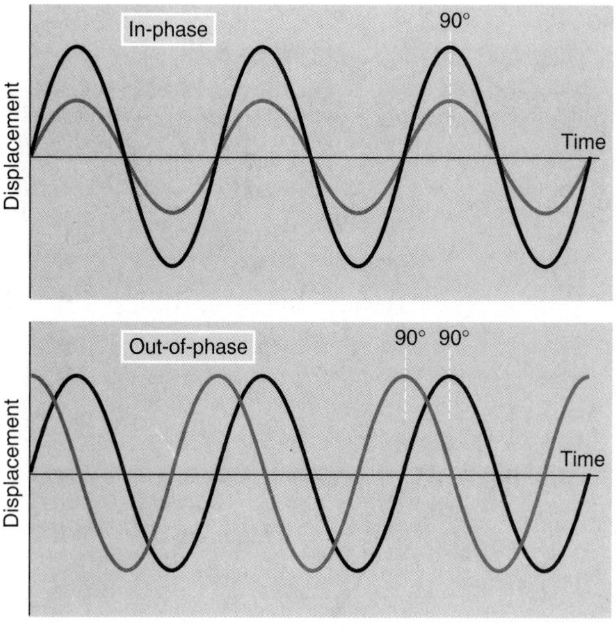

Figure 3.9. Two waveforms of the same frequency that are in-phase and out-of-phase.

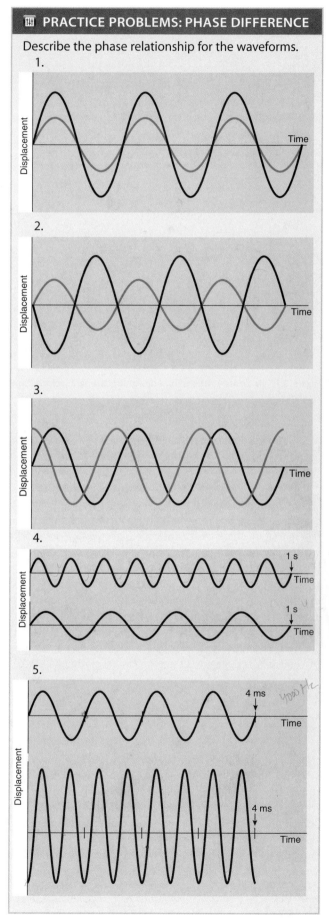

PRACTICE PROBLEMS: PHASE DIFFERENCE

Describe the phase relationship for the waveforms.

1.

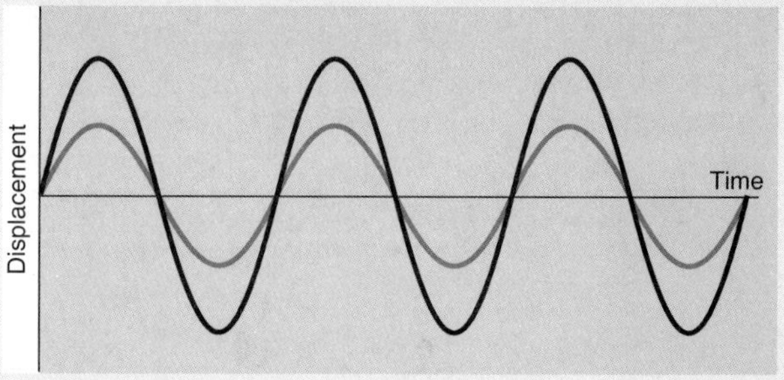

2.

3.

4.

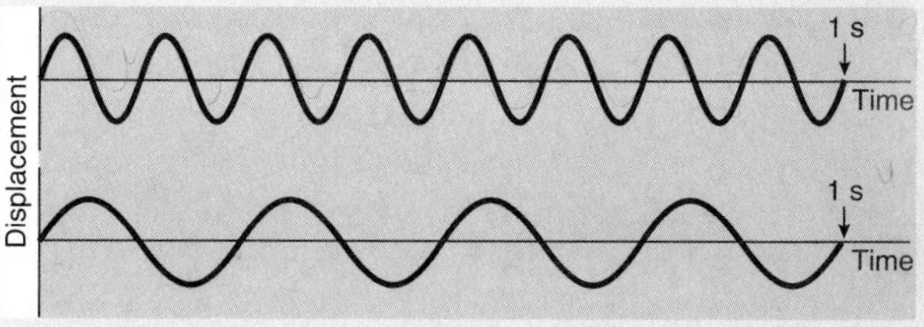

5.

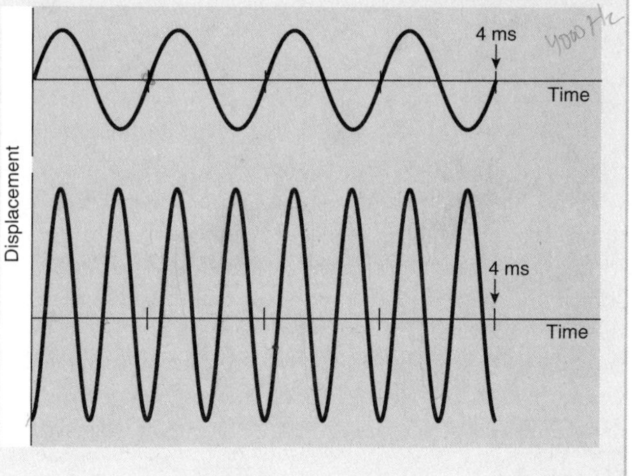

Answers (If you need help with these problems, consult the website.) **Link 3-3**

1. In-phase
2. 180° out-of-phase
3. 90° out-of-phase
4. In-phase
5. 90° out-of-phase

Magnitude and Amplitude

Recall from Chapter 2 that magnitude is a value that, along with a unit of measurement, specifies the quantity of something (e.g., 65 mpg, 20 m, or 0.1 J). A magnitude can be constant or it can vary in time. In a vibrating system, the magnitudes of displacement, velocity, and acceleration change across time. The magnitude of a variable quantity observed at any given moment of time is called the **instantaneous magnitude.** The maximum (peak) magnitude of a periodic waveform is called the **amplitude (*A*)**, and the whole range of magnitude changes within one period is called the **peak-to-peak magnitude** (or peak-to-peak value) (Fig. 3.10). In the case of simple harmonic motion the peak-to-peak value is twice as large as the waveform amplitude. In the case where a waveform is not symmetrical it may have different positive (+) and negative (–) amplitudes (peak magnitudes) and the peak-to-peak value is the difference between both amplitudes.

The amount of time during which harmonic motion (and most other waveforms) is at its peak magnitude is usually very small. Because of this, using the amplitude to describe the magnitude of harmonic motion does not usually do an adequate job of describing the changes in the magnitude of the motion across one cycle. For this reason, it is often useful to describe the magnitude of a waveform by a kind of an average value rather than its amplitude. Three of the ways to indicate the average magnitude of a waveform are shown in Figure 3.10. They are the average magnitude, the unipolar (rectified) average magnitude, and the root mean square (RMS) magnitude.

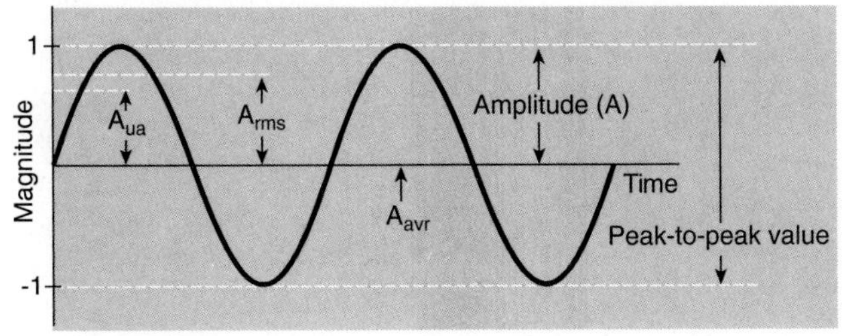

Figure 3.10. The magnitude of a sine wave. A, amplitude; A_{rms}, root mean square magnitude; A_{ua}, unipolar average magnitude; A_{avr}, average magnitude.

The **average magnitude (A_{avr})** is the average value of the magnitude calculated across the whole period of a waveform. Because the magnitude of simple harmonic motion is positive as often as it is negative, the average of the magnitude is always equal to zero. Some complex waveforms, however, may have an average magnitude that is other than zero. **Unipolar average magnitude (A_{ua})** (or rectified average magnitude) is the average magnitude calculated over the whole period of the waveform with the negative half of the waveform mirror imaged ("flipped up") on the positive side. If both halves of the waveform have the same duration and the same shape, the A_{ua} value can be calculated as the average magnitude across just the positive half-circle of the waveform. In the case of simple harmonic motion, the average unipolar magnitude is calculated using the following equation:

$$A_{ua} = \frac{2A}{\pi} \qquad (3.7)$$

where *A* is the amplitude of a waveform. From Figure 3.10, the amplitude is 1, so $2A/\pi = 0.637$.

None of the three magnitudes defined above represents the energy (power) of the waveform. Waveform energy, however, is an important consideration when describing systems that produce sounds. Therefore, another measure of waveform magnitude, one that represents the energy of the waveform, is the **root mean square (RMS) magnitude (A_{rms})**. The A_{rms} is defined as a *constant* magnitude (i.e., one value) that would produce the same power as the original quantity of the waveform (i.e., a magnitude that varies). The A_{rms} value is derived as the root of the mean of the squares of the instantaneous magnitudes calculated across the period of the waveform and indicates the power associated with the waveform. In the case of a sine wave, the RMS magnitude can be calculated by dividing the waveform amplitude by the square root of 2 or by multiplying the amplitude by 0.707:

$$A_{rms} = \frac{A}{\sqrt{2}} = A \times 0.707 \qquad (3.8)$$

For more information on the RMS magnitude, see the website. **Link 3-4** The website also contains additional information about the form factor and crest factor that describe the relationship between the peak value, average value, and RMS value of a waveform. **Link 3-5**

Example 3.2

What is the RMS magnitude of a sine wave with an amplitude of 6 volts? (Do not worry about the unit here; volts will be introduced in Chapter 13. Just get used to seeing it.)

Use Equation 3.8 to determine the RMS magnitude.

$$A_{rms} = 0.707 \times A \text{ volts}$$

$$A_{rms} = 0.707 \times 6 \text{ volts}$$

$$A_{rms} = 4.2 \text{ volts}$$

Answer: The RMS magnitude is 4.2 volts.

PRACTICE PROBLEMS: MAGNITUDE

Use the waveform below to answer the practice problems.

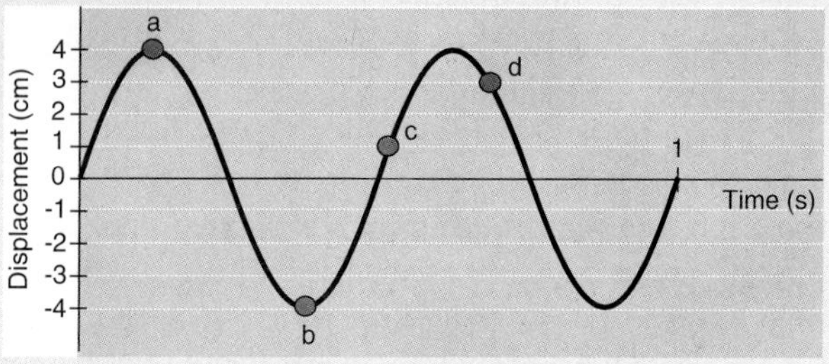

1. What is the instantaneous magnitude of the waveform at point a?
2. What is the instantaneous magnitude of the waveform at point b?
3. What is the instantaneous magnitude of the waveform at point c?
4. What is the instantaneous magnitude of the waveform at point d?
5. What is the amplitude of the waveform?
6. What is the unipolar average value of the magnitude of the waveform?
7. What is the average magnitude of the waveform?
8. What is the RMS magnitude of the waveform?

Answers (If you need help with these problems, consult the website.) **Link 3-6**

1. 4 cm
2. −4 cm
3. 1 cm
4. 3 cm
5. 4 cm
6. 2.55 cm
7. 0 cm
8. 2.83 cm

THE MASS-AND-SPRING SYSTEM

The simplest physical source of simple harmonic vibration that results from the interaction between the force of inertia and the force of elasticity is the mass-and-spring system shown in Figure 3.11. The system shown in Figure 3.11 consists of a mass located at the end of a spring suspended from an attachment point.*

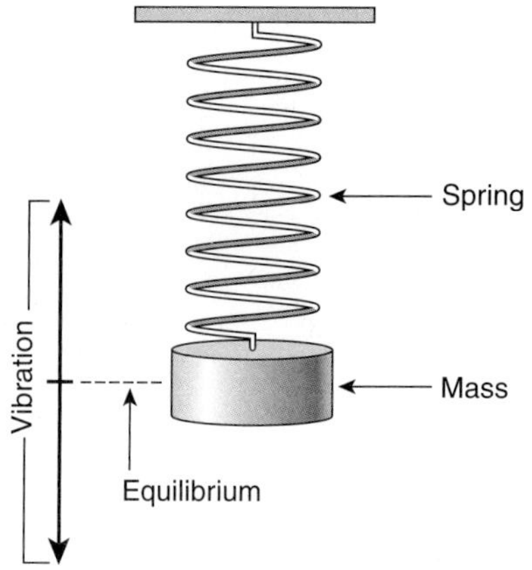

Figure 3.11. The mass-and-spring system.

In its equilibrium position the system has a certain potential energy and no kinetic energy, similar to the pendulum at rest.** When the mass is pulled away from its neutral (resting) position and released, it will move back toward equilibrium because of the restoring force provided by the elasticity of the spring. The elasticity of the spring has the same role in this system as the restoring force of gravity in the system of the pendulum. Similarly, like in the pendulum system, the mass will not stop once it has reached equilibrium, but will continue moving forward because of the inertia, that is, the acquired kinetic energy. The mass will vibrate back and forth in a simple harmonic motion because of the interaction between these two forces and the continuous flow of energy between its potential and kinetic forms. Figure 3.12 illustrates the displacement of a mass-and-spring system as a function of time.

Notice that the motion of the mass suspended on the spring represents the same simple harmonic (sinusoidal) motion as seen for the pendulum. Similarly, graphing velocity and acceleration associated with the mass-and-spring system would yield the same graphs as those seen for the velocity and acceleration of the pendulum. Let us now use the mass-and-spring system to take a closer look at factors affecting the motion of vibrating systems.

Elasticity and Inertia

In a pendulum swing, the initial displacement of the pendulum is determined by how far the pendulum is pulled away by an external force before it is released. In other words, it is determined by the amount of force applied to the system. Likewise, in the mass-and-spring system, the initial amplitude is determined by the force that is applied to the mass. If a small force is applied to the system (i.e., the mass is only pulled or pushed a small distance), the resulting amplitude

*The mass could also be connected to a spring attached to the wall and slide on a smooth surface, resulting in a horizontal movement of the system.

**The initial extension of the spring caused by the hanging mass compensates for the effect of the force of gravity acting on the mass, so both of these elements can be neglected in this examination.

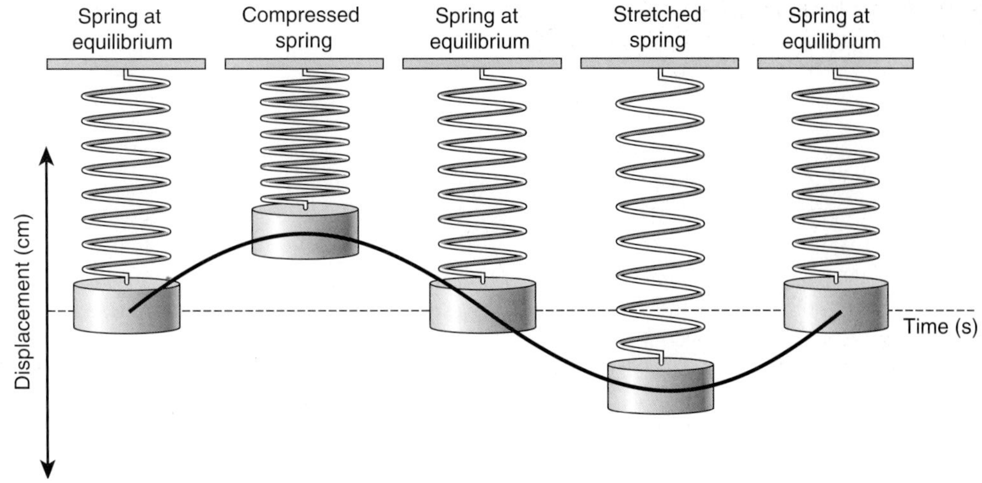

Figure 3.12. Displacement of a mass-and-spring system across time.

of vibration of the mass will be small. If the force applied to the system is larger, the amplitude of vibration will be larger, although limited to a certain stretching point beyond which the spring loses its original elasticity.

If the spring, or a similar elastic object, is stretched or compressed, it creates a force of elasticity that is trying to bring the system back to its original shape. This behavior is expressed by Hooke's Law of Elasticity, or in short, Hooke's Law. The farther the elastic object is stretched (or compressed), the greater the force of elasticity acting against the stretching (or compression). The law is named after the British mathematician and physicist Robert Hooke (1635–1703), who initially published it as the following phrase: "as the extension, the force." In its mathematical form, Hooke's law can be expressed as Equation 3.9:

$$F_e = -K \times d \tag{3.9}$$

Box 3.1 Hooke's Law of Elasticity

The force produced by an elastic object is linearly proportional to its extension.

where F_e is the force of elasticity, d is the displacement (extension or compression) of the elastic object creating the force F_e, and K is the stiffness of the elastic object in N/m. **Stiffness** is a mechanical property of an elastic object that describes its opposition to the change of its dimensions by an external force. Note the negative (−) sign on the right side of Equation 3.9 indicating that the force of elasticity acts in the opposite direction to the displacement, so if an elastic object is acted upon, the force of elasticity trying to bring the object to its normal (resting) position is acting against the external force.

Recall from Chapter 2 that elasticity is a form of potential energy. If an elastic object is stretched or compressed, it accumulates an energy that can be converted into kinetic energy as soon as the external stretching or compressing force is removed from the object and the object starts moving toward its initial (resting) position. Hooke's Law describes the force produced by the potential energy of an elastic object after the external force is removed. As the object moves closer to its resting position, the effect of the force of elasticity decreases, but the object increases its velocity because of the force of inertia. In a mass-and-spring system, if a spring is extended, the force of elasticity works against the extension (the spring "wants" to compress when it is extended). If the spring is compressed, the force of elasticity works against the compression. When the spring reaches its equilibrium position, the force of elasticity is equal to zero but the mass moves further due to the force of inertia (F_m). The force of inertia is a dynamic force produced by a moving object; this force was defined in Chapter 2 as equal to mass (m) times acceleration (a):

$$F_m = m \times a \tag{3.10}$$

The interaction between the forces of elasticity and inertia determines the frequency of the back-and-forth movement of the vibrating system. This frequency is called the resonance frequency of the system.

Resonance and Free Vibration

Thus far, we have described a vibrating system, such as a mass-and-spring system, to which a force is applied to pull an object away from equilibrium. If we leave the system alone, it will move back and forth, and its motion will continue forever. This motion represents the behavior of an ideal system called a closed system. A **closed system** is a system that does not exchange its energy with the environment, so it is forever exchanging its potential energy with kinetic energy and vice versa. In other words, once the system is set into vibration, there is absolutely no loss of energy in the system. Such "no-loss" systems only exist in theory and they are used to model the basic properties of physical systems. In reality, all systems are **open systems,** meaning that the system loses part of its energy to the surrounding environment due to the effect of friction. The presence of the force of friction in a vibrating system results in the transfer of kinetic energy to heat and the subsequent transfer of heat to the surrounding environment. As a result, the amplitude of vibration decreases over time and the system will eventually stop vibrating altogether.

The back-and-forth motion of the vibrating systems that exist after the external force has been removed from the system is called free vibration. **Free vibration** is the back-and-forth vibration of a system in which no additional energy is added to the system once it is initially set into motion. The frequency of free vibration is called the **resonance frequency** (f_r) of the system.* The resonance frequency of a system is also called the natural frequency of a system because it is the frequency at which a system will "naturally" vibrate back and forth when left alone to vibrate. Thus, **resonance** is the natural state of a vibrating system, the state in which it stays after being excited and left alone. Simple vibrating systems have one resonance frequency and complex systems may have several resonance frequencies. The resonance frequency is determined by the mass and stiffness of a closed (theoretical) system and by the mass, stiffness, and friction of an open (actual) system. The resonance frequency is also the frequency at which a system set into forced vibration will vibrate with its greatest magnitude. **Forced vibration** is a vibration in which a system is forced to vibrate by a continuously or periodically applied external force. This type of vibration will be discussed later in this chapter.

The resonance frequency of the ideal pendulum (no friction) depends on the length of the pendulum arm and can be calculated as:

$$f_r = \frac{1}{2\pi}\sqrt{\frac{g}{L}} \tag{3.11}$$

Here, L is the length of pendulum arm from the pivot point to the center of the pendulum's mass and g is the acceleration due to gravity (recall $g = 9.8$ m/s^2 for Earth). The general law of pendulum motion was discovered by Italian physicist and astronomer Galileo Galilei (1564–1642), who observed a chandelier hanging in a cathedral and noticed that the period of its swing did not depend on how far it swung to the side, but on the length of the chandelier arm. Equation 3.11 was derived later by a Dutch astronomer, Christiaan Huygens (1629–1695), who also built the first pendulum clock (e.g., grandfather clock). Note that Equation 3.11 describes the vibration of a closed system, but it can be used to calculate a relatively accurate resonance frequency of a simple real pendulum system (open system) if the angles of pendulum motion do not exceed 20°.

In a mass-and-spring system, the frequency of the system depends on the stiffness of the spring (also called the spring constant) and the amount of mass. A system with a large mass will have a lower resonance frequency compared with a system with a smaller mass. A system with a looser and longer spring will have a lower resonance frequency compared with a system with a stiffer and shorter spring. Figure 3.13 illustrates the effect of stiffness and mass on the frequency of the waveform. The lower frequency vibration shown on the top is produced by a system having a large mass or a loose spring. The higher frequency vibration shown at the bottom is produced by a system having a small mass or a tight spring. The resonance frequency (f_r) of a mass-and-spring system is calculated using Equation 3.12. See the website for a derivation of this equation. **Link 3-7**

$$f_r = \frac{1}{2\pi}\sqrt{\frac{K}{m}} \tag{3.12}$$

Note that the stiffness of the spring (K) is sometimes expressed by its inversion called **elasticity** or **compliance** (**C**), where $C = 1/K$, and Equation 3.12 is frequently written in acoustic and engineering books using this quantity instead:

$$f_r = \frac{1}{2\pi}\sqrt{\frac{1}{mC}} \tag{3.13}$$

As discussed above, the ideal pendulum system or ideal mass-and-spring system pulled away from the equilibrium position would never stop oscillating because no exchange of energy with the environment occurs. Real systems, however, gradually lose their energy to the surrounding environment due to the effects of friction; these vibrations are called damped vibrations.

Friction and Damped Vibration

According to Newton's First Law of Motion (Chapter 2), an object at rest will stay at rest and an object in motion will stay in motion until acted upon by an outside force. However, both the pendulum and the mass-and-spring system cease their motion after some time even if left to oscillate freely. This behavior is due to the presence of an additional force called friction. **Friction** is the force that opposes the relative motion (dynamic friction) or tendency to such motion (static friction) of two bodies in contact and causes the conversion of system energy into heat. In the case of the mass-and-spring system, friction is caused by the rubbing of parts of the vibrating system against surrounding surfaces and air particles. The amount of friction caused by two surfaces is characterized by the (dynamic) coefficient of friction. The **coefficient of friction** (r) is a unitless number that describes the resistance to sliding of two surfaces in contact with each other. The relationship between the force of friction (F_r) and the coefficient of friction is given by Equation 3.14.

*Hearing science textbooks often refer to the resonance frequency as the "resonant frequency"; however, Villchur (2000) pointed out that "a frequency cannot be resonant. One may refer to a resonant device or to its resonance frequency." In this text, we will defer to the wisdom of Villchur, using the term resonance frequency exclusively, and let other authors argue about which term is more correct and why.

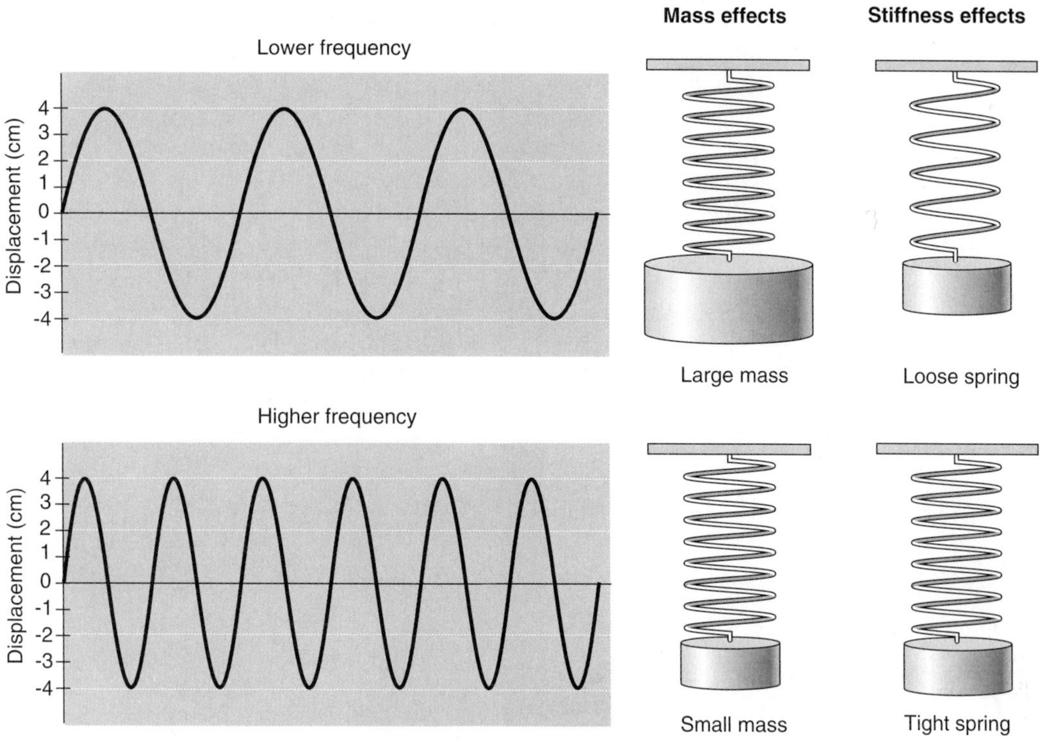

Figure 3.13. Mass and stiffness effects on the frequency of vibration.

$$F_r = r \times W \quad (3.14)$$

F_r is the force of friction, W is the weight of the object sliding on a given surface, and r is the coefficient of friction of the two surfaces.

Friction results in the transfer of energy from kinetic energy to thermal energy (heat). Heat is the energy of the vibrating system that is gradually transferred from the system to the environment until all of the system's energy is dissipated (transferred). The effect of friction on the amplitude of vibration is shown in Figure 3.14. Subsequent amplitudes become smaller and smaller in time until vibration ceases completely. The dashed lines indicate the **temporal envelope (waveform envelope)** which shows the overall shape of the waveform as it changes over time.

The effect of friction on a vibrating system is called damping and the resulting vibration is called **damped vibration. Damping** refers to the loss of energy in a vibrating system due to its dissipation to the surrounding environment, which causes a gradual decrease in the amplitude of motion. The presence of the force of friction and the resulting damping of the system's energy are natural and needed effects. Without friction, nothing could be held in place or moved from one place to another. Therefore, special damping elements are added to systems that should not have the tendency to oscillate but are prone to do so. A system is said to be a **minimally damped** (underdamped) **system** if there is very little friction in the system. A church bell is usually minimally damped and will vibrate for a fairly long time. A system is said to be a **heavily damped** (overdamped) **system** if there is a lot of friction in the system. A heavily damped system returns slowly to its neutral position without

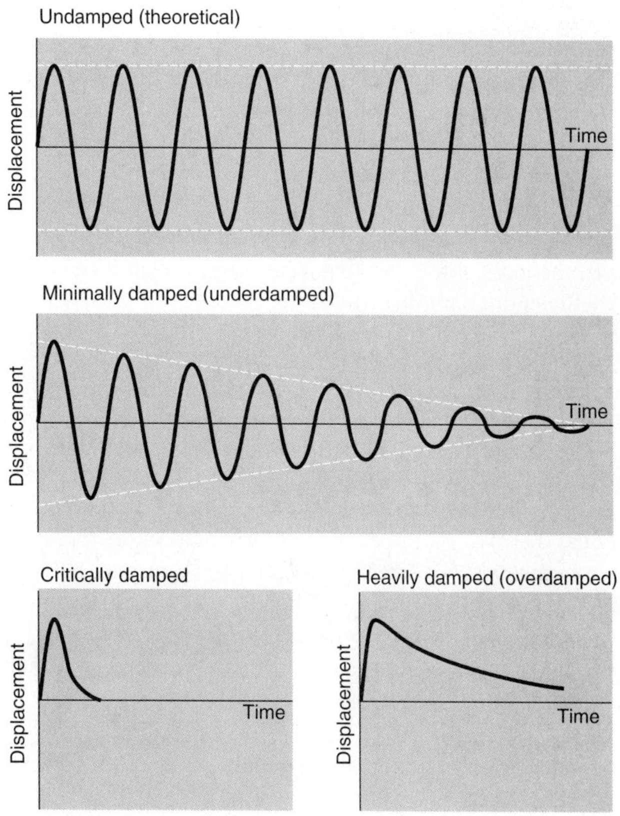

Figure 3.14. Undamped (theoretical), minimally damped (underdamped), critically damped, and heavily damped (overdamped) systems.

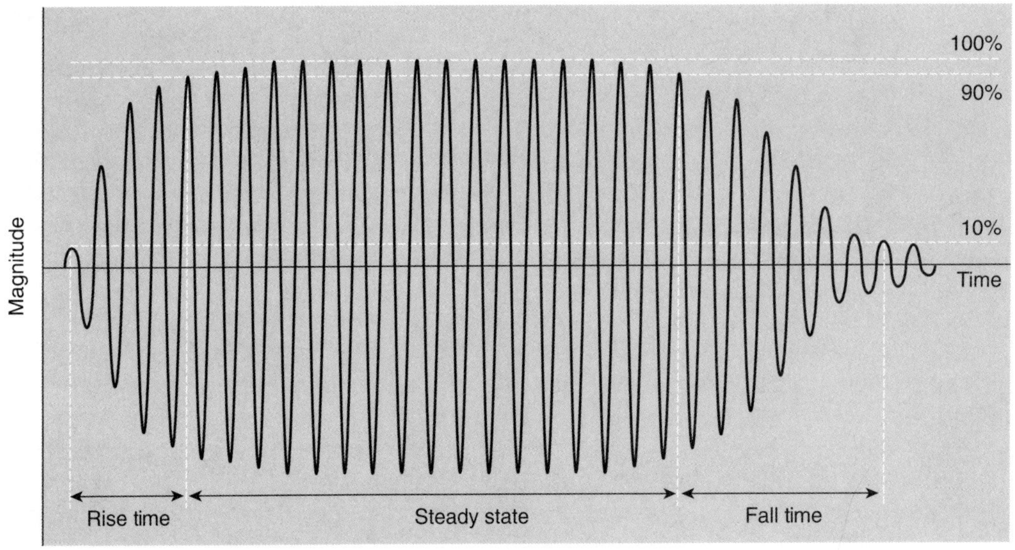

Figure 3.15. Rise time, fall time, and steady-state time illustrated on a waveform.

any oscillations. If an object is damped to the point that an object will make only one vibration and then return to its neutral position as fast as possible, this system is said to be a **critically damped system.** Critical damping indicates the most rapid response to a sudden change of force without overshooting past equilibrium. For example, a car suspension system should be critically damped to absorb frequent bumps on the road. This degree of damping is expected in a new car. As the shock absorbers wear down with time, the suspension system produces less damping and the car may start bouncing back after hitting a bump. Figure 3.14 illustrates the difference in the vibration patterns for three systems that differ in the amount of friction and, therefore, in the amount of damping. The rate of damping in the underdamped system is shown by the envelope of decreasing vibration amplitudes. The rate of damping depends on the relationship between the coefficient of friction and the mass of the vibrating system and is expressed by the **coefficient of damping (*a*):**

$$a = \frac{r}{2m} \tag{3.15}$$

where r is the coefficient of friction and m is the mass of the vibrating system. A reciprocal of the coefficient of damping is called the **time constant,** and it specifies the time (in seconds) after which the amplitude of vibration decreases by approximately 63%. If the coefficient of damping is large, then the vibrations cease quickly and the time constant is small. A vibrating system is considered to cease its vibrations after the elapse of three time constants,* which correspond to a 95% change in the magnitude of an initial displacement.

The presence of friction in a vibrating system affects not only the duration of vibration and its damping, but also the way the vibration starts, grows, and ceases to exist. The overall duration of each vibration can be divided into three time periods labeled the **rise time** (growth time, attack time), the **steady-state time** (sustain time), and the **fall time** (decay time, roll-off time) (Fig. 3.15). They are the three basic components of the waveform envelope. The rise time is typically defined as the time needed for a waveform to change from 10% to 90% of its peak value (e.g., full amplitude). Similarly, the fall time is defined as the time needed for a waveform to change from 90% to 10% of its peak value. Both the rise time and the fall time are called the **transients** of the waveform due to the fact that they are typically short events in time. The **initial transient** occurs at the beginning of the waveform and the **final transient** occurs at the end of the waveform; both have important effects on the physical and perceptual properties of the whole waveform.

Since friction exists in all real vibrating systems, the behavior of vibrating systems can be characterized by three forces: the force of elasticity (F_e), the force of inertia (F_m), and the force of friction (F_r). When the external force that initiated the motion is subsequently removed from the system, the motion of the vibrating system can be described by Equation 3.16.

$$F_e + F_m + F_r = 0 \tag{3.16}$$

Since forces acting in a vibratory motion are functions of time (their magnitudes change in time), the above equation contains all the information needed to determine the shape, frequency, and duration of damped vibrations of the system. In this context it is important to realize that the presence of friction not only affects the envelope of the waveform, but also reduces the natural resonance frequency of the vibrating system. The frequency of underdamped (minimally damped) real

*"Three time constants" refers to the three equal periods of time during which the signal decreases in intensity. For example, if the time constant is 100 ms, 100 ms after removing the driving force, the amplitude of vibration will decrease by 63%. After the next 100 ms, the amplitude will decrease by another 63% (86% total). After the third 100 ms, the amplitude of vibration decreases again by 63% (95% total). In other words, the amplitude of vibration will be 37%, 14%, and 5% of its original value at 100 ms, 200 ms, and 300 ms after removing the external force, respectively.

vibrations (f_d) can be determined by finding the coefficient of damping from Equation 3.16 and using the following formula:

$$f_d = \frac{1}{2\pi}\sqrt{4\pi^2 f_r^2 - a^2} \qquad (3.17)$$

where f_r is the resonance frequency of an ideal system (i.e., no friction) and a is the coefficient of damping. If the resonance frequency of the damped system (f_d) is equal to zero, the system is critically damped. If the expression under the square root is negative (which means it cannot be solved), it indicates that the system is overdamped and therefore f_d does not have a real value.

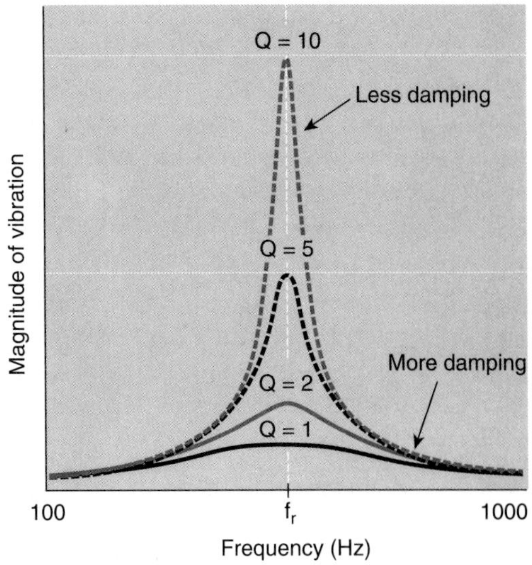

Figure 3.16. The magnitude of a forced vibration as a function of the frequency of the driving force for several systems with the same resonance frequency and different amounts of friction.

Forced Vibration

Thus far in the discussion of the pendulum and mass and spring, we have made an assumption that the system vibrates freely at its own resonance frequency. If a system is not allowed to vibrate freely, but instead is forced to vibrate by a continuous and periodic driving force, this vibration is called a forced vibration. The frequency of the external force is called the **driving frequency.**

In a forced mode of vibration, the system will vibrate back and forth at the frequency of the driving force. The magnitude of vibration of the system depends not only on the magnitude of the applied force, but also on the frequency of the periodic driving force. If a system is forced to vibrate close to or at its resonance frequency, the system will vibrate with a greater magnitude than if the same system is forced to vibrate at a frequency that is much lower or higher than the resonance frequency. For example, if a swing is pumped by a child at its natural frequency, it can swing quite high, but the same swing will not go as high if it is pumped at a higher or lower frequency. A frequently cited example of resonance that led to the destruction of a vibrating structure is the case of the Tacoma Narrows Bridge that collapsed due to bridge vibration caused by a strong wind. A movie showing the destruction of the Tacoma Narrows Bridge can be found at http://en.wikipedia.org/wiki/Tacoma_Narrows_Bridge. If this site is no longer active, this or another similar video can be easily located by searching the Internet for "Tacoma Narrows Bridge."

The dependence of the amplitude of vibration on the frequency of the driving force is called the **resonance curve** of the system. Recall that the closer the frequency of the driving force is to the resonance frequency of the system, the higher the magnitude of vibration. This means that the system responds with the highest magnitude of vibration when the frequency of the driving force is equal to the resonance frequency of the system. Examples of resonance curves are shown in Figure 3.16. These resonance curves have a bell-like (Gaussian, normal) shape with the greatest magnitude of vibration corresponding to the resonance frequency (f_r) of the vibrating system. This point indicates the greatest magnitude of the system response because at the resonance frequency, the system needs very little external energy to compensate for the loss of energy during vibration. At frequencies farther away (above and below frequency f_r), the system also vibrates, but with lower and lower magnitudes.

The height and shape of the resonance curve depend on the mechanical parameters of the system. The heavier the damping in the system, the lower and flatter the resonance curve is. Let us compare the two marked resonance curves in Figure 3.16. Both curves have the same resonance frequency but different amounts of damping. The lower the curve, the less responsive the system is to external forces. The narrower the curve, the more **selective** the system is in its response, in other words, the narrower the range of frequencies at which a system can be forced to vibrate with large amplitudes. The selectivity of a system is commonly expressed by its **quality factor (Q).** A more extensive discussion of Q and its role in sound production, transmission, and reception is included in Chapter 14.

Summary

Vibration creates sound. Vibration is the back-and-forth motion of a mechanical object around an equilibrium point. The pendulum and the mass-and-spring system are two common systems used to study vibration. Pendulum motion is the result of the interaction between inertia and the restoring force of gravity.

In mass-and-spring system vibration, vibratory motion is the result of the interaction between inertia and the restoring force of elasticity. Simple harmonic motion is a example of vibratory motion waveform, which shows changes in an object's position as a function of time. Characteristic elements of a waveform include frequency (the number of cycles of vibratory motion per second), period (the time required for the completion of one full cycle), phase (the particular stage of vibratory motion, using the angles of a circle), and amplitude (the maximum magnitude of the vibration). Frequency and period are affected in a mass-and-spring system by the inertia of the mass and the elasticity of the spring. In an ideal system (no loss of energy to other systems), the magnitude of vibration does not vary over time and is solely determined by the magnitude of the force that has displaced the mass from equilibrium. In a real system, the magnitude of vibration decreases over time as a result of friction (interaction with the environment). The effect of friction on the magnitude of vibration is described as damping. Various degrees of damping can be seen by examining the temporal envelope of a waveform. The temporal envelope (amplitude envelope, waveform envelope) is an imaginary line connecting the maximum instantaneous positive (or negative) magnitudes of a back-and-forth motion expressed as a function of time. For a system to vibrate for a long period of time, a continuous force must be applied to the system. Systems forced to vibrate will vibrate in synchrony with the frequency of the applied force rather than at the resonance frequency of the system. The amplitude of the forced vibration will depend on the frequency of the applied force and the damping of the system.

Key Points

- Oscillations and vibrations are back-and-forth motions of objects about an equilibrium point.
- When systems are set into oscillation/vibration by an outside force, they will oscillate/vibrate due to the interaction between inertia and a restoring force. The restoring force causing pendulum motion is gravity. The restoring force causing mass-and-spring vibration is elasticity.
- Periodic motion is motion that repeats itself in regular intervals.
- Simple harmonic motion is a motion described by a sinusoidal function. That is, when any characteristic of the simple harmonic motion (such as displacement, velocity, or acceleration) is graphed as a function of time, it has the shape of a sine wave.
- A waveform is a function representing changes in a characteristic of motion graphed as a function of time.
- Frequency (f) is the number of cycles per second. Period (T) is the time it takes to complete one cycle of vibration. Frequency and period are reciprocally (inversely) related such that $f = 1/T$ and $T = 1/f$. The frequency of vibration of a vibrating system is determined by the mass and stiffness characteristics of the system.
- The phase relationship describes the difference between the phases of two periodic waveforms as they cycle through time. When two waveforms have the same frequency and the same starting phase, their phase relationship is described as in-phase. If two waveforms have the same frequency and different starting phases, they are said to be out-of-phase.
- Amplitude is the maximum magnitude of a measured periodic quantity. The magnitude of vibration at any other time point is called the instantaneous magnitude. The root mean square (RMS) magnitude is a measure used to express the energy of a system. In simple harmonic motion, RMS magnitude is calculated by multiplying the amplitude by 0.707.

CHAPTER 4

Complex Vibrations and Waveform Analysis

Chapter Outline

Objectives

- To introduce the concept of complex vibration as the combination (synthesis) of various sinusoidal component waves
- To discuss types of complex vibration and the decomposition of complex motion into simple harmonic motions
- To discuss modes of vibration in strings, rods, membranes, and plates including the concepts of fundamental frequency and harmonics
- To discuss specific examples of complex waves created from a harmonic series
- To introduce the concept of impedance in a vibrating system

Key Terms

Admittance
Amplitude spectrum
Antinode
Aperiodic vibration
Bar
Chladni pattern (Chladni figure)
Circular mode of vibration
Complex inharmonic vibration
Complex vibration
Conductance
Continuous spectrum
Cycle
Elasticity
Fourier Theorem
Frequency domain
Fundamental frequency
Fundamental period
Greatest common factor
Harmonics
Impedance
Impedance matching
Line (discrete) spectrum
Load
Mass reactance
Mass susceptance
Mechanic impedance
Membrane
Missing fundamental
Mode
Node
Noise
Octave
Overtone
Partial
Periodic vibration
Periodicity
Phase spectrum
Plate
Power spectrum
Radial mode of vibration
Reactance
Resistance
Rod
Spectrum
Spectrum analysis
Spectrum component
Stiffness reactance
Stiffness susceptance
Time domain
Torsional vibration
Transient
Transverse vibration
Waveform analysis (Fourier analysis)
Waveform synthesis
White noise

COMPLEX VIBRATION

Simple harmonic motion (SHM), discussed in Chapter 3, is the most fundamental type of back-and-forth motion. This motion, when performed by a vibrating object, is called simple vibration.* Simple vibrations are rarely present in nature, as most natural vibrations are complex vibrations. **Complex vibration** is the sum of two or more simple vibrations. The simple vibrations that make up a complex vibration are called **frequency components** or **partials**.** In some cases, a complex vibration is the sum of only a few simple vibrations and in other cases a complex vibration is the sum of tens of thousands of simple vibrations. The fact that any complex waveform can be constructed from a number of sinusoidal waveforms is an important property of all vibratory motion and it is described by the Fourier Theorem (after French mathematician Jean Joseph Fourier, 1768–1830). The **Fourier Theorem** states that any complex oscillatory (vibratory) motion is the sum of various sinusoidal motions of varying amplitude, frequency, and phase. Examples of complex waveforms representing complex vibrations are shown in Figure 4.1. The appearance of a complex waveform can vary considerably depending on the number of sinusoidal components that are combined together to create the vibration and the frequencies, amplitudes, and temporal (time) envelopes of these components.

Complex vibration can be divided into two basic classes of back-and-forth motion: aperiodic vibration and periodic vibration. **Aperiodic vibration** is a vibration *without* a repeating pattern in time. A waveform illustrating typical aperiodic vibration is shown in Figure 4.1A. When looking at Figure 4.1A, notice the lack of a predictable pattern in the way the magnitude of displacement varies over time.

Periodic vibration is a vibratory motion in which an object returns to the same point in space periodically (at equal periods of time) during the motion. Knowing the period of a periodic vibration and the pattern of the motion within the period, one can predict the position of the object at any moment in time.

An example of a periodic waveform is shown in Figure 4.1B. Notice that in the periodic vibration a clearly repeating pattern is apparent in the way the magnitude changes over time. A single completed execution of this periodic pattern is called a **cycle.** The first cycle of the vibration shown in Figure 4.1B is outlined with a shaded box. Notice also that two complete cycles of the motion have occurred between 0 and 1 second and that four complete cycles are present in the figure.

The period of a complex vibration, called the **fundamental period (T_0)**, can be calculated by determining the duration of one cycle of complex periodic motion. This is the same concept as described in Chapter 3 in reference to simple harmonic motion.

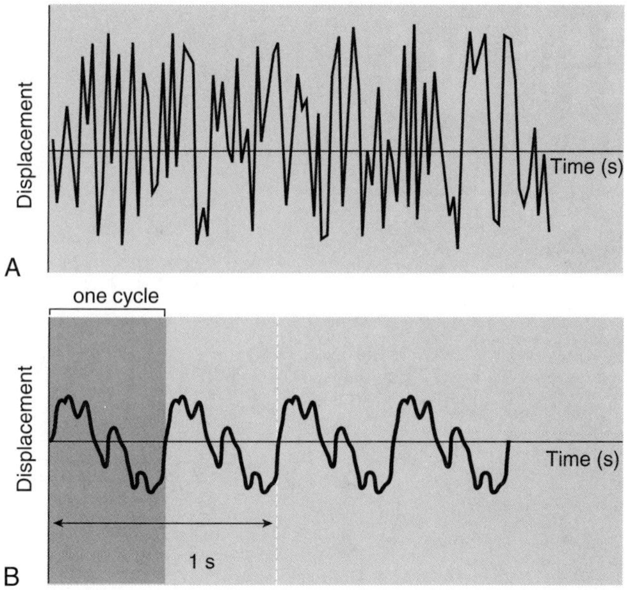

Figure 4.1. Complex aperiodic vibration **(A)** and complex periodic vibration **(B).**

Example 4.1

What is the fundamental period of the complex periodic waveform shown in Figure 4.1B?

In Figure 4.1B, two cycles of the vibration occurred in 1 second; therefore, the fundamental period (T_o) of the motion is equal to 0.5 second.

$$T_o = \frac{1 \text{ sec}}{2 \text{ cycles}}$$

$$T_o = 0.5 \frac{\text{sec}}{\text{cycle}}$$

When reporting the period, the "per cycle" portion of the units is disregarded (assumed) and the period is reported in a time unit only.

$$T_o = 0.5 \text{ s}$$

Answer: The fundamental period is 0.5 second.

The **fundamental frequency (f_o)** of a complex periodic motion is the inverse of the fundamental period (T_o) and can be calculated in hertz the same way it is for simple harmonic motion (Chapter 3). In a mathematical form it can be written as:

$$f_o = \frac{1}{T_o}$$

*A simple (sinusoidal) vibration converted into sound is called a pure tone. Sound examples of various pure tones are included in Chapter 5.

**The term *partial* is used primarily in music applications to mean a sinusoidal component of a vibration.

Example 4.2

What is the fundamental period of the complex periodic waveform from Figure 4.1B?

Using the formula $f_o = 1/T_o$, substitute known variables and solve. You know that T_o is 0.5 second.

$$f_o = \frac{1}{0.5 \frac{\text{sec}}{\text{cycle}}}$$

$$f_o = 2 \frac{\text{cycles}}{\text{sec}}$$

$$f_o = 2 \text{ Hz}$$

Answer: The fundamental frequency is 2 Hz.

PRACTICE PROBLEMS: COMPLEX WAVEFORMS

Use this waveform to answer questions 1 through 5.

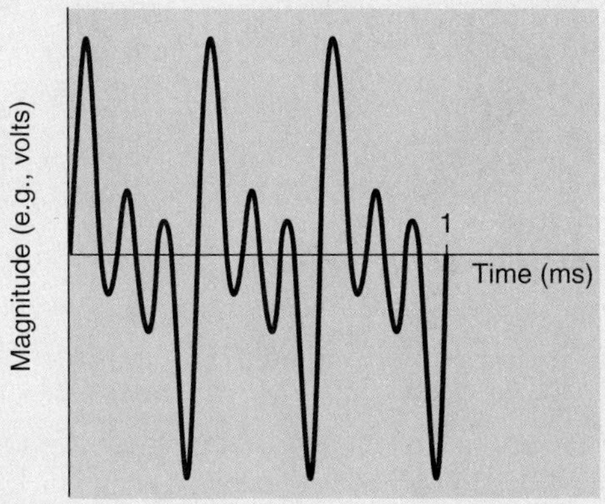

1. Is this a sinusoidal wave or a complex wave?
2. Is this an example of periodic or aperiodic vibration?
3. How many cycles of the motion are present on the graph?
4. What is the fundamental period (T_o) of the waveform?
5. What is the fundamental frequency (f_o) of the waveform?

Answers (If you need help with these problems, consult the website.) **Link 4-1**

1. Complex
2. Periodic
3. 3
4. T_o = 0.33 ms or 0.00033 second
5. f_o = 3000 Hz

The Composition of Complex Vibration

The process of combining several individual sinusoidal motions into a complex waveform is called **waveform synthesis.** This process is illustrated in Figure 4.2. In Figure 4.2, three simple vibrations that differ in frequency but that have the same amplitude and initial phase have been combined to form a complex vibration. Notice that by adding the instantaneous magnitudes of the sinusoids, the instantaneous magnitude of the complex waveform can be determined at any point in time. Only two such points are shown in Figure 4.2, but for every other time point, the same addition could have been shown also. This procedure can be applied regardless of the specific physical characteristic that is describing the vibrations as long as it is the same characteristic for all involved components. For example, the *y* axis in Figure 4.2 could display displacement, velocity, acceleration, and so forth, as long as the same characteristic is added for all of the components.

Assume, for example, that all of the waveforms in Figure 4.2 represent the amount of displacement in centimeters across time. If all three of these vibrations are combined into one complex vibration, the instantaneous values for the three component waves can be combined at any time point. For example, at time moment "a," the magnitudes are 2, 0, and 0 cm. Since 2 + 0 + 0 = 2, the instantaneous magnitude of the complex wave displacement at this point is 2 cm. At time moment "b," the instantaneous magnitudes of the three component vibrations are −2, 0, and 0 cm. Since −2 + 0 + 0 = −2, the instantaneous magnitude of the complex wave at this point is –2 cm. When the instantaneous displacements are summed together across the three component motions for all time points, the full shape of the complex vibration can be drawn (waveform D in Fig. 4.2).

The waveform synthesis shown in Figure 4.2 demonstrates an important property of complex periodic vibration: The frequencies of all of the frequency components of the complex waveform are whole-number multiples of the fundamental frequency. The fundamental frequency of the complex waveform shown in panel D is 4 Hz and the frequencies of the components are equal to 4 Hz, 8 Hz (i.e., 2 × the fundamental frequency), and 16 Hz (i.e., 4 × times the fundamental frequency). The complex vibration shown in panel D has maintained the periodic (repeating) character of the motion seen in sine waves A, B, and C (there are clearly four identical, repeated cycles in complex wave D); the shape of the waveform, however, is obviously different from a sinusoidal vibration. Notice again that in the presented example the fundamental frequency (4 Hz) and fundamental period (0.25 s) of the complex waveform are equal to the frequency (4 Hz) and period (0.25 s) of the lowest component of the waveform, respectively. The fundamental frequency, however, is not always equal to the lowest frequency component of the waveform, a situation that will be discussed later in this section.

When all of the components of a complex waveform are whole-number multiples of a certain frequency, they are

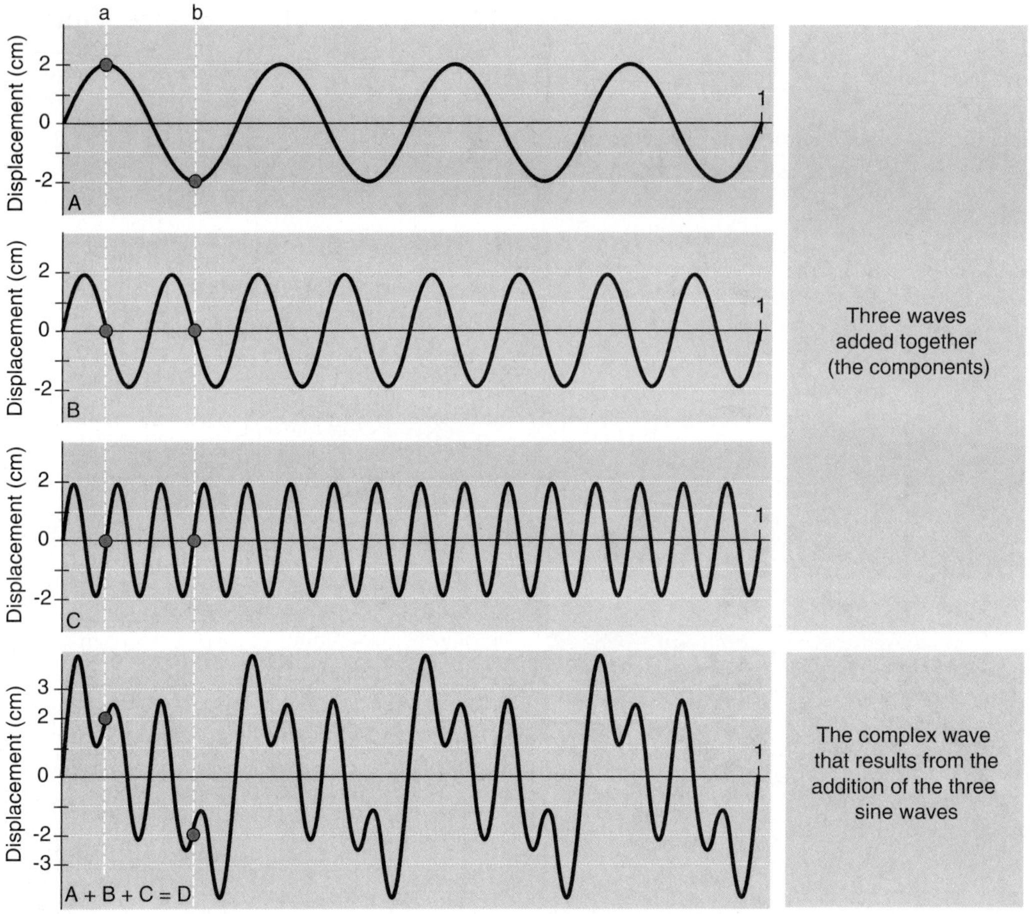

Figure 4.2. The process of adding together three simple vibrations **(A–C)** to form a complex vibration **(D)**.

called harmonics and the vibration resulting from their combination is periodic. Thus, **harmonics** are frequency components of a complex waveform that are whole-number multiples of its fundamental frequency. The fundamental frequency of this type of complex periodic waveform is called the first harmonic. A component that is two times the fundamental is called the second harmonic, a component that is three times the fundamental is called the third harmonic, and so forth. Sometimes, instead of the term *harmonic*, the term **overtone** is used (especially for musical applications). An overtone is a harmonic other than the fundamental frequency. Therefore, the second harmonic is the same as the first overtone, the third harmonic is the same as the second overtone, and so forth. Please note that the terms *fundamental frequency, component frequency, partial, harmonic,* and *overtone* apply to all complex waveforms regardless of their physical origin. Therefore, complex vibrations, complex sounds, and complex electric signals can be described using the same group of terms.

It is important to stress that the fundamental frequency of a complex vibration is not always equal to the frequency of its lowest frequency component. In Figure 4.2, the fundamental frequency and the frequency of the lowest frequency component were both 4 Hz. It is common, however, to have a complex periodic vibration in which none of the components has a frequency equal to the fundamental frequency of the complex waveform. Consider the following example.

Example 4.3

Imagine that four sinusoidal waveforms with frequencies of 1000 Hz, 1500 Hz, 2000 Hz, and 2500 Hz are combined into one complex waveform. Will the result be a complex periodic wave or a complex aperiodic wave?

In this case, the lowest frequency is 1000 Hz and two of the components (1500 Hz, 2500 Hz) are obviously not whole-number multiples of 1000 Hz, although all of the components are whole-number multiples of 500 Hz. Therefore, the complex waveform that results from the combination of these four components is periodic with a fundamental frequency of 500 Hz, even though 500 Hz is not an actual component of the waveform.

Answer: The waveform would be a complex periodic waveform.

Example 4.3 illustrates an important concept regarding the fundamental frequency. Specifically, the fundamental frequency of a complex vibration should be understood as the **greatest common factor** (GCF) of all the frequencies that make up the complex waveform, regardless of whether the fundamental frequency is an actual component of the complex waveform or not. A **common factor** is a number by which all the numbers in a given set can be divided without a remainder. The greatest common factor is the largest of the common factors. If a set of frequencies does not have a common factor, then their combination will result in an aperiodic wave instead of a periodic wave. If you would like to see an example of how to determine the GCF, see the website. **Link 4-2**

A complex periodic wave in which no component is equal to the fundamental frequency is said to have a **missing fundamental** (or phantom fundamental), because no energy is present at the fundamental frequency; in other words, the components do not include a frequency equal to the GCF. A number of sounds (including chimes and organ pipes) vibrate in complex periodic motion without a component equal to the fundamental frequency. The most interesting concept associated with the missing fundamental is that this frequency can often be perceived by a listener, even though no energy is present at that frequency. The physiologic implications that this frequency can be perceived by a listener are discussed in Chapter 9 and the auditory effect of the missing fundamental is described in Chapter 12.

The shape of a complex vibration is dependent not only on the frequency of the components, but also on the magnitude, phase, and duration of the components. For example, Figure 4.3 illustrates two examples where two sinusoidal vibrations with the same amplitude and frequency are added together. In Figure 4.3A the vibrations are added in-phase and in Figure 4.3B the vibrations are added 180° out-of-phase. Notice that the phase relationship between the vibrations makes a significant difference in the outcome. When the waves were combined in-phase, the amplitude doubled, but when the waves were combined 180° out-of-phase, the vibrations cancelled each other and the vibrating system became motionless.

As you can imagine, an infinite number of different complex waveforms can result when components with different amplitudes, frequencies, phases, and durations are combined. As each of these parameters changes, and as components begin and end, the complex wave changes. The concept of **periodicity** (i.e., the concept that a periodic wave keeps repeating itself for an infinite amount of time) assumes that all the vibrations that make up the wave continue forever. This is obviously only a theoretical concept. In reality, all vibrations have a beginning and an end and they need a certain amount of time to develop and to stop (see Chapter 3; Fig. 3.15). Therefore, the property of periodicity applies only to the time when the system is operating in an unchanging or steady state.

We have defined aperiodic vibration as a complex vibration with a pattern that does not repeat itself in time. Two main classes of events fall under this definition: noises and transients. **Noise** is a stochastic (random) sequence of events resulting from the combination of a

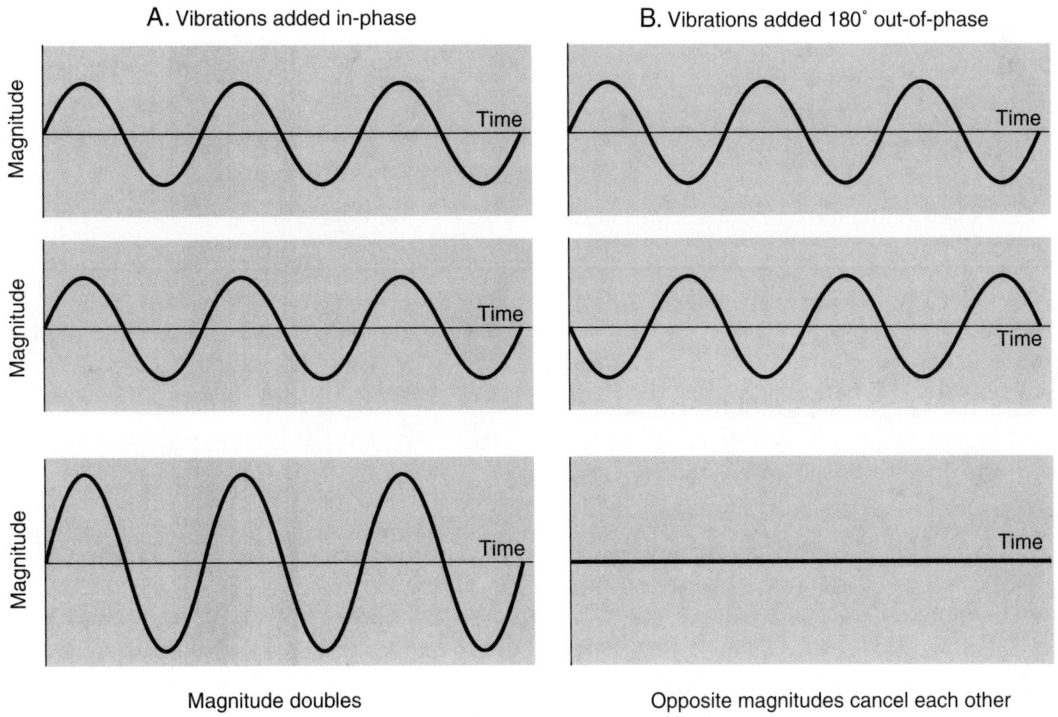

Figure 4.3. The addition of two simple vibrations with the same frequency and amplitude, but with different phase relationships: in-phase **(A)** and 180° out-of-phase **(B).**

very large (infinite) number of unrelated components. A **transient** is a brief single event that ceases to exist after a very short time (e.g., door slam). Another type of vibration, complex inharmonic vibration, could technically be classified as periodic (harmonic) or aperiodic (inharmonic) vibration, A **complex inharmonic vibration** can be defined as the sum of a finite number of components that does not repeat its pattern within a time period of observation. However, any vibration that consists of less than an infinite number of components is, as a matter of fact, a periodic vibration, although its fundamental frequency may be very low. For example, a complex vibration composed of 23 Hz, 71 Hz, and 237 Hz has a fundamental frequency of 1 Hz. Thus, the motion will repeat itself with a rate of 1 Hz and it is mathematically and logically a periodic motion.

The fact that a complex vibration is theoretically periodic is irrelevant in situations where the fundamental frequency is not perceived or observed. Consider, for example, that the human ear can only hear tones that have a frequency of 20 Hz ($T = 50$ ms) or higher. Therefore, we are unable to hear a fundamental frequency of 1 Hz ($T = 1$ s) in the example above and instead we will hear a mixture of three vibrations that are not harmonically related. In addition, if we observe the waveform of a recorded sample that is 300 ms long and the fundamental frequency is 1 Hz, the waveform will not repeat itself. Unfortunately, no consensus is found in the literature regarding how this type of vibration should be classified, although some authors differentiate physical periodicity (the repeating of the waveform) and perceptual periodicity (the perceived sound of the waveform) based on the sensation of pitch (Schwartz & Purve, 2004). In this book, we regard a complex vibration consisting of a limited number of components to be harmonic (periodic) even if it's fundamental frequency is lower than 20 Hz, which is the lowest frequency that can be heard by humans (Chapter 12). However, if the fundamental frequency is lower than 20 Hz, these vibrations may not be perceived as sound. Obviously, aperiodic and periodic vibrations can coexist together and these mixtures represent most real-world physical events.

PRACTICE PROBLEMS: COMPOSITION OF COMPLEX WAVES

1. Would the combination of four sinusoidal waveforms with frequencies of 100 Hz, 200 Hz, 700 Hz, and 4000 Hz result in a complex periodic waveform? Why or why not?
2. If the following four components were combined to form a complex periodic waveform: 50 Hz, 100 Hz, 200 Hz, and 300 Hz, would this waveform have a missing fundamental?
3. If the following components were combined: 1000 Hz, 2000 Hz, and 3000 Hz, what would be the fundamental frequency of the complex waveform?
4. If the following components were combined: 150 Hz, 500 Hz, and 675 Hz, what would be the fundamental frequency?
5. If the following components were combined: 500 Hz, 750 Hz, and 1000 Hz, would we describe the complex waveform that results as having a missing fundamental?
6. Would the combination of these three sinusoidal waveforms result in a complex periodic waveform? Why or why not?

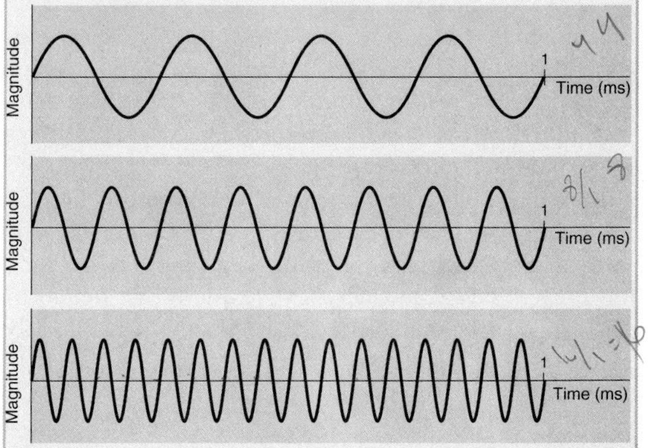

Answers (If you need help with these problems, consult the website.) **Link 4-3**

1. Yes. All of the sine waves are harmonically related because they are whole-number multiples of the fundamental frequency (f_o), which is 100 Hz.
2. No. The fundamental frequency of this complex waveform is 50 Hz.
3. 1000 Hz
4. 25 Hz
5. Yes
6. Yes. All of the components are harmonically related and they are whole-number multiples of the f_o.

WAVEFORM ANALYSIS AND SPECTRUM

In Chapter 3 we introduced the concept of a waveform as a function of vibratory motion over time. This concept was applied to simple harmonic motion but it also applies to all back-and-forth motions, regardless of whether the motion is

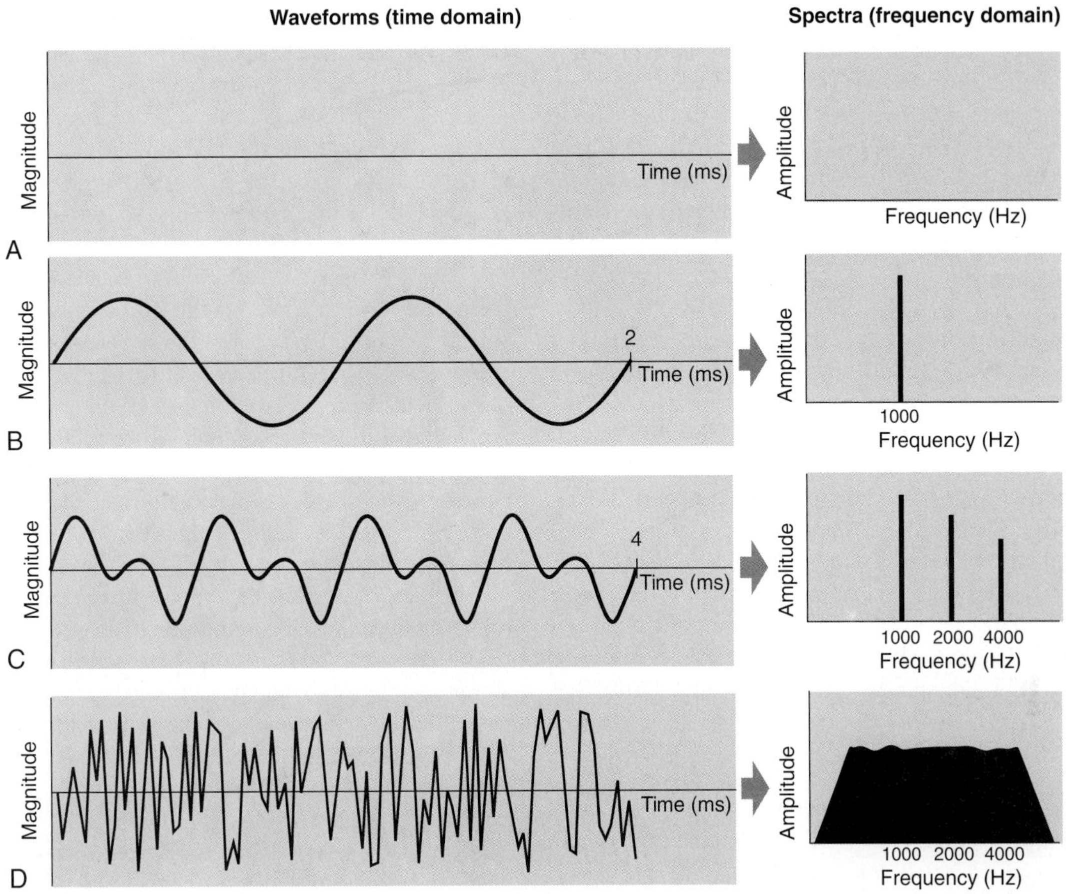

Figure 4.4. A comparison of the waveform (time domain) and spectrum (frequency domain). **Panel A** illustrates the coordinates (*x* axis and *y* axis) of the waveform and spectrum. **Panel B** shows a sine wave (1000 Hz) using a waveform and spectrum. **Panel C** illustrates complex periodic vibration composed of three sinusoids (1000 Hz, 2000 Hz, and 4000 Hz). **Panel D** illustrates complex aperiodic vibration composed of various sinusoids that are not harmonically related.

simple, complex, periodic, or aperiodic. To more closely examine a specific vibration, it is often necessary to break down a complex waveform and determine which components are present. In other words, instead of adding sine waves to form a complex waveform (waveform synthesis), it is often necessary to reverse the process and take a complex waveform and break it down into individual components. This process is called **waveform analysis.**

Breaking down a complex waveform into components is not as easy to illustrate as adding components together. Waveform analysis can be done electronically, using a variety of electronic analyzers (generally with a software package), or mathematically, using analytical tools based on Fourier's Theorem. Using waveform analysis (also known, depending on the application, as Fourier analysis, Fourier transform, spectrum analysis, and frequency analysis), a signal can be decomposed into its component sinusoidal waveforms, which are then called a Fourier series. This is exactly the reverse of the waveform synthesis process in which a number of components are combined to form a complex waveform. After a complex wave is analyzed, it is possible to see if just a few sine waves or thousands of sine waves are in the Fourier series and to examine the relationships among them.

Up to this point, a waveform (x axis = time; y axis = magnitude) has been used to display vibration as a function of time, that is, in what is called the **time domain.** When you are looking at a complex waveform, determining the specific frequency components that make up the waveform is generally not possible. Therefore, another form of graphic display is needed to illustrate the results of waveform analysis. This graphic display is called a spectrum (plural, spectra). A **spectrum** is a graphical representation of a complex waveform showing the waveform energy (amplitudes) of the individual components (y axis) arranged in order of frequency (x axis). Individual components, displayed as lines perpendicular to the x axis, are called **spectrum components** (spectral components, frequency components). Thus, the spectrum provides a graphical representation of the Fourier series of a complex vibratory motion.

The spectrum can be thought of as a display of a waveform in the **frequency domain.** Figure 4.4 illustrates the difference between the waveform (time domain) and the spectrum (frequency domain) for a sine wave, a complex periodic waveform, and a complex aperiodic waveform in the form of noise. Notice the change in the *x* axis between the waveform and spectrum from time to frequency (Fig. 4.4A). There is also a difference in the characteristic shown by the *y* axis. The *y* axis for the waveform indicates the instantaneous magnitude but the *y* axis for the spectrum indicates the amplitude of the components. Notice that the single sinusoidal waveform (Fig 4.4B) appears as a single vertical line on the spectral display because it has only one component (1000 Hz in this example). The spectrum of the complex periodic vibration (Fig. 4.4C) has three vertical lines corresponding to three components that combine to form the waveform (1000 Hz, 2000 Hz, and 4000 Hz in this example). The spectrum of noise (Fig. 4.4D) has so many different components that they no longer appear as separate lines on the spectrum. You are probably already familiar with a spectrum if you have used the "bars and line" features of Windows Media Player. See the website for an example of a spectrum that you may have seen outside of hearing science class. **Link 4-4**

When a complex waveform has been broken down into its individual components by waveform analysis and the resulting spectrum consists of one or more separate vertical lines (as in Figure 4.4B and C), this spectrum is called a **line spectrum** (discrete spectrum). The line spectrum characterizes both periodic and aperiodic vibrations that consist of a limited number of components.

Three specific complex periodic waveforms are frequently used in hearing science and acoustics: the sawtooth waveform, the square waveform, and the triangular waveform. Their temporal and spectral characteristics are shown in Figure 4.5. Notice that the sawtooth waveform is composed of all odd- and even-numbered harmonics decreasing in amplitude by $1/n$. In other words, the second harmonic is half the amplitude of the first harmonic, the third harmonic is one third the amplitude of the first harmonic, and so forth. The square wave is characterized by the presence of only odd-numbered harmonics with their amplitudes also decreasing by $1/n$. The triangular wave is composed of odd-numbered harmonics, similar to the square wave, but the harmonics decrease in amplitude with a rate of $1/n^2$. In other words, the amplitude of the second harmonic is one fourth of the first harmonic, the amplitude of the third harmonic is one ninth of the first harmonic, and so forth. The rate of decrease of $1/n$ and $1/n^2$ are also described in the hearing science literature as 6 dB/octave and 12 dB/octave on the decibel scale (the octave and the decibel will be discussed in Chapter 7).

The ideal waveforms that appear in Figure 4.5 are created only if all of the possible harmonics in the series are included. High-frequency harmonics in these series have very small amplitudes, however, and just a few lower frequency harmonics are needed to approximate the ideal shape.

In contrast to the line spectra shown in Figure 4.5, some spectra may contain thousands of components instead of just a few, as shown in Figure 4.4D. All noises are characterized by such spectra. If thousands of spectral components were drawn within a spectrum, they would not appear as individual lines because they would be too close together to

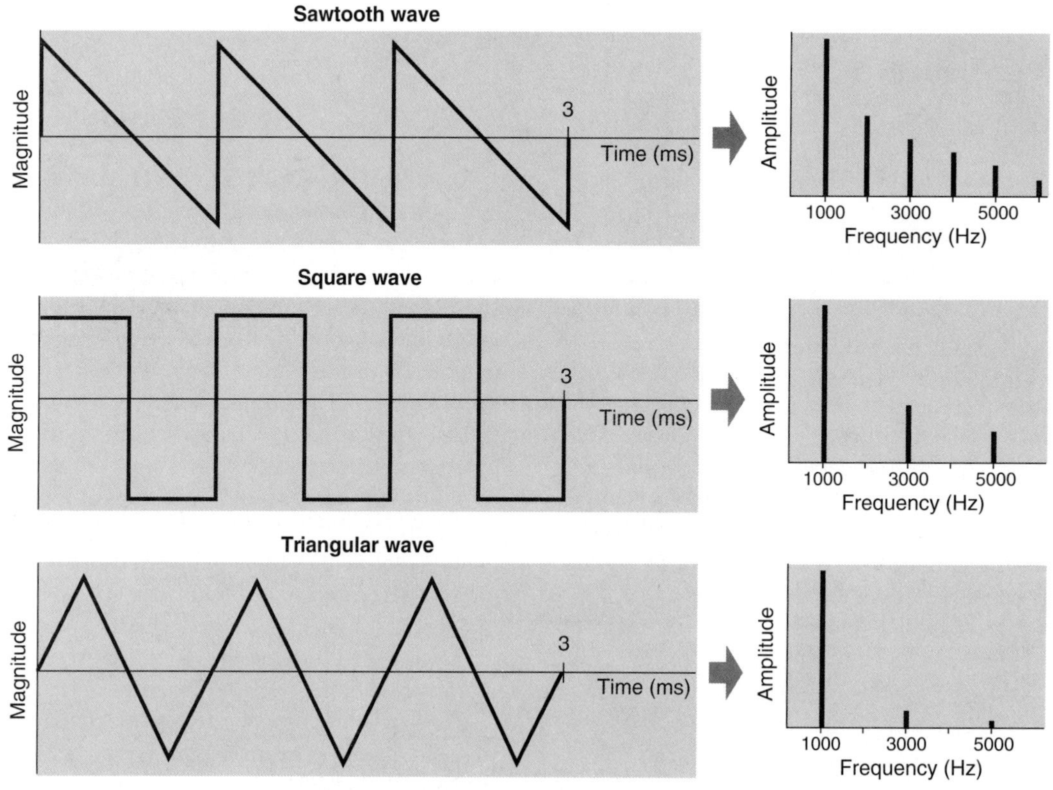

Figure 4.5. Sawtooth, square, and triangular waveforms and their spectra.

be differentiated from each other. Instead, the spectrum would appear as a filled area (e.g., the spectrum from Figure 4.4D). This type of spectrum is called a **continuous spectrum.** The upper border of the continuous spectrum is called the spectral envelope. A spectral envelope is a line connecting the maximum values (amplitudes) of all of the spectral components of the spectrum. A continuous spectrum represents a vibration with energy spread densely and evenly across a range of frequencies. For example, **white noise** has a spectrum consisting of an infinite number of sinusoidal components having the same amplitude but random phases, spread evenly across a wide frequency range (e.g., from 1 to 10,000 Hz). Many types of noise, such as pink noise and red noise, are of interest in hearing science; they will be discussed in Chapter 5.

In addition to dividing spectra into line spectra and continuous spectra based on the number of components, spectra can also be divided into amplitude spectra, power spectra, and phase spectra depending on the characteristic that is displayed on the *y* axis. An **amplitude spectrum** (frequency spectrum) displays the amplitude of various vector quantities associated with the components (e.g., velocity, displacement, force) and a **power spectrum** displays the energy (power) of the components. Recall from Chapter 2 that a vector quantity requires a magnitude and a direction (phase) to fully describe it. In the case of vibratory motion, the amplitude and phase of individual frequency components are both required for waveform summation. Therefore, the amplitude spectrum alone does not fully describe complex vibratory motion in the frequency domain and it must be supplemented with phase information. The phase information is provided by a **phase spectrum** that displays the initial ($t = 0$) phase angle of all the spectral components as a function of frequency. Thus, a pair of spectra—an amplitude spectrum and a phase spectrum—are needed to fully describe the complex waveform of a vector quantity in the spectral domain. In contrast, power does not depend on phase and the power spectrum does not require a phase spectrum to accurately describe the complex vibration. Therefore, the power spectrum is the most frequently reported spectrum used in waveform analysis. The amplitude spectrum alone is used in some cases when the phase differences are negligible or known a priori, such as in the harmonic spectrum of a vibrating string (described later in this chapter).

PRACTICE PROBLEMS: WAVEFORMS AND SPECTRA

1. Does this graph represent waveform or spectrum coordinates?

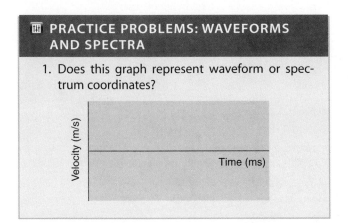

2. Does this graph represent waveform or spectrum coordinates?

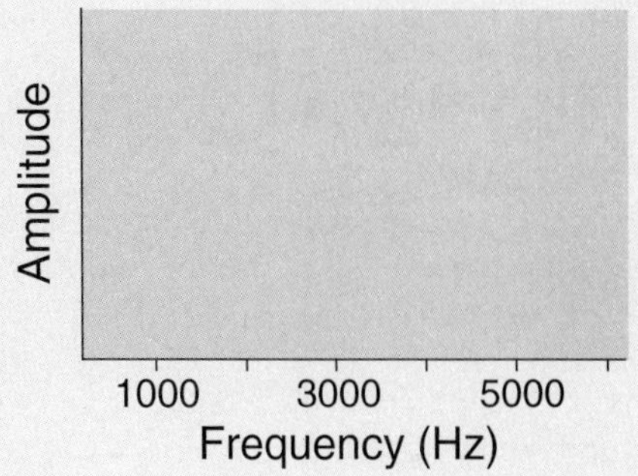

3. Is this a line spectrum or a continuous spectrum?

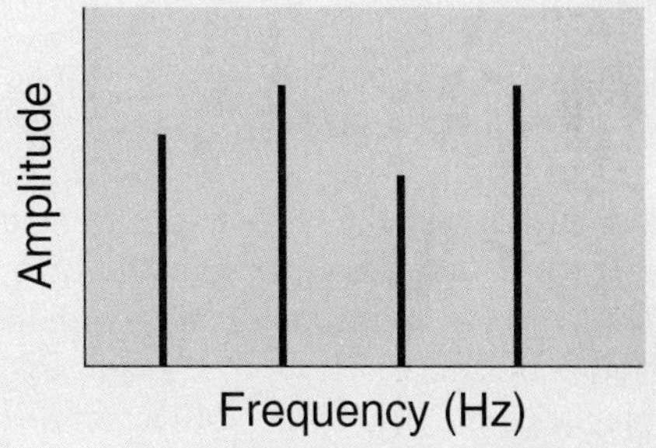

4. Sketch the spectrum of a sinusoidal waveform with a frequency of 3000 Hz and an amplitude of 4 (units unspecified).

5. Is this a line spectrum or a continuous spectrum?

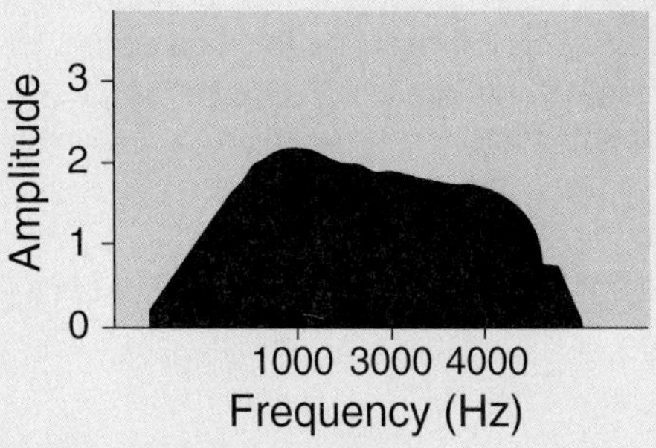

6. What is the amplitude of the spectral component (units unspecified) at 1000 Hz for the spectrum shown in problem 5?

Answers (If you need help with these problems, consult the website.) **Link 4-5**

1. Waveform
2. Spectrum
3. Line spectrum

4.

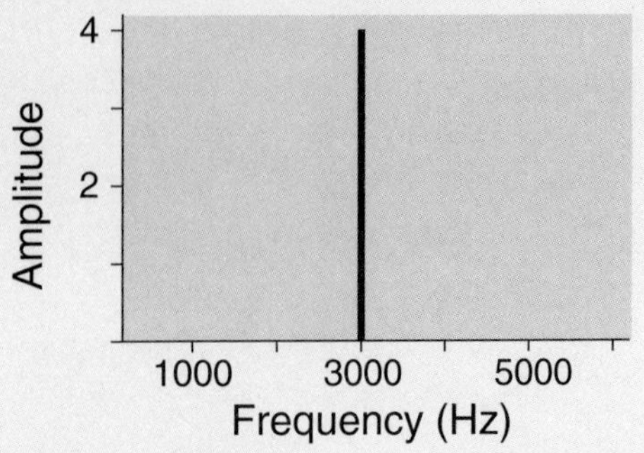

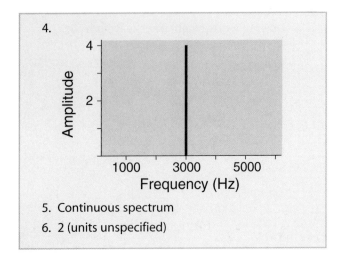

5. Continuous spectrum
6. 2 (units unspecified)

COMPLEX VIBRATING SYSTEMS

In Chapter 3, we discussed vibrating systems that have one resonance frequency. Such systems can be acoustic as well as mechanic. Regardless of whether we are considering an acoustic or a mechanic vibrating system, most vibrating systems have more than one resonance frequency. To understand the concept of multiple resonances, we need to expand beyond the simple vibrating system models we have examined in the previous chapter (e.g., the pendulum and the mass and spring) and explore in this chapter the patterns of complex mechanic vibration in strings, rods, plates, and membranes. Vibrations of acoustic systems such as Helmholtz resonators and air columns will be discussed in Chapter 6.

Strings, rods, plates, and membranes are all examples of mechanic systems that can simultaneously vibrate in many different sinusoidal motions, producing a vibration pattern that is complex. An exploration of complex vibration patterns in mechanic systems will create the foundation for understanding the operations of various sound sources and for the discussion of acoustic vibrating systems in subsequent chapters.

Strings

A string is a lightweight cord made of metal or plastic that is intended to be stretched across two points, as in a musical instrument or a bow. Let us consider the vibration pattern of a string fixed at both ends by examining the behavior of the strings on a guitar (Fig. 4.6). The guitar strings are stretched along the body and neck of the guitar and are fixed at the head nut and at the bridge nut. Both endpoints of each string are tightly fixed, so the string can only vibrate between these two points. The frequency of vibration of the string is determined by its length, mass, and stiffness (tension of the string). The six strings of the guitar are the same length, but they differ in thickness, mass, and stiffness and, thus, have different natural resonance frequencies.

When a guitar string is plucked, it vibrates up and down between the two endpoints (Fig. 4.7). At the endpoints themselves, there is no vibration. The points of the vibrating system at which displacement remains zero are called **nodes.** The points at which the vibration magnitude is greatest are called **antinodes.** For example, the center of the guitar string is the antinode for the fundamental **mode** of string vibration shown in Figure 4.7. A mode of vibration is the specific vibration pattern of a vibrating system associated with each resonance frequency of the system.

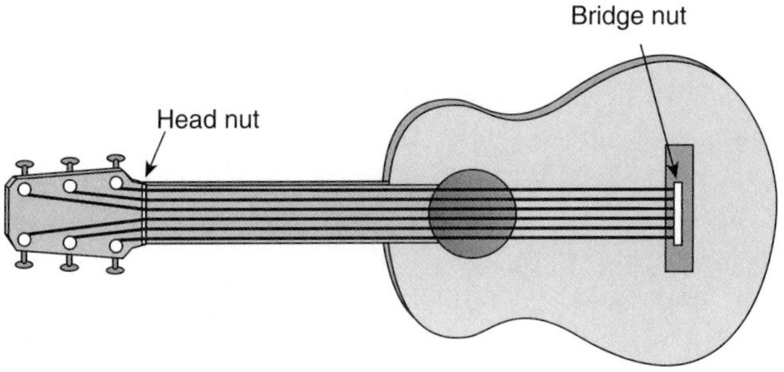

Figure 4.6. A six-string guitar.

Figure 4.7 illustrates only the lowest resonance frequency vibration for the guitar string. In reality, vibrating strings have multiple resonance frequencies and the actual shape of the string vibration is determined by where the string is plucked and the multiple resonances of the string. Figure 4.8 illustrates the vibration pattern of a string that is plucked at one fifth of its length to the left of center (the pluck point is the peak of the triangle shown in the top left panel). The vibration of this string creates a complex waveform that is composed of a harmonic series. In Figure 4.8, the left panel indicates the vibration modes associated with the first six resonance frequencies (harmonics) of the plucked string. The amplitude decreases for successive harmonics, as illustrated by the spectrum shown on the right of the figure. The fifth harmonic is missing since no node of vibration can be created at the activation (pluck) point on the string. Similarly, the 10th harmonic would be missing as well if the drawing was extended to include further harmonics.

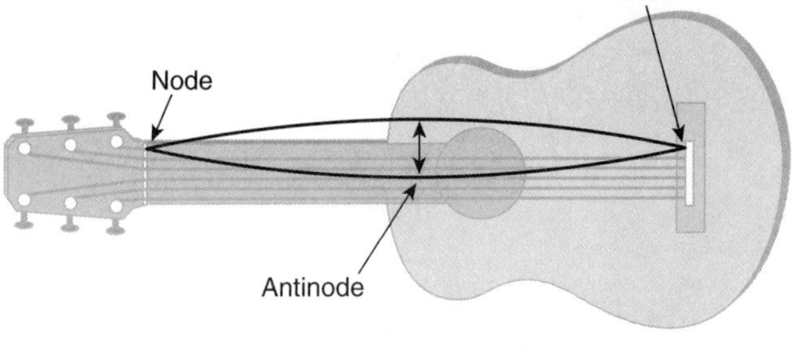

Figure 4.7. The main vibration mode of a guitar string.

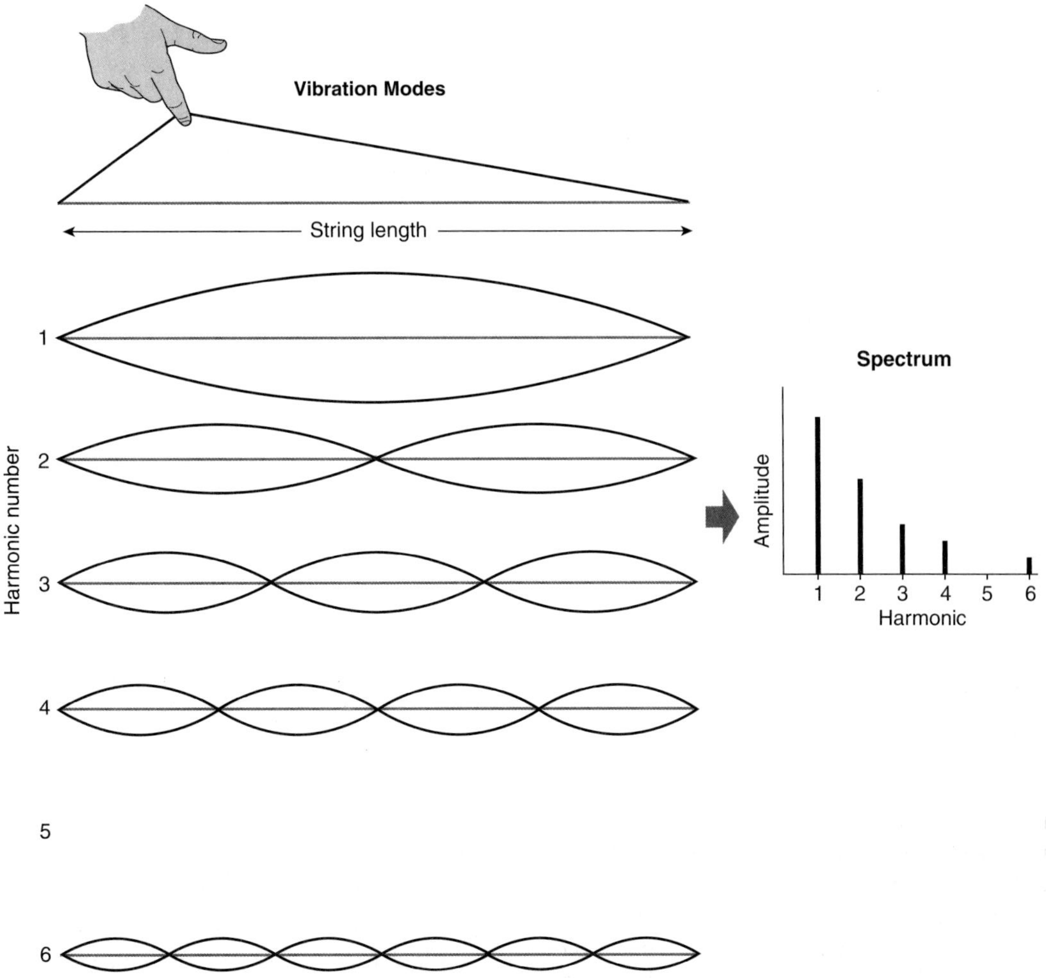

Figure 4.8. Modes of vibration and the spectrum of a plucked guitar string.

The lowest frequency of a vibrating string is its fundamental frequency (first harmonic); therefore, the fundamental frequency corresponds to the first mode of vibration. The terms *fundamental frequency* (denoted f_o) and *first harmonic* (denoted f_1) have the same meaning and may be used interchangeably; a consistent use of one or the other of these terms is strongly advised, however, since their subscripts differ. The other harmonics in the series are whole-number multiples of this lowest frequency. Thus, the second harmonic (f_2) corresponds to the second mode of vibration and is equal to two times the fundamental; the third harmonic (f_3) corresponds to the third mode of vibration, and so forth. Examine the second harmonic from Figure 4.8 and notice that instead of one antinode in the center of the string, which was seen for the first mode of vibration, the second mode of vibration has two antinodes. Also, in addition to the nodes at the head and bridge nuts, there is also a node in the center of the string. The pattern of vibration becomes more complex with higher modes of vibration. The number of harmonic modes with which a string fixed at both ends can vibrate is theoretically limitless; however, the amplitude of the harmonics decreases quite rapidly as the harmonic number increases.

The first harmonic (fundamental frequency) of the high E string (E_4) of a properly tuned guitar is 329.63 Hz. The second harmonic is 659.26 Hz (E_5), which is two times the frequency of the first harmonic ($f_2 = 2 \times f_1$). The doubling of frequency is called an **octave**, and this relationship will be described in greater detail in Chapter 7. The subsequent harmonics of the same string are 988.89 Hz, 1318.52 Hz (E_6), 1648.15 Hz, and so forth. The relationship between the specific frequency of vibration and the length of the string is given by Equation 4.1:

$$f_n = \frac{nv}{2L} \qquad \textbf{(4.1)}$$

where L is the length of the string in meters, v is the speed of vibration propagation through the string in m/s, and n is the number of the specific harmonic: $n = 1, 2, 3,$ etc. The speed of vibration propagation through the string is equal to:

$$v = \sqrt{\frac{TL}{m}} \tag{4.2}$$

where m is the mass of the string in kg and T is the tension of the string in kg × m/s^2. Inserting Equation 4.2 into Equation 4.1 allows us to write the final equation relating the frequency of vibration to the mechanic properties of the string as follows:

$$f_n = \frac{n\sqrt{\frac{TL}{m}}}{2L} = \frac{n}{2L}\sqrt{\frac{TL}{m}} \tag{4.3}$$

Equation 4.3 applies to an ideal string that is completely uniform along its length. Real strings, however, may not have a uniform thickness or density of string material along their lengths. Therefore, the actual frequencies produced by higher modes of vibration may not exactly follow a harmonic relationship. This is the reason that in music acoustics the frequencies above the fundamental are frequently referred to as overtones rather than the harmonics they approximate.

Example 4.4

Calculate the third harmonic of a vibrating violin string with length (L) = 0.3 m and mass (m) = 0.17 grams that is under a tension of T = 60 N. Assume that the mass and tension of the string are consistent along the length of the string.

First, you need to select an equation that will allow you to determine the harmonic given the length (L), mass (m), and tension (T) of the string; therefore, select Equation 4.3.

$$f_n = \frac{n}{2L}\sqrt{\frac{TL}{m}}$$

Substitute known variables.

$$f_3 = \frac{3}{2 \times 0.3\ \text{m}}\sqrt{\frac{60\text{N} \times 0.3\ \text{m}}{0.17\ \text{g}}}$$

Recall that 1 g = 10^{-3} kg and 1 N = kg × m/s^2 (Chapter 2), and substitute N and g with the basic SI units.

$$f_3 = \frac{3}{2 \times 0.3\ \text{m}}\sqrt{\frac{60\frac{kg \times m}{s^2} \times 0.3\ \text{m}}{0.17 \times 10^{-3}\ \text{kg}}}$$

Simplify the units.

$$f_3 = \frac{3}{2 \times 0.3\ \text{m}}\sqrt{\frac{60 \times 0.3\ \text{m}^2}{0.17 \times 10^{-3}\ \text{s}^2}}$$

Solve for f_3.

$$f_3 = \frac{3}{0.6\ \text{m}}\sqrt{105{,}882.35\frac{m^2}{s^2}}$$

$$f_3 = 1627 \times \frac{1}{s}$$

Answer: The third harmonic = 1627 Hz.

Example 4.4 is a realistic case for a steel violin string. The steel density (ρ) = 7800 kg/m^3 and the string tension can be quite high without breaking the string. Other strings such as gut, silk, and plastic (nylon) string have a much lower density (≈1300 kg/m^3) and therefore the string tension must be lower. If you are interested in seeing an example in which you need to calculate the tension of a plastic string to match the frequency of a steel string, see the website. **Link 4-6**

PRACTICE PROBLEMS: HARMONICS IN STRINGS

1. Calculate the second harmonic of a vibrating violin string with length (L) = 0.3 m and mass (m) = 0.17 grams that is under a tension of T = 60 N. Assume that the mass and tension of the string are consistent along the length of the string.
2. Calculate the second harmonic of a vibrating steel guitar string with length (L) = 0.64 m and mass (m) = 1.56 grams that is under a tension of T = 50 N. Assume that the mass and tension of the string are consistent along the length of the string.
3. Calculate the fourth harmonic of a vibrating steel bass string with length (L) = 1.22 m and mass (m) = 26.52 grams that is under a tension of T = 60 N. Assume that the mass and tension of the string are consistent along the length of the string.

Answers (If your answers do not agree with the answers provided, step-by-step solutions are provided on the website.) **Link 4-7**

1. 1084.65 Hz
2. 223.79 Hz
3. 86.13 Hz

Rods

A **rod** is defined as a rigid one-dimensional structure made of a material such as metal or wood that has a small cross section in comparison to its length. It is usually called a rod if it is round and a **bar** if it has a square or rectangular cross section. Both structures can have a straight shape or can be bent (e.g., a music triangle). An object can be classified as a rod or a bar if its predominant modes of vibration are along its length **(transverse vibrations)** or twisting around its axis **(torsional vibrations).** From the mechanic point of view, a rod can be considered a string that has a natural stiffness and does not need to be clamped (fixed) at both ends to vibrate. The internal stiffness of the rod provides a restoring force when the rod bends; thus, rods can vibrate by being fixed just at one place or by being supported just underneath at points close to its ends (like a xylophone). The vibration modes of a uniform rod or bar are typically highly inharmonic due to the way the natural stiffness limits the way the rod can bend. For example, the frequencies of the second, third, and fourth vibration modes of a simple vibrating bar with free ends (i.e., resting on a structure that does not firmly fix the bar to the support), are 2.76, 5.49, and 8.93 times higher, respectively, than the lowest frequency of bar vibration (Rossing, 1989). The rods and bars used in musical instruments can be shaped so that their modes of vibration are tuned and provide a more harmonized set of overtones.

An important example of a vibrating bar is a tuning fork. A tuning fork is a U-shaped metal bar with a central stem (foot, base, handle) extending from its bottom. The two arms of the tuning fork are called tines. When one of the tines is struck by a hard object, the tuning fork begins to vibrate and generates a sound. The tuning fork was invented in 1711 by John Shore, sergeant trumpeter to the British Royal Court (Ellis, 1880). The original purpose of the tuning fork was to serve as a reference tone for tuning musical instruments, but it is also widely used in hearing science for bone conduction testing (e.g., Weber Test, Rinne Test). Bone conduction is discussed in Chapter 11.

The vibration pattern of the tuning fork is illustrated in Figure 4.9. The primary vibration pattern is a simple back-and-forth vibration in which the tines alternate from both in (maximum negative displacement) through equilibrium to both out (maximum positive displacement) positions. Other vibration modes of the tuning fork resemble those of the bar clamped on one end; they are much weaker than the fundamental mode of vibration, however, and diminish quite quickly as the tuning fork continues to vibrate (Baccus, 1977). Therefore, the tuning fork can be considered to be a practical mechanic source of a simple harmonic vibration. The frequency of the tuning fork vibration depends on the mass and length of the tines and it decreases slightly with an increase in the temperature of the fork. The simple back-and-forth vibration of both tines results in a piston-like (up-and-down) movement of the handle that can be transmitted to other objects through direct contact.

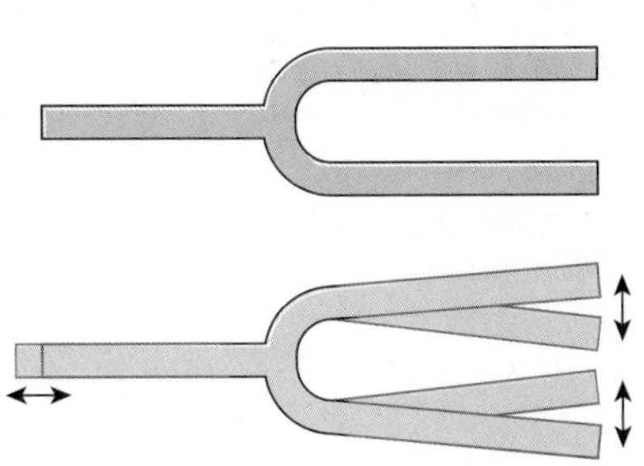

Figure 4.9. Primary vibration mode of a tuning fork.

Membranes and Plates

Membranes and plates are two-dimensional physical objects in which the thickness is much smaller than the length and width. A **membrane** is a thin sheet-like material (e.g., rubber) that needs to be stretched across and fixed along its edges to have some stiffness and produce vibration. Membranes can be flat or curved (a curved membrane is frequently conical). An example of a flat stretched membrane is the membrane of a drum and an example of a conical membrane is the membrane of a loudspeaker. A **plate** differs from a membrane in that it has its own stiffness and can vibrate without any structured support. Similar to membranes, plates can also be flat (e.g., a cymbal is relatively flat) and curved (e.g., bells). In hearing science, it is important to understand the unique vibration pattern observed in membranes and plates, because these vibration patterns are seen in various portions of the auditory system (e.g., the tympanic membrane [eardrum]; Chapter 8), in sound-generating equipment (e.g., the diaphragm of an earphone), and in various other instrumentation.

From the mechanic point of view, membranes and plates can be thought of as two-dimensional strings and rods and all of the discussion related to strings and rods applies also to membranes and plates. Similar to strings and rods, the vibration modes (resonance frequencies) of membranes and plates depend on their size, shape, mass, stiffness, and uniformity, although the vibration patterns of plates and membranes are far more complicated than the vibration patterns in strings and rods. For example, a common property of all round membranes and plates is the interaction between two series of vibration modes called radial modes and circular modes. The **radial mode** refers to nodes of vibration running across the plate or membrane, and the **circular mode** refers to modes of vibration that run in a circular manner in the plate or membrane. The main vibration modes of a round membrane and a rectangular membrane are shown in Figure 4.10. The white and shadowed parts in Figure 4.10 indicate the opposite directions of movement of the membrane in a specific mode of vibration. The solid lines indicate the nodes of vibration. Many of these modes of vibration are inharmonically related. Therefore, in some musical instruments (e.g., church bells) the membranes and plates must be specially treated to result in a harmonic sound. Some percussion instruments, such as cymbals, drums, and the triangle, produce inharmonic sounds, but these instruments are not used to play chords or melodies.

The nodes of vibration can be seen on plates after sprinkling fine sand over the plate and causing the plate to vibrate. The vibrations of the plate will move all the sand to the places that do not vibrate, thus arranging the sand in a pattern following the nodes of vibration. Touching the plate at some

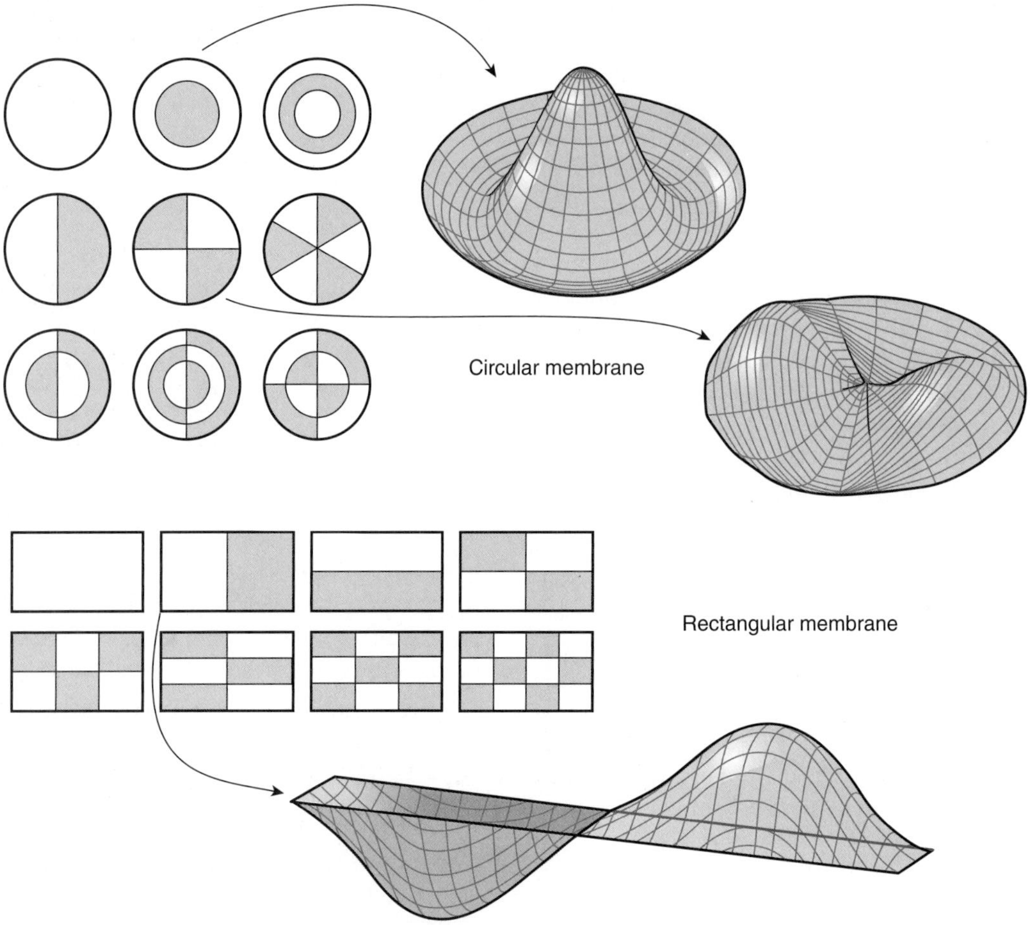

Figure 4.10. The main vibration modes of a round membrane and a rectangular membrane.

point with a finger prevents all the modes of vibration from developing except for those modes whose nodal lines pass through this point. Therefore, by touching the plate at various points one can activate and display various modes of vibration. This technique was developed by Ernst Chladni (1756–1827), a German physicist, and the nodal patterns displayed on the plates were named **Chladni figures** (Chladni patterns). An example of a Chladni figure of a highly complex mode of vibration of a square plate is shown in Figure 4.11.

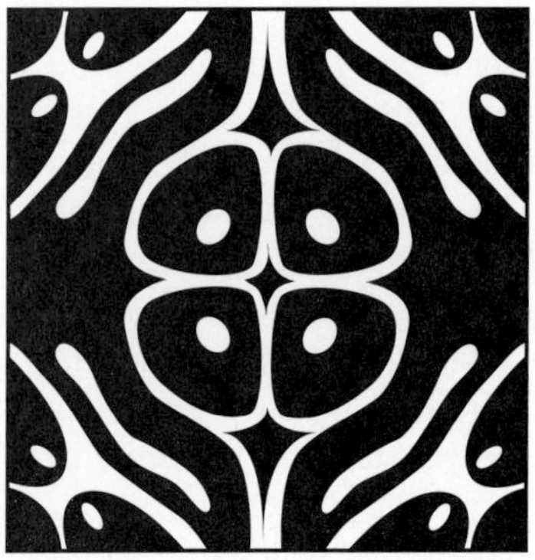

Figure 4.11. A Chladni pattern of a complex mode of vibration of a rectangular plate.

MECHANIC IMPEDANCE

For a system to vibrate, it needs a force that acts on the system. This means that to vibrate, a system needs to receive energy from another system either in the form of a single spike (impulse) of energy (e.g., a push of the pendulum) or a continuous supply of external energy (e.g., a periodic push of a swing). Thus, to complete the discussion of vibrating systems, it is important to discuss how this energy is transferred to the system and how different elements of the system affect the overall magnitude and phase of vibrations.

One example of energy transferred to a system is that of a person pushing a car. If the person pushes with sufficient force, the car will move with a certain velocity. If the force is increased, one would expect the car to move faster; thus, the force and the velocity of the system are closely tied. Other aspects of the system, however, may affect the relationship between force and velocity. Consider that when the car is empty, the person can push the car with a certain velocity, but if the same car is occupied by several passengers and the same person pushes it with the same force, the car will move more slowly or may not move at all. This means that for the same force applied to objects of various mass, the larger the mass of the object, the lower its velocity will be if all other conditions are kept the same. The same relationship applies to the friction and stiffness of an object. The rougher the surface on which the object is pushed and the more flexible (jelly-like) the object, the slower the movement caused by the same force. This means that for a given force (F) applied to a mechanic system, the complex mechanic characteristics of the system affect its velocity (v). These characteristics are represented by a property called **impedance (Z).** Impedance is the opposition to the flow of energy through a system or, in more broad terms, an opposition to any change in its state. Impedance is measured in ohms (Ω) and it relates the velocity of a system to the force acting on the system. This relationship is described by the following equation:

$$\text{Force } (F) = \text{Impedance } (Z) \times \text{Velocity } (v) \qquad (4.4)$$

or, in short,

$$F = Z \times v$$

In the case of mechanic objects, this impedance is called **mechanic impedance** and it depends on the mass, stiffness, and friction coefficient of the system. The unit of mechanic impedance is the mechanic ohm ($1\ \Omega = 1$ kg/s). If the system is acoustic or electric, this property is called acoustic impedance or electric impedance, respectively, and it depends on the respective acoustic or electric characteristics of the system. In all cases, the greater the impedance of a system is, the greater the amount of force that is needed to make the system move at a given velocity. Conversely, the lower the impedance of a system is, the lower the required force. For example, a system composed of a stiff spring and a large mass (large impedance) will move much slower than a system composed of a compliant (loose) spring and a small mass (small impedance) if all other things are kept equal.

Impedance consists of two parts, resistance and reactance (Fig. 4.12). **Resistance (R)** is the opposition of a system to movement caused by friction. **Reactance (X)** is the opposition of a system to a change in its state by the system's ability to store energy and prevent its transfer to or from another system. In mechanic systems, reactance is a result of the mass and stiffness of the system; therefore, it is divided into two parts: **mass reactance (X_m)** and **stiffness reactance (X_s).** Mass reactance is the ability of the mass to store energy, and stiffness reactance is the ability of the stiffness to store energy. For example, a large rolling stone is more difficult to stop from moving and a stiff spring is more difficult to compress than a small stone and a flexible spring, respectively. Mass reactance (X_m) can be calculated if the frequency (f) of the driving force and the mass (m) of the system are known using the following formula:

$$X_m = 2\pi \times f \times m \qquad (4.5)$$

Notice two things from Equation 4.5:

1. As the mass increases, the mass reactance increases
2. As the frequency of the driving force increases, the mass reactance increases

Stiffness reactance (X_s) can be calculated if the frequency (f) of the driving force and the compliance (C) of the system are known using the following formula:

$$X_s = \frac{1}{2\pi \times f \times C} \qquad (4.6)$$

Compliance (C), introduced in Chapter 3, is the inverse (reciprocal) of stiffness (K); that is, $C = 1/K$. Thus, a spring that is very stiff will have low compliance and vice versa. Think of stiffness and compliance as the two ends of the elasticity scale. Recall elasticity is the tendency of a stretched spring to return to its original shape. It is easy to stretch a spring that has low stiffness and it is easy to compress it. Thus, such a spring has a large compliance. If the spring is very stiff and difficult to stretch, the compliance is small. Note that the stiffness reactance is inversely proportional to both the frequency and the compliance. This means (1) as the frequency of the driving force increases, the stiffness reactance decreases and (2) as the compliance increases, the stiffness reactance decreases. The relationship between impedance and its components is graphically shown in Figure 4.12.

If mass reactance is greater than stiffness reactance, a system is said to be *mass dominated*, and if stiffness reactance is greater than mass reactance, the system is said to be *stiffness dominated*. According to Equations 4.5 and 4.6, mass reactance increases and stiffness reactance decreases with an increase in the frequency of the driving force. This means that the magnitude of vibration at high frequencies is dependent on the mass of the system, because the mass of the system is opposing the movement at high frequencies. Conversely, the magnitude of vibration at low frequencies is dependent on the stiffness of the system. Since the mass reactance and stiffness reactance are associated with the opposing forces of inertia and elasticity, they can cancel each other at a certain frequency when they become equal. In this case, when $X_m = X_s$, the system is said to be *resistance dominated* and it will vibrate at its maximum magnitude. It is important to note that the frequency of the driving force at which the system vibrates at its maximum amplitude is equal to the resonance frequency of the system (see Chapter 3).

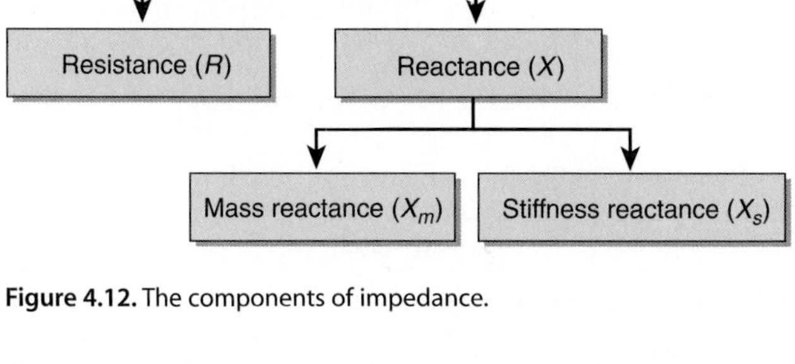

Figure 4.12. The components of impedance.

Impedance Calculations: Magnitude and Phase

The three components of impedance—resistance (friction), mass reactance, and stiffness reactance (all measured in

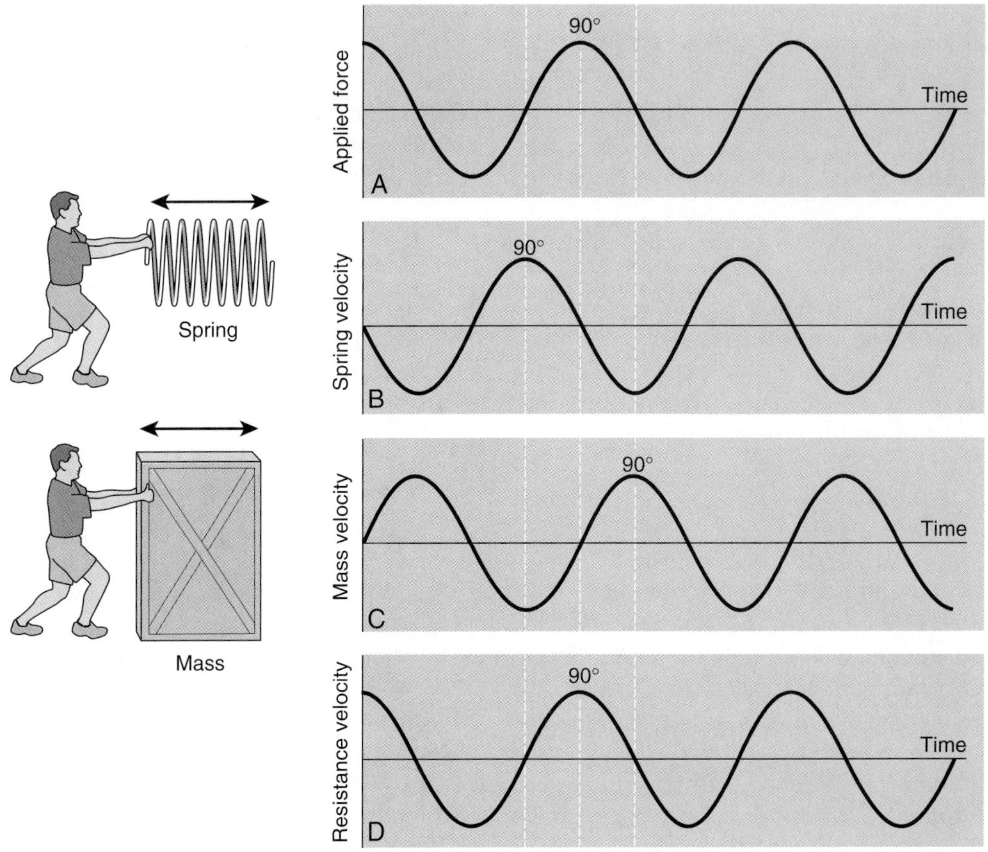

Figure 4.13. The relationship between the phase of an alternating applied force **(panel A)** and the phase of the stiffness reactance **(panel B),** mass reactance **(panel C),** and resistance **(panel D).**

ohms)—all contribute to the total impedance of a vibrating system. Since each of these components reacts in a specific direction, they are vectors and have both a magnitude and a phase angle (see Chapter 2). To understand the relationship between the phase of an applied alternating force and the resistance, mass reactance, and stiffness reactance, examine Figure 4.13. In the first drawing, the person is alternately pushing and pulling on a spring, forcing it to move back and forth between its compressed and expanded states, passing through equilibrium between each of these extremes. In this example, no mass is attached to the spring and we are just considering the effect of force on the velocity of the spring (i.e., on the ability of the spring to move). The applied alternating force is shown graphically in the right top panel (waveform A). The resulting velocity of the spring is shown graphically in the second panel (waveform B). Look at the relationship between waveform A and waveform B. The velocity of the spring is zero when the applied force is greatest (peak magnitude both positive and negative). This is due to the fact that when the force is at its maximum, the spring is maximally compressed or maximally expanded and it does not move anymore. Let us assume now that the spring is maximally extended, the acting force is at its maximum, and spring velocity is zero. When the amount of force decreases, the spring begins to move in the opposite direction to the acting force and extends back toward its equilibrium position. When the spring extension reaches its equilibrium point, the spring is in its resting position and makes no opposition to any external force. At this position the spring's ability to move is greatest and even the smallest force can make it move. This situation is shown as the minimum of force in waveform A and the maximum velocity in waveform B. The same mechanism is repeated when the spring is subsequently compressed and gradually allowed to return to its equilibrium position. Now examine the second picture on the left, that of a person applying an alternating force to a mass and making it move back and forth. Again, consider that the applied force is the same as shown by waveform A, but now examine the resulting mass velocity shown as waveform C. The velocity of the mass is zero when the mass is pulled all the way toward the person or pushed all the way away from the person because the mass does not go any further. When a person starts gradually pushing the mass away from his or her body, however, he or she transfers part of his or her energy to the mass, giving it some force of inertia; the resulting mass velocity is in agreement with the direction of the acting force. At the point when the pushing force drops to zero, the mass has accumulated its maximum possible energy and it "wants" to travel farther but the new pulling force starts slowing it down, bringing it to the rest at the maximum distance from the person's body. Please note that the spring velocity and mass velocity are both at their peak values when the force is not acting on the system but their directions are 180° out-of-phase. In other words, the maximum velocity of the mass occurs one fourth of a cycle after the maximum applied force, whereas the maximum velocity of the spring occurs one fourth of a cycle before the maximum applied force. Thus, the velocities of the mass element and the spring element are both 90° out-of-phase with the force that is making the system vibrate (−90° for spring, +90° for mass) and the movements of the mass element and the spring element are 180° out-of-phase with each other. The velocity of the system consisting of pure friction (waveform D) is in-phase with the applied force (waveform A) since friction resistance to movement is independent of the applied force.

The phase relationships described above are due to the properties of mass reactance, stiffness reactance, and friction resistance, which all, in different ways, oppose changes in the motion of a vibrating system. The phase relationship between the components of impedance is shown as a polar plot in Figure 4.14. This plot can be interpreted to indicate that the force of elasticity leads the instantaneous velocity of the vibrating system (i.e., stiffness acts first) and the force of inertia (mass) lags the instantaneous velocity of the vibrating system by 90° (i.e., mass acts last). The force of friction (resistance) is in-phase with the instantaneous velocity of the vibrating system (i.e., resistance does not cause any phase shift in the momentary velocity). This also means that the forces of elasticity and inertia act 180° out-of-phase with each other. This is nothing new, since we discussed these relationships in Chapter 3 as they relate to simple harmonic motion. However, the above discussion relates the phase differences observed between the direction of the different forces acting on a system to the specific properties (mass, stiffness, and friction) of vibrating systems and explains the vector properties of the individual elements of mechanic impedance.

Recall from Chapter 2 that vectors can be added by redrawing a vector beginning at the tail (arrow) of another

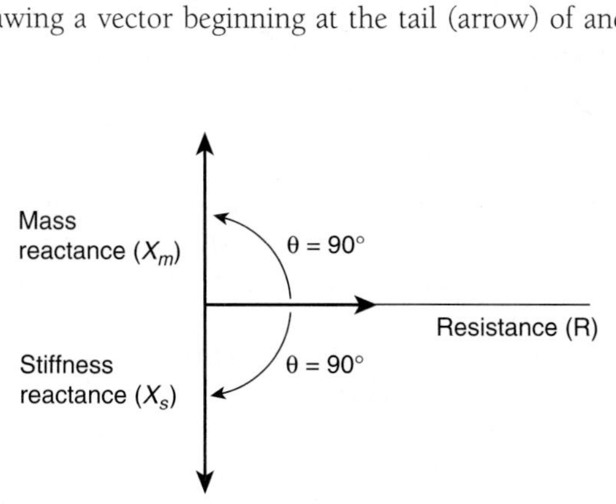

Figure 4.14. The phase relationship between the vectors of mass reactance (X_m), stiffness reactance (X_s), and resistance (R).

vector. They can also be added geometrically using the Pythagorean Theorem (Chapter 1). In the case of impedance, X_m and X_s are always 180° out-of-phase with each other and the total reactance is a simple subtraction of these two components, whereas resistance needs to be added with a 90° phase shift to the reactance. This can be stated mathematically as Equation 4.7. Since X_m and X_s are 180° out-of-phase, they are subtracted in this formula:

$$Z = \sqrt{R^2 + (X_m - X_s)^2} \tag{4.7}$$

Example 4.5

If the stiffness reactance (X_s) is 250 Ω and the mass reactance (X_m) is 500 Ω, what is the total reactance (X)?

Recall that X_m and X_s are vectors that are 180° out-of-phase as shown in Figure 4.14. Therefore, the magnitude of the total reactance is always the difference of the magnitudes of two individual components. To calculate these values, the second vector (X_s) can be repositioned by placing its origin at the tail of the first vector and added with negative phase to the first vector. The resultant total reactance has a magnitude of 250 Ω with the same direction as X_m (90°). This procedure is shown in the figure below.

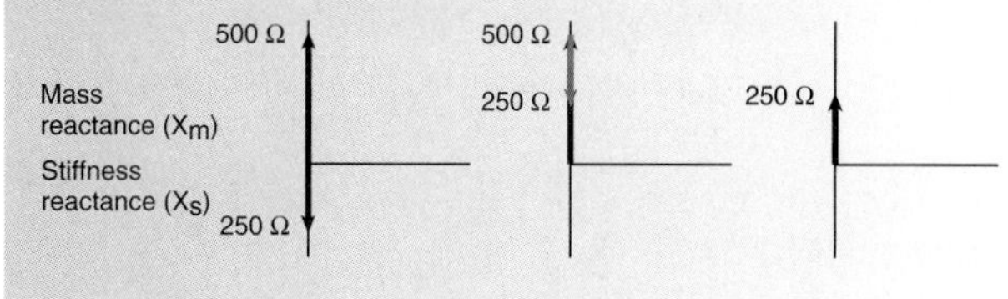

This example illustrates that the vector addition of mass reactance and stiffness reactance results in a magnitude equal to $X_m - X_s$. The direction (phase angle) of the resulting vector is determined by the one with the greater magnitude. If $X_m - X_s$ results in a positive number, the system has a greater mass reactance than stiffness reactance. If the difference is negative, it means that the system has greater stiffness reactance than mass reactance.

Next, let us consider the third vector, resistance. The direction of this vector is always shifted by ±90° in reference to the phase angle of the total reactance, so determining the magnitude and direction of the total impedance requires the use of the Pythagorean Theorem (see Chapter 1).

Example 4.6

If the total reactance (X) is 250 Ω (from Example 4.5) and the resistance (R) is 325 Ω, what is the magnitude of the impedance (Z)?

Consider the reactance and resistance as two vectors. The vectors can be repositioned in a similar manner as in

Example 4.5 so that one vector begins at the tail of the other vector (see drawing below). The resultant vector is equal to the total impedance (Z) of the system. Because the two vectors are at right angles (90°), the problem can be solved by considering the resultant vector to be the hypotenuse of a right triangle; therefore, you can use the Pythagorean Theorem to solve for Z.

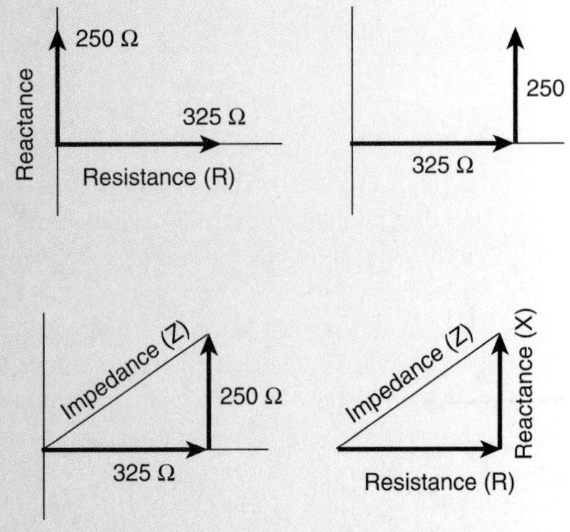

$$Z = \sqrt{(250)^2 + (325)^2}\ \Omega$$

$$Z = 410.03\ \Omega$$

Answer: The magnitude of the total impedance of the system is 410.03.

Notice that in Examples 4.5 and 4.6 we used vector addition concepts, graphic displays, and the Pythagorean Theorem to solve the problems and eventually found the value of Z. An easier way to determine the magnitude of the impedance, given X_s, X_m, and R, is to simply use Equation 4.5 to solve for the total impedance in one step.

Example 4.7

If the stiffness reactance (X_s) is 250 Ω, the mass reactance (X_m) is 500 Ω, and the resistance (R) is 325 Ω, what is the magnitude of the impedance (Z)?

Select Equation 4.7.

$$Z = \sqrt{R^2 + (X_m - X_s)^2}$$

Substitute known variables and solve.

$$Z = \sqrt{325^2 + (500 - 250)^2}$$

$$Z = \sqrt{105625 + 62500}$$

$$Z = 410.0304866714$$

Answer: The impedance = 410.03 Ω.

Vibrating systems often have multiple mass, spring, and friction elements. Therefore, the determination of the total impedance offered by a system can be quite complex, requiring multiple additions of a number of elements having various resistance and reactance. However, the basic concepts are the same; the components of the vibrating system must be considered as vectors and geometrically added. The resulting impedance vector will have its phase angle determined by whether the vibrating system is mass, stiffness, or friction dominated. Possible phase angles of the total impedance vector are shown in Figure 4.15.

The phase angle of the impedance can be calculated using vector addition techniques described and demonstrated in Chapter 1; one example for review follows.

Example 4.8

If the resistance (R) is 300 Ω, the mass reactance (X_m) is 245 Ω, and the stiffness reactance (X_s) is 125 Ω, what is the magnitude and phase angle of the impedance (Z)?

First, use Equation 4.7 to determine the overall impedance.

$$Z = \sqrt{R^2 + (X_m - X_s)^2}$$

$$Z = \sqrt{300^2 + (245 - 125)^2}$$

$$Z = \sqrt{300^2 + (120)^2}$$

$$Z = \sqrt{90000 + 14400}$$

$$Z = \sqrt{104400}$$

$$Z = 323.11$$

Next, determine the phase angle. First, find the Cartesian coordinates of the tip of the impedance vector. These coordinates can be determined quite easily because the distance along the x axis is the resistance (R), which in this problem is 300 Ω, and the distance along the y axis is given by the total reactance ($X_m - X_s$), which in this example is 120 Ω. Therefore, the Cartesian coordinates of the tip of the vector are (300, 120).

The phase angle can be calculated using Equation 1.11 from Chapter 1 for the conversion of Cartesian coordinates to polar coordinates. Since the length of the vector was already calculated in the first part of this example (323.11 Ω), we just need to find the angle θ

$$\theta = \tan^{-1}\left(\frac{y}{x}\right)$$

$$\theta = \tan^{-1}\left(\frac{120}{300}\right)$$

$$\theta = \tan^{-1}(0.4)$$

$$\theta = 21.80°$$

Answer: The magnitude of the impedance is 323.11 Ω and the phase angle of the impedance is 21.80°.

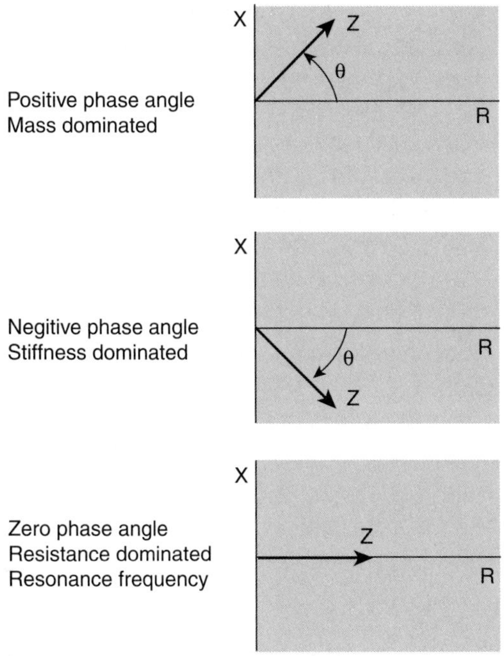

Figure 4.15. Impedance vectors for mass-dominated, stiffness-dominated, and resistance-dominated systems.

Please note that impedance problems can be provided using Cartesian (rectangular) notation or using polar coordinates. The differences between these two systems and a method for converting between Cartesian and polar coordinates for vector quantities was described in detail in Chapter 1.

PRACTICE PROBLEMS: IMPEDANCE

1. If resistance is 680 Ω, mass reactance is 400 Ω, and stiffness reactance is 340 Ω, what is the impedance? (Give magnitude and phase angle.)
2. If resistance is 500 Ω, mass reactance is 800 Ω, and stiffness reactance is 220 Ω, what is the impedance? (Give magnitude and phase angle.)
3. If resistance is 430 Ω, mass reactance is 25 Ω, and stiffness reactance is 890 Ω, what is the impedance? (Give magnitude and phase angle.)

Answers (If you need help with these problems, consult the website.) **Link 4-8**

1. The impedance magnitude is 682.64 Ω and the phase angle is 5.04°.
2. The impedance magnitude is 765.77 Ω and the phase angle is 49.24°.
3. The impedance magnitude is 965.98 Ω and the phase angle is –63.57°.

MECHANIC ADMITTANCE

Impedance (Z) was defined as the opposition the flow of energy through a system, in other words, an opposition to movement. Therefore, the inverse of the impedance indicates the mobility of a system, that is, the ability of a system to move. This inverse property of impedance (Z) is called admittance (Y). The relationship between impedance (Z) and admittance (Y) is shown in Equation 4.8.

$$Y = \frac{1}{Z} \tag{4.8}$$

Admittance (***Y***) is defined as the ease with which a system can vibrate due to an applied force. It is measured in a unit called the siemens (S), which is the reciprocal of the ohm.* To convert from impedance to admittance, simply insert the impedance into Equation 4.8.

Example 4.9

Determine the admittance of a system with an impedance of 50 Ω.

Use Equation 4.8, substitute known variables, and solve.

$$Y = \frac{1}{Z}$$

$$Y = \frac{1}{50}$$

$$Y = 0.02 \text{ S}$$

Answer: The admittance is 0.02 siemens.

Similar to mechanic impedance, mechanic admittance has different parts that correspond to mass, stiffness, and friction components of the system. Figure 4.16 lists the parts of admittance and the relationships among them. Admittance consists of conductance (G) and susceptance (B). **Conductance** (***G***) is the inverse (reciprocal) of resistance (R) and is the ease with which energy travels through a friction element in a system. **Susceptance** (***B***) is the inverse (reciprocal) of reactance (X) and is the ease with which energy travels through a mass or spring (stiffness) element in a system. Thus, susceptance is divided into two parts: **mass susceptance** (B_m) and **stiffness susceptance** (B_s).

Since conductance, mass susceptance, and stiffness susceptance are counterparts but reciprocal quantities to resistance, mass reactance, and stiffness reactance, the

*__Siemens (S)__ is the new unit of admittance (and all its parts) that replaced the old unit called mho (mho is *ohm* spelled backwards to indicate that admittance is the inverse of impedance). The name siemens was created in honor of Walter von Siemens (1816–1892), a German industrialist who invented the trolleybus and the moving-coil transducer. Note that siemens is both the singular and plural form of the unit.

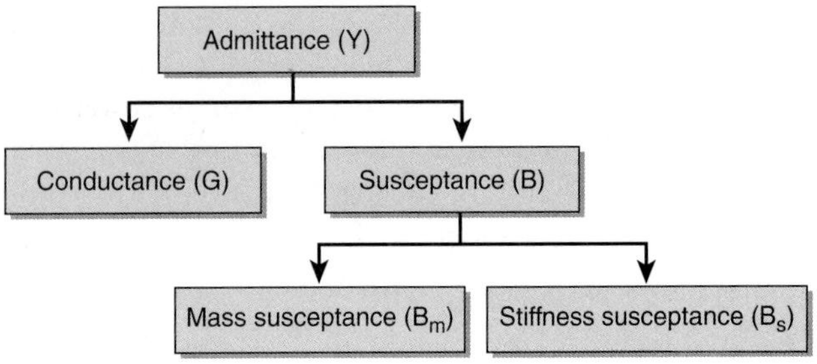

Figure 4.16. The components of admittance.

mathematical relationship between these quantities is as follows:

$$G = \frac{1}{R} \tag{4.9}$$

$$B_m = \frac{1}{X_m} \tag{4.10}$$

$$B_s = \frac{1}{X_s} \tag{4.11}$$

Similar to Equation 4.7 describing the magnitude of the total mechanic impedance, the total magnitude of the mechanic admittance can be determined by Equation 4.12.

$$Y = \sqrt{G^2 + (B_s - B_m)^2} \tag{4.12}$$

Example 4.10

If the conductance (G) is 0.2 siemens, the stiffness susceptance (B_s) is 0.5 siemens, and the mass susceptance (B_m) is 0.75 siemens, what is the magnitude and phase angle of the admittance (Y)?

Select Equation 4.12.

$$Y = \sqrt{G^2 + (B_s - B_m)^2}$$

Substitute known variables and solve.

$$Y = \sqrt{0.2^2 + (0.5 - 0.75)^2}$$

$$Y = \sqrt{0.04 + 0.0625}$$

$$Y = \sqrt{0.1025}$$

$$Y = 0.3202$$

Answer: $Y = 0.32$ siemens

The phase angle of the admittance can also be calculated in the same way as the phase angle was calculated for impedance. Because impedance and admittance have an inverse relationship, a positive phase angle for an impedance vector would be associated with a negative phase angle for the admittance vector.

PRACTICE PROBLEMS: ADMITTANCE

1. If the conductance (G) is 0.3 siemens, the stiffness susceptance (B_s) is 0.7 siemens, and the mass susceptance (B_m) is 0.4 siemens, what is the magnitude of the admittance (Y)?
2. If the conductance (G) is 1.0 siemens, the stiffness susceptance (B_s) is 0.5 siemens, and the mass susceptance (B_m) is 0.75 siemens, what is the magnitude of the admittance (Y)?
3. If the conductance (G) is 0.8 siemens, the stiffness susceptance (B_s) is 0.5 siemens, and the mass susceptance (B_m) is 0.5 siemens, what is the magnitude of the admittance (Y)?

Answers (If you need help with these problems, consult the website.) **Link 4-9**

1. $Y = 0.42$ siemens
2. $Y = 1.03$ siemens
3. $Y = 0.8$ siemens

The concepts of admittance, conductance, and susceptance are used for diagnostic and research purposes to measure the function of the middle ear system (tympanometry). In addition, the term *immittance* (Terkildsen & Thomsen, 1959) is often used for diagnostic purposes to indicate either impedance or admittance. However, this term blurs the difference between impedance and admittance and, in our opinion, should be abandoned. Most of the currently available systems for diagnostic assessment of middle ear function are admittance meters; therefore, the term *admittance* should be used to accurately report test results.

IMPEDANCE MATCHING

To make a system vibrate, some energy must be transferred to the system from another system. The transfer of energy between two systems is a complex concept, so we will begin the discussion with an analogy. Imagine a pool table containing two balls made of the same material but having very different sizes. If we push the small ball against the bigger one, the bigger ball will most likely be pushed forward a little and the small ball will be reflected back in the opposite direction. This means that one part of the energy contained in the small ball was transferred to the larger ball and another part was not transferred and caused the small ball to roll back after being reflected. If we push a large ball against a small ball, the small ball will most likely be pushed quite far but the large ball will not stop after the balls collide, but will continue its motion for some period of time. This means, again, that one part of the energy contained in the large ball was transferred to the small ball but another part could not be transferred and, instead, made the large ball move a little farther. This example illustrates the concept that when the impedances of two systems are very different, the energy transfer is not efficient. To transfer the greatest possible amount of energy from one system to another, the impedances of both objects—the **source** and the **load** (receiver of energy)—should be equal. In the previous example, the two balls should be identical for optimal transfer of energy. This requirement is called impedance matching.

Box 4.1 Impedance Matching

Impedance matching is the practice of making the impedance of the source of power equal to the impedance of the load to transfer as much energy as possible from the source to the load.

To further explain the principle of impedance matching, let us consider the case in which a moving ball (ball 1) hits a stationary ball (ball 2) with velocity v_{11} (v_{11} stands for the velocity of ball 1 before the collision). After the collision, the velocity of ball 1 is v_{12} and the velocity of ball 2 is v_{22}. Let the balls 1 and 2 have impedances Z_1 and Z_2, respectively, and let us also assume that there is no loss of energy due to friction when the balls are rolling. According to the Law of Conservation of Energy (Chapter 2), the total energy before and after collision must stay the same. Therefore:

$$E_o = E_1 + E_2 \tag{4.13}$$

where E_o is the energy originally carried by ball 1, E_1 is the energy carried by ball 1 after the collision, and E_2 is the energy carried by ball 2 after the collision.

The velocity of each ball after the collision can be determined using these equations:

$$v_{12} = v_{11}\left(\frac{Z_2 - Z_1}{Z_1 + Z_2}\right) \tag{4.14}$$

$$v_{22} = v_{11}\left(\frac{2Z_1}{Z_1 + Z_2}\right) \tag{4.15}$$

If you would like to know more about elastic collisions and how the above equations are derived, consult the website.

Link 4-10

In addition to the velocities of ball 1 and ball 2 after the collision, we can also calculate the power of ball 1 (P_1) and ball 2 (P_2) after the collision as well as the total power carried by both balls, which is $P = P_1 + P_2$. The power of each rolling ball is equal (Chapter 2, Equation 2.19) to:

$$P = F \times v \tag{4.16}$$

Since force is a product of velocity and impedance (Equation 4.4, $F = Z \times v$), Equation 4.16 can be rewritten in the form:

$$P = F \times v = v \times v \times Z = v^2 \times Z \tag{4.17}$$

that allows us to calculate powers P_1 and P_2 as well as the overall power $P = P_1 + P_2$ carried by balls 1 and 2 after the collision when we know the impedance and velocity of each ball.

The velocities of ball 1 and ball 2 and the powers of ball 1 and ball 2 after the collision are shown in Table 4.1 for an initial velocity (v_{11}) of 1 m/s for ball 1, an impedance (Z_1) for ball 1 of 100 Ω, and five different impedance values (Z_2) for ball 2 of 1, 10, 100, 1000, and 10,000 Ω. The data in Table 4.1 demonstrate the effect of the impedance ratio between ball 2 and ball 1 on the amount of power transmitted to ball 2.

The main columns of interest in Table 4.1 are column P_2 (W), which shows the absolute power delivered to the load, and column η (%), which shows the efficiency of the power transmission. The efficiency of power transmission is calculated as:

$$\eta(\%) = \frac{P_2}{P} \times 100\% \tag{4.18}$$

For example, notice in the first row that when $P_2 = 4$ W and $P = 100$ W, η (%) = 4/100 = 0.04 or 4%.

The numerical example shown in Table 4.1 illustrates the concept of impedance matching demonstrating that ball 2 receives the greatest power when the impedances of both balls are equal. Note that the delivery of the maximum absolute power (P_2) to the receiving ball coincides with the greatest transmission efficiency (η%). This is the characteristic property of systems that transmit a finite amount of energy and don't interact any longer. In the case of a mechanic system, this transmission is called an elastic collision. In systems where energy (power) is continuously drawn from a source, such as electrical systems, or during inelastic mechanic collisions where both objects (e.g., balls) travel together after the collision, the relationship between the maximum transmitted power and maximum transmission efficiency differs from the one described above. This case is discussed in Chapter 13.

Table 4.1. Power Distribution in a System Consisting of a Source (Z_1) and a Load (Z_2)

v_{11} (m/s)	Z_1 (Ω)	Z_2 (Ω)	v_{12} (m/s)	v_{22} (m/s)	P_1 (W)	P_2 (W)	P (W)	η(%)
1	100	1	−0.98	1.98	96.04	3.92	100	3.92
1	100	10	−0.82	1.82	67.24	33.12	~100	33.12
1	100	100	0	1	0	100	100	100
1	100	1000	0.82	0.18	67.24	32.4	~100	32.4
1	100	10000	0.98	0.0198	96.04	3.92	100	3.92

Summary

A complex vibration is composed of two or more simple vibrations. Complex vibrations can be divided into two basic classes of movements: aperiodic vibrations and periodic vibrations. The graphical representation of simple and complex oscillatory motion can be displayed in the time domain (waveform) or in the frequency domain (spectrum). The process of combining several individual sinusoidal motions into a complex waveform is called waveform synthesis, whereas the reverse process, taking a complex waveform and breaking it down into individual components, is called waveform analysis.

Most vibrating systems, including strings, rods, membranes, and plates, have more than one resonance frequency. The lowest resonance frequency of a vibrating system is called the fundamental frequency (f_o). Resonance frequencies that are whole-number multiples of the fundamental frequency are called harmonics.

Impedance (Z) is the opposition to the flow of energy through a system. Impedance consists of three vectors: resistance (R, friction), mass reactance (X_m), and stiffness reactance (X_s), which must be combined via vector addition to determine the magnitude and phase angle of the impedance. Admittance (Y) is the ease with which a system can vibrate due to an applied force. It is the reciprocal of impedance. To make a system vibrate, some energy must be transferred from one system called a source to a second system called a load. Impedance matching is the practice of matching the impedance of the power source to the impedance of the load. Maximum power transfer will occur if the impedance of the source and the impedance of the load are equal.

Key Points

- An aperiodic vibration is an oscillatory motion that does not repeat itself.
- Periodic vibration is an oscillatory motion in which an object returns to the same point in space periodically (at equal periods of time) during the motion.
- The period of the complex vibration is called the fundamental period (T_o).
- The fundamental frequency (f_o) is the reciprocal of T_o and can be determined using the formula $f_o = \frac{1}{T_o}$.
- When a spectrum consists of one or more separate vertical lines, this spectrum is called a line spectrum, and when a spectrum consists of energy spread across a large range of frequencies in a specific frequency range, this spectrum is called a continuous spectrum.
- The sinusoidal vibrations that make up a complex vibration are called spectral components or frequency components.
- If frequency components are harmonically related, that is, all components are whole-number multiples of the fundamental frequency (f_o), then the complex wave is periodic.
- Points of a vibrating system at which displacement remains zero at all times are called nodes. Points at which the vibration magnitude is greatest are called antinodes.
- The relationship between force (F), impedance (Z), and velocity (v) is described by the equation $F = Z \times v$, which means that the greater the impedance of a system is, the greater the amount of force that is needed to make the system move at a given velocity, or, conversely, the lower the impedance of a system is, the lower the required force needed to achieve the same velocity.

CHAPTER 5

The Nature of Sound

Chapter Outline

Objectives

- To introduce the fundamental aspects of sound, including the generation of sound by a disturbance in an elastic medium and propagation of sound waves through the medium via a series of compressions and rarefactions
- To introduce transverse and longitudinal wave motion
- To discuss how elasticity and density of a medium affect the speed of sound
- To introduce the concepts of sound pressure and sound intensity
- To introduce the concept of acoustic impedance and discuss the relationship between sound pressure and particle velocity
- To review the taxonomy (classification) of sounds and provide examples of various tones and noises

Key Terms

Acoustic impedance
Acoustic pressure
Amplitude distribution function
Audible sound
Auditory signal
Complex tone
Compression
Continuous noise
Deterministic sound
Dipole sound source (bidirectional)
Electromagnetic wave
Inverse square law
Longitudinal wave
Mechanic disturbance
Mechanic wave
Medium
Monopole sound source (omnidirectional)
Nonstationary noise
Overall sound power
Particle velocity (v)
Plane wave
Power spectrum density function
Propagation
Pure tone
Quadrupole sound source
Rarefaction
Sound
Sound energy (acoustic energy)
Sound field
Sound intensity
Sound pressure
Sound source
Sound wave
Speed of sound (c)
Spherical wave
Stationary noise
Stochastic (random) sound
Surface wave
Tone
Transverse wave
Wave (wave motion)
Wavefront
Wavelength (λ)

Oscillations and vibrations are periodic changes in the state of an object. These changes may be confined to the object itself or they may be transmitted to the surrounding space and travel farther and farther away from the object. The change traveling through the space is called a **wave motion** or a **wave.** After the wave motion is completed and the energy emitted by the object has been moved across the space, the space goes back to its original state. This means that energy was transferred but nothing in the space has been permanently moved. The process of conveying energy through space via a wave motion is called **propagation.** There are many different types of wave motions in nature but all of them can be grouped into two basic classes of motions: mechanic waves and electromagnetic waves.

A **mechanic wave** is the transfer of mechanic energy from one molecule to another. More information about molecules and particles is included on the website. **Link 5-1** For a mechanic wave motion to exist it requires a physical medium (plural: media) and a mechanic disturbance. A **medium** is a substance (matter) that occupies a space, and it can be a solid, fluid, or gas. A **mechanic disturbance** is any event that causes a change in a medium at a specific location. Examples of mechanic wave motions are sound waves, ocean waves, and earthquakes.

Examples of **electromagnetic waves** include light and radio waves. This type of wave motion does not require a medium. Electromagnetic waves will be discussed in greater detail in Chapter 13. In this chapter we will discuss only mechanic waves with the focus on sound waves, their basic physical properties, and the process of their generation.

MECHANIC WAVES

Two of the most common classes of mechanic waves are longitudinal waves and transverse waves. An example of a longitudinal wave is a sound wave; an example of a transverse wave is the "stadium wave" created by people moving sequentially up and down around a stadium during a sporting event. These two common forms of wave motion differ by the direction in which the particles of the medium move in relationship to the direction the wave moves.

Longitudinal waves are waves in which the particles of the medium are displaced in the same direction as the wave propagation through the medium. These waves are created by the back-and-forth motion of an object. A graphical representation of a longitudinal wave propagating through a medium is shown in Figure 5.1. Notice the alternating areas of **compression** (bunching of particles causing increased density) and **rarefaction** (spreading of particles causing decreased density). The alternating series of compressions and rarefactions in the medium are caused by the forward and backward movements of the acting force, in this case a piston, shown on the left side of the illustration. The vibrations of the piston are transmitted from one molecule to another, beginning at the piston and then traveling away from it. In the process of sound generation, the vibration of a sound source is conveyed to the surrounding molecules and from them the vibration is transmitted to molecules that are farther and farther away from the sound source. It is important to emphasize that individual molecules do not travel any significant distance due to the presence of the restoring force between the molecules (they only move around their natural rest positions), but the wave of disturbance may travel for miles.

The second common kind of wave motion is transverse wave motion. In **transverse wave** motion the particles of the medium are displaced in a direction that is perpendicular to the direction of the wave propagation through the medium. Recall that an example of a transverse wave is a "stadium wave" created by people moving sequentially up and down around a stadium. The direction of the wave is along the seats of the stadium, whereas the direction of the individual "particles" of the medium (i.e., the individual spectators) is up and down.

An example of transverse wave motion commonly seen in textbooks is the wave that travels across the top of bodies of water. Consider what happens when a stone is thrown into a pond. The stone hitting the water becomes the source of a water disturbance. This disturbance creates waves that spread out in a wider and wider circle across the water's surface, moving in a direction that is perpendicular to the

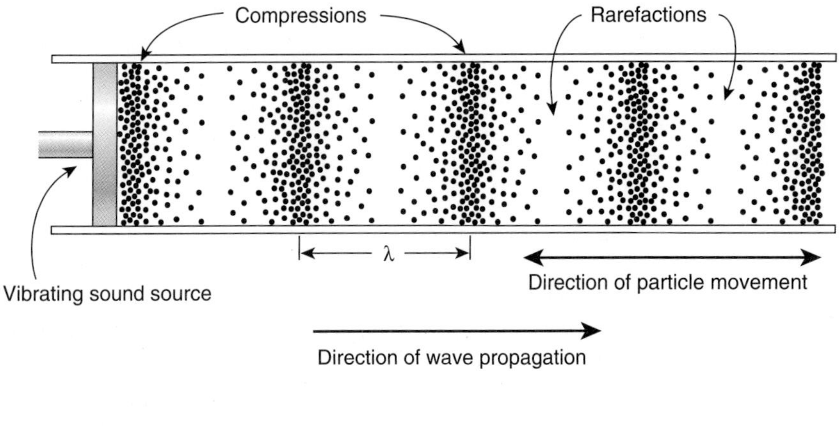

Figure 5.1. Instantaneous particle distribution in a longitudinal wave.

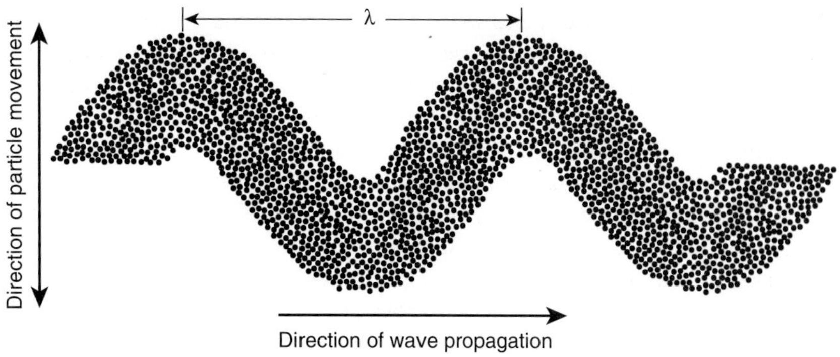

Figure 5.2. Instantaneous particle distribution in a transverse wave.

direction of the disturbance. If a bottle cork or a ping-pong ball is placed on the surface of the water, it is observed to move up and down, even as the wave moves outward from its epicenter. Thus, you can easily see that in transverse wave motion, the individual particles of the medium move up and down while the motion of the wave is contained in the horizontal plane (Fig. 5.2). Other examples of transverse waves are the movement of disturbance along a stretched rope, the vibration of a guitar string (Chapter 4), and the motion of the basilar membrane in the inner ear (Chapter 9).

Although waves on the surface of water are often used in the literature to explain the nature of the transverse wave motion, it must be understood that these water waves are somewhat different from true transverse waves. In fact, the kind of mechanic wave motion seen on the surface of water is actually called a surface wave. **Surface waves** are complex forms of wave motions created when a mechanic disturbance arrives at the border between two media having different densities, such as the surface of a lake, where water meets air. A surface wave is a combination of transverse and longitudinal wave motions causing the particles on the surface of the denser medium to move in an orbital (circular) motion, rather than a true up-and-down motion. Since the transverse component of the water wave is very visible, it is commonly used to explain the nature of the transverse waves. However, if you look very closely at the behavior of a floating object such as a cork on the surface of water when the wave is passing through its location, you will notice that it moves not only up and down (its dominant movement), but also slightly back and forth following a circular path. Other examples of surface waves are ocean waves created by the interaction between the force of wind and the force of gravity acting on the mass of the water, seismic (earthquake) waves, and mechanic waves in thin plates such as the cranial bones of the skull.

SOUND

The term **sound** has many meanings. In acoustics and hearing science it can mean (1) a disturbance in an elastic medium that propagates through the medium as a longitudinal wave motion, (2) a stimulus that causes an auditory sensation, and (3) an auditory sensation. This triple definition causes some ambiguity in interpreting the meaning of the word *sound*. A physicist would define sound using the first definition and a psychologist would define sound based on the second and third definitions. In physics, the term *sound* is synonymous with the term *acoustic*, referring to the propagation of longitudinal waves regardless of whether they can be heard or not. In this book both terms—*sound* (e.g., sound pressure) and *acoustic* (e.g., acoustic pressure)—are used. The term *sound* is used in general contexts, whereas the term *acoustic* is used in some cases when the focus is on the general physical phenomenon.

For a sound to occur as a mechanic event, three things are necessary: an energy source, a vibrating object, and an elastic medium. For example, the human voice requires the air pressure from the lungs (energy source), the vocal folds (vibrating object), and an elastic medium through which human voice travels (usually air). For a sound to be heard, two things are necessary: a stimulus arriving at a listener and a listener. The term *listener* means the physical presence of a person together with the person's ability and willingness to hear the stimulus. In this scenario, if the proverbial tree falls in the proverbial woods and no one is around who is able and willing to hear it, there would be no sound, because there is no one to acknowledge it. From the acoustic standpoint, there would be a sound in the woods because the falling of the tree would create a series of vibrations in the surrounding air.

A **sound wave** is a longitudinal wave motion caused by the mechanic disturbance of an elastic medium (Fig. 5.1). It is a back-and-forth motion of the particles of the medium propagating from the point of the disturbance to the surrounding particles and then farther and farther away from the point of origin. In other words, it is an organized movement of molecules caused by a disturbance in the medium (Olson & Carhart, 1967). The disturbance can be caused by a vibrating object (as described in Chapters 3 and 4) or by a brief event that creates a vibration in the medium, such as an explosion or thunder. A disturbance that produces a sound is called a **sound source.** A sound source can be a tuning fork, a bell, a drum, human vocal folds, and so forth. The medium through which sound travels can be air, helium, water, metal, or any other substance. The most common and natural elastic medium that keeps us alive and provides the typical environment for communication via spoken language is the air, a mixture containing mainly nitrogen (78%) and oxygen (21%) molecules. Therefore, most of the discussion of sound provided in this book assumes air as the medium for the generation, transmission, and reception of sound.

An undisturbed medium consists of molecules that are in constant random motion causing tiny pressure variations in the medium. The result of this random motion can be indirectly observed with the naked eye in the form of random movements of pieces of pollen on the static surface of a pond or as the random movement of dust particles in static air illuminated by a beam of sunlight. This phenomenon is called Brownian motion. If you would like to know more about Brownian motion, consult the website. **Link 5-2**

When a vibrating sound source is alternately pushing and pulling the surrounding particles creating regions with a greater concentration of particles (compressions) and regions with a lesser concentration of particles (rarefactions), the particles of the medium do not move in the unorganized motion seen in an undisturbed medium, but move in an organized manner that creates systematic changes in the density of the medium. The energy that is transferred from the vibrating object to the medium and propagates through the medium in the form of density changes is called **sound energy.**

ATMOSPHERIC PRESSURE

Sound needs a medium through which to travel. In the vacuum of space, which is a space without a medium, sound cannot travel because there are no molecules to transmit the sound energy. Sound can easily travel in Earth's atmosphere, however, where air molecules exist in abundance. Each cubic centimeter of air contains billions upon billions of air molecules. The number of air molecules per cubic centimeter in the atmosphere increases as one gets closer to the earth. At sea level and at a temperature of 15°C (59°F), air density is about 1.23 kg/m^3, and it drops to about 0.1 kg/m^3 at an altitude of 20 km above the earth and a corresponding temperature of −57°C (−70°F).* The low density of air surrounding the earth indicates that there are relatively few air molecules per specific volume of space. For example, at standard temperature and pressure conditions, each cubic centimeter of air contains 2.7×10^{19} molecules, but they only occupy 0.1% of the volume. This means that air is a very sparse gas with 99.9% of its volume being vacuum (Bannon, 1996).

*Note the simultaneous decreases in air density and air temperature at high altitude. They are both due to the decrease in atmospheric pressure. If the atmospheric pressure is kept constant, the decrease in temperature increases the density of air.

The decreases in air temperature and in air density with increasing altitude result from the decrease in the atmospheric pressure (density) at higher altitudes. When the sun's energy reaches the earth, the surface of the earth absorbs the sun's energy faster and more efficiently than the surrounding air. Consequently, the air in the troposphere (the atmosphere layer closest to the earth) is warmest at the surface of the earth. This warm air rises but it cools down as the altitude increases, because of air expansion. At higher altitudes, atmospheric pressure is lower than at the surface of the earth and the same amount of air is distributed over a larger volume of space, resulting in a lower air density and, therefore, a lower average temperature. The decrease in temperature with altitude is called the adiabatic* lapse rate or the thermal effect of the atmosphere and it is about 6°C per 1 km up to about 11 km above the surface of the earth.

Air (atmospheric) pressure is the result of the weight of the atmosphere acting on a specific surface. Atmospheric pressure can be measured in various units such as atmospheres (atm), millimeters of water (mm of H_2O), millimeters of mercury (mm Hg**), kilopascals (kPa), pounds per inch (psi), or bars (bar) using an instrument called a barometer. Due to the name of this instrument, atmospheric pressure is also referred to as barometric pressure.

Atmospheric pressure is the greatest at the Earth's low points (e.g., sea level) and lowest at the Earth's high points (mountaintops), decreasing further still at altitudes high above the earth's surface. To understand why the atmospheric pressure changes with altitude consider the analogy of a waiter carrying a tray that is empty compared to a tray loaded with other trays as shown in Figure 5.3. The downward pressure on the waiter carrying many trays is quite great compared with the downward pressure on the waiter who is not carrying any trays. Now consider the atmosphere surrounding the earth. If a cylinder of air is examined, it is clear that the air pressure close to the surface of the earth is considerably higher than the air pressure farther away from the surface because of all the air that is "stacked" above it.

Atmospheric pressure at sea level and a temperature of 15°C (59°F) is about 1 atm. This pressure is considered to be the normal pressure for human activities. The atmospheric pressure decreases by about 1 millibar per each 8 m of increase in altitude and is as low as 0.05 atm at an altitude of 20 km and a temperature −57°C (−70°F). Since during air travel at high altitudes the air pressure outside the airplane is very low, airplane cabins are pressurized to allow people to breathe air at a more typical and comfortable level. If the air pressure is too low, humans can become

*The adiabatic process is the thermodynamic process in which gas (e.g., air) changes temperature without any heat exchange with the surrounding environment. The change in temperature is due to gas expansion or concentration changing the amount of heat contained in a given volume of space.

**1 mm Hg is also called a Torr (1 mm Hg = 1 Torr) after Italian physicist and mathematician Evangelista Torricelli (1608–1647), the inventor of the barometer.

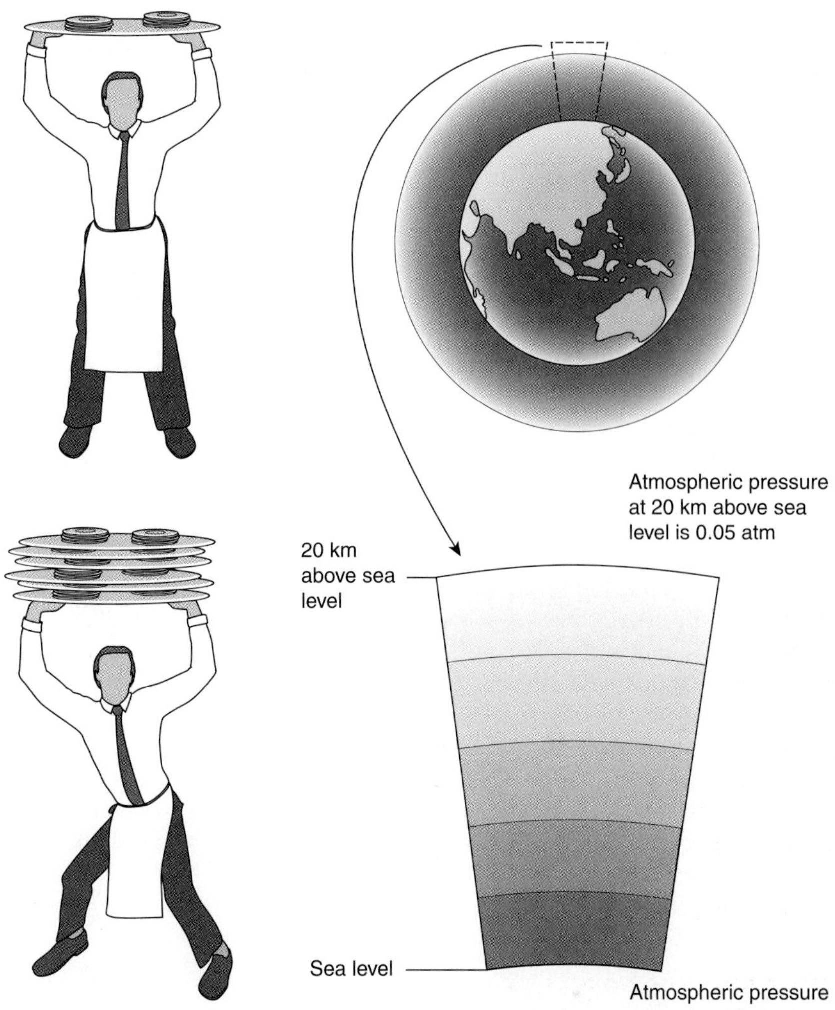
Atmospheric pressure
at 20 km above sea
level is 0.05 atm
20 km
above sea
level
Sea level
Atmospheric pressure
at sea level is 1 atm

Figure 5.3. The concept of atmospheric pressure.

dizzy, pass out, and even die. Air pressure also affects the speed with which sound travels through air.

SPEED OF SOUND

The rate at which sound travels (i.e., the rate at which energy propagates through a medium) is called the **speed of sound (*c*)**, where the symbol *c* has its origin in the Latin word *celeritas,* which means *speed*. The speed of sound depends on the density (ρ) and stiffness (K) of the medium through which the sound is traveling. Recall from Chapter 4 that the velocity of vibrations traveling through a string is determined with this equation (Equation 4.2):

$$v = \sqrt{\frac{TL}{m}} \tag{5.1}$$

where m is the mass of the string in kg, L is the length of the string in m, and T is the tension of the string (force acting on the string) in kg × m/s^2. Recall also from Chapter 2 that mass (m) is the product of density (ρ) and volume (V) (Equation 2.1). If you insert this equation into Equation 5.1 then it will take the form:

$$v = \sqrt{\frac{TL}{\rho V}} \tag{5.2}$$

The above equation can be further simplified by realizing that volume (V) is equal to area of cross section (A) and length (L); therefore:

$$v = \sqrt{\frac{T}{\rho A}} \tag{5.3}$$

The ratio of force (T) to the cross-sectional area (A) is the stiffness (K) of the medium. Therefore, this ratio can be replaced by the stiffness (K) of the medium and the speed of sound (c) in the medium can be described as:

$$c = \sqrt{\frac{K}{\rho}} \tag{5.4}$$

where c is speed of sound in m/s, K is stiffness of the medium in N/m^2 (or pascal), and ρ is density in kg/m^3. They, in turn, are affected by the temperature, pressure, and molecular composition of the medium. The relationship described by Equation 5.1 was one of the many discoveries made by Isaac Newton and described in his *Philosophiae Naturalis Principia Mathematica*.

Note that the unit of stiffness in Equation 5.4 is N/m^2. When we discussed stiffness in Chapter 3 (spring), we expressed stiffness in N/m. There is a difference, however, between the longitudinal (axial) stiffness of a solid object (a spring) and the bulk stiffness of a medium (a gas, fluid, or solid). Fluids and gases do not have their own shape; their shape is determined by their space boundaries. Each fluid and gas has the same stiffness in all three dimensions, and this stiffness is defined as the change in the pressure of the medium (in N/m^2) needed to produce a given relative change in volume (a unitless ratio). Therefore, the bulk stiffness of a medium is expressed in N/m^2 or pascals (Pa).

The bulk stiffness of gases and fluids is called the bulk modulus of elasticity (K), which is expressed in N/m^2. The situation is a little bit different in solid bodies that may have their stiffness dependent on the direction of the acting force. This means that a solid body may have a different modulus of elasticity depending on the direction of the acting force. This stiffness is characterized by Young's modulus of elasticity (E), which is the opposition of a solid body to a directional change in its shape. If the object is one-dimensional (e.g., spring, string, rod) and the force acts along its length, the longitudinal (axial) stiffness of the object is equal to the product of Young's modulus of elasticity and the ratio of the cross section of the object to its length, which is expressed in N/m.

The typical speed of sound in various solids, liquids, and gases and the corresponding value of Young's modulus (solids) or bulk modulus (fluids and gases) are listed in Tables 5.1 and 5.2. Notice that the values for Young's modulus and the bulk modulus of elasticity in Tables 5.1 and 5.2 are given in GPa (gigapascal), which is equal to 1×10^9 N/m^2.

According to Equation 5.4, the greater the stiffness and the lower the density of the medium, the faster the speed of sound is. This relationship seems difficult to reconcile with the commonly observed relationship that more dense media (e.g., metals such as steel and aluminum) transmit sound much faster than less dense media (e.g., air or other gases). Dense media are generally stiffer than less dense media, however, and the speed of sound is proportional to stiffness. Therefore, the higher speed of sound observed in denser materials is due not to their higher density, but to their greater stiffness. Solid materials are stiffer than fluids and fluids are stiffer than gases, so, in general, the speed of sound is fastest in solids, followed by fluids and then by gases; in other words, $c_{solids} > c_{fluids} > c_{gases}$. Thus, the fact that one material is denser than another does not

Table 5.1. Speed of Sound in Various Solids

Physical Matter	Speed of Sound (m/s)	Young's Modulus (GPa or $\times 10^9$ N/m^2)	Density (kg/m^3)
Aluminum	5128	71	2700
Brass	3500	104	8500
Cooper	3700	122	8900
Cork	500	0.05	200
Ice (0°C)	3230	9.6	920
Lead	1190	16	11,300
Iron (cast)	3780	110	7700
Steel	5100	200	7700
Glass (Pyrex)	5190	62	2300
Rubber (hard)	1445	2.3	1100
Rubber (soft)	70	0.005	950
Bone (cranial)	3160	19	1900
Concrete	3280	28	2600
Polystyrene	1825	3.5	1050
Rock (basalt)	4900	65	2700
Rock (granite)	5190	70	2600
Rock (sandstone)	3085	20	2100
Silicone	6485	98	2330
Soft tissue (muscle)	1545	2.5	1050
Soft tissue (fat)	1460	2	940
Wood (red oak)	3910	11	720

Table 5.2. Speed of Sound in Various Liquids and Gases

Physical Matter	Speed of Sound (m/s)	Bulk Modulus of Elasticity (GPa or $\times 10^9$ N/m^2)	Density (kg/m^3)
Alcohol (ethyl, 20°C)	1180	1.1	790
Mercury (20°C)	1435	28	13,600
Gasoline (20°C)	1335	1.3	740
Water (fresh, 20°C)	1485	2.2	998
Water (sea, 20°C)	1500	2.3	1026
Air (dry, no CO_2, 0°C)	332	0.000142	1.29
Air (dry, no CO_2, 20°C)	343	0.000142	1.21
Helium (20°C)	1025	0.00019	0.18

The values included in the table are typical for a given material. However, the properties of each of the materials may vary quite widely in various samples of material. The values for the speed of sound are rounded to the closest 5 m/s number, but the reader should be aware that these values will vary considerably.

Based on Kleppe J. Engineering Applications of Acoustics. Norwood, MA: Artech House, 1989:357, but substantially expanded.

necessarily mean that the sound travels faster through it. In several examples in Table 5.1, one medium has a greater density than another, but a lower stiffness. In this case, the speed of sound in more dense material may be lower. For example, air is denser than helium, but helium is stiffer than air, so sound travels about three times faster in helium than in air. Similarly, steel is denser than aluminum; however, aluminum is stiffer than steel, so aluminum conducts sound slightly faster.

Example 5.1

Imagine you had a metal with a Young's modulus of 113 GPa and a density of 5217 kg/m³. What would the speed of sound be through this material?

First, select the equation (Equation 5.4) that will allow you to determine the speed of sound given the elasticity and density.

$$c = \sqrt{\frac{K}{\rho}}$$

Next, substitute known variables. Here it is important to remember that the pascal (Pa) is equal to the N/m^2, so you can replace Pa with N/m^2. Furthermore, the prefix *giga* (G) is equal to 10^9 (from Chapter 2), so you can replace G with $\times\ 10^9$.

Make the unit conversion first.

$$\text{Young's modulus} = 113 \text{ GPa}$$

$$\text{Young's modulus} = 113 \times 10^9 \text{ N/m}^2$$

Next, substitute known variables into the equation.

$$c = \sqrt{\frac{113 \times 10^9 \text{ N/m}^2}{5217 \text{ kg/m}^3}}$$

Solve.

$$c = \sqrt{21659957.83 \frac{N \times m}{kg}}$$

Recall that the newton is equal to $\frac{kg \times m}{s^2}$, so substitute this for the unit N.

$$c = \sqrt{21659957.83 \frac{\frac{kg \times m}{s^2} \times m}{kg}}$$

Then reduce the units as follows:

$$c = \sqrt{21659957.83 \frac{m^2}{s^2}}$$

Simplify numbers and units.

$$c = 4654.0260 \text{ m/s}$$

Answer: The speed of sound is 4654.03 m/s.

One of the important characteristics affecting the speed of sound in gases and fluids is the temperature of the medium. Temperature has a relatively weak effect on the speed of sound through solids; however, it is an important factor in fluids and a dominant factor in gases since it greatly affects their density and, to a smaller degree, their stiffness. The relationships between the temperature, pressure, and volume of a gaseous matter are known as the gas laws. A gas law describes the relationship between two of the above quantities when the third quantity is held constant. If you would like to learn more about the gas laws, consult the website. **Link 5-3**

In discussing the relationship between the speed of sound and temperature, let us consider sound traveling through air, although the same reasoning applies to other fluids and gases as well. As the temperature increases (while holding pressure constant), the density of air decreases, so the speed of sound increases. Conversely, as temperature decreases, the density of air increases, so the speed of sound decreases. If the relationship between temperature and air density sounds counterintuitive, consider an air balloon. The heating of air expands the size (volume) of the balloon but the amount of air in the balloon remains constant, so air density decreases. If you would like to know more about the relationship between heat and temperature, consult the website. **Link 5-4**

The speed of sound in air can be determined easily given the temperature (in degrees Celsius) using Equation 5.5 (Bohn, 1988).

$$c_{air} = (331.45 + (0.6T)) \text{ m/s} \qquad (5.5)$$

where T is temperature in degrees Celsius. The value 331.45 m/s used in this equation is the value of the speed of sound at a temperature of 0°C and a pressure of 1 atm. These temperature (0°C) and pressure (1 atm) conditions are often used as a reference and are sometimes referred to in the literature by the acronym STP (standard pressure and temperature). At sea level (1 atm) and at the temperature of 15°C (59°F) sound travels at the speed of about 340 m/s (1225 km/hr). The speed of sound at 20°C and the same atmospheric pressure is 343 m/s (1235 km/hr). A sound created by an airplane flying at an altitude of 20 km above the earth with a temperature of about −57°C (−70°F) would travel at the speed of approximately 295 m/s (1062 km/hr).

Example 5.2

What is the speed of sound in air at a pressure of 1 atm and a temperature of 32°C?

Select the appropriate equation, here Equation 5.5.

$$c_{air} = (331.45 + (0.6T)) \text{ m/s}$$

Substitute known variables, in this case T, and simplify.

$$c_{air} = (331.45 + (0.6 \times 32)) \text{ m/s}$$

$$c_{air} = 350.65 \text{ m/s}$$

Answer: The speed of sound in air at 32°C and 1 atm is 350.65 m/s.

The derivation of Equation 5.5 is quite complex and is based on considering the volume, pressure, and temperature of gas media and an understanding of the Ideal Gas Laws. If you would like to follow the logical steps in the derivation of this equation or determine the speed of sound in air at a given temperature (assuming standard conditions for all other variables) using a speed of sound calculator, see the website. **Link 5-5 Link 5-6**

The speed of sound depends not only on temperature, but also to some degree on air humidity and the direction of the wind. The greater the relative air humidity (moist air is less dense than dry air), the greater the speed of sound is. This is because water vapor molecules have a lower molecular mass (*m*; m = 18) than both nitrogen (m = 28) and oxygen (m = 32) molecules. However, the actual amount of water vapor in the air is only a small fraction of the air mass even when relative humidity reaches 100%. In addition, the saturation point decreases with temperature. Therefore, the changes in air humidity have only a very small effect on the speed of sound in air.

The direction and speed of the wind have some effect on the speed of sound, but this effect is only practically important in the case of a very strong wind. However, even a relatively mild wind can have quite a large effect on the range of sound propagation (i.e., how far the sound can travel). The topic of wave propagation and the effects of humidity and wind on the range of propagation are covered in Chapter 6.

One more important property of the speed of sound is that it does not depend on the sound frequency. All waves of various frequencies produced by a sound source arrive at the observer at the same time.

PRACTICE PROBLEMS: SPEED OF SOUND

1. Imagine that you had a medium with a Young's modulus of 200 GPa and a density of 4289 kg/m^3. What would the speed of sound be through this medium?
2. Imagine that you measure the speed of sound at 5186 m/s in a medium with a bulk modulus of elasticity of 14.2 GPa. What is the density of the medium?
3. What is the speed of sound in air at a pressure of 1 atm and a temperature of 14.6°C?
4. What is the speed of sound in air at a pressure of 1 atm and a temperature of 78.6°F?

Answers (If you need help with these problems, consult the website.) **Link 5-7**

1. 6828.68 m/s
2. 528 kg/m^3
3. 340.21 m/s
4. 346.98 m/s

WAVELENGTH

Wavelength (λ) is the distance in space between two adjacent identical points of a propagating wave. In other words, it is the shortest distance between two points in space at which a propagating wave is in the same phase. Thus, the wavelength is the physical distance that is occupied by one period (one cycle) of a wave. In the case of a sound wave, it is the distance between two subsequent compressions (shown in Fig. 5.1) or two subsequent rarefactions of a longitudinal wave propagating through a medium. In the case of transverse or surface waves, it is the distance between the locations in space of two subsequent crests or two subsequent troughs of the waveform.

The wavelength depends on the speed of sound propagation through the medium and the frequency of stimulation. If a sound source vibrates with a frequency of 1 Hz and the sound wave propagates with a speed of 340 m/s, then in 1 second the wave will travel a distance of 340 m and the wavelength will be equal to 340 m. Similarly, if the sound source vibrates at 1000 Hz, then in 1 second the sound will create 1000 wavelengths and the wavelength will be 0.34 m. This relationship can be expressed in a more general form as:

$$\lambda = \frac{c}{f}[m] \qquad (5.6)$$

where λ is the wavelength in meters, c is the speed of sound in m/s, and f is the frequency of sound in Hz.

Example 5.3

What is the wavelength of a 500-Hz pure tone traveling through air at sea level and at a temperature of 15°C (59°F)?

First, select the appropriate equation. We need to find wavelength (λ), and we are given the frequency of the sound and clues as to the speed of sound (c), so select Equation 5.6.

$$\lambda = \frac{c}{f}[m]$$

Next, substitute known variables. We know that f = 500 Hz because it is given in the problem. We also known that c = 340 m/s at sea level at 59°F because it was discussed previously in the text. Thus:

$$\lambda = \frac{340\frac{m}{s}}{500\,Hz}$$

$$\lambda = \frac{340 \frac{m}{s}}{500 \frac{1}{s}}$$

$$\lambda = \frac{340\ m}{500}$$

Notice here that instead of the standard unit for frequency (Hz), we have replaced it with 1/s. This is a way to express that 1 (cycle) has occurred in 1 second. We can do this because "cycle" is assumed and it is not included in the unit for wavelength. These comments should explain the logic behind the unit conversion in the above equation leading to meters (m) as the unit for wavelength and not meters per cycle. Now, simplify the equation by dividing 340 by 500 and you arrive at:

$$\lambda = 0.686\ \text{m}$$

Answer: The wavelength (λ) is equal to 0.69 m.

PRACTICE PROBLEMS: WAVELENGTH

For practice problems 1 through 3, assume the sound wave is traveling in air, at 15°C and 1 atm, and therefore the speed of sound is 340 m/s. For practice problems 4 and 5, assume all conditions are the same except the temperature, which is specified in the problems. You can calculate the entire problem by hand or you can use the speed of sound calculator available on the website.

1. What is the wavelength of a 1000-Hz sound wave?
2. What is the wavelength of a 5000-Hz sound wave?
3. What is the frequency of a sound if it propagates with the wavelength of 6.8 m?
4. What is the wavelength of a 500-Hz sound wave traveling in air that is 100°F?
5. What is the wavelength of a 500-Hz sound wave traveling in air that is 0°F?

Answers (If you need help with these problems, consult the website.) **Link 5-8**

1. 0.34 m
2. 0.07 m
3. 50 Hz
4. 0.71 m
5. 0.64 m

TYPES OF SOUND SOURCES

As we discussed earlier in this chapter, any vibrating object surrounded by a medium can be a source of sound. The frequency and shape of the vibration of the sound source become the frequency and shape of the propagating wave. In addition, the directional pattern of the vibration will affect the flow of the wave in various directions. Although the specific vibration pattern will vary from sound source to sound source, all sound sources can be considered as simple or complex combinations of two basic types of sound source: a monopole (pulsating sphere) or a dipole (oscillating sphere) sound source. A monopole sound source is a sphere with a fixed center in space and a radius (r) that varies in a periodic pattern around it.

Figure 5.4A shows a model of a **monopole** (pulsating sphere) sound source. A pulsating sphere radiates sound energy equally well in all directions; therefore, this type of sound source is called an **omnidirectional** (nondirectional) sound source. An example of a sound source that acts as a monopole is lightning (causing thunder) or a gun shot. A practical realization of the monopole sound source using loudspeakers is the dodecahedron loudspeaker shown in Figure 5.5. A dodecahedron loudspeaker is a 12-sided solid with one loudspeaker located at each side of the solid sending

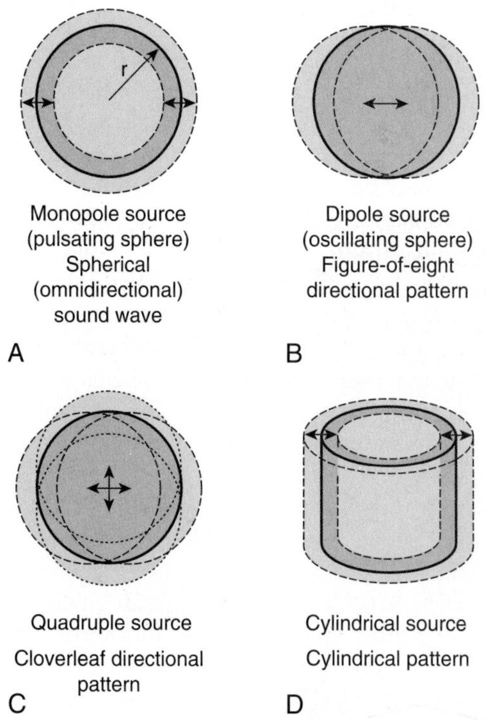

Figure 5.4. Sound sources with different vibration patterns including the two basic types of sound source: **(A)** a monopole source and **(B)** a dipole source. Two more complex sound sources are also shown: **(C)** a quadrupole source made up of four monopole sources working out-of-phase and **(D)** a cylindrical source created by multiple monopole sources lined up like a cylinder.

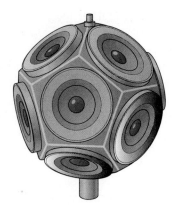

Figure 5.5. A dodecahedron (12-sided) omnidirectional loudspeaker (D 100). (Recreated from a photograph from Look Line, http://www.lookline.com/, with permission.)

a signal in all directions, thus creating an omnidirectional sound source.

A **dipole** sound source (oscillating sphere) is a set of two identical monopole sound sources pulsating out-of-phase and separated by a small distance as compared to the wavelength produced by the source. While one source expands, the other source contracts and the medium near the sources moves back and forth from one source (place) to another (Russell et al., 1999). The dipole sound source can also be imagined as an oscillating sphere that is moving back and forth along a straight line. The concept of a dipole (oscillating sphere) sound source is shown in Figure 5.4B. The radiation pattern of a dipole sound source is in the shape of a figure of eight, making the dipole a **bidirectional** sound source. Examples of sound sources behaving as a dipole are a tuning fork and a loudspeaker working without an enclosure that emits sound to the front and to the back.

The monopole and dipole are the two idealized forms of sound sources. Although some simple sound sources may behave in a way similar to these idealized sources, the vast majority of real sound sources act as complex combinations of these two basic forms. For example, four monopole sources forming a square with spheres at each corner working out-of-phase with respect to each other form a **quadrupole sound source** with a directional pattern that resembles a four-leaf clover (Fig. 5.4C). Similarly, a number of pulsating sound sources arranged in a line form a cylindrical sound source that creates a cylindrical sound wave (Fig. 5.4D).

The imaginary line connecting leading points (or connecting any other in-phase points) of a wave propagating through a medium is called the **wavefront.** If a sound source has the form of a pulsating sphere operating in an unlimited medium, the resulting sound wave propagates radially (outward from the center) in all possible directions and is called a **spherical wave.** This means that its wavefront has the form of a gradually expanding sphere. The wave produced by a dipole sound source will have a wavefront resembling a figure of eight and the wave produced by a cylindrical (linear) sound source will have the wavefront of an expanding cylinder. At a certain distance from a sound source, the wavefront of any wave is so large that locally it can be considered as a small piece of a straight surface. A wave with a wavefront that has a straight surface is called a **plane wave.** A plane wave is also generated by a sound source that has a large flat surface or by any sound passing through a narrow tube. As a matter of fact, the longitudinal wave shown in Figure 5.1 is a plane wave. It consists of a sequence of wavefronts with compressions and rarefactions that form parallel lines perpendicular to the direction of wave propagation. Since the sound source in Figure 5.1 is a piston occupying the whole left boundary of the space and the space is additionally limited to the form of a tube, the resulting wave can only propagate in one direction in the form of a plane wave.

A good understanding of the type of sound source that operates in a given environment is critical for understanding the type of sound field created in space. A **sound field** is any area where sound waves are present. The pressure created by sound waves varies throughout the sound field and its properties are highly dependent on the directional character of the sound source and space boundaries. Sound fields will be discussed in more detail in Chapter 6.

SOUND PRESSURE AND PARTICLE VELOCITY

A sound source has been defined as an object that emits sound energy into the surrounding environment. In the case of a monopole (pulsating sphere) sound source, this energy radiates outward from the sound source in the form of alternating compressions and rarefactions that spread in all directions over a larger and larger area like an expanding bubble. These compressions and rarefactions are temporary changes in the atmospheric pressure that are pushed through a medium. The magnitude of change in the local atmospheric pressure caused by the vibration of the sound source is called the **sound pressure** or **acoustic pressure.** Sound pressure is determined by the ratio of the alternating force provided by the sound source to the surface area over which the force is acting. In other words:

$$\text{Sound pressure } (p) = \frac{\text{Force (F)}}{\text{Area (A)}} \text{ [Pa]} \qquad (5.7)$$

Please note that both sound pressure and stiffness of a gas are expressed in the same units. This is because sound pressure is the result of overcoming gas stiffness.

Both the acting force and the sound pressure can be expressed in Equation 5.7 as peak values or root mean square (RMS) values (see Chapter 3). However, it is customary in hearing science to use RMS values in all sound-related calculations. Therefore, if the symbols have no subscripts or labels indicating to the contrary, the RMS values should be assumed.

Example 5.4

An alternating force ($F = 200$ N) acts over an area of 100 m^2. What is the sound pressure exerted by the acting force over this area?

First, select the appropriate equation (Equation 5.7).

$$p = \frac{F}{A}$$

Substitute known variables and solve. We know the force is 200 N and the area is 100 m^2.

$$p = \frac{200 \text{ N}}{100 \text{ m}^2}$$

$$p = 2\frac{\text{N}}{\text{m}^2}$$

$$p = 2 \text{ Pa}$$

Answer: The pressure is 2 pascals.

Notice in Example 5.4 that instead of using N/m^2, pressure has its own unit, the pascal (Pa), where 1 N/m^2 = 1 Pa. The units of force and pressure as well as the units of other physical magnitudes were discussed in Chapter 2.

When a sound source transfers its energy to the surrounding air molecules, it affects their displacement, velocity, and acceleration. The most important of these three characteristics is the molecule velocity, more commonly called the particle velocity, which is directly related to the kinetic energy of the moving sound. **Particle velocity (v)** is the velocity of a molecule vibrating at the frequency of the sound wave as it passes that place in space. It is important to realize that particle velocity is different from the speed of sound. The speed of sound (a scalar) is how fast the wave is traveling through a medium, whereas the particle velocity (a vector) is the velocity of individual vibrating particles that are excited by an applied energy and then carry this energy to the next particle. The speed of the sound wave depends on the properties of the medium, whereas the particle velocity does not. The particle velocity depends on the amount of sound energy traveling through the medium, whereas the speed of sound does not. Sounds with different energy (different sound pressure) travel at the same speed through a medium, but the particle velocity changes throughout the medium as the energy spreads out over a larger and larger area.

Assuming that the movement of an air particle is a simple back-and-forth vibration (sinusoidal motion) in the direction of the propagating wave, the graph of particle displacement and sound pressure will appear as sine waves that are out-of-phase by 90° (Fig. 5.6). Particle displacement indicates how far particles are displaced from their resting position. Sound pressure indicates how compressed or rarefied the particles are. In Figure 5.6, the compression indicates air pressure that is above the atmospheric pressure and the rarefaction indicates air pressure that is below ambient

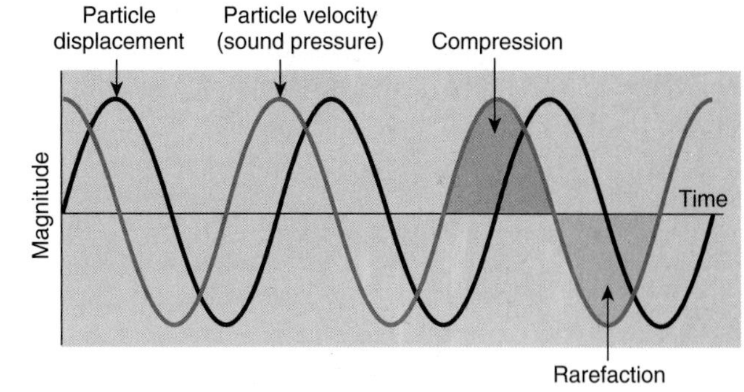

Figure 5.6. The relationship between air particle displacement and particle velocity (sound pressure).

pressure. You already learned in Chapter 3 that displacement and velocity are 90° out-of-phase. Because sound pressure is in-phase with velocity, particle displacement and sound pressure are also 90° out-of-phase.

ACOUSTIC IMPEDANCE

Recall from Chapter 4 that the relationship between force and velocity in vibrating systems is Force (F) = Impedance (Z) × Velocity (v) (Equation 4.4) and that this relationship is determined by the mechanic properties of the vibrating system, that is, its mechanic impedance. The same concept applies to a sound wave propagating through a medium. The opposition to the flow of sound energy through a medium is called **acoustic impedance** (specific acoustic impedance) and it is determined by the properties of the medium. The difference between mechanic and acoustic impedance lies in the fact that in vibrating systems the mechanic impedance of the vibrating object opposes the force acting in a specific direction, whereas during wave propagation the acoustic impedance of the medium opposes changes in pressure in all directions, i.e., pressure is spread out over an area and exerted on many individual particles. The acoustic impedance (Z) of a given medium determines the relationship between the sound pressure (p) and particle velocity (v) as follows:

$$p = v \times Z \qquad (5.8)$$

which is analogous to Equation 4.4. Both mechanic and acoustic impedances have the same internal structure. Mechanic impedance is determined by the combined effects of the mass, elasticity, and friction (resistance) of a vibrating system and acoustic impedance depends on the acoustic mass (M_a),* acoustic compliance (C_a),** and acoustic resistance (R_a).

There is one additional similarity between mechanic and acoustic opposition to motion if you consider fluid mechanics and hydraulic systems. In fluid mechanics there are two

*Acoustic mass is sometimes called inertance.

**The acoustic compliance (C_a) is the inverse of the stiffness ($C_a = 1/K$) of a propagating medium. Acoustic compliance is also called acoustic elasticity.

concepts of impedance: the mechanic impedance of the fluid itself and the flow impedance. The flow impedance is the opposition to fluid flow of a fluid through a pipe and it determines, for example, how fast water can flow from a water pipe into a bathtub (i.e., how fast you can fill the bathtub). Similarly, there are two impedances in acoustics: the specific acoustic impedance and the acoustic flow impedance. The specific acoustic impedance (described above) corresponds to the mechanic impedance described in Chapter 4, whereas the acoustic flow impedance corresponds to the mechanic flow impedance that opposes fluid flow in hydraulic systems. **Specific acoustic impedance** is the opposition of a medium to the propagation of sound energy *through* the medium. **Acoustic flow impedance** (acoustic impedance) is the opposition to the flow of energy from the surface of the sound source *to* the medium or through an acoustic system such as an air column. If you would like to know more about both types of acoustic impedance and how they are related, see the website. **Link 5-9**

SOUND INTENSITY

In Chapter 2 we defined power as energy expended over a certain period of time. When a sound source creates a disturbance, a certain amount of energy is transferred to the surrounding medium in a certain period of time. This power may be distributed over a very small area or over a very large area during wave propagation. The amount of sound power that travels through a specific area of the wavefront surface is called **sound intensity** (*I*). Sound intensity can be calculated as the ratio of the sound power (*P*) to the surface area (*A*) on which the power is acting.

$$\text{Sound intensity } (I) = \frac{\text{Sound power (P)}}{\text{Area (A)}} \qquad (5.9)$$

The standard unit used for sound intensity is the watt per square meter (W/m^2).

Example 5.5

If a sound source producing power ($P = 1000$ W) acts over an area of 100 m^2, what is the resulting sound intensity?

First, select the appropriate equation (Equation 5.9).

$$I = \frac{P}{A}$$

Substitute known variables and solve. We know the power of the sound source is 1000 watts and the area (*A*) is 100 m^2. Therefore:

$$I = \frac{1000 \text{ W}}{100 \text{ m}^2}$$

$$I = 10 \text{ W/m}^2$$

Answer: The intensity is 10 W/m^2.

Recall that if the sound source is a monopole (pulsating sphere), then energy radiates like a gradually growing sphere with a surface area that grows larger and larger. The surface area of a sphere is $A = 4\pi r^2$ and it depends entirely on the radius (*r*) of the sphere. Therefore, if we know the sound power provided by the sound source and the distance from the sound source to a specific point in space, we can calculate the sound intensity at the point of a sphere as:

$$I = \frac{P}{4\pi r^2} [\text{W/m}^2] \qquad (5.10)$$

This equation is identical to Equation 5.9 with the area of the sphere inserted into the denominator of the equation. Note that in the case of a spherical sound wave, sound intensity is inversely proportional to the square of the distance from the sound source (i.e., $I \propto \frac{1}{r^2}$; the symbol α means "proportional to"). This relationship is known as the **inverse square law** and it is one of the general laws of acoustics and wave propagation. The change in sound intensity along with distance from the sound source is shown in Figure 5.7.

Example 5.6

Imagine a monopole sound source producing 500 W of power. What is the intensity of the sound 3.4 m away from the source, assuming that the energy spreads equally in all directions?

Select Equation 5.10, substitute known variables, and solve.

$$I = \frac{P}{4\pi r^2} [\text{W/m}^2]$$

$$I = \frac{500}{4\pi (3.4)^2} [\text{W/m}^2]$$

$$I = \frac{500}{145.2672} [\text{W/m}^2]$$

$$I = 3.4419 \ [\text{W/m}^2]$$

Answer: The intensity is 3.44 W/m^2.

PRACTICE PROBLEMS: SOUND PRESSURE AND SOUND INTENSITY

1. If a 345-N force acts over an area of 1000 m^2, what is the resulting sound pressure?
2. If a 345-W power acts over an area of 1000 m^2, what is the resulting sound intensity?

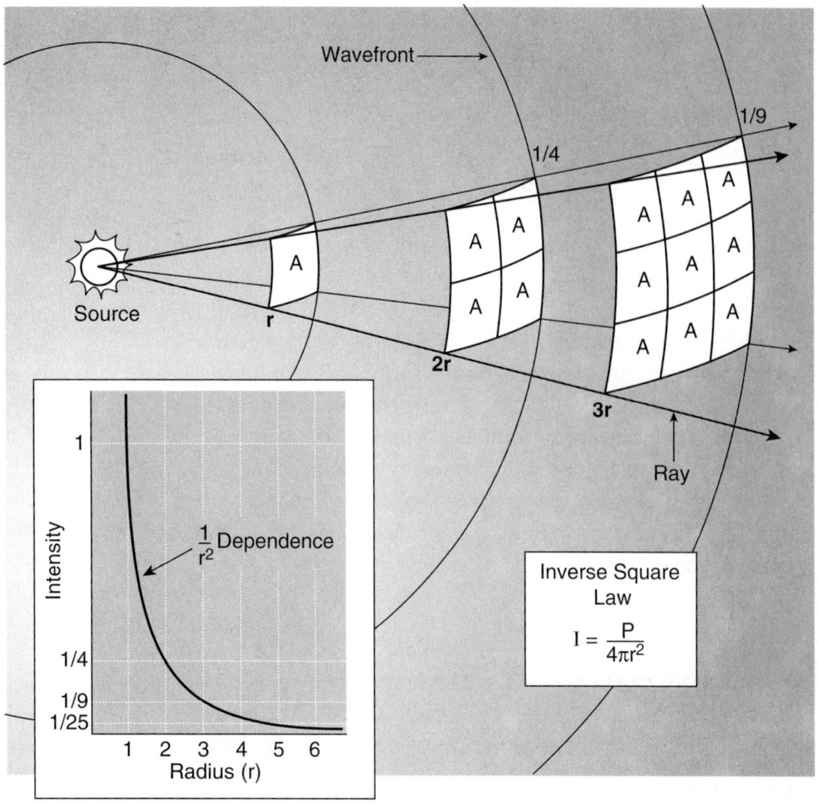

Figure 5.7. Propagation of a spherical wave and the inverse square law.

3. If a sound source acting with a force of 235.6 N produces a sound pressure of 0.41 Pa, what is the size of the area on which the sound source is acting?
4. If a 7.89×10^{2}-N force creates a pressure of 0.01 Pa, what is the size of the area over which the sound source is acting?
5. If a monopole sound source is producing 235 W of power, what is the intensity of the sound 2.8 m away from the source, assuming that the energy spreads equally in all directions?
6. Imagine a monopole sound source producing 9.32×10^{5} W of power. How far from the source are you if the sound intensity at your location is 4.98×10^{3} W/m^2?

Answers (If you need help with these problems, consult the website.) **Link clip 5-10**

1. 0.35 Pa
2. 0.35 W/m^2
3. 574.63 m^2
4. 78900 m^2
5. 2.39 W/m^2
6. 3.86 m

THE RELATIONSHIP BETWEEN SOUND INTENSITY AND SOUND PRESSURE

You know from the previous two sections of this chapter that sound pressure indicates how compressed or rarefied the particles are and sound intensity indicates how much sound power is transferred from the sound source to the surrounding area. Therefore, it should be obvious that sound power and sound pressure are related: A powerful sound source will produce a greater sound pressure than a weak source. In fact, sound intensity and sound pressure can be thought of as two different ways to represent the strength of sound.

If you compare the equations for sound intensity (5.9) and sound pressure (5.7), you will notice that the sound intensity depends on the sound power and the sound pressure depends on the force:

$$\text{Sound intensity (I)} = \frac{\text{Sound power (P)}}{\text{Area (A)}}$$

$$\text{Sound pressure (p)} = \frac{\text{Force (F)}}{\text{Area (A)}}$$

This means that to understand how sound intensity and sound pressure are related, we need to review the relationship between power and force. Recall from Chapter 2 that power is equal to the product of force and velocity.

$$\text{Power } (P) = \text{Force } (F) \times \text{velocity } (v) \qquad (5.11)$$

In the case of sound, force is the product of sound pressure and area ($F = p \times A$); thus:

$$P = p \times A \times v \quad (5.12)$$

where v is the particle velocity. Subsequently, we can insert the right side of the above equation into the equation describing sound intensity ($I = P/A$) and express sound intensity as:

$$I = \frac{p \times A \times v}{A} = p \times v \quad (5.13)$$

According to Equation 5.13, sound intensity is equal to the product of sound pressure and particle velocity. Recall further from the previous section of this chapter that sound pressure and particle velocity are not independent and their relationship depends on the specific acoustic impedance of the medium. If we isolate particle velocity (v) from Equation 5.8 (i.e., $v = p/Z$) and insert it into Equation 5.13, it will show the relationship between sound intensity and sound pressure.

$$I = \frac{p^2}{Z} \quad (5.14)$$

Notice from this equation that the sound intensity is proportional to the square of the sound pressure. We will revisit this relationship in Chapter 7 when we discuss the decibel.

TAXONOMY OF SOUNDS

Taxonomy is a scientific classification system that acts to divide a large number of objects or concepts into a number of different classes on the basis of certain properties. A typical taxonomy is hierarchical (multilevel) in nature and expands from global to detailed descriptors. One of the most common examples is the division of living species into different categories based on kingdom, phylum, class, order, family, genus, and species. The purpose of taxonomy is to organize a large group of objects into smaller and more manageable groups. This may seem to be a simple task, but there is actually no ideal taxonomy. All taxonomies have some overlap and a number of exceptions.

There are a large number of taxonomies of sounds that can be used independently or mixed together. Sound is a common name for all acoustic events whether they are intended to be heard or not. However, if the word *sound* comes without any qualifier, most people assume it means an **audible sound** (a sound that can be heard) or **auditory signal** (a signal that is intended to be heard). The primary parameter (apart from sound intensity) characterizing whether sound can be heard or not is frequency; therefore, one basic sound taxonomy divides sounds into three classes based on the frequency content: infrasound, sound (audible sound), and ultrasound (Table 5.3). The frequency boundaries for this taxonomy are based on human hearing and cannot be applied to other species, which may be able to hear sounds at higher or lower frequencies than humans or may have a more limited frequency range for hearing. Even in humans this classification scheme is only related to sounds perceived through the ear, since sounds perceived by bone conduction stimulation may have a frequency as high as 50 kHz (Corso, 1963; Lenhardt et al., 1991; Fujimoto et al., 2005).

▸ **Table 5.3.** Taxonomy of Sounds Based on Frequency

Infrasound	Very-low-frequency sounds that cannot be heard (typically below 20 Hz)
Sound (audible sound)	Sounds in the frequency range of normal human hearing (typically in the 20-Hz to 20,000-Hz range)
Ultrasound	Very-high-frequency sounds that cannot be heard (typically above 20 kHz)

The above taxonomy is very straightforward if the sounds have just one or very few similar frequency components (Chapter 4). Sounds that consist of a small number of distinct frequency components are called **tones.** Tones that have only one frequency component are called **pure tones** and tones that have more than one component are called **complex tones.** To hear pure tones (sine waves) of various frequencies, see the website. The website has demonstrations of pure tones commonly used for hearing testing (see Figure 5.8) and several other pure tones that are lower and higher than those used in conventional audiometry. **Audio clip 5-1**

Complex tones can be divided into several subgroups based on their complexity (number of components and the relationship among components) and temporal envelope. If the components that make up the complex tone follow a specific frequency and intensity relationship, then the complex waveform will have a characteristic shape that can be used as a sound descriptor. For example, the sound waveform may have the shape of a square, sawtooth, or triangular wave (Chapter 4); a rectangular wave; or a pulse train (a sequence of spikes). To hear complex tones that differ in their complexity

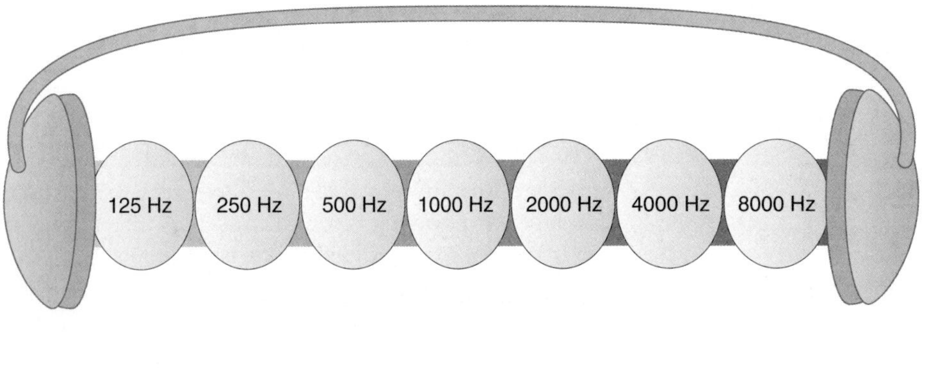

Figure 5.8. Examples of pure tones used in audiometric testing.

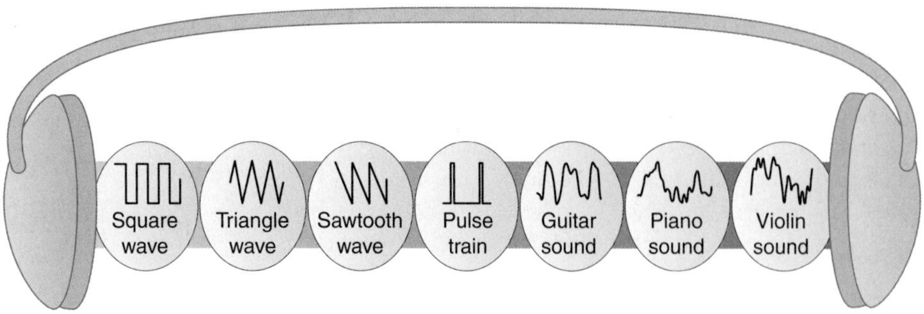

Figure 5.9. Examples of complex tones.

(and therefore in their waveform shape), see the website. The website has demonstrations of several basic complex tones (see Fig. 5.9). **Audio clip 5-2**

If we know the behavior of a steady-state tone within a single period of its waveform, we know its behavior at any point in time. Sounds that repeat their behavior, period after period, or are in some other way predictable (mathematically) are called deterministic sounds. **Deterministic sounds** are sounds in which the magnitude at different points in time can be predicted exactly.

Sounds in which the behavior cannot be predicted exactly are called **stochastic sounds** (random sounds). Stochastic sounds are sounds in which the future behavior of the sound wave cannot be predicted or can only be predicted with some probability. These sounds are called noises. We have already defined noise in Chapter 4 as a vibration that contains a very large (infinite) number of frequency components that appear as a continuous spectrum in the frequency domain. This spectrum can extend across the entire frequency scale or can be limited to a specific frequency band.

The same concepts of periodicity, inharmonicity, transient, and noise introduced in Chapter 4 as forms of vibration apply to sound. Similar to the term *sound*, the term *noise* also has multiple meanings: physical and psychological (perceptual). The definition of noise listed above is the physical definition of noise. The psychological definition describes noise as any unwanted sound.* Throughout most of this book we use the term *noise* in its physical meaning. When we refer to its psychological meaning, this meaning is clearly indicated (e.g., in Chapter 12).

*In this sense the term *noise* can also refer to other sensations and activities, indicating any stimulus that is unwanted and interferes with the performance of a task.

Pure tones and noises are at the extreme opposite ends of signal complexity, which is the basis for the taxonomy of sounds presented in Figure 5.10. The taxonomy shown in Figure 5.10 classifies sounds as tones and noises. Further, tones are classified as pure tones and complex tones. Noises can also be classified into two main categories: continuous noise and impulse noise. **Continuous noise** is noise that consists of a large number of random acoustic events connected together into one continuous stream. Continuous noise can also be characterized as the noise that is present in the environment for an extended period of time, exceeding the period of interest (observation). Continuous noise can further be divided into two general classes: nonstationary and stationary noise. A **stationary noise** is a random sound that has average acoustic properties that do not vary much over time. Conversely, if the noise content and the intensity change randomly over time and the noise's average properties cannot be reasonably predicted, this noise is called **nonstationary noise.** Street noise, music, and speech are examples of nonstationary sounds that vary unpredictably and quite considerably over time. Examples of stationary noises include white noise, pink noise, speech-spectrum noise, and any noise produced simultaneously by a large number of similar sound sources (e.g., applause). Please note that we described music in this paragraph as a nonstationary noise. While a single music sound is usually a complex tone, a long sequence of such sounds played on various instruments (e.g.,

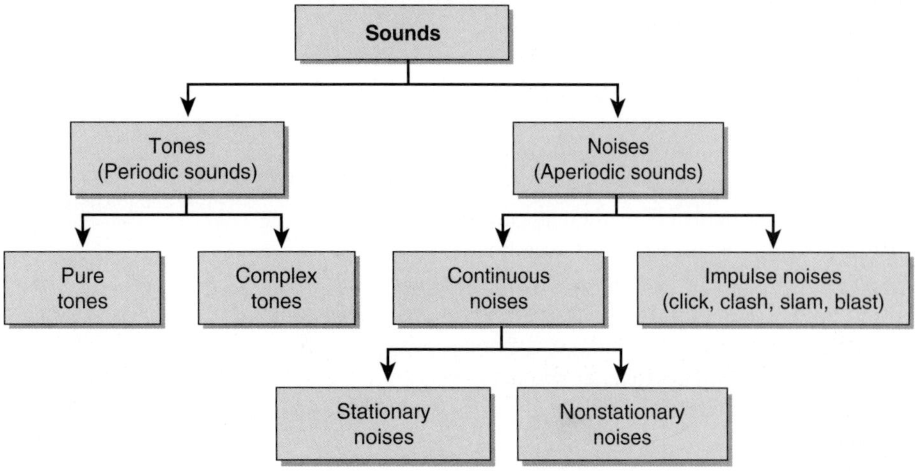

Figure 5.10. Sound complexity taxonomy.

a symphony) has the form of a nonstationary noise when averaged together and presented as an average spectrum. The same applies to speech, although some speech sounds are short-term noises themselves.

An impulse noise is a single brief event with a large peak value and short duration. An impulse noise has a peak value that exceeds its RMS magnitude by thousands of times (e.g., a gun shot). **Audio clip 5-3** Some relatively short sounds, such as tone bursts **Audio clip 5-4** and noise bursts, **Audio clip 5-5** also have a short duration but their peak values are comparable with their RMS values, so they are not impulse noises, even though they can be very short. However, they do not continue for an extended period of time, so they are not continuous tones or continuous noises either. Obviously, these sounds can be classified as short-term tones and short-term noises and can be assigned to their own classes in an expanded taxonomy, but there is no taxonomy that would ideally organize each and every acoustic event.

In Chapter 3 we defined several measures that can be used to describe the magnitude of a waveform. These measures are directly applicable to periodic sounds (deterministic sounds), but noise (random, stochastic sounds) can only be described in terms of the expected magnitude and the variability of the magnitude. Although tones can be described as having specific frequency components, overall intensity, and intensity of its components, the same is not true of noises. Noises, instead, are characterized by their expected values in both the time domain, using an **amplitude distribution function** (described on the website **Link 5-11**), and in the frequency domain, using a **power spectrum density function.**

The power spectrum is the amount of sound power in the sound wave that is distributed across all frequency components. This spectrum was already discussed in Chapter 4. The power spectrum density function is an average power spectrum characterizing noises and other long-term stochastic (random) sounds (e.g., speech or piece of music) where the concept of sound power at discrete frequencies has to be replaced by an average power in a bandwidth (usually in a bandwidth of 1 Hz). A bandwidth is a range of frequencies listed from low to high (e.g., an octave bandwidth could range from 1000 Hz to 2000 Hz and a 1-Hz bandwidth could range from 1000 Hz to 1001 Hz).

Some examples of power spectrum density functions for various noises are shown in Figure 5.11.

The **overall sound power** is the amount of power in the entire sound, that is, in the overall frequency range (bandwidth) of the sound. The sound power in various bandwidths can be calculated mathematically (e.g., by Fourier analysis; Chapter 4) or measured experimentally by filtering the sound with narrow band filters and registering the filters' output values (Chapter 14). Filtering allows us to look at different "spectral pieces" (bands) of the noise. Thus, we can look at the entire noise (overall sound power) or we can look at the power contained within a specific bandwidth of the noise.

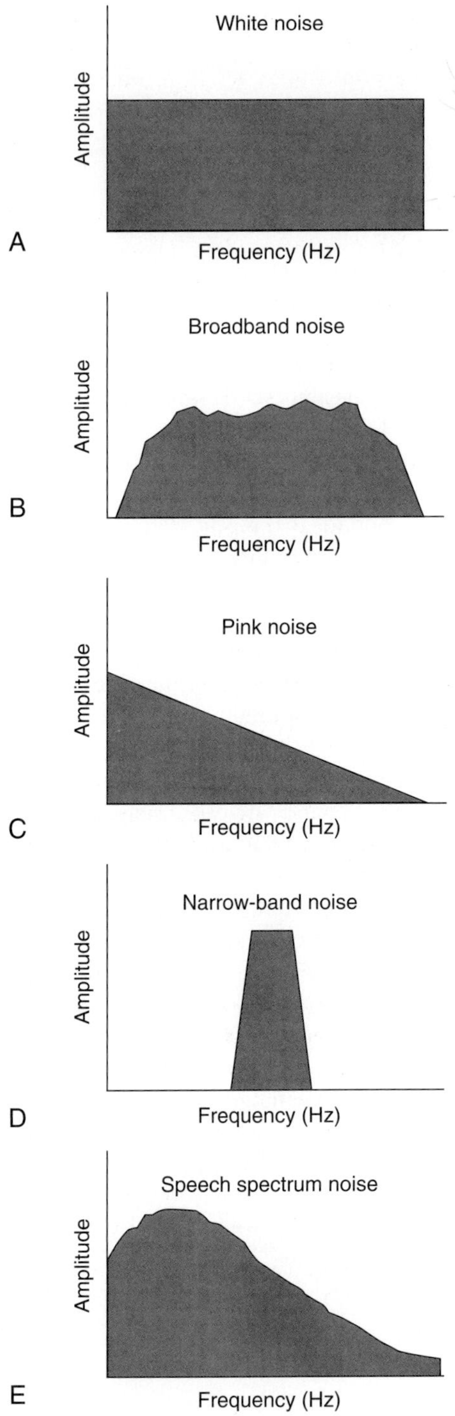

Figure 5.11. The power spectra of some common noises: **(A)** white noise, **(B)** broadband noise, **(C)** pink noise, **(D)** narrowband noise, and **(E)** speech spectrum noise. The vertical axis represents amplitude of sound intensity and the horizontal axis is the frequency of the components.

To understand the concept of a noise being divided into "spectral pieces," imagine that you have a box of 64 crayons that are used to different degrees and you want to know how much coloring you can still do with the set. You could measure the combined length of all 64 crayons and get the overall length of all the crayons put together. If you compare this length with the total length of a new set of crayons, you can get some idea how much they have been used and how much "coloring power" is still left in them. Alternately, you could compare the lengths of individual crayons and determine how much "coloring power" they have in relationship to each other. For example, you could determine that the cherry-red crayon is much longer than the aquamarine crayon so you could color with the cherry-red crayon much longer (i.e., it has much more "coloring power"). A box of crayons is a good analogy to a broadband noise that contains many frequency components. If we use a filter and measure (e.g., how much power is contained in a band of noise between 1000 Hz and 1001 Hz and another band of noise between 2000 and 2001 Hz), then we have the acoustic equivalent of a comparison between the "coloring power" of a cherry-red and aquamarine crayon. In other words, filtering allows us to look at individual bands ("colors") of the noise spectrum. Depending on the type of filter, the bands of noise used in the above analysis may be very narrow (1 Hz wide) or quite broad (1 octave wide). In addition, various natural noises may be narrowband or broadband themselves. The differences between various types of noise can be easily observed by comparing their continuous spectra.

All of the noises included in Figure 5.11 are wideband noises except for one narrowband noise (panel D). White noise (panel A) is a synthetic noise that has equal energy in every 1-Hz-wide band of noise across the entire bandwidth. White noise is analogous to white light in which all of the wavelengths of the visible spectrum are present and have equal energies. Keep in mind, however, that when white noise is presented to a listener by an earphone or loudspeaker, the spectrum of the white noise is modified by the limitations of the earphones or loudspeaker system and the actual noise may be less than an ideal white noise and is instead a broadband noise (panel B). Notice that the amplitudes of the components in the broadband noise shown in Figure 5.11 decrease in magnitude at both very low and very high frequencies and that there is some fluctuation in amplitude across the entire spectrum. Pink noise (panel C) is noise in which the amplitudes of individual components decrease as frequency increases. For this reason, pink noise is also called 1/*f* noise because as frequency increases, intensity decreases. There are also other color-named noises that have different spectral shapes such as red noise and blue noise. If you would like to know more about color-named noises, consult the website. Please note that the online text entitled "The Color of Noise" uses the concept of the decibel. If you are not yet familiar with this concept, you may want to read Chapter 7 before using this link. **Link 5-12**

Octave band noise is one of the most common examples of narrowband noise (panel D). Octave band noise has a bandwidth of one octave; that is, its highest frequency is twice as large as its lowest frequency. The concept of the octave is discussed in detail in Chapter 7. Speech spectrum noise (panel E) is a synthetic noise that has an amplitude spectrum similar to that of the long-term average spectrum of speech. Notice that the amplitude of individual components decreases as frequency increases. This is because the low-frequency sounds of speech (e.g., sounds created with vocal fold vibration like /a/ and nasal resonance like /m/) have more power than the high-frequency sounds of speech (e.g., the sounds created without vocal fold vibration like /s/ and /sh/). To hear samples of various wideband noises, such as those shown in Figure 5.12, see the website. **Audio clip 5-6**

The taxonomies presented in Table 5.2 and Figure 5.10 are just two taxonomies that can be used to classify sounds. They are based on sound frequency and sound complexity and were used to differentiate between basic properties of ideal tones and noises. However, these taxonomies are not sufficient to classify the whole body of real-world sounds. First, most real-world sounds are not just ideal tones or ideal noises; they usually include elements of both. Second, real-world sounds may have energy in both the audible and inaudible ranges. Third, any real-world taxonomy should greatly depend on its practical purpose and different taxonomies may be useful to different people. One may need to classify natural sounds and synthetic sounds, another may need to classify speech, music, and sound effects, and yet another may need a taxonomy based on types of music sounds. Some taxonomies may be very simple, whereas others may need an extensive hierarchical structure to be useful. Therefore, the general taxonomies shown in Table 5.2 and Figure 5.10 should be considered as two examples out of many possibilities. Other taxonomies can be found in the literature.

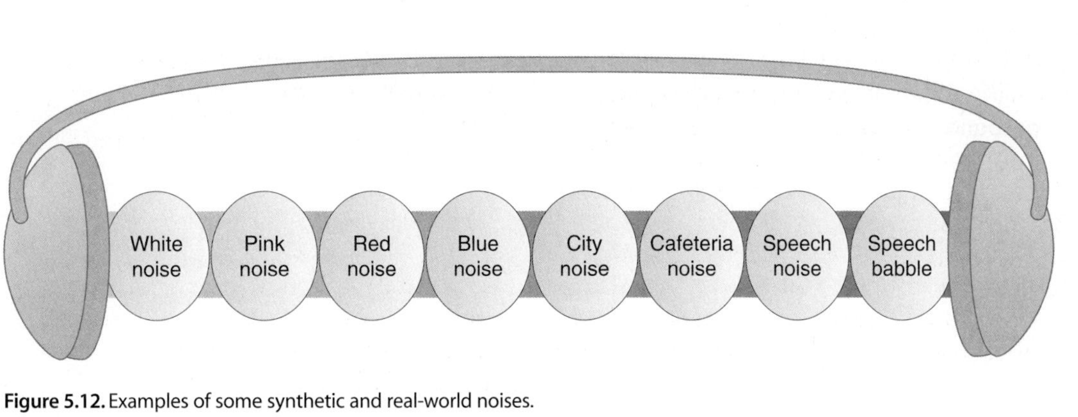

Figure 5.12. Examples of some synthetic and real-world noises.

Summary

Sound is created when a vibrating object, called a sound source, causes localized pressure changes within an elastic medium, such as air. Sound waves are the alternating regions of increased density, called compressions, and decreased density, called rarefactions, propagating through a medium. Two types of wave motion are transverse and longitudinal wave motion. Sound waves are examples of longitudinal wave motion, meaning that the vibration pattern of the medium particles is parallel to the direction of wave motion. Two basic types of sound source are monopole and dipole. The speed of sound is affected by the stiffness and density of the medium through which the sound is traveling. Sound moves much more quickly through very stiff materials, such as metal, compared to less stiff materials, such as air. The speed of sound in air increases as temperature increases because the temperature inversely affects air density. The wavelength of a sound is the distance in space between two consecutive compressions or two consecutive rarefactions, and it is determined by the speed and frequency of the sound. Sound pressure is equal to the force of vibration over the area of vibration, and sound intensity is equal to the power of the vibration over the area of vibration. The inverse square law states that the sound intensity of a spherical sound wave decreases proportionally to the square of the distance from the sound source. Acoustic impedance is the property of a medium opposing sound propagation and it affects both sound pressure and particle velocity. Sounds can be classified based on a variety of different taxonomies (classification systems). One common taxonomy breaks sounds into tones (pure tones, complex tones) and noises (continuous and impulse).

Key Points

- A systematic pressure disturbance through an elastic medium created by alternating regions of compression and rarefaction is called a sound (acoustic) wave.
- The energy transferred from a sound source to a medium is called sound energy.
- Two common types of wave motion are transverse wave motion and longitudinal wave motion. In transverse wave motion, the particles of the medium vibrate in a direction perpendicular to the direction of wave propagation, and in longitudinal wave motion (sound waves), the particles of the medium vibrate parallel to the direction of wave propagation.
- The speed of sound (c) is affected by the density and stiffness of the medium through which it is traveling. The stiffer the medium, the faster the speed of sound is.
- The wavelength (λ) of a sound is the distance in space between identical points in the cycle of adjacent waves. Wavelength depends on the speed of sound and the frequency of vibration.
- Sound sources are simple or complex combinations of monopole (pulsating sphere) and dipole (oscillating sphere) sources. Monopole sources are omnidirectional and dipole sources are bidirectional.
- Sound pressure is equal to the force of vibration over the area of vibration, and sound intensity is equal to the power of vibration over the area of vibration.
- Noises can be continuous or impulse, depending on their duration. Continuous noises can be further broken down into stationary and nonstationary noises, depending on whether the sound varies considerably over time.

CHAPTER 6

Sound Propagation

Chapter Outline

Objectives

- To describe the effects of wave absorption, refraction, reflection, and diffraction that occur as sound waves travel through a sound field
- To describe the sound wave interference that occurs when sound waves meet in a sound field, including the presence of standing waves and beats
- To describe various sound field phenomena created by moving sound sources, including the Doppler effect and the sonic boom
- To relate the effects of wave absorption, refraction, reflection, interference, and diffraction on sound intensity distribution and sound decay in rooms
- To describe the behavior of sound vibration in a Helmholtz resonator and in an air column

Key Terms

Absorption
Absorption coefficient
Acoustic effect
Acoustic shadow
Acoustic system
Anechoic chamber
Beat frequency
Beats
Boundary
Closed space
Constructive interference
Critical distance
Destructive interference
Diffraction
Diffuse field
Direct field
Dispersion (diffusion)
Doppler effect
Echo
End correction
External absorption
Far field
Free field
Helmholtz resonator
Incident wave
Indirect field
Interference
Internal absorption
Mach number
Near field
Open space
Reflected wave
Reflection
Reflection coefficient
Refracted wave
Refraction
Reverberation
Reverberation chamber
Reverberation time
Shadow zone
Shock wave
Signal-to-noise ratio
Snell's Law
Sonic boom
Sound field
Sound interference
Sound propagation
Standing wave
Temperature gradient
Thermal effect
Total internal reflection
Wind shear

Sound is a wave phenomenon in which an elastic disturbance in the atmosphere spreads throughout a medium. As a sound wave travels across a medium, its energy is spread over a larger and larger area and its sound intensity gradually decreases. The decrease in sound pressure due to the spherical spreading is predictable based on the inverse square law stating that for every doubling of distance from a sound source, the intensity decreases four times. The inverse square law was discussed in Chapter 5.

In addition to this predictable change in sound intensity with the distance from the sound source, **sound propagation** is affected by a number of wave phenomena that affect the speed, direction, intensity, and phase of sound waves. These phenomena are due to properties of the medium through which the sound wave travels and the presence of the boundaries of the space within which the sound is traveling. The **boundaries** of the space are the surrounding walls and other obstacles that affect the way that sound waves travel. The main phenomena affecting sound wave behavior in space are absorption, refraction, reflection, interference, and diffraction of sound energy. These phenomena apply in various degrees to all mechanic and electromagnetic (e.g., light) waves and are generally called wave effects. The wave effects discussed in this chapter are limited to acoustic waves and are referred to as **acoustic effects.**

The relative impact of various acoustic effects on the sound wave depends on the type of space in which the sound is propagating. The two basic types of acoustic spaces are **open space** (outdoor space) and **closed space** (indoor space). Very small closed spaces, such as the inside of a loudspeaker box, a musical instrument body, and the ear canal (when it is closed by an earphone), where the dimensions of the space are smaller or comparable to the wavelength of the propagating sound wave, are called **acoustic systems.** Acoustic systems are characterized by standing waves rather than traveling waves. **Standing waves** are the modes of vibration created in vibrating systems such as strings (described in Chapter 4). They can also exist in acoustic systems and will be discussed in greater detail in this chapter as they relate to sound. Acoustic systems have the ability to greatly modify sound energy or even to create sound when properly excited by mechanic energy. The material included in this chapter covers the acoustic effects seen during sound wave propagation, discusses different types of sound fields, and offers several examples of acoustic systems.

ACOUSTIC EFFECTS

Sound Absorption

A sound wave propagating through a medium will ultimately lose all its energy because of **sound absorption** by the medium and surrounding boundaries. Sound absorption by the medium is the result of the **internal friction** within the medium, which converts sound energy into heat as sound passes through a medium. Sound absorption by space boundaries is the result of the transfer of sound energy from one medium to another as sound arrives at the boundary between two media. Thus, the resulting loss of sound energy in a medium can be due to **internal absorption** (absorption by the medium) and **external absorption** (absorption by space boundaries). Internal absorption is the dominant factor in sound energy dissipation in open spaces and in large sports arenas. External absorption is affected by the size and physical properties of the surfaces surrounding the space within which the sound wave propagates. External absorption is the dominant factor in the sound decrease in enclosed spaces such as auditoriums, theaters, living rooms, classrooms, and audiometric booths.

The ability of the medium and its boundaries to absorb the energy of sound waves is characterized by a quantity called the **absorption coefficient.** The total amount of sound energy absorbed by a medium itself during wave propagation is an exponential function of the distance from the sound source and the physical properties of the medium. This relationship is expressed mathematically in Equation 6.1 (Porges, 1977, p. 86):

$$I = I_o \times e^{-2mx} \qquad \textbf{(6.1)}$$

where I is the sound intensity at the distance x from the sound source, I_o is the sound intensity at the sound source, $e = 2.718281$ (the base of the natural logarithm), and m is the absorption coefficient of the medium. The absorption coefficient of the medium is analogous to the coefficient of damping in a vibrating system discussed in Chapter 3 and described by Equation 3.15. It is the ratio of the internal friction coefficient of the medium to the effective mass of the vibrating medium, which depends on the molecular structure of the medium. It is also frequency dependent ($m \sim f^2$). The average coefficient of absorption for air is about two magnitudes higher than for water. Therefore, a high-intensity sound wave with a frequency of about 100 Hz is completely absorbed by air in less than a 500-km distance, whereas in water it can travel almost halfway around the world (Weston, 1997).

The absorption of sound by a medium is greatly affected by the presence of obstacles and impurities (Harris, 1966). For example, absorption of sound energy by the air depends on the amount of dust particles in the air and by the humidity of the air. Humid air contains a larger number of water vapor molecules compared with dry air and water vapor molecules are larger and lighter than air molecules (Bohn, 1988). This mixture makes it more difficult for the sound wave to travel through.

The effect of humidity (the amount of water in the air) on sound wave propagation is usually described as an effect of relative humidity. Relative humidity is the amount of water in the air calculated as a percentage of the total amount of water that could be held in the air at this specific temperature. The effect of changes in relative humidity on the absorption

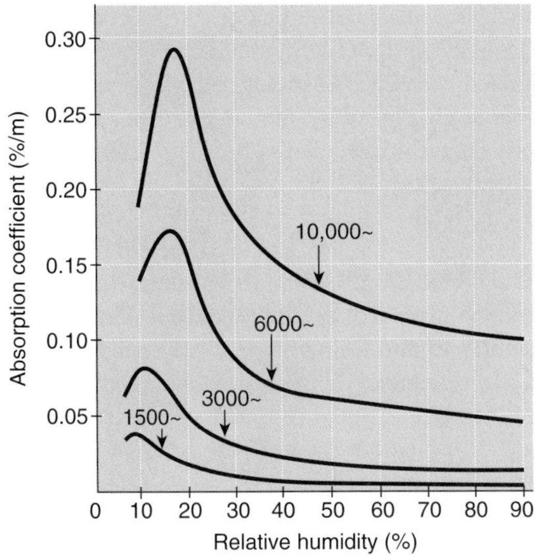

Figure 6.1. Absorption of sound in air at 20°C as a function of relative humidity. (From Knudsen VO, Harris CM. Acoustical Designing in Architecture. New York, NY: John Wiley & Sons, Inc., 1950:69. Used with permission of the American Institute of Physics.)

coefficient of moist air for sound waves of different frequencies is illustrated in Figure 6.1. Consider, for example, the effect of relative humidity on the absorption coefficient for a 10,000-Hz sound. The greatest air absorption of sound energy occurs when the relative humidity is at about 20%, and it decreases by two to three times for dry air (0% humidity) and highly saturated air (90% humidity). Frequencies lower than 10,000 Hz demonstrate a similar pattern, with maximum absorption coefficients existing at a lower relative humidity with decreasing sound frequency. At high temperatures the air can hold more water before being saturated. Therefore, the higher the temperature, the lower the relative humidity is for the same amount of water dispersed in the air. This means that at higher temperatures, the attenuation of sound by moist air can be greater even if the relative humidity stays the same.

In humid air, water vapor molecules uniformly mix with the air molecules and uniformly affect the propagation of sound waves. In contrast, the presence of rain, snow, or fog has less of an effect on sound absorption in the air because of the uneven distribution of water molecules, unless a heavy fog or lasting rain or snow affects the air humidity. Thus, the relative effect of precipitation on sound propagation can be considered minimal. This may sound counterintuitive, because, for example, when it is snowing everything sounds quieter. However, snow on the ground is highly absorbent and, in addition, there is often less activity in the environment; thus, the environment itself is quieter.

Similar to the concept associated with precipitation, strings, ropes, and loosely woven fabrics provide less attenuation to sound than thinner but more uniform barriers. For example, a wet handkerchief attenuates sound better than a 1-cm layer of a dry and loose felt (Tyndall, 1867). In general, precipitation and sparse obstacles have a negligible effect on sound propagation. Humidity has a larger effect and it needs to be considered in cases involving long distances and high-frequency sounds (Harris, 1966).

In contrast to outdoor environments (open space), in which the internal absorption is dominant, in indoor environments (closed spaces) sound travels much shorter distances and is mostly absorbed by the surfaces surrounding the sound field. In the case of a sound arriving at a space boundary, the absorption coefficient (α) for the boundary can be calculated using Equation 6.2:

$$\alpha = \frac{I_{abs}}{I} \tag{6.2}$$

where I is the sound intensity arriving at the specific area of the boundary and I_{abs} is the amount of energy absorbed by this area. The value of the absorption coefficient varies on a scale from 0 to 1 and depends on the frequency of the propagating sound, the thickness and structure of the walls (boundaries), the amount of wall surface, and the type of wall material (i.e., its molecular structure, density, uniformity, and temperature). For example, sound arriving at a soft material such as a thick carpet would be absorbed more easily than the sound arriving at a hard surface, such as a tile floor. The values of the coefficients of absorption for sounds of different frequencies for selected materials used for walls, ceilings, floors, and so forth are listed in Table 6.1.

As a general rule, sound absorption increases with sound frequency (Porges, 1977, p. 85); however, this dependence

Table 6.1. Coefficients of Absorption of Selected Materials as a Function of Frequency (Typical Values)

	Frequency (Hz)					
Material	125	250	500	1000	2000	4000
Carpet on concrete	0.02	0.06	0.14	0.37	0.60	0.65
Carpet on foam backing	0.08	0.24	0.57	0.69	0.71	0.73
Ceiling (acoustic tile)	0.45	0.55	0.60	0.90	0.86	0.75
Concrete (unpainted)	0.36	0.44	0.31	0.21	0.39	0.25
Concrete (painted)	0.10	0.05	0.06	0.07	0.09	0.08
Drapes (heavy velour)	0.14	0.35	0.55	0.72	0.70	0.65
Glass (window)	0.35	0.25	0.18	0.12	0.07	0.04
Plywood paneling	0.28	0.22	0.17	0.09	0.10	0.11
Upholstered seat (empty)	0.19	0.40	0.60	0.68	0.61	0.58
Upholstered seat (occupied)	0.49	0.66	0.80	0.88	0.82	0.7
Wallboard (gypsum)	0.29	0.10	0.05	0.04	0.07	0.19
Wooden floor	0.15	0.11	0.10	0.07	0.06	0.07

is affected by the presence of impurities, the shape of the barriers or objects that are made of this material, and their ability to vibrate. Notice in Table 6.1 that an upholstered seat, which is made of a soft, porous material, has much higher absorption coefficients at all frequencies than glass, which is a hard, nonporous material. However, notice also that the glass has a higher absorption coefficient for low-frequency sounds compared with high-frequency sounds, which is the reverse of the upholstered seat, in which the absorption coefficient is higher for high-frequency sounds. Glass and other objects that can vibrate easily can absorb more low-frequency energy than high-frequency energy. Porous material, such as concrete, can become less absorptive when its surface is painted since the paint becomes an additional, less porous, and more reflective layer on its surface.

Sound propagation outdoors is affected not only by the medium itself (i.e., air), but also by the absorption of sound by the ground, and it depends on various terrain features such as berms of earth, ruts in the ground, variations in the type of soil, and vegetation. For sound waves traveling close to the ground, this type of absorption may have a greater effect on wave absorption than the molecular absorption by the medium itself.

Sound Reflection

When a sound wave strikes the surface of a space boundary, part of its energy is absorbed by the boundary medium, whereas the remaining part of the sound energy is reflected back to the space. The reflective property of the boundary material is characterized by the **reflection coefficient (β)**, which is defined as:

$$\beta = \frac{I_{ref}}{I} \qquad (6.3)$$

where I is the sound intensity arriving at the space boundary and I_{ref} is the amount of energy reflected back from the boundary to the space. Similar to the absorption coefficient, the value of the reflection coefficient varies on a scale from 0 to 1 and depends on the frequency of the arriving sound wave and the molecular structure, density, uniformity, and temperature of the space boundary. Since the whole sound energy arriving at a specific surface is either absorbed (I_{abs}) or reflected (I_{ref}), then the total sound intensity at the surface of the boundary must be equal to the sum of the two:

$$I = I_{abs} + I_{ref} \qquad (6.4)$$

If you consider both Equations 6.2 and 6.3, it is obvious that the reflection coefficient (which varies from 0 to 1) and the absorption coefficient (which also varies from 0 to 1) must equal 1. In other words:

$$\alpha + \beta = 1$$

The fact that different materials have different abilities to absorb and reflect sound energy is used in architectural acoustics to control the amount of energy in specific acoustic spaces such as concert halls, classrooms, churches, hospitals, libraries, and so forth. Highly reflective walls also help to isolate one space from another by containing all the sound energy within the original space.

The energy of a wave arriving at a wall is reflected back to the space at an angle that is the mirror image of the angle at which the wave arrived. This effect is discussed in the next section of this chapter. If the wall is flat and smooth, all of the sound energy arriving at a specific angle is reflected in the same direction. If the wall is curved and rough, the sound energy reflected from different places on the wall may be reflected in different directions. Such spreading of reflections is called **dispersion** (diffusion). Thus, depending on the orientation and shape of the space boundaries and the smoothness of their surfaces, the reflected energy can be dispersed (scattered) throughout the space or reflected sounds can be focused in one or several specific areas. Dispersed sound is an important requirement in designing concert halls and other public listening spaces, so that reflected sounds are dispersed throughout the hall, rather than focused in a loud and clearly audible way in certain places in the room. In contrast, sometimes focused reflections are used for purposely channeling sound between two places in space, which make a talker located in one place clearly audible in another location. This situation is illustrated in Figure 6.2.

Situations like the one shown in Figure 6.2 exist in various "whispering galleries" that can be found in some old castles, royal gardens, science centers, and houses of worship. The walls of these rooms are specially angled or curved so that speech whispered at one place in the room can be clearly heard at another distant place of the room. Well-known "whispering galleries" include Statuary Hall in the U.S. Capitol, the Whispering Gallery in St. Paul's Cathedral in London, and the spherical Mapparium in the Christian Science Complex in Boston (Bate, 1938; Spotts, 2006).

Sound Refraction

When a sound wave strikes the surface of a wall, part of its energy travels through the surface and is absorbed by the wall material. As the sound enters the new medium, the speed of sound will change because the speed of sound is affected by

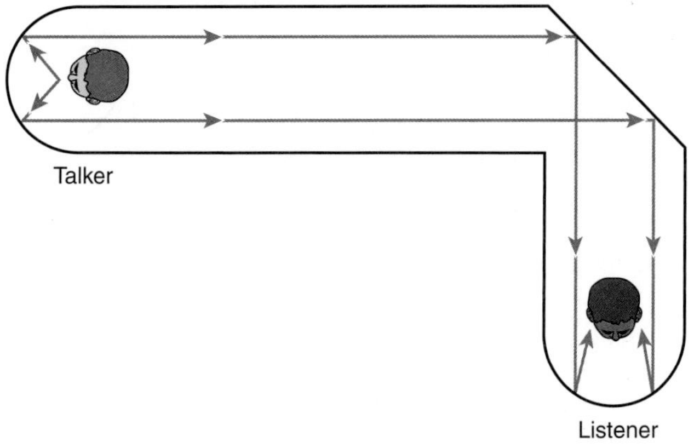

Figure 6.2. Example of a design directing reflected waves toward a specific point in space.

the stiffness and density of the new medium (Chapter 5). The sound frequency in the new medium remains the same, but since the speed of sound is different, the wavelength of the sound wave will change. In addition, the direction of the sound wave propagation in the new medium may change. The phenomenon of sound wave bending (changing direction) when the sound encounters a medium with a different density (and stiffness) is called **sound refraction.** To understand why sound refraction occurs, imagine a toy car traveling across a wooden floor and encountering a carpet. If one wheel of the car hits the carpet earlier than the other one, it will start moving more slowly due to the greater friction offered by the carpet's surface. At the same time, the other wheel will still travel at its original speed, moving over a larger distance on the wooden floor. The different speeds of the left and right wheels will make the car turn toward the wheel that is moving at a lower speed. An illustration of sound wave refraction is shown in Figure 6.3. The line that is

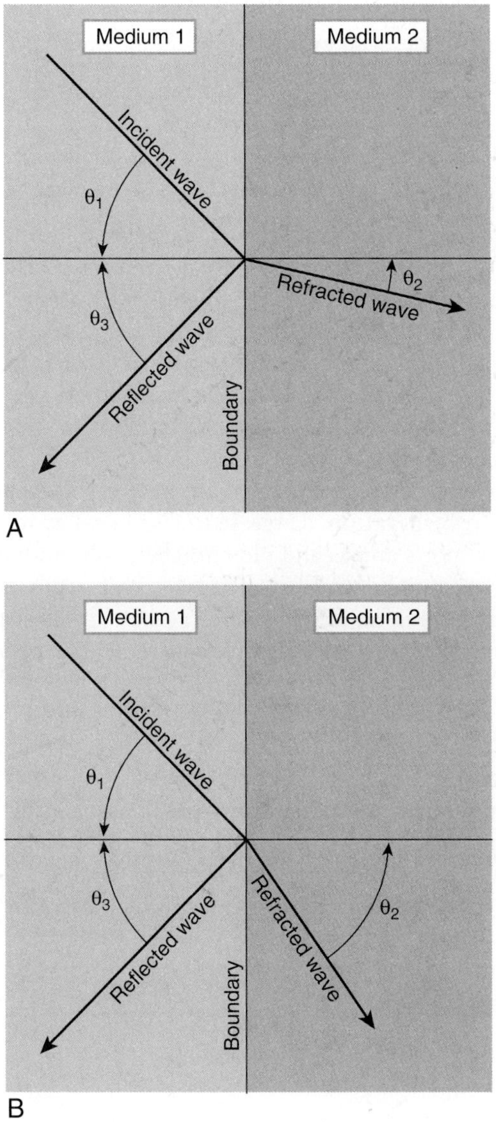

Figure 6.3. Sound wave refraction at the boundary of two media.

perpendicular to the boundary between medium 1 and medium 2 is the reference line. The **incident wave** is the original incoming sound wave. The incident wave approaches the boundary at a certain angle compared with the reference line. This is called the **angle of incidence** (θ_1). The **refracted wave** is the sound wave after it has entered the barrier. It also travels through the second medium at a certain angle (θ_2, the **angle of refraction**) compared to the perpendicular line. The **reflected wave** is the sound wave that has "bounced" off the wall into the original medium (with angle θ_3) in the opposite direction but at the same angle as the incidence angle (i.e., $\theta_1 = \theta_3$). Since the incidence wave and the reflected wave are traveling in the same medium, that is, at the same speed, the angles of incidence and reflection will be the same.

If a sound wave enters another medium where the speed of sound is lower than in the first medium (i.e., $c_1 > c_2$), then the sound wave will bend toward the reference line, that is, away from the boundary between the two media (Fig. 6.3A). In contrast, if the sound speed in the second medium is greater than in the first medium (i.e., $c_2 > c_1$), then the sound wave will bend away from the reference line, that is, toward the boundary between the two media (Fig. 6.3B). The relationship between the speed of wave propagation and the angle of refraction is known as **Snell's Law** after the Dutch mathematician Willebrord Snell (1580–1626). Snell's Law is usually stated using the Snell Equation:

$$\frac{\sin\theta_1}{c_1} = \frac{\sin\theta_2}{c_2} \tag{6.5}$$

where θ_1 is the angle of the incident wave in the first medium, θ_2 is the angle of the refracted wave in the second medium, and c_1 and c_2 are the speeds of sound in medium 1 and medium 2.

The phenomenon of refraction is very important in optics and everywhere else where energy travels in the form of a concentrated beam (ray) or as a plane wave. In acoustics, this effect explains the existence of specific "acoustic channels" in oceans and the behavior of ultrasound beams in medical and other applications. In hearing science, this effect is important for understanding sound behavior in rooms and outdoors. First, note that Snell's Law defines the relationship between the angle of the wave arriving at the reflective surface of a space and the angle of the reflected wave. Since the speed of sound of the arriving wave is the same as the speed of sound of the reflected wave but the directions are opposite, it means that $c_1 = -c_2$ and $\sin\theta_1 = -\sin\theta_2$. This means that the angle of the reflected wave is the mirror image of the angle of the arriving wave in respect to the dashed reference line shown in Figure 6.3.

Second, note that due to the effect of refraction, a sound wave entering a boundary with a denser medium and traveling at a sufficiently large angle of incidence may be bent at an angle past the boundary (i.e., greater than 90° from the reference line in Fig. 6.3). This means that the energy entering the second medium will actually re-enter the first medium, making the boundary 100% reflective for this angle of incidence. This phenomenon is known as **total internal reflection (TIR).** The smallest angle of incidence for which this effect occurs is called the **critical angle of incidence.** The critical angle of incidence (θ_{cr}) can be calculated using the Snell Equation (Equation 5.5) in which $\theta_2 = 90°$ (so $\sin\theta_2 = \sin 90° = 1$). Therefore:

$$\sin\theta_{1c} = \frac{c_1}{c_2} \tag{6.6}$$

To understand the phenomenon of total internal reflection, consider waves traveling from air to water. If the incident wave is perpendicular to the surface of the water, it will continue into the water at the same angle, staying perpendicular to the water's surface. If the incident wave then changes gradually away from perpendicular, the refracted wave will bend more and more toward the boundary. Beyond a certain angle of incidence (e.g., about 13° for air to water), the wave will bend so much that the wave will not enter the barrier but will be totally reflected back into air.

Sound wave bending occurs not only when sound waves enter two entirely different media, but also when they are traveling through a single medium that changes in its density, such as when sound travels through air that changes temperature. In the evening, the air just above the ground is warm and the temperature decreases with altitude. The opposite effect takes place in the morning where the air near the ground is cooler and the air temperature increases farther above the ground. This change in temperature with altitude is called a **temperature gradient.** Temperature gradients are also observed in water, where deeper water tends to be cooler than water at the surface. Since the speed of sound in warmer air is greater than the speed of sound in cooler air, sound waves bend toward the cooler air and away from the ground. This effect is illustrated in Figure 6.4. Notice in the figure that when warmer air is closer to the ground and colder air is above it, sound waves bend away from the ground; therefore, there is less sound energy arriving at the listener. This is called the **thermal effect.** In contrast, when cold air is closer to the ground and warmer air is above it, sound waves bend toward the ground; therefore, there is more sound energy arriving at the listener. This is called the **inverse thermal effect.** The two described thermal effects illustrate the fact that the changes in the audibility of sound waves in open space during the day and at night are the natural result of changes in sound refraction.

Sound and Wind

The presence of wind affects the speed of sound in the environment in a similar manner as the temperature gradient. In other words, changes in wind speed with height above the ground can result in sound refraction that affects the distance that sound can travel.*

The wind speed generally increases as altitude increases, causing a **wind shear** phenomenon, which acts similarly to the temperature gradient. This means that when the wind is blowing, the speed of sound is greater higher in the atmosphere than it is just above the ground. When a sound originates downwind (wind blowing from the sound source toward the listener), sound waves are bent toward the ground by the wind, increasing the distance that the waves can travel and still be heard. When a sound originates upwind (wind blowing from the listener toward the sound source), the sound waves are bent upward and dispersed in the atmosphere, limiting the distance that the waves can travel and creating an extended **shadow zone** (Heimann, 2003). A shadow zone is an area into which sound waves do not enter or in which the sound intensity is significantly decreased. The effects of wind on sound wave propagation downwind and upwind are shown in Figure 6.4.

Reverberation Time and Echo

The discussion of sound reflections in the previous sections focused on the amount of energy that is reflected and the angle of reflection. However, it is very important to realize that the reflected wave is also delayed in time compared to the direct wave. The time delay due to sound reflection is illustrated in Figure 6.5.

Consider the situation shown in Figure 6.5. The direct sound of the talker's speech needs to travel the distance d_o in order to reach the listener, whereas the reflected sound needs to travel the distance $d = d_1 + d_2$. This is just an example of a single sound reflection in a room in which there are thousands of reflections from many walls. However, this example demonstrates the basic concept of a sound delay.

The reflected sound energy within an enclosed space is called **reverberation.** Large spaces with reflective walls, such as sports arenas and old churches, will produce a lot of reverberation, while small spaces with walls covered with absorbing material, such as audiometric test booths and anechoic rooms, will produce very little reverberation. A common measure of the amount of reverberation is the reverberation time. **Reverberation time (RT)** is the duration of time needed for a sound pressure to decrease 1000 times (i.e., by 60 dB; see Chapter 7) after the sound source ceases its operation. The reverberation time depends on the volume and shape of the space and the reflective properties of the surrounding boundaries. It can be calculated using the Sabine Equation, named in honor of American physicist Wallace Sabine (1868–1919), who experimentally derived this formula. The Sabine Equation states:

$$RT = k\frac{V}{A} \tag{6.7}$$

where k is a constant that depends on the temperature of the air (e.g., $k = 0.161$ for $T = 22°C$), RT is reverberation time (in seconds), V is the volume of the room (or space) in m^3,

*Wind has a negligible effect on the perceived frequency (wavelength) of a sound wave because the speed of sound is much faster than the speed of the wind.

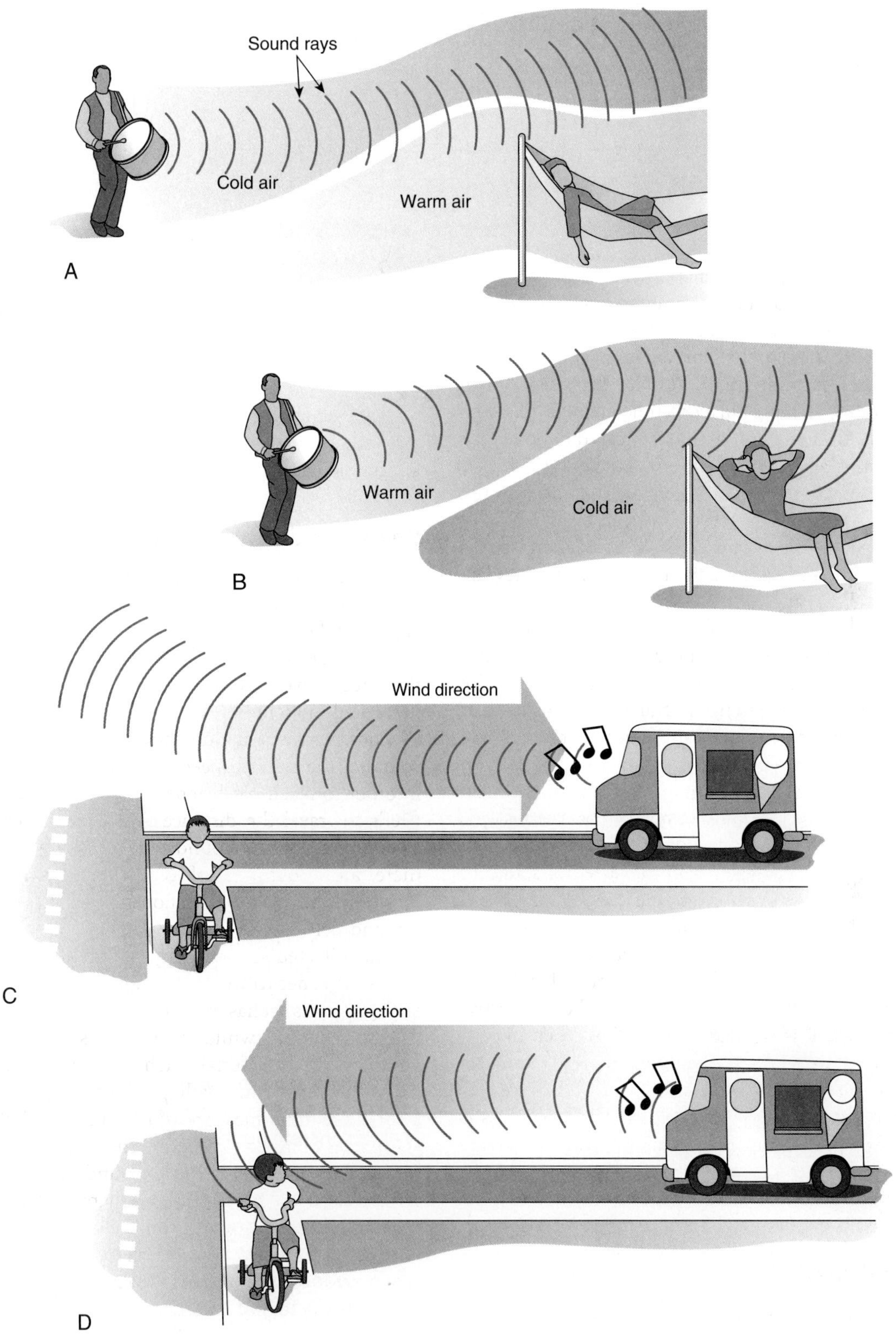

Figure 6.4. Refraction of sound waves due to the thermal and wind effects.

and A is the total absorption of the space boundaries. The total absorption (A) is calculated as:

$$A = S_1\alpha_1 + S_2\alpha_2 + S_3\alpha_3 + \cdots + S_n\alpha_n \quad (6.8)$$

where S_1 through S_n are the surfaces of the walls, floor, and ceiling surrounding the space and α_1 though α_n are the absorption coefficients of the individual surfaces. The total absorption of space boundaries (A), also called room absorption, is frequently expressed in units called *sabins* (m^2). Note also that reverberation time changes with the frequency of sound since the absorption coefficients of the space boundaries are frequency dependent.

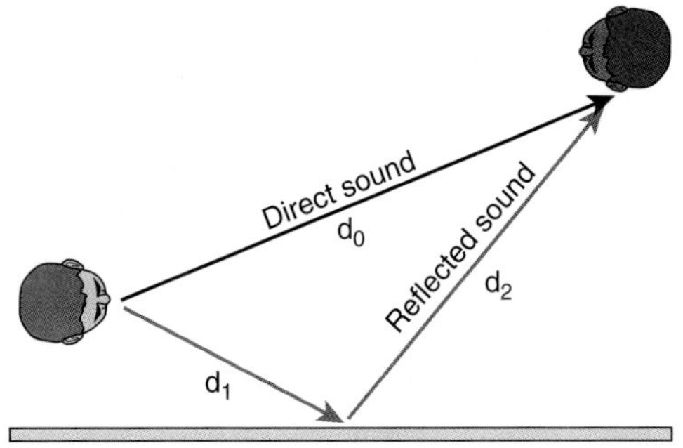

Figure 6.5. Direct and reflected sound in a closed space.

Example 6.1

Estimate the reverberation time for a 2000-Hz tone in a room that is 7 m (long) × 5 m (wide) × 4 m (tall) with gypsum wallboard covering the floors and ceiling, no windows, a 2 m × 1 m door made of plywood, and a carpet over concrete.

First, determine the surface area of each part of the room that is made of different materials including the door, the floor, the walls, and the ceiling.

$$\text{Door (plywood)} = 2 \times 1 = 2 \text{ m}^2$$

$$\text{Walls (wallboard): Two long walls: } 7 \times 4 = 28 \times 2 \text{ walls} = 56 \text{ m}^2$$

$$\text{Two shorter walls: } 5 \times 4 = 20 \times 2 \text{ walls} = 40 \text{ m}^2$$

$$\text{All four walls minus the door} = 56 + 40 - 2 = 94 \text{ m}^2$$

$$\text{Ceiling (wallboard): } 7 \times 5 = 35 \text{ m}^2$$

$$\text{All wallboard areas (walls and ceiling): } 94 + 35 = 129 \text{ m}^2$$

$$\text{Floor (carpet over concrete): } 7 \times 5 = 35 \text{ m}^2$$

Second, determine the absorption coefficient of each type of surface for 2000 Hz from Table 6.1.

$$\text{Door (plywood)} = 0.10$$

$$\text{Walls and ceiling (gypsum wallboard)} = 0.07$$

$$\text{Floor (carpet over concrete)} = 0.6$$

Third, determine the absorption (A) of the room using Equation 6.8.

$$A = S_1\alpha_1 + S_2\alpha_2 + S_3\alpha_3 + \cdots + S_n\alpha_n$$

$$A = (2 \times 0.10) + (129 \times 0.07) + (35 \times 0.6)$$

$$A = 30.23$$

Fourth, calculate the volume of the entire room (Chapter 2).

$$\text{Volume of a rectangle} = \text{length} \times \text{width} \times \text{height}$$

$$\text{Volume} = 7 \times 5 \times 4 = 140 \text{ m}^3$$

Fifth, select Equation 6.7 to calculate the reverberation time of the room.

$$RT = 0.161\frac{V}{A}$$

Substitute the variables you determined in steps 3 and 4.

$$RT = 0.161\frac{140}{30.23}$$

$$\text{RT} = 0.75 \text{ seconds}$$

Answer: The reverberation time of this room is 0.75 seconds.

Note that the Sabine Equation was experimentally derived and it does not work equally well for all listening conditions. It predicts RT well for rooms with highly reflective walls but is less accurate for rooms that are highly damped. For example, if all of the absorption coefficients in a room are equal to 1, then the RT should equal 0; however according to the Sabine Equation, the RT can never equal zero. Other theoretically derived estimates of RT, which work well for highly damped rooms, were proposed later by several authors and are available in books on room acoustics. Two of the most widely used formulas are the Norris-Eyring Equation and the Millinton-Sette Equation.

PRACTICE PROBLEMS: SABINE EQUATION

1. Estimate the reverberation time for a 1000-Hz tone in a room that is 3.1 m × 3.1 m × 3.1 m with gypsum wallboard covering the floors and ceiling, no windows, a 3.3 m × 0.8 m door made of plywood, and a carpet on a foam backing.
2. What would be the effect on the reverberation time from problem 1 if the foam backing was not used and the carpet was put directly on the concrete floor?
3. Estimate the reverberation time for a 2000-Hz tone in a room that is 4 m × 5 m × 3.5 m with painted concrete walls, 4 square meters of widows, a 3.3 m × 0.8 m door made of plywood, a wooden floor, and a ceiling with acoustic tile.

Answers (If you need help with these problems, consult the website.) **Link 6-1**

1. 0.55 s
2. The RT increased to 0.84 s.
3. 0.52 s

Reverberation time can vary from practically zero (no reflections) to several seconds in large and reflective spaces. For example, Lord Rayleigh (1877) observed an RT of 12 seconds in one of the churches in Pisa. This is an extremely long RT, since RTs longer than 2 seconds are considered long for most applications. Large empty classrooms or similar spaces with a lot of highly reflective surfaces have an average* RT of about 1.0 to 2.0 seconds. These rooms are frequently referred to as "live" rooms. An empty, tiled bathroom and a high school cafeteria are examples of "live" rooms. Medieval churches, domes, and large warehouses may have RTs on the order of 3.0 to 5.0 seconds or more. A small concert hall with an RT around 1.5 seconds is good for playing chamber music and concert halls with an RT of about 2.0 to 2.5 seconds are good for classical and romantic music. For example, Carnegie Hall in New York and the Symphony Hall in Boston have an average RT of about 1.7, and the Kennedy Center in Washington, DC, has an RT of about 2.2 seconds (Beranek, 1962). In order to direct sounds from the stage to the audience in such spaces, strong but diffuse reflections from the walls and the ceiling are needed. The floor and the seats (the audience) in the theaters and concert halls are usually considered 100% absorptive.

Rooms with a lot of highly absorbing surfaces and soft furniture may have average RTs as low as 0.3 to 0.5 seconds. Such rooms are often called "dead" rooms. Control rooms in recording studios are generally "dead" rooms, so the monitored recorded music is not affected by the acoustic properties of the room. Libraries also tend to have small RTs to limit the background noise level for reading and studying purposes.

Of great importance in hearing science is the acoustics surrounding the design of classrooms. Classroom environments in which there is a high level of background noise from heating, ventilating, and air condition (HVAC) systems; electronic instructional equipment (e.g., overhead projectors); multitalker noise; and so forth are not conducive to learning. A high level of reverberation has a negative effect on the learning environment, since it can enhance the background noise and additionally affect the perception of a teacher's voice even in a quiet classroom. Classrooms with a high RT have reflected speech sounds that overlap and mask (cover) the teacher's speech. This decreases the ability of all children (and especially children with hearing loss) to hear a clear signal and it negatively affects their academic achievement. An American National Standard (ANSI S12.60-2002) suggests that the RT in core learning spaces should be less than 0.6 second for small classrooms (<283 m^3) and less than 0.7 second for moderate-sized classrooms (between 283 and 566 m^3). For larger classrooms (e.g., gymnasiums) the RT is not specified; however, the standard lists guidelines for the control of reverberation via the percentage of wall, floor, and ceiling space that should contain absorptive materials and guidelines for the types of materials that should be used.

Closed spaces with highly reflective surfaces that do not absorb arriving sounds are called **reverberation chambers** (reverberation rooms). Reverberation chambers are built to create a diffuse sound field in which the same amount of sound energy is arriving from each direction. In the ideal reverberation room, the sound intensity at a specific point in space is independent of the specific location of the sound source in the room, so no matter where you are in the room, the sound intensity is the same. Well-designed reverberation rooms for scientific purposes have highly reflective nonparallel walls, floors, and ceilings and a number of additional reflective objects that help to diffuse reflected sounds.

When the difference between distance d_0 and distance $d_1 + d_2$ in Figure 6.5 is small, direct and reflected sounds arrive at the listener at about the same time and practically overlap in time, making the total sound more intense (louder). When the difference in time between d_0 and $d_1 + d_2$ becomes slightly larger, the delayed reflected sound will overlap part of the original sound, making the resulting sound last slightly longer and causing the sound to be less clear. Above a certain time delay, the reflected sound will arrive so late that it will be a repetition rather than a continuation of the original sound. This effect is called an **echo.** An echo is the repetition of an original sound caused by reflected sound waves. An echo is perceived when the distinct (strong) reflected sound arrives about 50 ms or more after the original sound. This time difference corresponds to about 17 meters of additional distance traveled by the sound waves (assuming a speed of sound of 340 m/s). Acoustic engineers and architects who design theaters, opera houses, concert halls, and courts must carefully consider this distance in their designs to avoid potential echoes from the walls and ceiling. A special case of an echo is the flutter echo, which is a series of multiple echoes created by reflections between parallel walls. Thus, larger spaces in which flutter echo can be audible should avoid parallel walls. If you would like to hear examples of sound reflections, go to the website. **Audio clip 6-1**

In contrast to the highly reflective reverberation chambers, specialized rooms with very soft walls, ceilings, and floors that absorb most of the arriving sound are called **anechoic chambers** (anechoic rooms). In the ideal anechoic chamber all of the sound energy arriving at the walls, ceiling, and floor is absorbed and there are no sound reflections off the room boundaries. Anechoic chambers are designed to simulate a reflection-free sound propagation condition in which sound propagates, like in the outdoors, far away from the ground.

The word *anechoic* is a Greek word that means "without echo," but almost all rooms are "without echo." While there are often reflections from the walls of most rooms, most of the reflections are not greater than 50 ms (the minimum time required for a true echo). True echoes are common in caverns and canyons and near mountains, but not in living rooms or classrooms. Therefore, note that an anechoic room

*The average RT means the RT measured at 500 Hz (typically) or 1000 Hz.

should actually be called "a room without reverberation" since this is a room with very little or no reflected energy. In our opinion, the lingering use of the word *echo* to mean any reflection (reverberation) is incorrect. If you would like to listen to sounds produced in various reverberant spaces, go to the website. **Audio clip 6-2**

Sound Diffraction

When a sound wave propagating through the air arrives at an obstacle that partially blocks the path of the wave, the behavior of the sound wave depends on the relationship between the wavelength (λ) of the sound and the smallest dimension (d) of the obstacle that is facing the direction of the propagating wave. Two such situations are shown in Figure 6.6. For cases where the dimensions of the obstacle are *much larger* than the wavelength, that is $d >> \lambda$, the wave will be reflected from the obstacle, creating an **acoustic shadow**, which is an area behind an obstacle that the direct sound wave does not enter (Fig. 6.6A). If the dimensions of the obstacle are *much smaller* than the wavelength, that is $d << \lambda$, the sound waves enter the area behind the obstacle and an acoustic shadow does not exist. When the dimensions of the obstacle are comparable with the wavelength, that is, $d \cong \lambda$, part of the sound energy enters the area behind the obstacle (i.e., it bends around the obstacle) and decreases the size of the acoustic shadow, but some area of the shadow will still remain (Fig. 6.6B).

The phenomenon of sound waves bending around objects and through openings in boundaries is called **sound diffraction.** This term was coined by Italian physicist Francesco Grimaldi (1618–1663), who first described this phenomenon. The amount of diffraction (the degree of bending) increases as the wavelength of the sound wave increases. The theory of wave diffraction has its origin in the Huygens' Principle published in 1678 by the Dutch physicist Christian Huygens (1629–1695). The Huygens' Principle states that each point on the wavefront becomes the source of a new spherical wave, called a wavelet, which is a small, localized spherical wave with the same wavelength but a reduced intensity compared to the original wavefront. After a certain time (Δt) one new wavefront is created from all the secondary waves. A graphic representation of the Huygens' Principle is shown in Figure 6.7.

According to the Huygens' Principle, a sound wave arriving at the edge of an object creates a new spherical wave that can enter the area behind the object. The longer the wavelength, the easier it is for the wave to enter the space behind the obstacle, the stronger the effect of diffraction, and the smaller the acoustic shadow behind the object. Similarly, a sound wave arriving at an opening in a boundary that is much smaller than the wavelength of the propagating wave can expand beyond the opening due to the effect of diffraction, becoming the source of a new spherical wave.

Diffraction of sound waves around obstacles is the physical reason for people hearing sound sources located on the

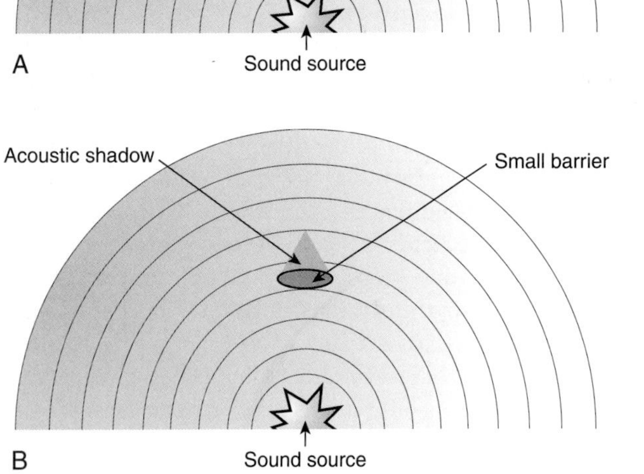

Figure 6.6. Sound diffraction around **(A)** a large barrier resulting in an acoustic shadow and **(B)** a small barrier resulting in a much smaller acoustic shadow.

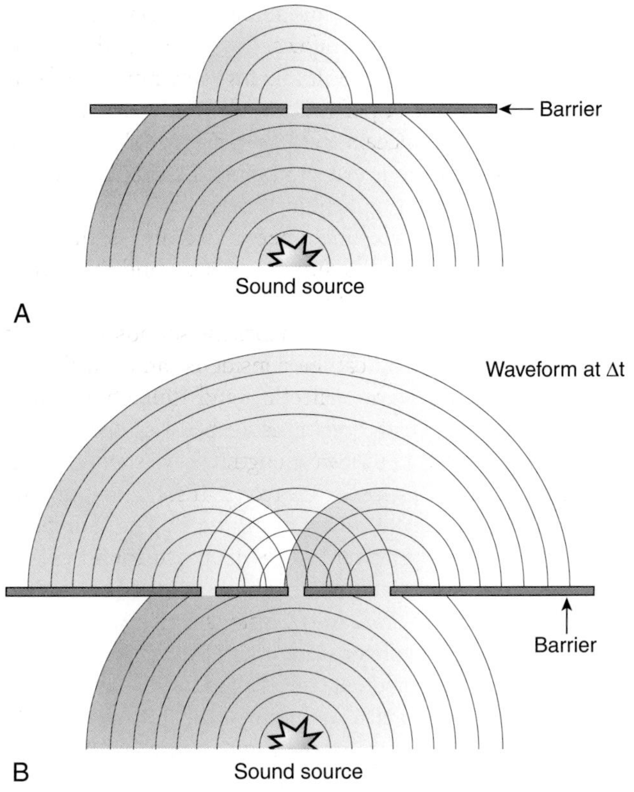

Figure 6.7. Illustration of sound diffraction through **(A)** a single hole in a barrier and **(B)** multiple holes in a barrier. Notice in frame B that after a certain period of time (Δt), the wavefront of the whole wave is reconstructed from the individual wavelets based on Huygens' Principle.

other side of barriers or around the corner of a building. Imagine a marching band walking along a street and approaching a road crossing. If you are standing on a perpendicular street you will hear the drums and other low-frequency instruments long before the band enters the cross section. Gradually, the higher frequency (higher pitch) instruments become audible and finally you see the marching band and hear all of the frequencies. You will hear the drum first because low frequencies have the longest wavelengths and are diffracted (bent) most efficiently around the corners. However, you may not hear the triangle, flute, or piccolo until you can actually see the musicians playing these instruments. This is because their frequencies may be so high that they are not diffracted at all.

Diffraction and sound reflections are also the reason that it is very difficult to localize a heavy vehicle (such as a dump truck or tank) moving in a city. The truck produces a lot of low-frequency sounds, which diffract around corners and are reflected from buildings. You hear the sound from a large distance but the direction is not clear because sounds have been reflected and bent around obstacles rather than arriving via a straight pathway. The effect of sound diffraction also helps low-frequency sounds travel a longer distance in a forest where high-frequency sounds are easily attenuated and dispersed by the absorption and reflection of sound by trees and bushes.

A good understanding of the effect of diffraction is needed for engineers designing screens and barriers that protect people from harmful sounds or provide some amount of privacy in open offices. For example, the sound walls or berms placed adjacent to a highway must be of sufficient height to protect people living behind them from the low-frequency noise of cars and trucks diffracted around the top of the barriers. Note that the cars and trucks on a highway create a lot of low-frequency noise, and if the barriers are not high enough or the berms are not sufficiently absorbent, the sound will simply diffract around the barrier and enter into the space behind it.

The effect of diffraction also shapes the sounds arriving at our ears. A human head can be considered an obstacle to a propagating sound wave, reflecting and diffracting sound energy depending on the relationship between the dimensions of the head and the wavelength of the sound. High-frequency sounds, with short wavelengths, do not diffract around the head and therefore enter the farther ear with a lower intensity than the ear that is nearer to the incoming sound. Low-frequency sounds have wavelengths that are much longer than the head dimensions and arrive at both ears with similar intensity; however, their arrival time may be different. These differences in sound between the right and left ears provide the auditory system with important cues for locating the direction of sound (Chapter 8).

Sound Interference

When two or more sound waves propagate in the same medium, they travel independently and can pass through each other. In regions where they overlap, their pressures add together and their individual behaviors become disturbed. This effect is called **sound interference.** Sound interference is the combination (superposition) of two or more propagating waves. Sound interference can be observed between sounds generated by different sound sources, by the same sound diffracted around an obstacle, or between the original sound and its reflection off a boundary. For example, sound reflected from a wall or an object interacts with the original sound when the original wave and reflected waves pass each other.

If two overlapping waves of the same wavelength are in-phase (i.e., their compressions and rarefactions coincide), their interference is called **constructive interference.** In general, constructive interference is any interference that results in a wave having a larger amplitude than both of the component waves. If the two waves are out-of-phase and the resulting wave has lower amplitude than at least one of the component waves, their interference is called **destructive interference.** If both waves have identical frequencies and amplitudes and are 180° out-of-phase, they cancel each other out completely. As a general rule, when the two sound waveforms differ in one or more characteristics (e.g., frequency, amplitude, phase, waveform), the shape of the resulting overlapping waveform can be determined by applying the rules of waveform synthesis described in Chapter 4 to sound.

An example of an interference of two waves generated at two different points in space is shown in Figure 6.8. This is an interference of two waveforms created by the diffraction of one original wave passing through two small openings in a space boundary. The arrows in Figure 6.8 indicate the points where the compressions from one wave meet compressions from the other wave and where the rarefactions from one wave meet the rarefactions from the other wave. At these points, constructive interference occurs and the combination of the maximum positive magnitudes or maximum negative magnitudes from the waves will result in an increased magnitude at those points. Other arrows indicate the points where the compressions from one wave meet the rarefactions from the other wave. At these points, destructive interference occurs. Obviously, there will also be interference at all of the other places in the space, with varying amounts of constructive and destructive interference, depending on the magnitude and phase of each sine wave across the space and time.

The interference pattern in the space can be quite complex and it depends on the number of sound sources, the number of reflective surfaces, and the direction of propagation of individual waves. Most importantly, this pattern changes in time as each of the contributing waves continues its propagation.

Standing Waves

A standing wave (stationary wave) is a special case of wave interference when the sound is bouncing between two

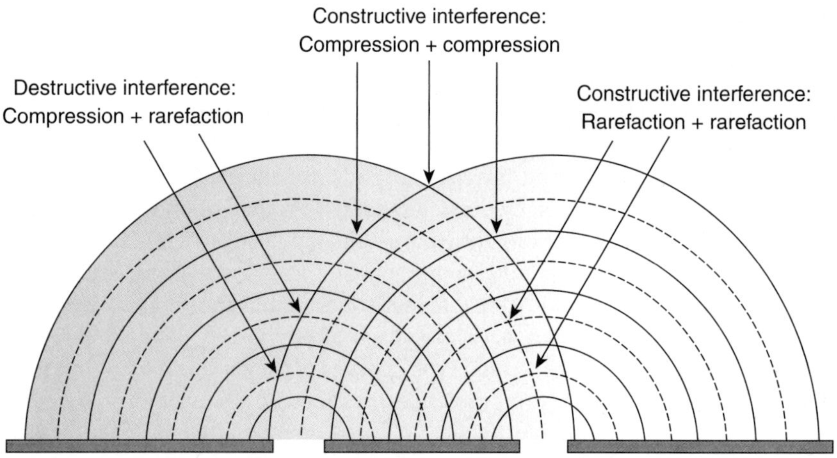

Figure 6.8. The interference of two sounds of the same frequency. The solid lines represent the maximum compressions of each wave and the dashed lines represent the maximum rarefactions of each wave. The points at which compressions meet compressions and rarefactions meet rarefactions will increase the amplitude of the wave (constructive interferences). The points at which a compression meets a rarefaction will decrease the amplitude (destructive interference).

reflected parallel surfaces producing nodes and antinodes that are identical in nature to those observed in the mechanic systems from Chapter 4 (e.g., strings, rods, and plates). This means that a standing wave is an interference that is stationary and does not propagate in a space. In both mechanic and acoustic systems, the observed behavior of standing waves is identical and the only difference is the type of medium. Standing waves can also be generated in pipes and tubes with open ends (e.g., the ear canal).

The frequency of a standing wave is the resonance frequency of a system (Chapter 4). Recall that the resonance frequency is the natural frequency of a system (i.e., the frequency at which a system would vibrate in free vibration or the frequency at which a system will vibrate at its greatest amplitude when the system is forced to vibrate). Standing waves in the resonator box of a musical instrument are an important part of musical instrument design because they amplify the energy produced by the vibrations of the instrument at certain frequencies. A well-designed musical instrument has its resonator (i.e., the body of the instrument) tuned in such a way that its resonance frequencies (i.e., standing waves) equally support all of the musical notes played on the instrument. However, standing waves are a real nuisance in architectural acoustics and room acoustics since they produce areas of increased and decreased intensity across the space. If a room has a standing wave with a wavelength that is comparable with the size of the human head, a person can move his or her head slightly to the left and to the right and hear the sound only in the left or in the right ear.

The potential for creating standing waves in an audiometric test room (hearing test room) is the reason that sound signals generated by loudspeakers for hearing testing should be complex signals rather than pure tones. If a pure tone is presented through a loudspeaker to determine a patient's hearing threshold, it is possible that one of the test frequencies may be one of the standing wave frequencies of the room. This means that in different places in the room the test tone may be much louder or softer than intended, and that will result in an inaccurate hearing test. For this reason, the signals used for sound field testing should be complex signals such as warble tones (tones that fluctuate in frequency) and narrow bands of noise.

Beats

Beats represent a special case of sound interference. **Beats** are slow periodic amplitude fluctuations caused when two sine waves that are very close in frequency interfere with one another. They occur due to the periodically changing phase relationship between the two pure tones. The difference in frequency between the tones must be less than about 30 Hz. Let us consider two tones having frequencies of 200 Hz and 208 Hz propagating together in space. When the sounds are combined, the interference results in a new waveform with a basic frequency (f_o), which is the mean frequency of the two component frequencies (f_1 and f_2):

$$f_o = \frac{f_1 + f_2}{2}$$

For 200 Hz and 208 Hz tones the average frequency is 204 Hz. The number of times per second that the amplitude of the combined sound wave fluctuates, that is, the number of beats (pulses) that occur per second, is called the **beat frequency** and it is equal to the difference between the two frequencies.

$$f_{beats} = f_2 - f_1$$

In the present example, f_1 is 200 Hz and f_2 is 208 Hz, so the beat frequency is 208 − 200 = 8 Hz (you can't have a negative number of beats, so always subtract the lower from the higher frequency). Two component waveforms and the combined waveform are shown in Figure 6.9. If you would like to listen to beats of various frequencies, go to the website. **Audio clip 6-3**

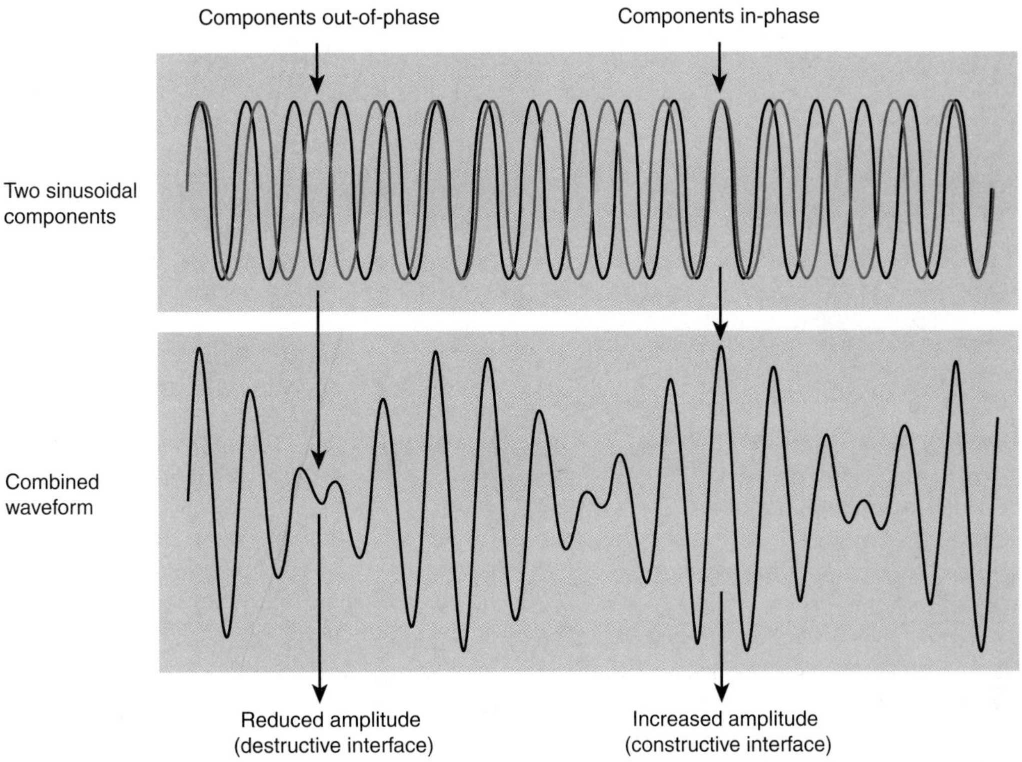

Figure 6.9. Two sinusoidal components that have close (but not identical) frequencies combined to form beats.

Doppler Effect

The **Doppler effect** is a shift in the frequency of a sound wave resulting from the movement of a sound source, the movement of a listener, changes in the medium, or a combination of these factors. The effect is named after the Austrian physicist Christian Doppler (1803–1853), who originally described this effect in 1842. The Doppler effect is heard as an increase in the frequency of an approaching sound source (e.g., train whistle, ambulance siren) followed by a similar decrease in frequency when the sound source passes the listener and is moving away. A similar effect can be observed when a listener is in a car passing a stationary sound source.

In order to explain the physical bases of the Doppler effects, let us recall from Chapter 5 that the wavelength of sound is described by the equation:

$$\lambda = \frac{c}{f} \tag{6.9}$$

where c is the speed of sound, f is the frequency of the sound generated by the sound source, and λ is the resulting wavelength of the sound. This equation applies to a situation in which both the sound source and the listener are stationary. Let us now consider situations in which the listener moves toward the sound source or a sound source moves toward the listener.

Listener Moving Toward a Sound Source

When a listener is moving toward a sound source, the actual speed of sound affecting the listener is equal to the sum of the speed of sound in air (c) and the velocity of the listener (v_l). Thus, the frequency of the sound arriving at the listener is equal to:

$$f = \frac{c + v_l}{\lambda} \tag{6.10}$$

If we replace the wavelength (λ) in Equation 6.10 with Equation 6.9 (i.e., $\frac{c}{f}$) and then simplify the equation, we can relate the frequency of the sound received by the listener (f_l) moving toward the sound source to the frequency (f) generated by the sound source as follows:

$$f_l = f\left(\frac{c + v_l}{c}\right) \tag{6.11}$$

When the listener moves away from the sound source, then Equation 6.11 takes the following form:

$$f_l = f\left(\frac{c - v_l}{c}\right) \tag{6.12}$$

Example 6.2

If a listener is moving with a velocity of 20 m/s toward a sound source producing a 2000-Hz tone, what is the sound frequency perceived by the listener (assuming that the speed of sound is 340 m/s)?

First, select Equation 6.11 because the listener is moving toward the sound source.

$$f_l = f\left(\frac{c + v_l}{c}\right)$$

Substitute known variables and solve.

$$f_l = 2000\left(\frac{340 + 20}{340}\right)$$

$$f_l = 2117.647059$$

Answer: The perceived frequency by the listener is 2117.65 Hz.

Sound Source Moving Toward a Listener

When the listener is moving toward the sound source, the listener's speed affects the sound frequency, but the actual sound wavelength in the medium is not affected. However, when the sound source moves toward the listener, the wavelength of sound in the medium is affected and it gets shorter. A sound with a shorter wavelength has a higher frequency. This effect is schematically shown in Figure 6.10. Let us assume that a sound source moves toward a listener with velocity (v_s). The wavelength of the sound in air is determined by the difference between the speed of sound and the speed of the sound source:

$$\lambda = \frac{c - v_s}{f} \tag{6.13}$$

Equation 6.9 ($\lambda = \frac{c}{f}$) can be rewritten by isolating the frequency as follows:

$$f = \frac{c}{\lambda} \tag{6.14}$$

If you replace λ in Equation 6.14 with Equation 6.13, the relationship between the original frequency made by the sound source (f) and the frequency heard by the listener (f_l) can be determined:

$$f_l = f\left(\frac{c}{c - v_s}\right) \tag{6.15}$$

Similarly, when the sound source is moving away from the listener, Equation 6.14 takes this form:

$$f_l = f\left(\frac{c}{c + v_s}\right) \tag{6.16}$$

All four equations (6.13, 6.14, 6.15, and 6.16), considered together, explain the Doppler effect mathematically. In order to determine the Doppler effect, one needs to consider the direction of motion and if the sound source or the listener is moving. In general, if the listener and the sound source are getting closer together, the listener hears a higher frequency; when they move apart, the listener hears a lower frequency.

Example 6.3

If a 1000-Hz sound source travels toward a listener with a velocity of 45 mph, what is the shift in the frequency of the sound heard by the listener (assuming that the speed of sound is 340 m/s)?

First, convert 45 mph into m/s. Since 1 mile = 1609 meters and there are 3600 seconds in an hour, then 45 mph is equal to about 20 m/s. Next, select the appropriate

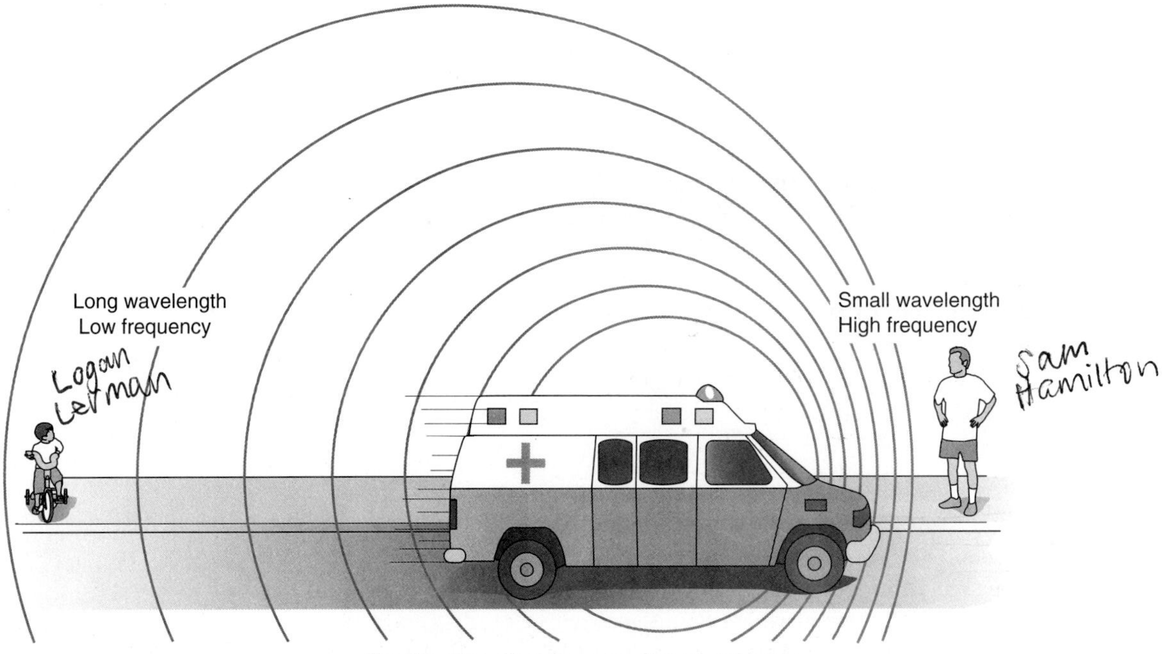

Figure 6.10. The Doppler effect is the perception of increased pitch caused by shorter wavelengths reaching the listener.

equation, which is Equation 6.15, because the sound source is traveling toward the listener.

$$f_l = f\left(\frac{c}{c - v_s}\right)$$

Substitute known variables into the equation and simplify.

$$f_l = 1000\text{ Hz}\left(\frac{340\text{ m/s}}{340\text{ m/s} - 20\text{m/s}}\right)$$

$$f_l = \frac{340{,}000}{320}$$

$$f_l = 1063\text{ Hz}$$

The question asks not about f_l but about the shift, so subtract:

$$1063 - 1000 = 63$$

Answer: The resulting shift in frequency is 63 Hz.

This shift equals about a 6% change in the original frequency of the sound (which corresponds to a musical semitone).

In some cases both the sound source and the listener move simultaneously. In such cases, Equations 6.11 or 6.12 and 6.15 or 6.16, depending on the directions of movement, need to be combined together to determine perceived sound frequency. The universal Doppler effect equation is written as follows:

$$f_l = f\left(\frac{c \pm v_l}{c \mp v_s}\right) \tag{6.17}$$

where the top signs apply to the case when the source and the listener move toward each other and the bottom signs apply to the situation when they move away from each other. If you would like hear an example of the Doppler effect, go to the website. **Audio clip 6-4**

PRACTICE PROBLEMS: DOPPLER EFFECT

Assume for these problems that the speed of sound is 340 m/s (speed of sound in air under standard conditions).

1. If a listener is moving with a velocity of 10 m/s toward a sound source and the sound source is producing a 1000-Hz tone, what is the sound frequency perceived by the listener?
2. If a listener is moving with a velocity of 5 m/s toward a sound source and the sound source is producing a 2000-Hz tone, what is the sound frequency perceived by the listener?
3. If a sound source is moving with a velocity of 50 m/s toward a listener and the sound source is producing a 3000-Hz tone, what is the sound frequency perceived by the listener?
4. If a sound source is moving with a velocity of 43 m/s away from a listener and the sound source is producing a 500-Hz tone, what is the sound frequency perceived by the listener?
5. If a listener is moving with a velocity of 10 m/s toward a sound source producing a 2000-Hz tone and simultaneously the sound source is moving toward the listener with a velocity of 20 m/s, what is the perceived frequency as the sound source passes the listener?

Answers (If you need help with these problems, consult the website.) **Link 6-2**

1. 1029.41 Hz
2. 2029.41 Hz
3. 3517.24 Hz
4. 443.86 Hz
5. 2187.5 Hz

Shock Waves and Sonic Boom

The Doppler effect applies to situations in which the velocity of a moving object is lower than the speed of sound. However, modern airplanes and space vehicles can move with a velocity that exceeds the speed of sound.* Bullets and other projectiles also fly faster than the speed of sound. As a matter of fact, the ratio of the speed of an aircraft to the speed of sound is used in aerodynamics to describe an important aircraft characteristic called the **Mach number** (M), where Mach 1 (M = 1) denotes the speed of sound. Aircrafts are classified into subsonic (M $<$ 1), transonic (M $\cong$ 1), supersonic (1 $<$ M $<$ 5), and hypersonic (M $>$ 5) categories. For example, the French-British commercial aircraft Concorde could fly with a speed just over 2 M, the SR-71 Blackbird military aircraft can fly at over 3 M, and the space shuttle re-enters Earth's atmosphere with a speed of about 25 M. In contrast, a Boeing 747 has a top speed of about 0.8 M. The Mach number was named in honor of the Austrian physicist Ernest Mach (1838–1916), who first deduced and mathematically confirmed the existence of a special medium deformation called a **shock wave** during the supersonic motion of a projectile.

In cases where a moving object travels at or faster than the speed of sound it compresses the medium in front of itself and takes this compressed waveform with it. This compressed clump of air is called a shock wave and it is a source

*Recall that at high altitudes the speed of sound is less than at the ground. For example, at the altitude of 12 km, speed of sound is about 290 m/s. Therefore, an aircraft flying at this altitude with a speed higher than 290 m/s is traveling faster than sound.

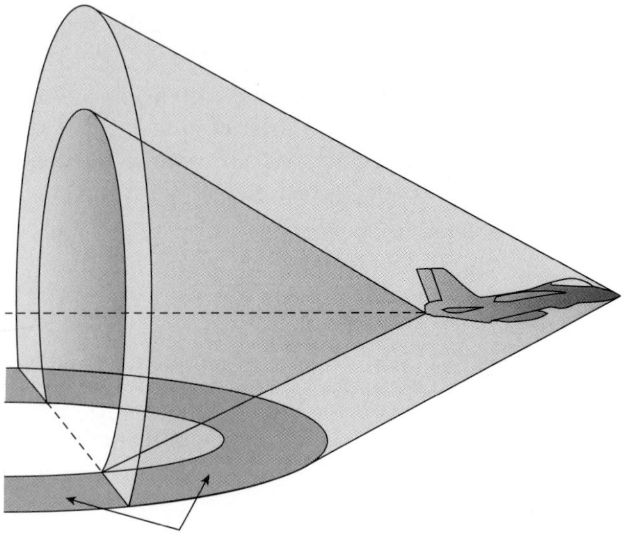

Figure 6.11. The shock wave zone created by a supersonic aircraft. The sonic boom is created by the beginning and the end of the zone.

of sound when it reaches a listener. Other examples of shock waves are deformations in air density produced by lightning strikes and explosions. One other example of a shock wave is the movement at the tip of a bullwhip, which moves faster than sound and creates a "cracking" noise. A **sonic boom** is heard as a very loud "thunder," "thud," or "thump" noise. If an object travels with the speed of sound, the shock wave travels with the object and a listener located in front of the moving object will hear nothing until the object arrives.

A supersonic aircraft moving through air actually produces two shock waves. The aircraft produces a sudden increase in medium pressure at its nose, which decreases gradually to a negative pressure at the aircraft tail and returns suddenly back to normal. This wave pattern is similar to the wave pattern at the bow and stern of a moving boat, and it is frequently referred to as an N wave (N-shaped wave). Thus, the N wave created by the supersonic aircraft is a series of two shock waves (positive and negative) that usually produces two sonic booms resulting in a double thump. The concept of the sonic boom created by the N-shaped shock wave of a supersonic aircraft is shown in Figure 6.11.

SOUND FIELD

A **sound field** is a term commonly used to describe a space containing sound waves. The same space is also called an acoustic space, a soundscape, or an acoustic environment depending on the type of literature and the focus of the author. The character of the sound field is dependent on the medium, the boundaries, and the sound sources operating in the space. Close to the sound source, the sound field is composed of several different direct sound fields produced by the various parts of the vibrating source. For example, if you examine the pressure disturbance very close to a vibrating membrane, the various parts of the membrane create different sound fields that interfere with each other. In addition, the sound wave produced by one part of the membrane may be absorbed or reflected by another part of the membrane. The resulting variations in sound pressure near the sound source are referred to as the **near field** of the sound source. The near field is characterized by large and nonuniform local maxima and minima in acoustic pressure that gradually disappear into a more uniform signal with increasing distance from the sound source.

As we move farther away from the source, the nonuniform changes in the sound field gradually disappear and the resulting sound field becomes more uniform and there is a gradual decrease in sound pressure following the inverse square law as one moves away from the source. The region of uniformly decreasing sound pressure ($1/r$) observed far away from the sound source is called the **far field.** The boundary between the near and far fields is located at the point of the farthest local maximum of sound pressure beyond which the sound pressure decreases smoothly following the inverse square law (Chapter 5). It can be said that outside the near field the sound source can be considered as a small radiating object (point source). The distance between the sound source and the boundary between the near and far fields depends on the size of the sound source and the wavelength of the radiated sound and it can be calculated as $2d^2/\lambda$, where d is the largest dimension of the sound source and λ is the wavelength of the radiated sound (Lecklider, 2005). In most practical applications, the border between the near field and far field can be considered to be at a distance that is about three times the length of the largest dimension of the sound source. For example, if the cone of an unmounted loudspeaker is 50 cm across, the boundary between the near field and far field is 150 cm from the sound source. For small sound sources, the distance between the sound source and the boundary between the near field and the far field is typically less than 1 meter. Therefore, a 1-meter distance is commonly used as a standardized distance for measuring sound properties in the far sound field for hearing research.

The concept of near field and far field applies to a situation in which a sound source radiates its energy in a uniform open space with no boundaries and the sound field created by the sound source depends only on the sound source behavior. The sound field created by a sound source in an unbound space is called the **direct sound field.** This ideal direct sound field is called a **free field.** The ideal free field is a theoretical concept because there will always be some space boundaries (e.g., obstacles, walls, the ground) affecting sound propagation. However, if the sound source is far away from space boundaries and the reflections from the space boundaries are relatively weak, we can consider the direct sound field of a sound source to be a reasonably free field.

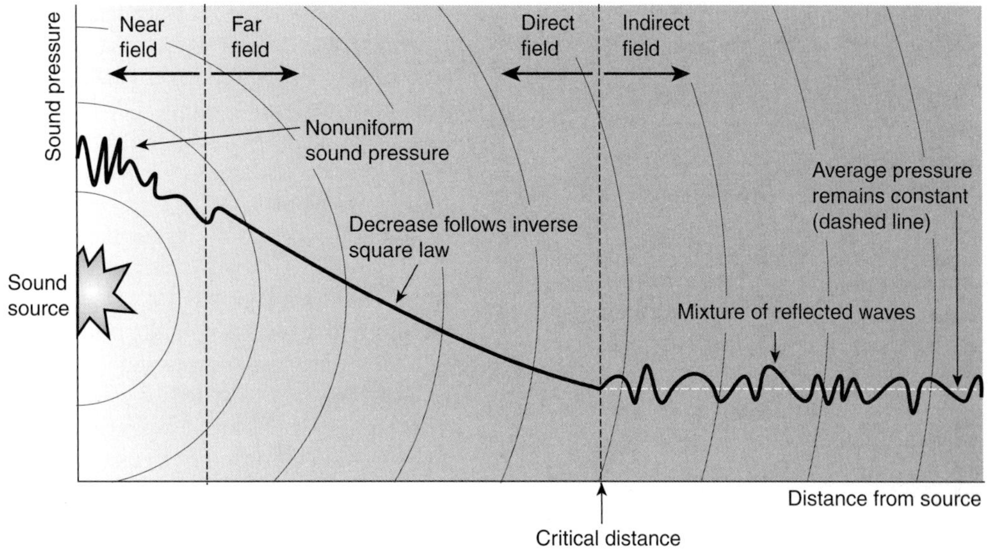

Figure 6.12. The relationship among sound source, near field, far field, direct field, and diffuse field in a closed space.

Closer to space boundaries and other reflective surfaces the sound field becomes a mixture of direct waves and reflected waves, and this is called the **indirect sound field** (or reverberant sound field). The indirect sound field develops naturally in closed spaces such as rooms and halls. An idealized type of reverberant field in which there is almost no variability in sound pressure is called a diffuse sound field. A **diffuse sound field** is an area filled with sound energy from random reflections coming from all possible directions and in which the sound pressure level is the same at all locations (Hirschorn, 1989). This type of field can only exist in a highly reflective multisurface environment and far away from the sound source(s). Similar to the ideal free field, the perfect diffuse field is a theoretical concept, but as long as the sound pressure in a specific area is relatively constant with sound reflections coming from all possible directions, we can consider such a field to be a diffuse field. The relationship between near, far, direct, and indirect sound fields is shown in Figure 6.12.

As seen in Figure 6.12, a typical sound field is a room with a combination of a direct field and an indirect (reverberant) field. Close to the sound source the sound field is dominated by the direct field of the sound source, whereas close to the space boundaries it is dominated by reflections. The distance from the sound source where the intensity of both fields is about equal is called the **critical distance** (d_c). That is:

$$d_c = \text{distance at which } I_{direct} = I_{reverb}$$

The critical distance depends on the power of the sound source, the directional pattern of its vibration (Chapter 5), sound frequency, the distance to space boundaries, and the reflective properties of the space boundaries. The critical distance is a very important design parameter in planning classrooms, auditoriums, and other spaces where speech understanding and sound clarity are critical. If a listener is located within the critical distance of a talker, speech communication is clear and relatively free from room reflections. However, when a listener is located beyond the critical distance of a talker, the talker's speech becomes smeared by room reflections and becomes less intelligible. This effect, in addition to the presence of background noises, determines the feasibility of various spaces for speech communication. The concept of the critical distance is shown in Figure 6.12.

The terms *free field* and *direct field* as well as *indirect (reverberant) field* and *diffuse field* used in this chapter may sound like pairs of synonyms and frequently they are considered as such in various publications. However, these individual terms focus on different aspects of the sound field, that is, on how ideal the sound field is (free field and diffuse field) or how relatively close to the sound source the specific point of the sound field is (direct field and indirect field).

SIGNAL-TO-NOISE RATIO

A very important concept in acoustics and hearing science is the **signal-to-noise ratio** (SNR). The signal-to-noise ratio is the ratio of the intensity of a signal, such as speech, to the intensity of a noise, such as ambient (background) noise. The term *signal* means a message, that is, useful information that is carried by the sound energy. The term *ambient noise* (from the Latin term *ambire* meaning "to go around") indicates the noise that is created by all internal and external sound sources that are not considered to be the sources of the signal and that do not change considerably in time and space. In other words, it is a continuous noise that is uniformly distributed in a specific area of space.

If we consider SNRs in relationship to the direct and indirect sound fields discussed in the previous section of this chapter, the direct sound can be considered as the "signal' and reflected sounds as the "noise." In this case the SNR is the ratio of the two respective sound intensities and the critical distance can be defined as the location where the SNR is equal to 1. SNR values are usually expressed in decibels, which will be discussed in Chapter 7.

ACOUSTIC SYSTEMS

Acoustic systems are masses of medium that do not propagate sound waves but instead vibrate themselves, creating standing waves within an enclosed space filled with the medium. Thus, acoustic systems include vibrating, air-filled resonance boxes of musical instruments such as the violin, oboe, or piano filled with vibrating air. Acoustic vibrations are triggered by a mechanic or aerodynamic force applied either as an impulse (e.g., plucking a string in a guitar) or continuous excitation (e.g., bow movement in a violin, blown air in a flute). Plucking a guitar string and bowing a violin string are mechanic forces, and the air flow across the flute is an example of an aerodynamic force. Another example of an aerodynamic force is a kettle whistle, in which heated water produces steam that passes through narrow openings and creates sounds.

Helmholtz Resonator

The simplest acoustic system with a single resonance frequency is a **Helmholtz resonator.** The Helmholtz resonator was named after German acoustician Hermann von Helmholtz (1821–1894), who described its properties in 1862. However, the properties of Helmholtz resonators (tuned ceramic or bronze vases) were known already by the ancient Greeks, who used them to correct acoustic deficiencies in their amphitheaters (Vitruvius, 1999). The same type of resonators were also used by the Romans (in amphitheaters) and in old Russian orthodox churches (Brüel, 1946; Vitruvius, 1999).

A Helmholtz resonator is an enclosure, generally round with rigid walls and with a small neck as shown in Figure 6.13. It is an acoustic system that consists of an acoustic mass (M_a; the mass of the air in the neck), an acoustic elasticity (C_a; the volume of the air in the enclosure), and an acoustic resistance (R_a; friction in the neck).

When a change in air pressure acts on the neck of the resonator it pushes the air mass (M_a) contained in the neck inward toward the volume (V). This movement compresses the air occupying the volume (V) of the main enclosure. Subsequently, the elasticity of the compressed air in the volume (V) pushes outward on the air mass (M_a). The outward movement of the mass (M_a) lowers the pressure in the enclosure to a value below the external pressure and the mass (M_a) is pulled back toward the enclosure. This back-and-forth movement of the mass (M_a) is analogous to the movement of the mass in a mass-and-spring system (Chapter 3). Both systems are resonance systems that can produce very large vibrations when excited by a periodic force at the resonance frequency. The resonance frequency (f_o) of a Helmholtz resonator can be calculated as:

$$f_o = \frac{c}{2\pi}\sqrt{\frac{A}{hV}} \qquad (6.18)$$

where c is the speed of sound in a medium filling the resonator, A is the cross-sectional area of the neck, h is the height (length) of the neck, and V is the volume of the enclosure in cubic meters.

You can create a working version of a Helmholtz resonator using a commonly available water bottle (e.g., your average plastic springwater bottle from about 8 to 24 ounces in size). Just take off the cap, drink some of the water, and blow directly across the top of the open bottle (this may take some practice). If you are successful at creating a "hooting" type of sound, you are now using a force (your breath) to cause the air in the bottle to vibrate at its resonance frequency. If the bottle has a lot of water in it, it will have a very small air space to act as a spring, so the frequency of vibration will be high. If the bottle has very little water in it, it will have a much larger air space, thus a looser spring, and the frequency of vibration will be lower.* If you can locate a rigid cylinder

*A set of glass containers (e.g., wine glasses) having the same shape but various amounts of water can be tuned to create a musical scale and various melodies can be played by simply touching (striking) individual glasses.

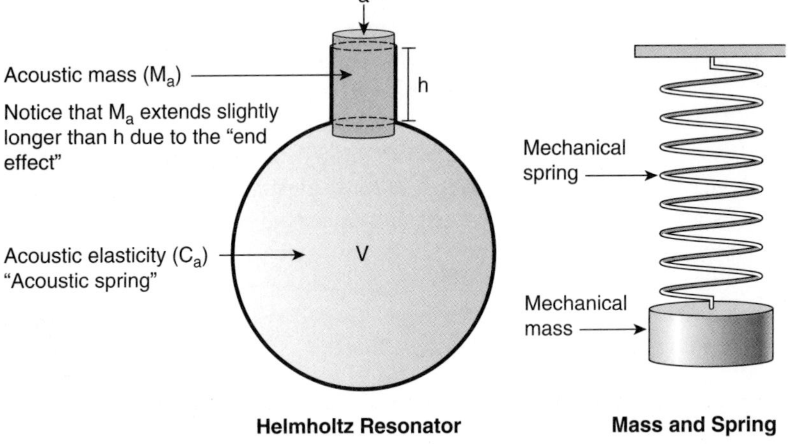

Figure 6.13. A Helmholtz resonator, which is the acoustic equivalent of a mass-and-spring system.

that is about the same diameter as the bottle neck and you attach it to the neck of the bottle, extending its length, you can increase the size of the mass element of the resonator and thus decrease the frequency of the "hoot."

PRACTICE PROBLEMS: THE HELMHOLTZ RESONATOR

1. What is the resonance frequency (f_o) of a Helmholtz resonator with a volume of 0.5 liters when the neck has a cross-sectional area of 0.02 m^2 and a length of 0.03 m (assuming that the speed of sound is 340 m/s)?
2. What is the resonance frequency (f_o) of a Helmholtz resonator with a volume of 0.5 liters when the neck has a cross-sectional area of 0.002 m^2 and a length of 0.03 m (assuming that the speed of sound is 340 m/s)?
3. What is the resonance frequency (f_o) of a Helmholtz resonator with a volume of 0.5 liters when the neck has a cross-sectional area of 0.02 m^2 and a length of 0.003 m (assuming that the speed of sound is 340 m/s)?
4. What is the resonance frequency (f_o) of a Helmholtz resonator with a volume of 0.05 liters when the neck has a cross-sectional area of 0.02 m^2 and a length of 0.03 m (assuming that the speed of sound is 340 m/s)?
5. If the resonance frequency (f_o) of a Helmholtz resonator is 500 Hz and the neck has a cross-sectional area of 0.01 m^2 and a length of 0.003 m, what is the volume of the enclosure (assuming that the speed of sound is 340 m/s)?

Answers (If you need help with these problems, consult the website.) **Link 6-3**

1. 1975.92 Hz
2. 624.84 Hz
3. 6248.39 Hz
4. 6248.39 Hz
5. 39 liters or 0.039 m^3

Air Columns

In Chapter 5, we discussed transverse vibratory motion in a vibrating guitar string and in this chapter we have discussed standing sound waves in air. It is easy to picture the up-and-down vibrations of the string, but it is rather difficult to picture the vibration pattern of air molecules in a column. We cannot see the air particles move since the amplitude of their vibration is very small and air particles are invisible to the naked eye as they move along the air column. However, the basic principle of vibration modes from strings that was shown in Chapter 4 can be used to understand vibration modes in air. Imagine a straight tube (pipe) containing air. Similarly to mechanic systems, the resonance properties of the air column depend on the dimensions of the vibrating element and the endpoints of the system. Therefore, the resonance frequencies of the air column will depend on the length of the column and whether the tube is open at both ends (open/open), closed at both ends (closed/closed), or open at one end and closed at the other (closed/open).

Consider the effect of a tube closed at both ends to be the same as the effect of a string fixed at both ends. In other words, if the tube is closed, that end must contain a node of vibration, because air particles cannot vibrate back and forth through a wall. The particle *displacement* for the first two modes of vibration for the three basic types of tubes is shown in Figure 6.14. Remember that particle displacement and acoustic (sound) pressure are 90° out-of-phase; thus, wherever there is a particle node, there will be a pressure antinode and vice versa. The vibration patterns in Figure 6.14A illustrate the first mode of vibration and they are similar to the

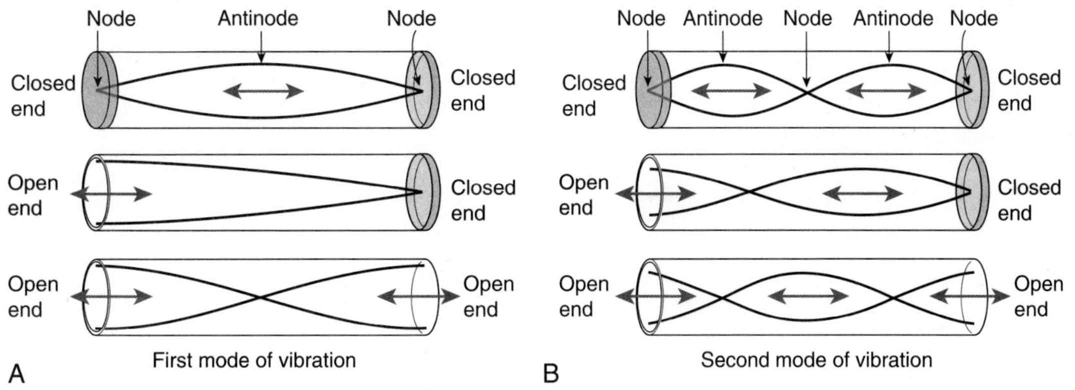

Figure 6.14. The first **(A)** and second **(B)** vibration modes of a tube that is closed at both ends, open at one end and closed at the other, and open at both ends.

illustration that was used to describe the first mode of vibration in a vibrating string. However, the particles of air are *not* vibrating in transverse motion like the string (shown in Figure 6.14 for demonstration purposes only), but in longitudinal motion (*horizontal arrows* in figure), and the perpendicular displacement is only shown to facilitate understanding for the location of the nodes and antinodes. Similar to the string vibration, other modes (standing waves) of vibration also exist in the column of air. The second vibration mode for each type of air column is shown in Figure 6.14B.

The main difference between the Helmholtz resonator and the vibrating column of air is that the vibrating column of air has several resonance frequencies and can vibrate in more than one mode, whereas the classic Helmholtz resonator has only one vibration mode. The resonance frequencies (f_n) of an air column can be calculated quite easily if the length of the tube containing the column is known. The lowest resonance frequency of a tube open on both ends (open/open) or closed on both ends (closed/closed) has a wavelength twice the length of the tube. Practical examples of such tubes are open organ pipes and a flute. The formula to calculate resonance frequencies for such tubes is the same as for the vibrating string (Chapter 4) and has the form:

$$f_n = \frac{nc}{\lambda} = \frac{nc}{2l} \qquad (6.19)$$

where f_n is the nth resonance frequency of the air column, c is the speed of sound in the column, l is the length of the column, and n is the sequential number. For example, the first four resonance frequencies of an air column contained with a 34-cm-long tube closed (or open) on both ends (assuming that speed of sound [c] = 340 m/s) are equal to:

$$f_1 = \frac{1 \times 340 \text{ m/s}}{2 \times 0.34 \text{ m}} = 500 \text{ Hz}$$

$$f_2 = \frac{2 \times 340 \text{ m/s}}{2 \times 0.34 \text{ m}} = 1000 \text{ Hz}$$

$$f_3 = \frac{3 \times 340 \text{ m/s}}{2 \times 0.34 \text{ m}} = 1500 \text{ Hz}$$

$$f_4 = \frac{4 \times 340 \text{ m/s}}{2 \times 0.34 \text{ m}} = 2000 \text{ Hz}$$

In the case of the tube that is open on one end and closed on another end (open/closed or closed/open), the standing waves will need to have a node and an antinode at the ends of the tube and their resonance frequencies can be calculated as:

$$f_n = \frac{(2n - 1)c}{\lambda} = \frac{(2n - 1)c}{4l} \qquad (6.20)$$

The lowest resonance frequency of a tube open at one end and closed at the other end (open/closed or closed/open) has a wavelength four times the length of the tube. The higher resonance frequencies will be only the odd-numbered harmonics of the fundamental frequency. Practical examples of such tubes are all brass and woodwind (reed) music instruments (e.g., tuba, trombone, trumpet). The four lowest resonance frequencies of a 34-cm-long tube open on one end are equal to:

$$f_1 = \frac{1 \times 340 \text{ m/s}}{4 \times 0.34 \text{ m}} = 250 \text{ Hz}$$

$$f_2 = \frac{3 \times 340 \text{ m/s}}{4 \times 0.34 \text{ m}} = 750 \text{ Hz}$$

$$f_3 = \frac{5 \times 340 \text{ m/s}}{4 \times 0.34 \text{ m}} = 1250 \text{ Hz}$$

$$f_4 = \frac{7 \times 340 \text{ m/s}}{4 \times 0.34 \text{ m}} = 1750 \text{ Hz}$$

Note that in both Equations 6.19 and 6.20 the resonance frequencies of the vibrating air column are independent of the diameter and shape of the column cross section. However, this is actually only true in the case of a tube closed on both ends. When the tube is open at one or both ends, the resonating air column does not stop at the end of the tube but continues for a bit farther like air in the neck of the Helmholtz resonator. Thus, to calculate the exact resonance frequency of an open air column, the length of the tube needs to be extended by some amount called the **end correction** that is dependent on the width of the tube. In Chapter 8 we will discuss the end correction that needs to be added to the actual length of the ear canal to estimate the resonance frequency of the ear canal.

PRACTICE PROBLEMS: CONTINUOUS VIBRATING SYSTEMS

For these problems, assume that the speed of sound is 340 m/s and neglect the end correction.

1. What is the lowest frequency resonance of a tube open at both ends that is 0.6 m long?
2. What is the lowest frequency resonance of a tube of air open at one end and closed at the other that is 2 cm long?
3. What are the lowest three resonance frequencies of a tube 15.5 cm long that is open at one end and closed at the other?
4. What are the lowest three resonance frequencies of a tube 0.02 m long that is open at both ends?

Answers (If you need help with these problems, consult the website.) **Link 6-4**

1. 283.33 Hz
2. 4250 Hz
3. 548.39 Hz, 1645.16 Hz, and 2741.94 Hz
4. 8500 Hz, 17,000 Hz, and 25,500 Hz

Summary

The traveling of sound waves through a medium is called sound propagation and the space filled with propagating waves is called a sound field. As sounds propagate, they are affected by sound field effects including absorption, refraction, reflection, interference, and diffraction. Sound waves propagating through a medium will eventually lose all of their energy due to internal and external absorption. Internal absorption is energy loss due to the acoustic properties of the medium through which sound waves are traveling and external absorption is energy loss due to the presence of boundaries or objects, such as walls, pillars, and so forth, that absorb part of the wave energy. The amount of energy absorbed by a boundary is measured by the absorption coefficient. Sound refraction is the change in the direction of sound wave propagation as the sound wave passes between two different media at an oblique angle, or through a single medium of varying density (temperature). Sound reflection, quantified by the coefficient of reflection, is the bouncing of sound waves off of a boundary. The reflected sound wave from a source arrives at the listener with varying time delay compared with the direct sound. If the time delay is greater than about 50 ms, the reflected sound is perceived as an echo.

The sound field close to the sound source is called a direct sound field and the sound field far away from the sound source and made up of reflected waves is called an indirect (reverberant) sound field. The phenomenon of sound waves bending around objects and through openings in boundaries is called sound diffraction. The amount of diffraction increases as the wavelength of the sound wave increases. Sound interference is the combination of two or more propagating waves. If overlapping waves of the same wavelength are in-phase, constructive interference occurs. If the two waves are out-of-phase, destructive interference occurs. Interference phenomena include standing waves and beats. The phenomenon of standing waves indicates that the whole mass of the medium vibrates at a specific frequency, making the behavior of the medium similar to that of a mechanic system. This type of vibrating medium together with its boundaries is called an acoustic system. Examples of acoustic systems are Helmholtz resonators and air column resonators. The resonance properties of an air column depend on the length of the column and whether the tube is open at both ends, closed at both ends, or open at one end and closed at the other. The lowest resonance frequency of a tube that is open or closed at both ends has a wavelength twice the length of the tube. The lowest resonance frequency of a tube open at one end and closed at the other end has a wavelength four times the length of the tube.

Key Points

- The nonuniform vibration pattern seen close to the source of a sound is referred to as the near field of the sound source, whereas the more uniform vibration pattern seen farther from the sound source is called the far field of the sound source.
- A free field involves the radiation of energy from a sound source into a uniform open space with no boundaries. The opposite of a free field is a diffuse field, which is the result of multiple sound wave reflections.
- The difference between the angle at which a wave approaches a boundary, called the angle of incidence, and the angle at which the wave travels through the second medium, called the angle of refraction, depends on the density and stiffness of the two media.
- The total amount of reflected energy is called reverberation. Reverberation time is the amount of time it takes for a sound to decrease in sound pressure by 1000 times (60 dB).
- A standing wave is a special case of wave interference when the sound is bouncing between two reflected parallel surfaces producing nodes and antinodes.
- Beats are periodic amplitude fluctuations caused when two sounds that are very close in frequency are played together. The beat frequency is the number of beats that occur per second, and it is

equal to the difference between the frequencies of two component sounds (f_1 and f_2).

- The Doppler effect is a shift in the frequency of a sound wave resulting from the movement of a sound source, a listener, or both.
- A sonic boom is created by an object moving faster than the speed of sound and creating a zone of compressed air.
- The simplest acoustic system with a single resonance frequency is called a Helmholtz resonator.

Chapter Outline

CHAPTER 7

The Decibel

Diana C. Emanuel, Szymon Letowski, and Tomasz Letowski

Objectives

- To introduce the concepts of relative and absolute units of measurement
- To discuss the practical application of logarithmic scales
- To review the rationale for and a brief history of the development of the decibel scale
- To apply basic math skills from Chapter 1 in the calculation of sound pressure level and sound intensity level for a given sound pressure and sound intensity
- To demonstrate problem-solving skills using the dB IL and dB SPL scales when sound pressure and sound intensity change

Key Terms

Absolute difference	Level	Relative measurement
Absolute measurement	Octave	Sound intensity level
Bandwidth (Δf)	Power level	Sound pressure level
Bel (B)	Reference point	Spectrum level
Decibel (dB)	Relative difference	Zero level

The decibel's a tricky thing
In size it doth increase
But not in any normal way
Instead your brow will crease
When you find the decibel's
In league with ol' base 10
Expanding logarithmically
Again and again and again . . .

—From *The Decibel*, by Tom Farley

The most frequently used unit of measurement in hearing science is the decibel. It is a unit related to physical power, but it is unlike all the units you learned about in Chapter 2. First, it does not truly measure a specific physical characteristic. Rather, it describes the relationship between the magnitude of one physical measurement and the magnitude of another physical measurement. In other words, it indicates the ratio between two measurements. Second and more importantly, it is a nonlinear unit based on the logarithm, which is what actually makes working with decibels so different. This chapter will start by introducing the difference between absolute and relative measurement and go on to introduce the decibel and explain the logic behind the use of the decibel in hearing science. The last part of the chapter will provide a detailed discussion of how the decibel scale is used in making sound intensity and sound pressure measurements, including step-by-step instructions on how to solve most of the decibel problems you will encounter in hearing science.

ABSOLUTE AND RELATIVE MEASUREMENT

The concept of physical measurement was introduced in Chapter 2. This discussion was followed by an introduction to the metric system and the International System of Units. Given any two measurements of the same physical characteristic, there are two natural ways for them to be compared quantitatively. We can calculate either their absolute difference or their relative difference. The **absolute difference** tells us *how much* greater one measurement is than another and it is expressed in the number of units that one value is larger than the other. The **relative difference** tells us *how many times* greater one measurement is than another. Calculating absolute difference involves subtraction, while determining relative difference involves division. In the scientific literature these two types of comparison are called **absolute measurement** and **relative measurement.**

Sometimes the absolute difference is more meaningful, and sometimes it makes more sense to use the relative difference. For example, when parents talk about a growing child, they talk about the absolute difference between two height measurements; for example, "Devon has grown 4 inches over the past year." Have you ever heard anyone say, "My son grew 20% since last January"? On the other hand, if we were comparing U.S. state areas, relative difference would be more informative. The fact that Mississippi is twice as large as West Virginia is much more telling than the fact that it is 62,807 km^2 larger.

One situation where relative difference becomes particularly important is when we are concerned with human perception. Our response to physical stimuli is far from linear. A given absolute quantity may mean a little or a lot depending on the situation. For example, it is easy for a person to differentiate between an object with a mass of 1 kg and an object with a mass of 2 kg. This 1-kg difference is, however, much less obvious when comparing a 10-kg mass to an 11-kg mass and even less obvious when comparing 100 kg to 101 kg. This fact illustrates a general rule of human perception, namely that humans do not respond to absolute differences in physical properties (e.g., a 1-kg change in mass) but rather to relative differences in these properties (e.g., a 10% change in mass). In the example above, the 1-kg absolute difference represented a relative difference of, respectively, 100%, 10%, and 1% of the initial mass. Clearly, it is easiest to perceive the 100% change in mass and most difficult to detect the 1% change.

Perception of weight is just one of many examples of human reaction to physical stimuli. Most human reactions are in response to a relative, not absolute, change in the stimulus. Relative measurements and relative units are, therefore, of great importance in all domains concerned with human interaction with the physical world. Human response to physical stimuli will be discussed in greater detail in the psychoacoustics chapter, once the necessary foundation skills have been reviewed.

LOGARITHMIC UNITS

The decibel is a relative unit based on a logarithmic scale. In the previous section we dealt with the first of the two aspects of the decibel, namely its relative nature. In this section, we will investigate the second of these—its logarithmic basis. If you are not familiar with logarithms, go back to the mathematics chapter and review the logarithm and antilog sections. We will begin the discussion of logarithmic scales with a relative scale that is familiar to most people, one that is known by anyone who has ever taken music lessons—the music scale and its fundamental unit, the **octave.**

The octave is the fundamental building block of all of Western music scales. Given that music is intrinsically tied to human perception, it should come as no surprise that the octave measures relative difference. More to the point, the octave is a relative unit of frequency, with one octave representing a doubling in frequency. For example, middle A has a frequency of 440 Hz. The A one octave above middle A has a frequency of 880 Hz (2 × 440 Hz) and the A one octave below middle A has a frequency of 220 Hz (0.5 × 440 Hz). Note that the absolute difference in frequency between octaves is not the same in both cases: 880 Hz − 440 Hz = 440 Hz and 440 Hz − 220 Hz = 220 Hz. So each time a note is raised by one octave, its frequency does *not* increase by a constant absolute value; rather, its frequency goes up by a constant relative factor, specifically by a factor of two. Therefore, in music, we are primarily concerned with the relative difference in frequency and not the absolute difference.

If we take the sequence of all the A notes on the piano and consider the relative difference in frequency between the first (lowest) A and each successive A, we form the following progression of ratios in frequency: 2:1, 4:1, 8:1, 16:1, 32:1, 64:1, and 128:1. The second A note in the sequence is one octave above the initial A, so its frequency is twice as great (i.e., the ratio of 2:1). The next A has a frequency again twice as great, so the relative difference between it and the initial

A becomes 2 × 2:1 = 4:1. We continue in this fashion until the final A. Since each doubling of frequency corresponds to an octave, the sequence of ratios listed above is equivalent to the sequence of one, two, three, four, five, six, and seven octaves. This range of seven octaves is smaller than the whole audible range of sound, which extends for about 10 octaves in young normal-hearing human ears (20 Hz to 20 kHz).

The use of frequency ratios in music rather than frequencies themselves is dictated by our perception. However, the use of octaves rather than frequency ratios is dictated by a need for simplicity. Since the octave is the basic measure of perceived changes in frequency, it is much more natural and easier to talk about octaves than about frequency ratios when discussing music. For example, we typically say that a singer has a three-octave range, rather than an 8:1 frequency range, and that a piano spans seven octaves, rather than that it spans a 128:1 frequency ratio.

Please note that the number of octaves (one, two, three, four, five, six, seven) is the logarithm (base 2) of the ratios (2:1, 4:1, 8:1, 16:1, 32:1, 64:1, 128:1). This relationship is shown in Table 7.1.

If you take a look at the third column in Table 7.1, you will notice that the frequency ratio is equal to the base 2 raised to a power equal to the number of octaves. For example, 64:1 = 2^6:1; thus, a relative difference in frequency of 2^6 is equal to six octaves. Mathematically, this relationship can be expressed in the following way.

$$MINT = \log_2\left[\frac{f_2}{f_1}\right][\text{octave}] \qquad (7.1)$$

where *MINT* is the relative difference between the two frequencies, f_1 and f_2. The acronym MINT stands for the term *music interval*. It describes how far apart two frequencies are in music and it is used to construct music scales and chords. Each music interval can be expressed as a fraction or a multiple of an octave or it may have its own musical name. You may have heard of common intervals such as thirds or fifths. They are simply fractions of an octave. As you can see from Equation 7.1, they, like the octave, simply represent specific ratios of frequencies.

It is important to understand why a base of 2 is used for the octave. An octave indicates a relationship between frequencies that have similar musical quality. This relationship was determined to be the doubling of frequency. However, humans did not start out with the concept of frequency doubling and then decide to call it an octave. Instead, the concept of an octave was used long before frequency was even a measurable characteristic. Once frequency was measured, it was found that the octave was equal to a doubling of frequency. Thus, the logarithm base 2 is a reflection of the relationship between the physical characteristic and our perception of it. If you would like to hear linear steps on the frequency scale, see the website. **Audio clip 7-1** You will notice that logarithmic octave steps **Audio clip 7-2** sound more equal to your ears than linear steps.

A similar nonlinear relationship between the power of a signal and its perceived effect is the reason for using a base 10 logarithmic scale for describing changes in signal intensity. The unit of this scale is the decibel.

Table 7.1. A Comparison of the Frequency Ratio to the Octave*

Frequency Ratio	Octave	Base 2 and Logarithm
2:1	1	2^1
4:1	2	2^2
8:1	3	2^3
16:1	4	2^4
32:1	5	2^5
64:1	6	2^6
128:1	7	2^7

**The associated logarithm is also included.*

THE DECIBEL

Soon after the advent of the telephone in 1876, a definite relationship was noted between power loss in a signal being transmitted over a telephone line and the loudness of the transmitted message. Since power loss is a relative measure, telephone operators needed a relative unit of power to describe the contributions of different elements of the telephone network to the final power at the output. Therefore, they were searching for a relative measure of power that would correlate with the loudness of the received message (Martin, 1924).

Until the early 1920s the loss of signal power was measured with a unit known as the standard cable mile (SCM). The SCM indicated how far in terms of miles of cable the signal could travel and still have sufficient power to be heard. This was a linear unit and so it was not very useful for dealing with the effect of power loss on the loudness of the transmitted signal. Therefore, in 1924, the engineers at Bell Laboratories proposed a logarithmic unit of power loss to replace the SCM. They called it the **bel** (B) in honor of Alexander Graham Bell and their laboratory. It was defined as follows (Martin, 1929):

$$L = \log_{10}\left(\frac{P_2}{P_1}\right)[\text{B}] \qquad (7.2)$$

The variable L in Equation 7.2 denotes a relative difference in power, measured in bels (B). The symbols P_1 and P_2 denote the two magnitudes of power being compared. Thus, the bel is a logarithmic unit of power equal to the logarithm base 10 of the ratio of two powers.

The logarithm used in Equation 7.2 is base 10 for two reasons. First, defining the bel in this way gave the engineers a clear and simple way of predicting the effect of power loss on speech loudness. That means that they could relate equal changes in power in bels to similar changes in loudness.*

*This relationship was shown later not to be exact. The relationship between sound power and its loudness will be discussed in Chapter 12.

Second, as you will recall, the number 10 is the basis for the entire metric system of units. Thus, it is also the most convenient base for doing any logarithmic calculations on measurements.

An important benefit of using a logarithmic unit, such as the octave or the bel, is that it compresses a large range of magnitudes into a much smaller range, which eliminates the need to work with very small and very large numbers. To see how this works in the case of the bel, consider the following range of powers:

$$1 \times 10^{-12}\ \text{W to } 1 \times 10^{6}\ \text{W}$$

Translated into standard notation, this range is equal to:

$$0.000000000001\ \text{W to } 1{,}000{,}000\ \text{W}$$

This is a very large range with a tedious number of zeros to write whenever a linear power measurement is made. But if we take their logarithms (base 10), then the range becomes much smaller:

$$\log_{10}(1 \times 10^{-12}) = -12$$
$$\log_{10}(1 \times 10^{6}) = 6$$

So, the range of values we need to be concerned with now extends only from −12 to 6. This is a much more manageable range of numbers. The extent to which the range of numbers is compressed into a smaller range of numbers is determined by the base of the logarithm used: The greater the base is, the greater the compression. The octave, discussed in the previous section, does not compress the range of numbers as much as the bel, because the octave is base 2 and the bel is base 10. The octave only needs to compress the frequency range of music instruments, which is relatively small compared to the power range associated with human hearing.

The base 10 used in the definition of the bel adequately captures the underlying connection between a physical stimulus and the human response, relating the power of a signal to its resulting loudness. However, the compression created by the bel turned out to be too large for practical purposes. To hear consecutive one-bel steps in sound level, see the website. **Audio clip 7-3**

In order to decrease the amount of scale compression, the base of the logarithm could be lowered or the unit could be divided into smaller fractional units. The second solution is much better because it preserves both the perceptual and the decimal character of the scale. Therefore, in 1929 the bel was replaced by the **decibel** (dB), which as you might guess from the deci- prefix is one tenth of a bel (Martin, 1929). The decibel has all the same properties as the bel except that it is 10 times smaller; that is, 10 dB = 1 B. To hear consecutive one-decibel and three-decibel steps in sound level, see the website **Audio clip 7-4** and contrast them with one-bel steps heard previously.

To convert Equation 7.2 from bels to decibels, the right-hand side of the equation just needs to be multiplied by 10:

$$L = 10 \times \log\left(\frac{P_2}{P_1}\right) [\text{dB}] \qquad (7.3)$$

In Equation 7.2 the base (10) was explicitly shown, but in Equation 7.3 notice that the number 10, indicating the base of the logarithm, has been omitted. This omission is in agreement with the standard convention that if the base of a logarithm is not specified, base 10 should be assumed. This standard convention will be followed from this point on throughout the rest of the book. So, every time you see "log" written without any base number, it means "$\log_{10}$."

To hear the perceptual effects of equal linear (W/m^2) and logarithmic (dB) changes in sound intensity, see the website. **Audio clip 7-5**

It is important to stress that the decibel as defined in Equation 7.3 does not measure a physical property in the way that a meter measures length or a gram measures mass. It specifies the relative difference between two measurements of a single physical property, like a percent. Just as we can describe relative difference in length or mass using percent, we use decibels to describe a relative difference in power or other related characteristic. In other words, we specify the level of one power above another one. Therefore, when a value is expressed in dB, the measured property is called a **level.** For example, the characteristic specified by Equation 7.3 is the **power level.** The main examples of level-type scales used in hearing science are **sound intensity level** and **sound pressure level.**

In summary, the decibel is a very attractive unit that is used to measure the amount of stimulation acting on humans and to express changes in the signal strength in communication fields because of its three related properties:

1. It allows for the numerical representation of physical magnitudes in a manner that correlates to human perception.
2. It allows for the compression of a large range of physical values to a much smaller and more manageable range.
3. It supports the metric system by using the base 10 logarithm.

It is important to stress that the decibel is not the only logarithmic unit that is used in physical sciences to express the *amount* of a given property. Other similar logarithmic units have also been proposed and are used in some applications (e.g., the neper), but the fact that the decibel is the base 10 logarithmic unit makes it the logarithmic unit of choice. Note that in some areas of science it is natural to use base 2 logarithmic scales (e.g., the music scale based on an octave interval and the binary scale based on a yes–no decision), but these scales are not useful for the intensity of sound.

The decibel and the level-based scales based on the decibel are most frequently used in electronics, telecommunications, hearing science, and acoustics. They are used to express the relative difference (ratio) of powers (e.g., electric power, solar power, acoustic power, etc.) and power-related characteristics such as magnetic field, sound pressure, mechanic force, and voltage. In the next section, we will focus on the two level-based scales that are the most important in hearing science: the sound intensity level and the sound pressure level scales.

SOUND INTENSITY LEVEL AND SOUND PRESSURE LEVEL

Propagation of sound in the environment is characterized by its sound intensity (I) and sound pressure (p). Both of these magnitudes were introduced and discussed in Chapter 5. Recall that sound intensity is the density of acoustic power across the area of radiation ($I = \frac{Power}{Area}$). Therefore, if we keep the area the same, the ratio of two sound intensities is the same as the ratio of two powers and it can be expressed in decibels as:

$$L = 10 \times \log\left(\frac{I_2}{I_1}\right)[\text{dB}] \qquad (7.4)$$

where I_1 and I_2 are the two sound intensities under consideration. Following the convention introduced in the previous section, the quantity defined by Equation 7.4 is known as the sound intensity level (IL).

Recall also from Chapter 5 that sound intensity is proportional to the square of sound pressure (i.e., $I \propto p^2$). So, if we replace the sound intensities (I_1 and I_2) in Equation 7.4 with sound pressure squared and simplify the equation, then we can rewrite Equation 7.4 as Equation 7.5:

$$L = 10 \times \log\left(\frac{p_2^2}{p_1^2}\right)[\text{dB}]$$

$$L = 10 \times \log\left(\frac{p_2}{p_1}\right)^2[\text{dB}]$$

$$L = 20 \times \log\left(\frac{p_2}{p_1}\right)[\text{dB}] \qquad (7.5)$$

The L value in Equation 7.5 is the same sound intensity level calculated in Equation 7.4, but since it is expressed in Equation 7.5 by sound pressures, it is called the sound pressure level (SPL).

Box 7.1 Important Point

Sound intensity level and sound pressure level are two different names of the same logarithmic scale of sound intensity.

If the sound pressures and sound intensities in Equations 7.4 and 7.5 represent the same pair of sounds, the quantities defined by both equations must be numerically identical. Therefore, the sound intensity level and sound pressure level for the same pair of sounds are just two different ways of reporting the same relationship. To prove this point consider the following two sound pressures: $p_1 = 2 \times 10^{-3}$ Pa and $p_2 = 2 \times 10^{-2}$ Pa. The difference in their sound level is equal to 20 dB as shown below:

$$L = 20 \times \log\left(\frac{p_2}{p_1}\right)[\text{dB}]$$

$$L = 20 \times \log\left(\frac{2 \times 10^{-2}\ Pa}{2 \times 10^{-3}\ Pa}\right)[\text{dB}]$$

$$L = 20 \times \log(10)[\text{dB}]$$

$$L = 20 \times 1[\text{dB}]$$

$$L = 20 \text{ dB}$$

Now, let us consider their related sound intensities. The sound intensity corresponding to a sound pressure of $p_1 = 2 \times 10^{-3}$ Pa is $I_1 = 10^{-8}$ W/m², and the sound intensity corresponding to a sound pressure of $p_2 = 2 \times 10^{-2}$ Pa is $I_2 = 10^{-6}$ W/m². Upon inserting these values into Equation 7.4, we will conclude that:

$$L = 10 \times \log\left(\frac{I_2}{I_1}\right)[\text{dB}]$$

$$L = 10 \times \log\left(\frac{10^{-6}\ \frac{W}{m^2}}{10^{-8}\ \frac{W}{m^2}}\right)[\text{dB}]$$

$$L = 10 \times \log(100)[\text{dB}]$$

$$L = 20 \text{ dB}$$

Indeed, both equations provided the same answer of 20 dB, which proves the earlier point that *the sound intensity level and the sound pressure level produced by the same sound are numerically identical.* Thus, when we talk about a *change* in sound level we do not really need to specify whether we mean sound intensity or sound pressure. We can just simply say, referring to the example discussed above, that the **sound level** changed by 20 dB. This means that the sound pressure changed 10 times and the sound intensity changed 100 times.

REFERENCE POINT AND ZERO LEVEL

Recall that the number of decibels by itself only describes a ratio. It does not provide any indication as to whether the specific ratio (e.g., 10:1) is between small (e.g., 1 and 10) or large (e.g., 1000 and 10,000) magnitudes. It simply indicates how many times greater (or smaller) the second number is than the first number. If one wants to describe the relative change in a sound, then the number of decibels by itself is perfectly sufficient, and it is enough to say, for example, that the sound level increased by 20 dB or decreased by 6 dB. However, in these cases, we do not know anything about the actual values of the sound intensity and sound pressure that have been changed.

If one would like to know the actual values of sound intensity and sound pressure for the values expressed on the level scale (decibel scale), some kind of a reference magnitude needs to be known and the number of decibels must refer to this magnitude. This magnitude is known as the **reference point** and it can be arbitrarily selected, although it is usually standardized to minimize potential confusion that could result from the use of several reference points. The standardized reference point for sound pressure has been selected to be **20 μPa.** This sound pressure is equal roughly to the lowest sound pressure that can be heard by the human ear in the midfrequency range.

A sound pressure of 20 μPa results from a sound intensity of **10^{-12} W/m²**, which is the standardized reference point for sound intensity. The range of sound pressures (and sound intensities) that are of interest to hearing science extends from this reference point to 20 Pa (1 W/m²), which is the threshold of pain, and further to 2×10^4 Pa (10^6 W/m²), which is the sound pressure (sound intensity) created by explosions and artillery fire.

The reference values 20 μPa and 10^{-12} W/m² are denoted in this book as p_r and I_r, where the *r* indicates that the value is a reference point value. Please note that some older sources express reference points using CGS units rather than MKS units (see Chapter 2); consult the website for a description of the use of the CGS system in hearing science problems. **Link 7-1**

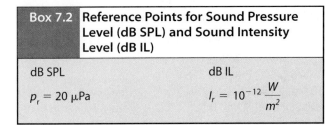

Box 7.2 Reference Points for Sound Pressure Level (dB SPL) and Sound Intensity Level (dB IL)

dB SPL	dB IL
$p_r = 20\ \mu\text{Pa}$	$I_r = 10^{-12}\ \dfrac{W}{m^2}$

Following this convention, sound intensity level (7.4) and sound pressure level (7.5) equations can be written as:

$$L = 10 \times \log\left(\frac{I}{I_r}\right) = 10 \times \log\left(\frac{I}{10^{-12}}\right)[\text{dB IL}] \quad (7.6)$$

and

$$L = 20 \times \log\left(\frac{p}{P_r}\right) = 20 \times \log\left(\frac{p}{20\ \mu Pa}\right)[\text{dB SPL}] \quad (7.7)$$

Notice in Equations 7.6 and 7.7 the addition of the letters IL and SPL after the dB unit. Since decibels are used with a variety of physical characteristics, when we express a certain value in decibels in relationship to a specific reference point, an indication of the reference point must be specified. A standardized method of referring to a specific reference point in mathematical expressions is to add information about the reference point after the dB symbol using the letters "re:" (meaning *re*ference), for example, 40 dB re: 20 μPa. The reference point can also be specified with a label. The standardized labels used for 20 μPa and 10^{-12} W/m² are SPL (sound pressure level) and IL (intensity level), respectively. The labels should be written as dB SPL and dB IL. In some textbooks and other publications, other forms of labeling the reference points are used such as dBSPL, dB (SPL), or dB_{SPL}. They are not standardized notations and in our opinion, they should be avoided. Please pay special attention to the space that needs to exist between the dB symbol and the reference point label. It is a very important space because it separates the unit from its reference point. In the case of dB SPL and dB IL, the unit is the same (dB) but the reference points are different. If there were no spaces between the dB and the respective labels, it would indicate that the dB, dBSPL, and dBIL were three different units, which is not the case. It has to be stressed also that each and every time a dB value is expressed in reference to a specific reference point, this reference point needs to be identified to prevent potential confusion. However, the reference label is not used when a specific characteristic changes its value and we report the amount of change (e.g., that the sound pressure level increased by 3 dB). A list of common reference points used in hearing science and telecommunication and their associated abbreviations is available on the website. **Link 7-2**

Let us consider now the sound intensity level and sound pressure level of a sound at the reference point. It should be obvious that if we compare something against itself, there is no difference to speak of; in other words, there is a 0% change. Thus, for a sound having an intensity of 10^{-12} W/m², compared to a reference point of 10^{-12} W/m², the sound intensity level will be 0 dB, indicating no difference between sound intensity and the reference point. If you recall that log (1) = 0 (Chapter 1), this is easy to see. The calculation using sound intensity level is shown below by selecting Equation 7.6, substituting 10^{-12} for *I*, and simplifying:

$$L = 10 \times \log\left(\frac{I}{10^{-12}}\right)[\text{dB IL}]$$

$$L = 10 \times \log\left(\frac{10^{-12}\frac{W}{m^2}}{10^{-12}\frac{W}{m^2}}\right)[\text{dB IL}]$$

$$L = 10 \times \log(1)\ [\text{dB IL}]$$

$$L = 10 \times 0\ [\text{dB IL}]$$

$$L = 0\ \text{dB IL}$$

Similarly, for a sound having a sound pressure of 20 μPa, compared to a reference point of 20 μPa, the sound pressure level will be 0 dB, indicating no difference in the sound pressure level compared to the reference point. Mathematically, this is shown by substituting 20 μPa for *p* in Equation 7.7.

$$L = 20 \times \log\left(\frac{p}{20 \mu Pa}\right)[\text{dB SPL}]$$

$$L = 20 \times \log\left(\frac{20\ \mu Pa}{20\ \mu Pa}\right)[\text{dB SPL}]$$

$$L = 20 \times \log(1)[\text{dB SPL}]$$

$$L = 20 \times 0\ [\text{dB SPL}]$$

$$L = 0\ \text{dB SPL}$$

Since every reference point clearly corresponds to 0 dB on the level scale, this point is also frequently referred to as the **zero level.**

Box 7.3 Points to Remember

Sound pressure reference 20 μPa	=	Sound pressure level 0 dB SPL
10^{-12} W/m² Sound intensity reference	=	0 dB IL Sound intensity level

It is important to note that 0 dB SPL and 0 dB IL do not signify the absence of sound. It is possible to have negative decibel values (e.g., −6 dB, −10 dB). These values represent sound intensities or sound pressures below the reference point.

Table 7.2 shows several examples of sound pressures with their associated sound pressure levels. As you can see, the range of values shown for the linear scale is much larger than that of the logarithmic scale. Recall that this is one of the advantages of using decibels. The sound pressure levels corresponding to various common sounds are listed on the website. **Link 7-3**

In order to convert from sound intensity (W/m²) to sound intensity level (dB IL), we use Equation 7.6, and to convert from sound pressure (μPa) to sound pressure level (dB SPL), we use Equation 7.7. These equations have included the reference points for the intensity level scale (10^{-12} W/m²) and sound pressure level scale (20 μPa) as constants so the measured sound intensities and sound pressures are calculated in reference to the zero level. Here are two examples illustrating the conversion from sound intensity to sound intensity level and from sound pressure to sound pressure level.

Example 7.1

Convert a measured sound intensity of 10^{-9} W/m² to sound intensity level.

First, select the correct formula. Since the question gives the sound intensity and asks for the sound intensity level, select the sound intensity level equation.

$$L = 10 \times \log\left(\frac{I}{10^{-12}\frac{\mathrm{W}}{\mathrm{m}^2}}\right) [\text{dB IL}]$$

Second, substitute known variables. Here, the sound intensity output of the sound source (I) is given in the problem; it is 10^{-9} W/m².

$$L = 10 \times \log\left(\frac{10^{-9}\frac{W}{m^2}}{10^{-12}\frac{W}{m^2}}\right) [\text{dB IL}]$$

Third, solve for L by using the order of operation skills you learned in Chapter 1. First do the operation within the parenthesis. Recall the log rule from Chapter 1, $\frac{x^a}{x^b} = x^{a-b}$.

$$L = 10 \times \log(10^{(-9)-(-12)}) [\text{dB IL}]$$

$$L = 10 \times \log(10^3) [\text{dB IL}]$$

Next, perform the log calculation. Recall that a log is just an exponent, so the log of 10^3 is simply 3.

$$L = 10 \times 3 [\text{dB IL}]$$

$$L = 30 \text{ dB IL}$$

Answer: The sound intensity level is 30 dB IL.

Example 7.2

If sound pressure is 10 μPa, what is the sound pressure level?

First, select the correct formula. Since the question gives the sound pressure and asks for the sound pressure level, select the sound pressure level equation.

$$L = 20 \times \log\left(\frac{p}{20\ \mu Pa}\right) [\text{dB SPL}]$$

Second, substitute known variables. Here, the sound pressure of the sound source (p) is given in the problem; it is 10 μPa.

$$L = 20 \times \log\left(\frac{10\ \mu Pa}{20\ \mu Pa}\right) [\text{dB SPL}]$$

Next, solve for L.

$$L = 20 \times \log(0.5) [\text{dB SPL}]$$

Notice that the log of 0.5 is a negative number, −0.3. You will find a negative log whenever the ratio within the parenthesis is less than one.

$$L = 20 \times (-0.3) [\text{dB SPL}]$$

$$L = -6 \text{ dB SPL}$$

Answer: −6 dB SPL

▶ Table 7.2. Comparison of Sound Pressures With Sound Pressure Levels

Sound Pressure (Linear Scale)	Sound Pressure Level (Logarithmic Scale)
2 μPa	−20 dB SPL
20 μPa	0 dB SPL
200 μPa	20 dB SPL
2000 μPa	40 dB SPL
20,000 μPa	60 dB SPL

PRACTICE PROBLEMS: CONVERTING FROM SOUND PRESSURE TO SOUND PRESSURE LEVEL AND FROM SOUND INTENSITY TO SOUND INTENSITY LEVEL

1. If sound pressure is equal to 10 μPa, what is the corresponding sound pressure level?

2. If sound pressure is equal to 2453 μPa, what is the corresponding sound pressure level?
3. If sound intensity is equal to 10^{-10} W/m^2, what is the corresponding sound intensity level?
4. If sound intensity is equal to 2.3×10^{-9} W/m^2, what is the corresponding sound intensity level?
5. If sound pressure is equal to 3.54×10^{7} μPa, what is the corresponding sound pressure level?
6. If sound intensity is equal to 2,570,000 W/m^2, what is the corresponding sound intensity level?
7. What is the sound pressure level if sound pressure is equal to 3×10^{2} μPa?
8. What is the sound intensity level if sound intensity is equal to 4.2×10^{-3} W/m^2?

Answers (If you need help with these problems, consult the website.) **Link 7-4**

1. −6 dB SPL
2. 41.77 dB SPL
3. 20 dB IL
4. 33.62 dB IL
5. 124.96 dB SPL
6. 184.10 dB IL
7. 23.52 dB SPL
8. 96.23 dB IL

It has to be stressed again that for a specific sound, the dB IL and dB SPL values are the same values expressed on the same logarithmic scale of sound intensity. Keeping this relationship in mind, we can explore various practical situations where the sound level produced by a single sound source or by a group of sound sources needs to be calculated.

OPERATIONS ON SOUND INTENSITY AND SOUND PRESSURE LEVELS

To express a change in sound intensity as a *change* in sound level, either Equation 7.4 or Equation 7.5 can be used depending on whether the calculations are based on sound intensity or sound pressure values. To express sound intensity in reference to the sound intensity reference (10^{-12} W/m^2), use Equation 7.6. To express sound pressure in reference to the sound pressure reference (20 μPa), use Equation 7.7. In order to get proficient in operations involving decibels, begin by inspecting Table 7.3, which presents the sound pressure levels of four selected sound pressures starting with the reference point value of 20 μPa.

Table 7.3. The Effect of Sound Pressure Doubling on the Sound Pressure Level

Sound pressure	20 μPa	40 μPa	80 μPa	160 μPa
Sound pressure level	0 dB SPL	6 dB SPL	12 dB SPL	18 dB SPL

You should notice that the selected sound pressures are doubled from column to column and their corresponding sound pressure levels increase by 6 dB. In other words, doubling sound pressure results in a 6-dB increase in sound pressure level. Compare, for example, the sound pressures of 40 μPa and 20 μPa. According to Equation 7.5:

$$L = 20 \times \log\left(\frac{40\ \mu Pa}{20\ \mu Pa}\right)[\text{dB}]$$

and subsequently:

$$L = 20 \times \log\left(\frac{2}{1}\right)[\text{dB}]$$

$$L = 20 \times \log(2)\ [\text{dB}]$$

$$L = 20 \times 0.3\ [\text{dB}]$$

$$L = 6\ \text{dB}$$

Every time the pressure is doubled, that is, the ratio of two sound pressures is 2:1 (e.g., 160 μPa and 80 μPa), the resulting change in sound pressure level will be 6 dB. This example demonstrates a very handy and commonly used sound pressure level rule. Whenever the sound pressure is doubled, the sound pressure level increases by 6 dB.

Box 7.4 Decibel Rule #1

When the sound pressure doubles, the sound pressure level increases by 6 dB. In other words:

New sound pressure level = Original sound pressure level [dB SPL] + 6 dB

Example 7.3

If a sound source has a sound pressure level of 80 dB SPL and the sound pressure is doubled, what is the new sound pressure level?

First, select the appropriate equation. Recall from decibel rule #1 that when the sound pressure doubles, the sound pressure level increases by 6 dB.

New sound pressure level = Original sound pressure level [dB SPL] + 6 dB

Substitute known variables. We know the sound pressure level of the original sound source was 80 dB SPL.

New sound pressure level (L) = 80 dB SPL + 6 dB

$$L = 86\ \text{dB SPL}$$

Answer: 86 dB SPL

This rule holds true only for a doubling of *sound pressure*. Let us now take a look at what happens when the *intensity* of a signal is doubled. Remember that a doubled value is a 2:1 ratio compared to the original value and this ratio can also be expressed in fraction form as $\frac{2}{1}$. So, following the same approach as for sound pressure, we can enter this fraction into Equation 7.4 and determine the change in sound intensity level that corresponds to a doubling of sound intensity:

$$L = 10 \times \log\left(\frac{I_2}{I_1}\right) [\text{dB}]$$

$$L = 10 \times \log\left(\frac{2}{1}\right) [\text{dB}]$$

$$L = 10 \times \log(2)\ [\text{dB}]$$

$$L = 10 \times 0.30\ [\text{dB}]$$

$$L = 3\ \text{dB}$$

Thus, a 3-dB increase in the intensity level occurs when the sound intensity doubles. No matter what the original sound intensity level is, whenever the sound intensity is doubled, add 3 dB to it to arrive at the new sound intensity level.

Box 7.5 Decibel Rule #2

When the sound intensity doubles, the sound intensity level increases by 3 dB. In other words:

New sound intensity level = Original sound intensity level [dB IL] + 3 dB

Example 7.4

If the intensity of a signal with an original sound intensity level of 46 dB IL is doubled, what is the new sound intensity level?

First, select the appropriate equation. Recall from decibel rule #2 that when the sound intensity doubles, the sound intensity level increases by 3 dB.

New sound intensity level (L) = Original sound intensity level [dB IL] + 3 dB

Substitute known variables. We know the sound intensity level of the original sound source was 46 dB IL.

New sound intensity level (L) = 46 dB IL + 3 dB

L = 49 dB IL

Answer: 49 dB IL

Next, let us consider what happens to the sound pressure level when the sound pressure is increased by a factor of 10. Just as doubling the sound pressure didn't double the sound pressure level, increasing the sound pressure 10-fold will not result in a 10-fold increase in the sound pressure level. Before we calculate the actual increase, think about how many times you need to double a value to make it 10 times greater than it was originally. The first time we double it, it becomes twice as large. The second time, it becomes four (2 × 2) times as large. The third time, it becomes eight (2 × 2 × 2) times as large. After the fourth time we double it, it has become 16 times (2 × 2 × 2 × 2) as large. So if we double a value three times, we have almost increased it 10-fold, but if we double it a fourth time, we go too high. So we should expect the increase in the sound pressure level for a 10-fold increase in sound pressure to be a little higher than the increase caused by doubling the sound pressure three times, but less than that caused by doubling it four times. Since the sound pressure level increases by 6 dB each time the sound pressure is doubled, a 10-fold increase in the sound pressure should result in an increase of between 18 (3 × 6) dB and 24 (4 × 6) dB in the sound pressure level.

Now, let us determine the actual increase. Following the same method as in the previous examples, we enter the fraction corresponding to the ratio of the increase in the sound pressure into the sound pressure level equation. A 10-fold increase signifies a 10:1 ratio, which is represented by the fraction $\frac{10}{1}$. The steps needed to calculate the exact sound level increase are presented in the following example.

Example 7.5

If the sound pressure of a signal is increased 10-fold, by how much does the sound level increase?

Since the question asks about the increase in the sound pressure, use the sound pressure level equation.

$$L = 20 \times \log\left(\frac{p_2}{p_1}\right) [\text{dB}]$$

Substitute known variables. The increase of sound pressure is 10:1; therefore:

$$L = 20 \times \log\left(\frac{10}{1}\right) [\text{dB}]$$

Solve for L as you did in the previous examples.

$$L = 20 \times \log(10) [\text{dB}]$$

$$L = 20 \times 1\ [\text{dB}]$$

$$L = 20\ \text{dB}$$

Answer: 20 dB

A 10-fold increase in sound pressure will always result in a 20-dB gain in the sound pressure level. This is another commonly used rule for calculating sound pressure levels.

Box 7.6 Decibel Rule #3

When the sound pressure increases by a factor of 10, the sound pressure level increases by 20 dB. In other words:

New sound pressure level = Original sound pressure level [dB SPL] + 20 dB

Example 7.6

If the sound pressure of a signal having a sound pressure level of 48 dB SPL is increased by a factor of 10, what is the new sound pressure level?

First, select the appropriate equation. Here, use decibel rule #3.

New sound pressure level (L) = Original sound pressure level [dB SPL] + 20 dB

Substitute known variables. The original sound pressure level is 48 dB SPL.

$$L = 48 \text{ dB SPL} + 20 \text{ dB}$$

$$L = 68 \text{ dB SPL}$$

Answer: 68 dB SPL

Our last task, then, in this section will be to examine the effect of a 10-fold increase in sound intensity on the sound intensity level. Recall that doubling the sound intensity results in a 3-dB increase in the sound intensity level, so recalling our previous discussion, a 10-fold increase in sound intensity should cause an increase of between 9 (3 × 3) dB and 12 (4 × 3) dB in the sound intensity level.

To calculate the actual increase, we simply need to enter the fraction $\frac{10}{1}$ into the sound intensity equation (Equation 7.4). The steps involved in this calculation are outlined in Example 7.7.

Example 7.7

If the sound intensity of a signal is increased 10-fold, by how much does the sound level increase?

First, select the appropriate equation. Since the question asks about an increase in sound intensity level, select the sound intensity equation:

$$L = 10 \times \log\left(\frac{I_2}{I_1}\right)[\text{dB}]$$

and insert a 10:1 ratio into the formula:

$$L = 10 \times \log\left(\frac{10}{1}\right)[\text{dB}]$$

Simplify using the same steps you used in the other examples.

$$L = 10 \times \log(10)[\text{dB}]$$

$$L = 10 \times 1\ [\text{dB}]$$

$$L = 10 \text{ dB}$$

Answer: 10 dB

A 10-fold increase in sound intensity will always result in an increase of 10 dB in the sound intensity level. No matter what the initial sound intensity level, whenever the intensity is increased 10-fold, add 10 dB to it to arrive at the new sound intensity level. This is the last of the four commonly used decibel rules.

Box 7.7 Decibel Rule #4

When the intensity increases by a factor of 10, the sound intensity level increases by 10 dB. In other words:

New sound intensity level = Original sound intensity level [dB IL] + 10 dB

Example 7.8

If the sound intensity of a signal having a sound intensity level of 50 dB IL is increased by a factor of 10, what is the new sound intensity level?

First, select the appropriate equation. Here, use decibel rule #4.

New sound intensity level (L) = Original sound intensity level [dB IL] + 10 dB

Substitute known variables and solve.

New sound intensity level (L) = 50 [dB IL] + 10 dB

$$L = 60 \text{ dB IL}$$

Answer: 60 dB IL

The final example is a little bit more complicated.

Example 7.9

If we double the sound pressure of a sound source producing a level of 90 dB SPL, what sound intensity level does the sound source now produce?

This problem can be solved in two steps.

Step #1: The question states that the sound pressure is doubled. Whenever the sound pressure doubles, use decibel rule #1.

New sound pressure level (L) = Original sound pressure level [dB SPL] + 6 dB

$$L = 90 \text{ dB SPL} + 6 \text{ dB}$$

$$L = 96 \text{ dB SPL}$$

Step #2: The second part of the problem is to report the sound intensity level that the sound source now produces. Since sound pressure level and sound intensity levels are two names of the same quantity:

$$96 \text{ dB SPL} = 96 \text{ dB IL}$$

Answer: 96 dB IL

In summary, increasing the sound pressure and sound intensity will increase the sound pressure level and the sound intensity level. Since sound pressure (μPa) and sound intensity (W/m^2) are measured on a linear scale while sound pressure level (dB SPL) and sound intensity level (dB IL) are measured on a logarithmic scale, the numerical increase in dB SPL or dB

▶ **Table 7.4.** General Rules of Sound Pressure and Intensity Increases

	Sound Pressure (μPa)	Sound Intensity (W/m²)
Doubling (×2)	Add 6 dB	Add 3 dB
Tenfold increase (×10)	Add 20 dB	Add 10 dB

IL will be much smaller than the numerical increase in μPa and W/m². When the *sound pressure is doubled*, the sound pressure level increases by 6 dB (and the sound intensity level increases by 6 dB). When the *sound intensity is doubled*, the sound intensity level increases by 3 dB (and the sound pressure level increases by 3 dB). When the sound pressure increases by a factor of 10, the sound pressure level increases by 20 dB (and the sound intensity level increases by 20 dB). Finally, when the sound intensity increases by a factor of 10, the sound intensity level increases by 10 dB (and the sound pressure level increases by 10 dB). These four basic rules are summarized in Table 7.4. See the website for an extended version of this table, which makes it easy to estimate any decibel change. **Link 7-5**

PRACTICE PROBLEMS: INCREASING AND DECREASING SOUND PRESSURE AND SOUND INTENSITY

1. What is the sound intensity level produced by a sound source emitting 65 dB IL if the sound intensity is doubled?
2. What is the sound pressure level produced by a sound source emitting 50 dB SPL if the sound pressure is doubled?
3. If the sound intensity of a sound source producing 40 dB IL is increased 10 times, what is the resulting sound intensity level?
4. If the sound pressure of a sound source producing 53 dB SPL is increased 10 times, what is the resulting sound pressure level?
5. The sound pressure of a sound source producing 100 dB SPL is increased eight times. What is the new sound pressure level produced by this sound source?
6. The sound pressure of a sound source producing 65 dB SPL is decreased by a factor of five. What is the new sound pressure level produced by this sound source?
7. If the sound pressure of a sound source producing 62 dB SPL is decreased by a factor of 10, what is the resulting sound pressure level?

Answers (If you need help with these problems, consult the website.) **Link 7-6**

1. 68 dB IL
2. 56 dB SPL
3. 50 dB IL
4. 73 dB SPL
5. 118.06 dB SPL
6. 51.02 dB SPL
7. 42 dB SPL

Combining Sound Levels: Equal Sound Levels

Recall that the doubling of sound pressure produced by a sound source increases sound pressure level and sound intensity level by 6 dB and the doubling of sound intensity produced by a sound source increases sound pressure level by 3 dB. Consider now a situation in which instead of doubling the sound pressure or sound intensity of a single sound source, a second sound source producing the same sound level is added to the first one.*

Sound pressure is a vector quantity (see Chapter 2). So in the case of combining the sound pressure from two separate sources, the overall sound pressure depends on the phase relationship between the outputs of the two sources. For example, if the two separate sound sources are in-phase, the sound pressure will double (i.e., a 6-dB increase); if the two sources are 180° out-of-phase, the sound pressure of the two speakers will cancel each other; and if the two sources are 90° out-of-phase, the result is a 3-dB increase in sound level (based on vector addition; Chapter 2). If the phase relation changes randomly in time, this will also produce a 3-dB increase in sound level since the outputs will differ, on average, by 90°. Thus, any two sound sources that are phase independent (i.e., do not have a fixed phase relationship) produce together a sound level that is 3 dB higher than the sound level of a single source. Since in most cases separate sound sources are phase independent, in all other examples and practice problems that have multiple sound sources we assume that the sound sources are phase independent.

Note further that a 3-dB increase in sound level means a doubling in sound intensity. In other words, combining two independent sound sources producing the same sound level doubles the sound intensity produced by a single source. This is the basic rule used in combining sounds of the same intensity (pressure) produced by various sound sources together.

Box 7.8 Decibel Rule #5

Doubling the number of equal intensity sound sources results in a doubling of sound intensity, not a doubling of sound pressure.

*In the problems dealing with multiple sound sources, assume that all the sources are located in the same place.

Example 7.10

If two loudspeakers produce a sound intensity level of 30 dB IL each:

(a) What is the total sound intensity level?
(b) What is the total sound pressure level?

First, note that both sound sources produce the same sound intensity level of 30 dB IL. You know from the previous examples that this means each sound source also has a sound pressure level of 30 dB SPL. Second, recall our discussion that separate sound sources are phase independent. Therefore, when the two sources are combined, their sound intensity is doubled (decibel rule #5). Thus, select the intensity equation to determine the result of combining two separate, but equal, sound sources.

New sound intensity level = Original sound intensity level [dB IL] + 3 dB

L = 30 [dB IL] + 3 dB

L = 33 dB IL

Answer to part a: 33 dB IL

Since the second question of this example was about the combined sound pressure level, convert the numeric result from dB IL to dB SPL.

33 dB IL = 33 dB SPL

Answer to part b: 33 dB SPL

Example 7.11

If one loudspeaker produces 80 dB IL and we add a second loudspeaker, also producing 80 dB IL, what is the total sound intensity level?

Select the appropriate equation. Remember, when working with separate sound sources, always use the intensity level rules and equations. Two equal loudspeakers create double the intensity compared to the intensity of one loudspeaker.

New sound intensity level (L) = Original sound intensity level [dB IL] + 3 dB

L = 80 [dB IL] + 3 dB

L = 83 dB IL

Answer: The new level is 83 dB IL.

Example 7.12

If the sound pressure produced by one loudspeaker is measured at 90 dB SPL and we add a second loudspeaker also producing 90 dB SPL, what is the total sound pressure level?

First, recall that dB SPL is equal to dB IL.

90 dB SPL = 90 dB IL

Second, remember to use the intensity level equation for separate sound sources.

New sound intensity level (L) = Original sound intensity level [dB IL] + 3 dB

L = 90 [dB IL] + 3 dB

L = 93 dB IL

The new sound intensity level is 93 dB IL.

Convert back to dB SPL.

93 dB IL = 93 dB SPL

Answer: The total sound pressure level is 93 dB SPL.

The previous two examples involved two loudspeakers, but their number may be much larger. Consider, for example, a group of 10 loudspeakers. It is no more difficult to calculate the total sound intensity level in this situation than in the case of two loudspeakers. Hopefully, you have not forgotten decibel rule #4.

Example 7.13

If a loudspeaker produces 80 dB IL, what would the total sound intensity level be for an array of 10 such loudspeakers?

Select the appropriate equation. Here, recall decibel rule #4.

New sound intensity level = Original sound intensity level [dB IL] + 10 dB

L = 80 dB IL + 10 dB

L = 90 dB IL

Answer: The total sound intensity level is 90 dB IL.

In general, if there are more than two sound sources, the following formula can be used to calculate the total sound intensity level. Since sound intensity level and sound pressure level are numerically equivalent for any single sound source, we can apply this formula (Equation 7.8) regardless of whether we are provided with or asked for the sound intensity level in dB IL or the sound pressure level in dB SPL:

$$\text{Total level} = \text{Level of single source [dB Ref]} + [10 \times \log(\text{number of sources})]\ \text{dB} \quad (7.8)$$

where Ref can be either SPL or IL and refers to the reference label identified in the problem.

Example 7.14

If there are three loudspeakers each producing 76 dB IL, what is the total sound intensity level?

Select the appropriate equation. Here, use Equation 7.8.

$$\text{Total level} = \text{Level of single source [dB Ref]} + [10 \times \log(\text{number of sources})]\ \text{dB}$$

Substitute known variables. Here, the level of a single source is 76 dB IL and there are three sources. Therefore:

$$L = 76 \text{ dB IL} + [10 \times \log(3)] \text{ dB}$$

Simplify the equation.

$$L = 76 \text{ dB IL} + [10 \times 0.48] \text{ dB}$$

$$L = 76 \text{ dB IL} + 4.8 \text{ dB}$$

$$L = 80.8 \text{ dB IL}$$

Answer: 80.8 dB IL

Example 7.14 could be restated as follows: If there are three loudspeakers each producing 76 dB SPL, what is the total sound pressure level? The calculation would be exactly the same as above with the exception of the units. Notice here the use of dB SPL instead of dB IL.

$$\text{Total level} = \text{Level of single source [dB Ref]} + [10 \times \log(\text{number of sources})] \text{ dB}$$

$$L = 76 \text{ dB SPL} + [10 \times \log(3)] \text{ dB}$$

$$L = 80.8 \text{ dB SPL}$$

Answer: 80.8 dB SPL

Remember, regardless of whether the problem specifies dB SPL or dB IL, if separate sound sources are being combined, you should always use the formula for combining sound levels produced by equal intensity sound sources, which is based on the intensity rules for changes in level.

PRACTICE PROBLEMS: COMBINING SEPARATE SOUND SOURCES

1. If two loudspeakers work together, each of them producing a sound pressure level of 62 dB SPL, what is their combined sound pressure level?
2. If three loudspeakers produce 85 dB IL each, what is the combined intensity level produced by the whole group?
3. A single loudspeaker produces 72 dB SPL. What would be the sound pressure produced by a group of five such loudspeakers?
4. A sound system has four loudspeakers. Each of these loudspeakers produces 32 dB IL. What is the total sound intensity level produced by the system?
5. If a choir has 16 sopranos and each of them produces a sound pressure level of 75 dB SPL, what is the overall sound pressure level produced by the whole group of sopranos?
6. What is the total sound pressure level produced by a group of 40 Canada geese if each of them quacks at 64 dB SPL?
7. If the outputs of 100 loudspeakers producing a sound intensity level of 8 dB IL each are added together, what is their combined sound intensity level?
8. If 10 people speaking simultaneously at 49 dB IL each produce a speech babble, what would be the overall sound intensity level of the babble?

Answers (If you need help with these problems, consult the website.) **Link 7-7**

1. 65 dB SPL
2. 89.77 dB IL
3. 78.99 dB SPL
4. 38.02 dB IL
5. 87.04 dB SPL
6. 80.02 dB SPL
7. 28 dB IL
8. 59 dB IL

Extracting the Sound Level of a Single Sound Source

The objective of the previous sections was to find the overall sound level produced by a group of sound sources emitting sounds of the same intensity. In this section we will consider the reverse problem and determine the sound level produced by a single sound source given the total sound intensity level (or sound pressure level) produced by a group of sound sources. As before, we will use the Formula for Combining Equal Sound Levels. However, in this case our unknown is the "level of a single source" instead of the "total level" as in the preceding section.

Example 7.15

If 58 loudspeakers (each producing the same sound intensity level) combine to produce an overall intensity level of 130 dB IL, what is the individual intensity level of each loudspeaker?

First, select the appropriate equation and as before select the Formula for Combining Equal Sound Levels.

$$\text{Total level} = \text{Level of single source [dB Ref]} + [10 \times \log(\text{number of sources})] \text{ dB}$$

Substitute known variables. In this case, the total intensity level and the number of sources are known. The unknown quantity is the intensity level of a single source.

$$130 \text{ dB IL} = L + [10 \times \log(58)] \text{ dB}$$

Simplify.

$$130 \text{ dB IL} = L + [10 \times 1.76] \text{ dB}$$

$$130 \text{ dB IL} = L + 17.6 \text{ dB}$$

Next, isolate L on one side by subtracting 17.6 dB from both sides of the equation.

$$\{130 \text{ dB IL}\} - 17.6 \text{ dB} = \{L + 17.6 \text{ dB}\} - 17.6 \text{ dB}$$

$$112.4 \text{ dB IL} = L$$

Answer: Each loudspeaker has an intensity level of 112.4 dB IL.

Example 7.16

If 14 loudspeakers (all at the same sound pressure level) combine to produce an overall sound pressure level of 100 dB SPL, what is the sound pressure level of each loudspeaker?

First, select the appropriate equation. Remember to use the Formula for Combining Equal Sound Levels regardless of whether it is intensity level or pressure level that is specified.

$$\text{Total level} = \text{Level of single source [dB Ref]} + [10 \times \log(\text{number of sources})] \text{ dB}$$

Substitute known variables. The total pressure level and the number of sources are known. The unknown quantity is the pressure level of a single source.

$$100 \text{ dB SPL} = L + [10 \times \log(14)] \text{ dB}$$

Simplify.

$$100 \text{ dB SPL} = L + [10 \times 1.15] \text{ dB}$$

$$100 \text{ dB SPL} = L + 11.5 \text{ dB}$$

Next, solve for L by subtracting 11.5 dB from both sides of the equation.

$$\{100 \text{ dB SPL}\} - 11.5 \text{ dB} = \{L + 11.5 \text{ dB}\} - 11.5 \text{ dB}$$

$$88.5 \text{ dB SPL} = L$$

Answer: Each loudspeaker has a sound pressure level of 88.5 dB SPL.

PRACTICE PROBLEMS: DETERMINING SOUND PRESSURE AND SOUND INTENSITY GIVEN SOUND PRESSURE LEVEL AND SOUND INTENSITY LEVEL

1. If 100 loudspeakers (each producing the same sound intensity level) produce an overall sound intensity level of 100 dB IL, what is the sound intensity level produced by each loudspeaker?
2. If six ducks (each of them quacking at the same intensity level) produce an overall sound intensity level of 86 dB IL, what is the sound intensity level produced by each duck?
3. If 54 violinists (each playing at the same sound intensity level) produce an overall sound intensity level of 98 dB IL, what is the sound intensity level produced by each violinist?
4. If eight vacuum cleaners (all making noise at the same sound intensity level) produce an overall sound intensity level of 53.78 dB IL, what is the sound intensity level produced by each vacuum cleaner?
5. If two dishwashers (each making noise at the same sound intensity level) produce an overall sound intensity level of 77 dB IL, what is the sound intensity level produced by each dishwasher?
6. If 11 loudspeakers (each producing the same sound pressure level) produce an overall sound pressure level of 65 dB SPL, what is the sound pressure level produced by each loudspeaker?
7. If 90 loudspeakers (each producing the same sound pressure level) produce an overall sound pressure level of 19 dB SPL, what is the sound pressure level produced by each loudspeaker?
8. If eight weaving looms (each generating the same sound pressure level) produce an overall sound pressure level of 54 dB SPL, what is the sound pressure level produced by each loom?

Answers (If you need help with these problems, consult the website.) **Link 7-8**

1. 80 dB IL
2. 78.22 dB IL
3. 80.68 dB IL
4. 44.75 dB IL
5. 73.99 dB IL
6. 54.59 dB SPL
7. −0.54 dB SPL
8. 44.97 dB SPL

Combining Sound Levels: Groups With Equal Sound Levels

Frequently, the total sound intensity level of multiple sound sources is known but an additional group of sound sources (each producing sound of equal intensity) needs to be added. Consider, for example, a choir with 20 singers to which four new singers are added. This section shows how to calculate the new sound level with the additional singers.

Example 7.17

In a textile manufacturing plant, a room contains 15 working looms producing a total intensity level of 100 dB IL. If the textile manufacturer purchases and installs four additional looms (each making the same sound), what will the total sound intensity level be in the room? (Note: Other factors, such as differences in location of individual looms and the reflection of sound waves within the room [Chapter 6], should also be considered, but we will focus in this chapter only on the simple combination of sounds produced by multiple sound sources).

The addition of four looms would bring the total number of looms in the room to 19 looms. If the noise created by 19 looms is compared with the noise created by the original 15 looms, this becomes a 19:15 ratio. We are interested in the increase in sound intensity level that would result from a 19:15 ratio change in the linear scale. Recall the original sound intensity level equation.

$$L = 10 \times \log\left(\frac{I_2}{I_1}\right) [\text{dB}]$$

For this example, substitute the ratio 19/15 into the equation.

$$L = 10 \times \log\left(\frac{19}{15}\right) [\text{dB}]$$

Simplify.

$$L = 10 \times \log(1.2667) [\text{dB}]$$

$$L = 10 \times 0.1027 [\text{dB}]$$

$$L = 1.0267 [\text{dB}]$$

$$L = 1.03 \text{ dB}$$

The result, 1.03 dB, is the amount added to the overall intensity level created by 15 looms. The result is the new overall intensity level with 19 looms.

New sound intensity level = Original sound intensity level + 1.03

$$L = 100 + 1.03$$

$$L = 101.03$$

Answer: 101.03 dB IL

PRACTICE PROBLEMS: COMBINING GROUPS OF SOUND SOURCES

1. If 54 loudspeakers (each one producing an equal sound intensity level) produce together 58 dB SPL and 54 additional loudspeakers are added (each one producing an equal intensity level compared with the first group), what is the new sound pressure level?
2. If 29 loudspeakers (each one producing an equal sound intensity level) produce together 60 dB IL and 17 additional loudspeakers are added (each one producing an equal intensity level compared with the first group), what is the new sound intensity level?
3. If 34 loudspeakers (each one producing an equal sound intensity level) produce 60 dB IL and 12 loudspeakers are added (each one producing equal intensity levels compared with the first group), what is the new sound intensity level?
4. If nine loudspeakers (each one producing an equal sound intensity level) produce 24 dB SPL and nine additional loudspeakers are added (each one producing an equal sound intensity level compared with the first group), what is the new sound pressure level?
5. If 100 loudspeakers (each one producing an equal sound intensity level) produce 54 dB SPL and three additional loudspeakers are added (each one producing an equal sound intensity level compared with the first group), what is the new sound pressure level?
6. If 14 loudspeakers (each one producing an equal sound intensity level) produce 5 dB SPL and seven additional loudspeakers are added (each one producing an equal sound intensity level compared with the first group), what is the new sound pressure level?
7. If 50 loudspeakers (each one producing an equal sound intensity level) produce 42 dB SPL and 15 loudspeakers are turned off, what is the new sound pressure level?
8. If 11 loudspeakers (each one producing an equal sound intensity level) produce 58 dB SPL and five are turned off, what is the new sound pressure level?

Answers (If you need help with these problems, consult the website.) **Link 7-9**

1. 61.01 dB SPL
2. 62.00 dB IL
3. 61.31 dB IL
4. 27.01 dB SPL
5. 54.13 dB SPL
6. 6.76 dB SPL
7. 40.45 dB SPL
8. 55.37 dB SPL

Combining Sound Levels: Unequal Sound Levels

The decibel operations described in the previous three sections involved sound pressure level or sound intensity level produced by a single sound source or by a group of sources all emitting sound at the same level. In this section the above relationship will be expanded to situations where the sound levels produced by different sound sources are not equal. Consider two loudspeakers (A and B), working together, with the louder loudspeaker A producing a sound intensity level of 50 dB IL. The closer the sound intensity of loudspeaker B is to the sound intensity of the louder speaker A, the greater the effect loudspeaker B will have on the total sound intensity level.

A (louder) + B (quieter)

If loudspeakers A and B each produce 50 dB IL, the combined intensity will be double the intensity of each loudspeaker individually, so the total intensity level would increase by 3 dB from 50 dB IL to 53 dB IL. The lower the sound intensity level of the quieter loudspeaker (B) is, the less effect it has on the total sound intensity level. However, even if loudspeaker B was unplugged, the total intensity level for both loudspeakers could not be less than 50 dB IL because loudspeaker A is producing 50 dB IL by itself. Therefore, the combined intensity level must be somewhere between 50 and 53 dB IL. To think of this situation another way, imagine riding on the subway. In the subway car one person has a boom box that is turned up to its maximum volume and another person with a smaller radio gets on the subway car. The sound from the smaller radio will not have a large effect on the overall amount of sound in the subway car. The quieter the small radio gets, the less effect the sound has on the total intensity in the subway car. However, even if the small radio is turned off, the total amount of sound produced by the small radio plus the boom box will not be less that the sound level produced by the boom box by itself. In summary, when two sound sources are combined, the total sound intensity level cannot be less than the intensity level of the louder one and it cannot be more than 3 dB greater than the louder one.

Example 7.18

Give a ballpark estimate of the combined sound intensity level that would result if source A produces a sound intensity level of 60 dB IL and source B produces a sound intensity level of 40 dB IL.

Remember that the louder source is 60 dB IL, so the total cannot be less than 60 dB IL. If the second source were 60 dB IL, the total intensity level would be 63 dB IL.

Answer: The total sound intensity level will be somewhere between 60 and 63 dB IL.

However, there is a much more precise way to determine the overall intensity level when combining different intensity sound sources than the procedure described above. If a group of *n* sound sources works together, then you can use the equation for combining unequal sound levels produced by different sound sources, which is the equation expressed below:

$$L = 10 \log(10^{L_1/10} + 10^{L_2/10} + \cdots + 10^{L_n/10})[\text{dB IL}] \quad (7.9)$$

where L_1 = the level of the first source, L_2 = the level of the second source, and so forth up to L_n, which is the last source to be combined. If you would like to see the derivation of this equation, see the website. **Link 7-10** It is actually quite easy to apply this formula if you take it step by step.

Example 7.19

What is the total sound intensity level when three sources of sound produce 20 dB IL, 25 dB IL, and 30 dB IL?

First, select the appropriate equation. Use the equation for combining unequal sound levels produced by different sound sources.

$$L = 10 \log(10^{L_1/10} + 10^{L_2/10} + \cdots + 10^{L_n/10})[\text{dB IL}]$$

Second, substitute known variables into the equation. From the problem, we know that there are three levels to be considered: $L_1 = 20$, $L_2 = 25$, and $L_3 = 30$.

$$L = 10 \log(10^{20/10} + 10^{25/10} + 10^{30/10})\ [\text{dB IL}]$$

Next, simplify the equation. First, simplify the logs by dividing by 10.

$$L = 10 \log(10^2 + 10^{2.5} + 10^3)\ [\text{dB IL}]$$

Next, simplify the log problems within the parenthesis.

$$L = 10 \log(100 + 316.2 + 1000)\ [\text{dB IL}]$$

Next, add the numbers within the parenthesis.

$$L = 10 \log(1416.2)\ [\text{dB IL}]$$

Next, find the log of 1416.2.

$$L = 10 \times 3.2\ [\text{dB IL}]$$

Simplify.

$$L = 32 \text{ dB IL}$$

Please note that combining two other sound sources with lower sound intensity levels (i.e., 20 and 25 dB IL) to the sound source producing 30 dB IL only slightly changed the overall sound intensity level.

PRACTICE PROBLEMS: COMBINING SEPARATE SOUND SOURCES OF DIFFERENT INTENSITY

1. Loudspeakers producing 23, 42, 33, 38, and 40 dB SPL operate together. Use the equation for combining unequal sound levels to determine the total sound pressure level.
2. Loudspeakers producing 45, 43, and 22 dB SPL operate together. Use the equation for combining unequal sound levels to determine the total sound pressure level.
3. Loudspeakers producing 42, 31, 85, 24, and 12 dB SPL operate together. Use the equation for combining unequal sound levels to determine the total sound pressure level.

Answers (If you need help with these problems, consult the website.) **Link 7-11**

1. 45.4 dB SPL
2. 47.14 dB SPL
3. 85 dB SPL

CONVERTING SOUND LEVELS INTO SOUND PRESSURE AND SOUND INTENSITY

The final sound level calculation that is used in solving practical problems involves mathematical concepts that have already been discussed. Sometimes we need to determine sound intensity (W/m^2) or sound pressure (μPa) knowing the sound intensity level (dB IL) or sound pressure level (dB SPL). To determine these values, use Equations 7.6 and 7.7 introduced at the beginning of the chapter and isolate the unknown variable.

Example 7.20

What is the sound pressure that is equal to 9.6 dB SPL?

First, select the appropriate equation. Since the problem involves dB SPL and a specific sound pressure (p), use the sound pressure level equation.

$$L = 20 \times \log\left(\frac{p}{20\ \mu Pa}\right)$$

Next, substitute known variables. In this problem, the sound pressure level of the sound source is 9.6 dB SPL.

$$9.6 = 20 \times \log\left(\frac{p}{20\ \mu Pa}\right)$$

Solve by using reverse order of operations (from Chapter 1). First, divide each side by 20.

$$\frac{9.6}{20} = \frac{20 \times \log\left(\frac{p}{20\ \mu Pa}\right)}{20}$$

$$0.48 = \log\left(\frac{p}{20\ \mu Pa}\right)$$

Next, take the antilog of both sides.

$$antilog\ \{0.48\} = antilog\left\{\log\left(\frac{p}{20\ \mu Pa}\right)\right\}$$

$$3 = \frac{p}{20\ \mu Pa}$$

Last, multiply both sides by 20 and simplify.

$$20 \times 3 = \frac{p}{20\ \mu Pa} \times 20$$

$$60 = p$$

Answer: 60 µPa

PRACTICE PROBLEMS: FINDING SOUND PRESSURE AND SOUND INTENSITY GIVEN SOUND PRESSURE LEVEL AND SOUND INTENSITY LEVEL

1. If the sound pressure level is 60 dB SPL, what is the sound pressure?
2. If the sound pressure level is 83 dB SPL, what is the sound pressure?
3. If the sound intensity level is 100 dB IL, what is the sound intensity?
4. If the sound pressure level is 99 dB SPL, what is the sound pressure?
5. If the sound intensity level is −14.76 dB IL, what is the sound intensity?

Answers (If you need help with these problems, consult the website.) **Link 7-12**

1. 20,000 µPa (or 2.0×10^4 µPa)
2. 282507.51 µPa (or 2.82×10^5 µPa)
3. 0.01 W/m^2 (or $1.0 \times 10^{-2}\ W/m^2$)
4. 1782501.88 µPa (or 1.78×10^6 µPa)
5. $3.34 \times 10^{-14}\ W/m^2$

APPLICATIONS OF THE DECIBEL SCALE

The decibel scale has many practical uses across the fields of hearing science, audiology, acoustics, and engineering. The most common applications include audiologic (hearing) testing, background noise and signal-to-noise ratio measurements for assessment of classroom acoustics (Chapter 6), and the measurement and comparison of sound spectra using waveform analysis (Chapter 4) or similar analytical tools.

Audiologic testing includes various types of sounds presented at various levels. Since human perception of sound is frequency dependent, the sounds that are presented to the listener at different frequencies must be at different sound pressure levels in order to provide information about a patient's hearing. The level of sound that a patient hears, that is, the patient's threshold of hearing, is actually reported not in dB SPL, but using a different point of reference called hearing level (HL), which indicates how closely a patient's hearing is to average normal hearing at a given frequency (see Chapter 12). Some tests also require the use of still another point of reference called sensation level (SL), which indicates how much louder or softer a tone is compared to the quietest sound a patient can hear at a given frequency. The next five chapters in this book will discuss more about how the ear receives and processes sound.

The hearing level and sensation level scales are examples of weighted scales. A weighted scale is a scale in which the reference level changes with frequency. Some other examples of weighted scales are scales dB (A), dB (B), and dB (C) that are used to predict how loud and damaging a given sound is to the human ear. When using a weighted scale, some of the spectral components of the sound are given a weight smaller than 1, whereas some others are given a weight larger than 1 in order to simulate the frequency dependence of the human ear at a given sound level. Detailed descriptions of weighted scales used for sound measurement can be found in books on industrial audiology and noise control. Another industrial and military application of the decibel scale is in the calculation of the noise reduction rating (NRR) of hearing protection devices. The NRR indicates how much sound is attenuated (blocked out) by an earmuff, earplug, or other hearing protection device. Note that the NRR gives only one attenuation value, but the attenuation provided by hearing protection devices varies across frequency.

Classroom acoustics were discussed in Chapter 6. Assessment of various listening conditions and comparisons between listening environments are best done using the decibel scale. For example, reverberation time (RT) is calculated as the amount of time it takes for a sound to decrease in intensity by 60 dB. Another commonly used concept in the evaluation of listening conditions is that of the signal-to-noise ratio (SNR). If a teacher speaks at a level of 70 dB SPL and an air conditioner is making a noise of 60 dB SPL, this creates a signal-to-noise ratio of 70 − 60 dB = 10 dB SNR. This is not an optimal listening environment; however, it is better than a signal-to-noise ratio of 0 dB SNR or even −10 dB SNR (where the signal has an intensity level 10 dB lower than the noise.)

An additional domain where the decibel is commonly used is sound analysis. In Chapter 4 we discussed spectrum density and used waveform analysis to determine the components that make up a complex wave. The decibel is frequently used as the relative measure when reporting both the overall level of the sound and the level of the components. The intensity level of each spectral component that is 1 Hz wide is called the **spectrum level** (L_o). The L_o can be determined if the overall intensity level (L) and the **bandwidth** (Δf) of a sound are known. The bandwidth is the frequency range of the sound. Conversely, the overall intensity level (L) can be determined if both the bandwidth (Δf) and the spectrum level (L_o) are known using the following equation:

$$L = L_o + 10 \log (\Delta f) \quad (7.10)$$

Example 7.21

What is the overall intensity level (L) of a sound having a spectrum level (L_o) of 10 dB IL and a bandwidth (Δf) of 10,000 Hz?

First, select Equation 7.10.

$$L = L_o + 10 \log (\Delta f)$$

Substitute known variables and solve.

$$L = 10 + 10 \times \log (10{,}000) \text{ [dB IL]}$$

$$L = 10 + (10 \times 4) \text{ [dB IL]}$$

$$L = 10 + 40 \text{ [dB IL]}$$

$$L = 50 \text{ dB IL}$$

Example 7.22

What is the spectrum level of a sound with a bandwidth of 10,000 Hz if the overall intensity level is 95 dB SPL?

Use Equation 7.10.

$$L = L_o + 10 \log (\Delta f)$$

Substitute known variables. Here you will solve for L_o instead of L.

$$95 \text{ dB SPL} = L_o + 10 \log (10{,}000)$$

$$95 \text{ dB SPL} = L_o + 40$$

$$55 \text{ dB SPL} = L_o$$

PRACTICE PROBLEMS: OVERALL SOUND PRESSURE LEVEL AND SPECTRUM LEVEL

1. What is the overall sound pressure level of a sound having a spectrum level of 23 dB SPL and a bandwidth of 8000 Hz?
2. What is the overall sound pressure level of a sound having a spectrum level of 56 dB SPL and a bandwidth of 7000 Hz?
3. What is the spectrum level of a sound with a bandwidth of 5000 Hz if the overall sound pressure level is 100 dB SPL?
4. What is the spectrum level of a sound with a bandwidth of 10,000 Hz if the overall sound pressure level is 78 dB SPL?

Answers (If you need help with these problems, consult the website.) **Link 7-13**

1. 62.03 dB SPL
2. 94.45 dB SPL
3. 63.01 dB SPL
4. 38 dB SPL

Summary

The decibel is a relative unit of measurement that measures the ratio of two physical measurements. Relative units tell us how many times one value is greater than another. This information is particularly relevant when dealing with human response to physical stimuli, as we respond to relative and not absolute changes in the environment. A logarithmic unit of measurement is a unit that uses the logarithm of a measured quantity instead of the quantity itself. The use of a logarithmic unit is helpful when the possible quantities cover a large range of values, because the logarithmic transformation compresses the range into a much smaller and much more manageable range.

The decibel is a logarithmic unit that is equal to the logarithm base 10 of the ratio of two powers or power-like quantities. Measurements expressed in decibels are called levels. Two fundamental forms of level calculations are $L = 10 \times \log\left(\frac{I_2}{I_1}\right)$ [dB] and $L = 20 \times \log\left(\frac{P_2}{P_1}\right)$ [dB]. If these formulas refer to the specific reference points of 10^{-12} W/m^2 and 20 μPa, they are called the sound intensity level and the sound pressure level scales, respectively. Numerous forms of these equations are used to calculate relative levels of sound in various applications.

Key Points

- Most human reactions are in response to a relative, not absolute, change in a stimulus.
- The decibel is a relative measurement and a logarithmic unit with base 10.
- Logarithmic units allow for the numerical representation of physical magnitudes in a manner that correlates to human perception and allow for the compression of a large range of physical values into a much smaller and more manageable range.
- Sound pressure can be converted to sound pressure level using the equation:

$$L = 20 \times \log\left(\frac{p}{20\ \mu Pa}\right) \text{ [dB SPL]}$$

- Sound intensity can be converted to sound intensity level using the equation:

$$L = 10 \times \log\left(\frac{I}{10^{-12}\frac{w}{m^2}}\right) \text{ [dB IL]}$$

- Sound intensity level and sound pressure level of the same sound are by definition the same, that is, 100 dB IL = 100 dB SPL.

PART III

Hearing

Chapter Outline

CHAPTER 8

Outer Ear and Middle Ear

Objectives

- To review outer and middle ear anatomy
- To provide students with an understanding of outer and middle ear physiology including how sound entering the ear canal is changed by the cavities and structures within the outer and middle ear
- To review concepts of impedance as they relate to the physiology of the middle ear

Key Terms

Acoustic reflex
Aditus ad antrum
Annular ligament
Annulus
Anterior ligament of the malleus
Antihelix
Antitragus
Antrum
Auricular tubercle (Darwin's tubercle)
Azimuth estimation
Binaural
Binaural localization cues
Cartilaginous portion of the ear canal
Catenary lever (buckling effect)
Cavum concha
Cerumen
Chorda tympani
Concha
Cone of light
Crura of the antihelix
Crus of the helix
Cymba concha
Distance estimation
Elevation estimation
Epitympanum
Eustachian tube (auditory tube, pharyngotympanic tube)
External auditory canal
External auditory meatus
Helix
Hypotympanum
Incudostapedial joint
Incus
Inner ear
Interaural
Interaural intensity difference (IID)
Interaural phase difference
Interaural time difference (ITD)
Intertragal notch
Isthmus
Lenticular process of the incus
Levator veli palatini muscle
Lobule (ear lobe)
Localization
Localization cues
Malleus
Manubrium of the malleus
Mastoid air cells
Mesotympanum
Middle ear
Monaural
Monaural localization cues
Nasopharyngeal cavity (nasopharynx)
Notch of Rivinus
Obturator foramen
Osseous portion of the ear canal

Ossicles	Pressure transformer	Tragus
Ossicular chain	Pyramidal eminence	Transducer
Ossicular lever	Scaphoid fossa	Triangular fossa
Otoscope	Stapedius muscle	Tympanic cavity
Outer ear	Stapes	Tympanic membrane
Pars flaccida	Tegmen tympani	Tympanic sulcus
Pars tensa	Temporomandibular joint	Tympanosclerosis
Pinna (auricle)	Tensor tympani muscle	Tympanum
Posterior ligament of the incus	Tensor veli palatini muscle	Umbo
		Valsalva maneuver

The ear is the organ for hearing and balance. The ear structure consists of three major parts: the **outer ear**, the **middle ear**, and the **inner ear**, which are shown in Figure 8.1. The outer ear and the middle ear collect and transmit sounds. The inner ear contains the vestibulocochlear organs, which convert sound (cochlea) and body movements (vestibular system) into neural impulses that can be interpreted by the brain for the perception of sound and maintenance of balance. The outer ear, the middle ear, and the inner ear work together to convert sound from its original form (sound waves in air) to a bioelectrical energy that can be transmitted to and interpreted by the brain. In the process of energy conversion, sound enters the outer ear in the form of sound waves propagating in the air and it is converted by the mechanical motion of the tympanic membrane and the ossicular chain (middle ear) into fluid waves in the inner ear. The fluid motion of the inner ear affects the behavior of the auditory receptor cells, which convert the mechanical motion into electrochemical energy for transmission by the nervous system to the brain. The main functions of the outer and middle ear structures are to receive acoustic energy, convert this acoustic energy into mechanical energy, and deliver it to the inner ear.

OUTER EAR ANATOMY

The outer ear, also called the external ear, is the most familiar part of the ear because it is visible from the outside of the body. The outer ear consists of the **pinna** (**auricle**) and the **external auditory canal** (ear canal). The external auditory canal terminates at the **tympanic membrane** (eardrum), which separates the outer ear from the middle ear.

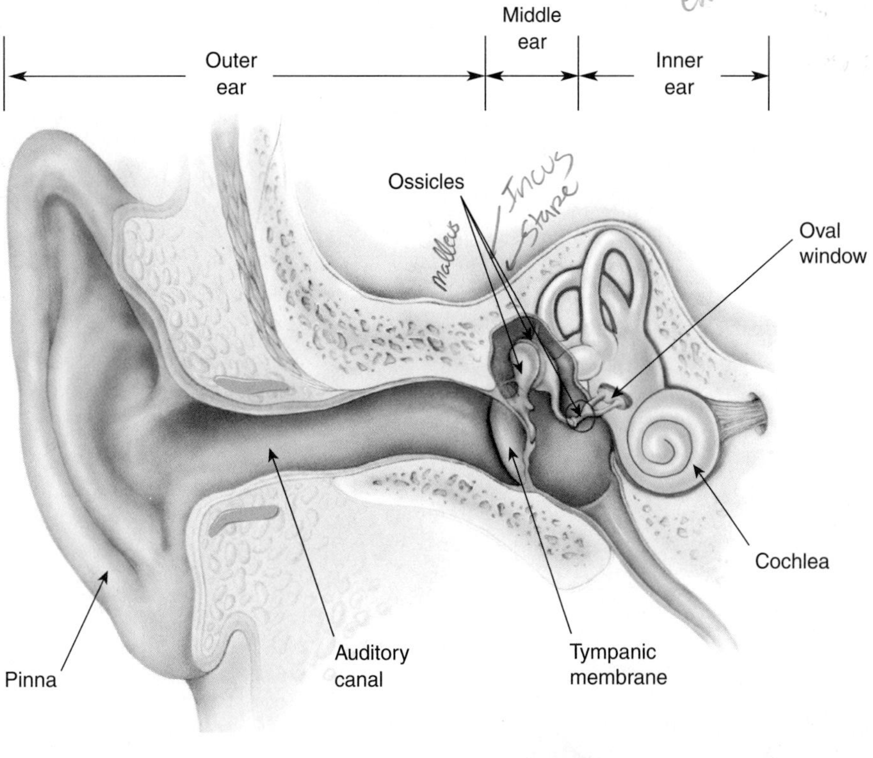

Figure 8.1. Cross section of the ear. (Modified from Bear MF, Connors BW, Parasido MA. Neuroscience—Exploring the Brain. 2nd Ed. Philadelphia: Lippincott Williams & Wilkins, 2001.)

Pinna

The pinna is the structure of the outer ear that extends out from the side of the head at about a 30° angle around the **external auditory meatus** (opening) of the ear canal (Glasscock & Shambaugh, 1990). The convoluted shape of the pinna is created by an internal frame made of cartilage and fibrous tissue that is quite flexible when manipulated. A number of distinctive landmarks on the pinna are identified in Figure 8.2.

The lowest part of the pinna is the **lobule** (ear lobe). The lobule is composed of skin and fat, but there is no cartilage in this portion. If you feel your earlobe with your finger, you can identify where the cartilage begins at the edges of the earlobe. The **helix** is the outer fold of the pinna that curves around the outside edge and ends at the **crus of the helix** (*crus* means "leg"). Sometimes there is a bump of extra tissue along the edge of the helix called an **auricular tubercle** (or Darwin's tubercle). Underneath the curve of the helix is a groove called the **scaphoid fossa.** The second ring of cartilage is the **antihelix.** At the top of the pinna, the antihelix spreads into two separate folds called the **crura of the antihelix** (*crura* is the plural of crus) forming a triangle-shaped indentation called the **triangular fossa.** Notable projections at the bottom of the pinna include the **tragus** and the **antitragus,** and the groove between them is called the **intertragal notch.** The deepest groove in the pinna, a bowl-shaped depression called the **concha,** is approximately 10 to 20 mm in diameter and leads directly into the opening of the ear canal. The concha is often described as having two parts, the **cavum concha,** which is closest to the external auditory meatus, and the **cymba concha,** which is the upper part of the concha that curves up and between the crus of the helix and the inferior crus of the antihelix. The complex shape of the pinna structure helps in locating the direction from which sound is coming (localization).

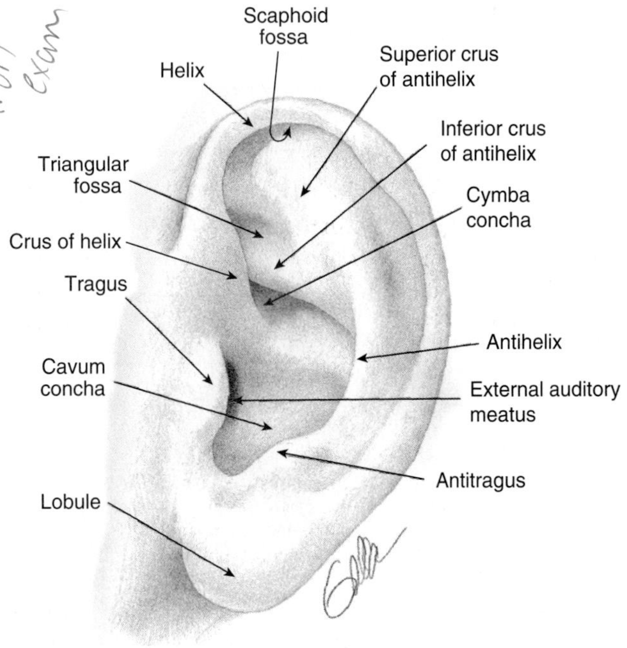

Figure 8.2. The pinna. (Modified from Janfaza P, Nadol Jr JB, Galla R, et al. Surgical Anatomy of the Head and Neck. Philadelphia: Lippincott Williams & Wilkins, 2001.)

External Auditory Canal

The cartilage that creates the frame of the pinna also lines the outer one third of the ear canal (Fig. 8.1). This part of the ear canal is called the **cartilaginous** portion. The inner two thirds of the ear canal does not contain a layer of cartilage and is referred to as the **osseous** or bony portion of the ear canal. The cartilaginous portion of the ear canal contains a relatively thick layer of skin (0.5 to 1 mm thick) containing hairs and glands that create **cerumen** (ear wax), whereas the osseous portion of the ear canal contains a thinner layer of skin (about 0.2 mm thick) without hairs or ceruminous glands (Lucente, 1995). About 4 mm from the tympanic membrane, the ear canal forms an **isthmus** (narrowing). The **temporomandibular joint** (the jaw joint) is anterior to (in front of) the ear canal. If you put your finger in your ear canal and open and close your jaw, you can feel a change in the size and shape of the ear canal as the jaw moves.

The length of the external auditory canal in adults is approximately 2.5 cm long (Alvord & Farmer, 1997). The canal forms an S-shaped curve ending at the tympanic membrane, which forms the border between the outer ear and the middle ear. The effective acoustic length of the canal is about 25% longer due to the "end effect" of the concha (Teranishi & Shaw, 1968). The "end effect" is an effective acoustic elongation of the anatomic length of the ear canal due to the flare-like opening of the ear canal at the concha and the stiffness of the air. The volume of the ear canal is about 1.4 cm^3 (Liu & Chen, 2000). The cross-sectional area of the ear canal has an oval-like shape and changes along its length with average horizontal and vertical diameters of 6.5 mm and 9 mm, respectively (Wever & Lawrence, 1954). The typical diameter of the ear canal at its concha end is about 7 mm (Gelfand, 1990). The ear canal is terminated at its medial (toward the body) end by the tympanic membrane, which is at an oblique (40°) angle to the axis of the ear canal (Alvord & Framer, 1997). The angle of the tympanic membrane is easy to visualize if you imagine that your right tympanic membrane is a compact disc (CD). If you hold the CD in front of you perpendicular to the floor so you can see just the narrow edge, then tilt the *top* of the CD to the right slightly and tilt the *front* of the CD to the left slightly, you will have an approximation of the tilt of the right tympanic membrane (the left ear is a mirror image). The tympanic membrane is not flat like the CD but is cone shaped, with the tip of the cone (**umbo**) pulled about 2 mm toward the middle ear (Alvord & Farmer, 1997) and with an apex angle of about 120° (Fumagalli, 1949).

OUTER EAR PHYSIOLOGY

The main function of the outer ear is sound transmission, although it also provides protection for the middle ear. The sound transmission function involves the selective amplification of sounds, based on sound frequency and direction, and the delivery of sound to the tympanic membrane. The differences in sound arriving from various directions provide information regarding the location of a sound in space. The outer ear protection function involves guarding the middle ear against foreign objects, stabilizing environmental conditions at the input to the middle ear, and protecting the middle ear from the effects of wind and physical trauma.

Sound Transmission Function

Sound Amplification

Some species—like dogs—can move their pinnae toward the direction of an incoming sound, increasing its loudness and clarity. People do not have this ability but can create an artificial extension of the pinna by cupping a hand around the ear to increase the sound intensity coming from specific directions during difficult listening situations. Cupping the outer ear, as shown in Figure 8.3, boosts mid- to high-frequency sounds by as much as 8 dB (Barr-Hamilton, 1983).

The ear canal is the main resonance cavity in the auditory chain. The sound entering the ear canal is preprocessed by diffraction and reflection of sound waves by the human body and by the resonance (sound-enhancing) properties of several pinnae cavities; however, the resonance properties of the ear canal serve as the major enhancer for speech sounds. The ear canal acts primarily as a one-quarter wavelength resonator. A one-quarter wavelength resonator is a tube that is open at one end (external meatus) and closed at the other (tympanic membrane), as described in Chapter 5. A one-quarter wavelength resonator will enhance the sound pressure at its closed end for a sound wave that has a wavelength four times the length of the tube and at odd whole-number multiples of this frequency. The frequency of the resonances can be calculated easily using the following equation:

$$f_n = \frac{(2n - 1)c}{4l} \quad (8.1)$$

Here, f_n is a resonance frequency of the resonator, c is the speed of sound, l is the length of the tube (in this case the average effective length of the ear canal, 0.03 m), and n is a natural number from 1 to ∞ (infinity). To calculate the first resonance frequency of a system, substitute the number 1 for n in the equation, to calculate the second resonance frequency of a system, substitute the number 2 for n in the equation, and so forth. The speed of sound (c) varies with the temperature of the air (Chapter 5); however, it is usually assumed to be 340 m/s in air unless it is specifically stated otherwise. This is the speed of sound in air at 15°C.

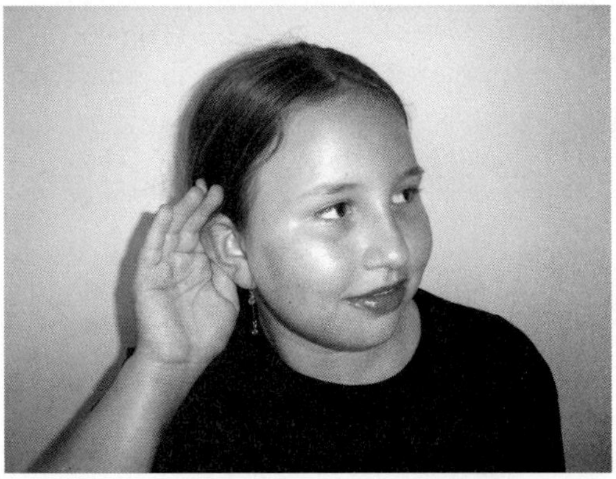

Figure 8.3. Additional amplification of sound by cupping the outer ear.

Example 8.1

The effective length of the ear canal is approximately 3.0 cm long (0.03 meters). Predict the lowest resonance frequency of the ear canal.

First, select the appropriate equation. The ear canal acts like a one-quarter wavelength resonator, so select equation 8.1 for calculating resonance frequencies for a one-quarter wavelength resonator.

$$f_n = \frac{(2n - 1)c}{4l}$$

Substitute known variables. We know the length of the tube (l) is 0.03 m and the speed of sound is 340 m/s. Since we are trying to find the lowest resonance, n is equal to 1.

$$f_1 = \frac{(2 \times 1 - 1) \times 340}{4 \times 0.03}$$

$$f_1 = \frac{340}{0.12}$$

$$f_1 = 2833.33 \text{ Hz}$$

Answer: We would predict that the lowest resonance of the ear canal is 2833.33 Hz.

If the ear canal were a hard-walled tube (instead of a tube covered with soft tissue) with a uniform diameter (instead of bends and an isthmus), the tube would resonate at 2833 Hz. Various factors influence the exact frequency and intensity of the ear canal resonance, however, including the impedance of the tympanic membrane and the shape and the cross-sectional area of the ear canal. The overall impact of these factors is relatively small; therefore, the theoretically calculated frequency is a good estimate of the real frequency. The resonance created by the outer ear can be measured using a probe tube microphone inserted into the ear canal. If you would like to read more about probe tube microphone measurement, see the website. **Link 8-1**

Figure 8.4 shows the modifications in sound intensity caused by various parts of the human body in response to sound. The transfer functions displayed in this figure show that the resonance properties of the concha cavity increase the intensity of the incoming sound around 5000 Hz and

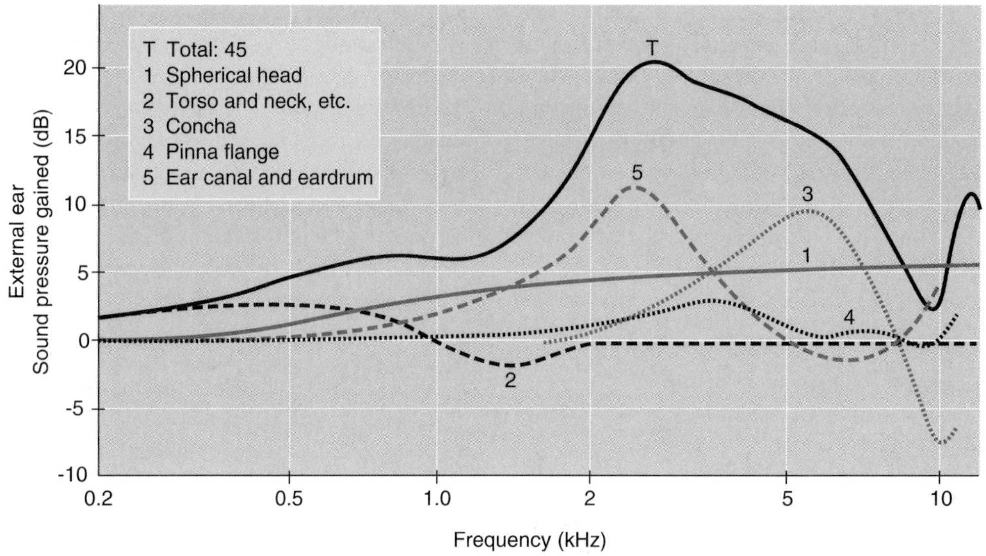

Figure 8.4. Resonances of the outer ear. (From Shaw EAG. The external ear. In: Keidel WD, Neff WD [eds.]. Auditory System: Anatomy Physiology [Ear]. Berlin: Springer-Verlag, 1974. With kind permission of Springer Science and Business Media.)

the helix and antihelix increase the intensity by about 3 dB across a broader range of frequencies around 4000 Hz. The largest increase in the intensity of the incoming sound is created by the ear canal resonance, which enhances sound by over 10 dB between 2000 and 3000 Hz. Altogether (Fig. 8.4, *line T*), the peak of the resonance of the outer ear occurs close to 3000 Hz.

Directional Function of the Ear

The magnitude of change in the sound pressure caused by the body and outer ear varies as a result of the direction of the incoming sound. The transfer function that results from sound arriving at three different azimuths is illustrated in Figure 8.5. Sound approaching from 45° results in the greatest gain in the mid- to high-frequency region compared with a signal directly from the front (0°), directly from the side (90°), or from just behind the ear (135°). The fact that the spectrum of the sound arriving at the tympanic membrane depends on the direction of the incoming sound is one of the important factors permitting localization of sound sources. This factor, together with the differences between sounds arriving at the left and right ears of a listener, constitutes the bases of directional properties of human hearing.

Localization is the process of determining the location of a sound source in space and it includes two components: azimuth estimation and elevation estimation. Recall from Chapter 1 that the word *azimuth* means the angle (θ) that represents direction on the horizontal plane. Similarly,

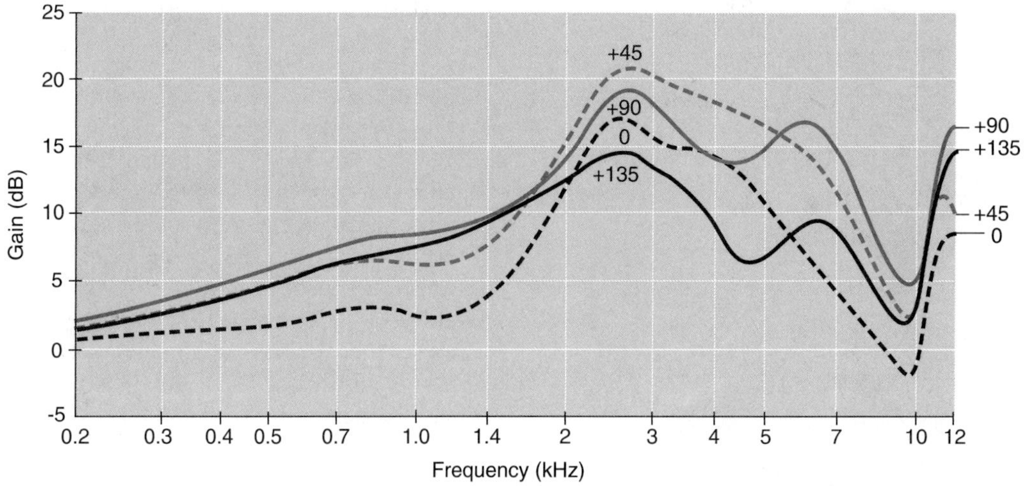

Figure 8.5. Intensity gain as a function of frequency for different azimuths. (From Shaw EAG. The external ear. In: Keidel WD, Neff WD [eds.]. Auditory System: Anatomy Physiology [Ear]. Berlin: Springer-Verlag, 1974. With kind permission of Springer Science and Business Media.)

the word *elevation* means the angle (φ from Chapter 1, although θ is also used in this context) that represents direction on the vertical plane. **Azimuth estimation** is the process of determining the direction on the horizontal plane at which a sound is arriving at the listener. It involves differentiation between front, right, back, and intermediate directions. **Elevation estimation** is the process of determining the angle between the horizontal plane passing through the ears of the listener and the direction in the vertical plane from which the sound is arriving. It involves differentiation between sounds coming from various angles above and below the listener's ears. **Distance estimation** is the process of determining how far we are from a sound source. Distance estimation clues include sound intensity and the amount of sound energy reflected from space boundaries.

The specific properties of the received sounds that are used to determine the direction of a sound source in space are called **localization cues.** Localization cues that are created by the reflection and refraction of sound by the folds, cavities, and ridges of each outer ear are called **monaural** (one ear) **localization cues.** Localization cues created by differences between sounds arriving at the right ear and left ear are called **binaural** (two ear) **localization cues.**

Monaural localization cues are the primary cues for localization of sound sources in the vertical plane (elevation estimation). They play a smaller role in azimuth estimation, and are primarily used to differentiate sounds coming from the front versus the back of the head. When sound waves reach the pinna, the sound waves can be reflected off the various folds of the pinna (Fig. 8.6), so the sound entering the ear canal consists of the original sound wave that reaches the ear and reflected waves. The reflection of sound waves in this manner causes subtle changes in the spectrum of the sound when it approaches a listener from above or below compared

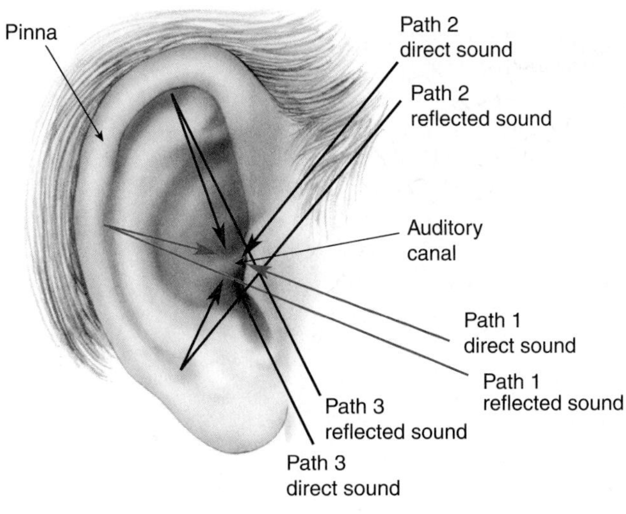

Figure 8.6. Reflections from surfaces of the pinna. (From Bear MF, Connors BW, Parasido MA. Neuroscience—Exploring the Brain. 2nd Ed. Philadelphia: Lippincott Williams & Wilkins, 2001.)

to sounds approaching on the same level as the listener's ear. These spectral differences are interpreted by the central auditory nervous system as differences in the elevation of the sound source, thus helping people localize sound in the vertical plane.

Binaural localization cues are the dominant auditory cues for localization of sound sources on the horizontal plane. These cues are **interaural** (between ear) differences in the intensity and phase (arrival time) of sounds arriving at the left ear and the right ear. The differences in *intensity* between the ears result in **interaural intensity difference** (IID) cues and the differences in *phase* between the ears result in **interaural phase difference** (IPD) cues or, more generally, **interaural time difference** (ITD) cues. The IID and ITD cues reflect the fact that sound arriving from the left side will be more intense (louder) in the left ear and will arrive earlier at the left (nearer) ear than at the right (farther) ear. The opposite is true for sounds arriving from the right side.

The effects of the outer ear, human torso, IIDs, and ITDs on the sound arriving at the human ear from a specific direction are represented by the head-related transfer function (HRTF) of the human head. The HRTF is the direction- and frequency-dependent ratio of the sound pressure arriving at the ear of a listener to the sound pressure that would exist at this location if the listener was not present. Two HRTFs, measured for the left and right ears, are needed to account for all of the information used by the listener to identify the location of a sound source. Obviously, every specific sound source location results in a different pair of HRTFs. Thus, to reconstruct directional hearing across the entire sphere surrounding the head, numerous HRTFs need to be measured and combined to represent a specific listener (individualized HRTFs) or population (nonindividualized HRTFs). HRTFs are primarily used to create acoustic spatial environments (three-dimensional sound) for virtual reality applications and to study how various anatomic and physical factors (e.g., the size of pinna, the type of headgear) affect a person's ability to localize sound sources. Processing of localization cues by the central nervous system and psychoacoustic aspects of directional perception of sound localization are discussed in Chapters 10 and 12.

Ear Protection Function

In addition to the sound transmission function, the outer ear performs a second important function by protecting the tympanic membrane and the middle ear mechanism from physical damage and abuse. The small ear canal opening, curved and relatively long ear canal, and narrow isthmus provide a protective mechanism to keep wind and larger objects away from the tympanic membrane. This is normally sufficient protection against natural environments, but these protective features can be bypassed with a sufficiently long, hard, and narrow object. Very small objects that enter the ear (e.g., particles of dust) are trapped by the small hairs growing at the walls of the ear canal and the ear wax (cerumen) produced by the ear canal glands that provide a lubricating protective layer for the skin in the ear canal. Rather than flaking off like the skin from the arm, the skin in the ear canal migrates out of the ear canal. At the junction between the bony and cartilaginous portions of the ear canal, the skin begins to wrinkle and dead skin cells, cerumen, and debris make their way out of the ear canal. Normally, this process provides a self-cleaning mechanism so that the ear canal does not become blocked. The removal of cerumen is only necessary for ears that have an unusually large collection of cerumen that can harden and block the canal.

MIDDLE EAR ANATOMY

The middle ear is an air-filled cavity (about 2 cm^3 in volume) called the **tympanic cavity** (or **tympanum**) (von Békésy, 1960). The tympanic cavity contains the three smallest bones in the body: the **malleus** (hammer), **incus** (anvil), and **stapes** (stirrup, the smallest bone in the body). These are collectively called the **ossicles** or **ossicular chain.** The lateral (outside) wall of the middle ear is formed by the tympanic membrane (eardrum), which is attached around most of its circumference by a ring-shaped ligament called the **annulus** to a ring-shaped groove in the temporal bone called the **tympanic sulcus.** The ring has a small discontinuity at its top to accommodate a tiny interruption in the tympanic sulcus called the **notch of Rivinus.** At the other side of the tympanic cavity, the medial (toward the middle) wall of the tympanic cavity is the bony wall that divides the middle ear from the inner ear.

A conceptual model of the tympanic cavity is shown in Figure 8.7 as if the middle ear were a box with the front wall removed. The superior wall of the tympanum, called the **tegmen tympani,** is a thin plate of bone separating the middle ear from the cranial cavity (brain cavity). In the posterior (back) bony wall of the tympanum, a narrow bony passageway, called the **aditus ad antrum,** connects the tympanum to the **antrum,** a small chamber within the mastoid portion of the temporal bone. This is also shown in Figure 8.8 in an adult and in an infant. The antrum is surrounded by **mastoid air cells,** which are air pockets that look like a honeycomb within the mastoid portion of the temporal bone.

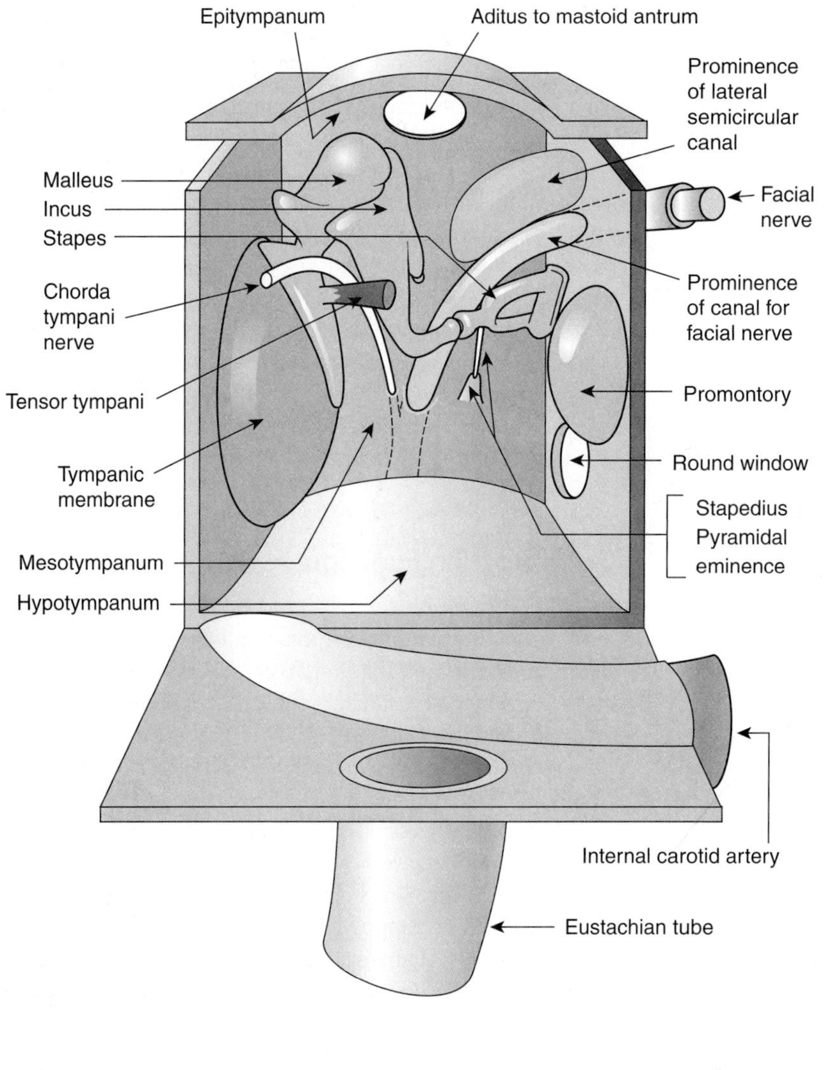

Figure 8.7. A model of the middle ear seen from the front. (Modified from Moore KL, Dalley AF [eds.]. Clinical Oriented Anatomy. 4th Ed. Baltimore: Lippincott Williams & Wilkins, 1999.)

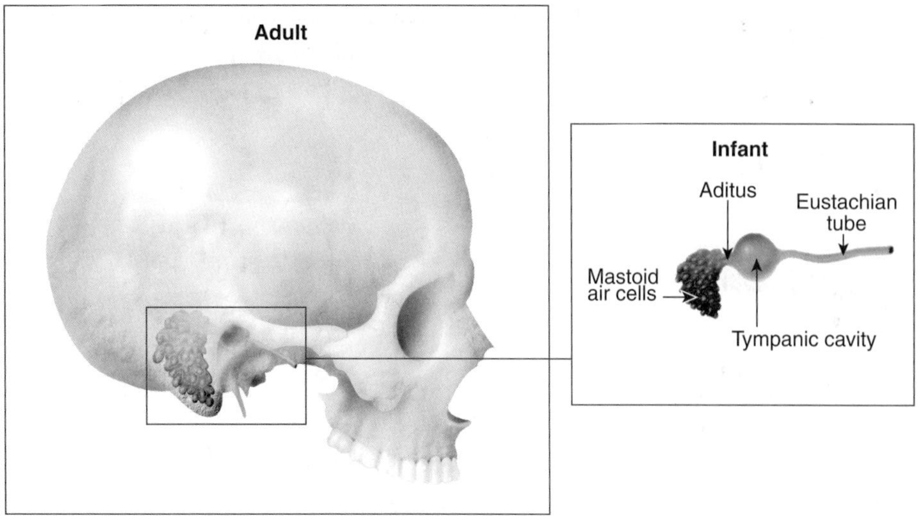

Figure 8.8. The orientation of the middle ear cavity including the mastoid air cells and eustachian tube in an adult and an infant. (Image from Anatomical Chart Co.)

The posterior wall also contains a bony projection called the **pyramidal eminence**, which contains a tunnel from which the tendon of the stapedius muscle emerges. The **stapedius muscle** itself is located within the posterior wall of the tympanic cavity. The anterior (front) wall of the middle ear contains the opening of the **eustachian tube** (after Bartolomeo Eustachi, 1513–1574), also called the **auditory tube** or **pharyngotympanic tube**, which connects the middle ear cavity with the **nasopharyngeal cavity (nasopharynx)** of the upper part of the throat (behind the nasal cavity). The eustachian tube is a bony canal for about one third of its length as it exits the middle ear and is cartilaginous for about two thirds of its length as it approaches the nasopharynx. In adults, the middle ear opening of the eustachian tube is 20 to 25 mm higher than the nasopharyngeal opening, which facilitates middle ear drainage. In infants, the tube position is closer to the horizontal position (Fig. 8.8), which makes fluid drainage less efficient. The anterior wall of the middle ear also contains the canal from which the tendon of the tensor tympani muscle emerges to connect with the malleus. The **tensor tympani muscle** itself is located within the anterior wall of the middle ear. Also anterior to the middle ear, the internal carotid artery* runs through a bony tunnel called the carotid canal. Another major blood vessel, the internal jugular vein,** travels in the bone near the posterior/inferior wall of the middle ear through the jugular foramen, a bony opening in the floor of the skull.

The medial wall of the middle ear (which separates the middle and inner ears) contains two openings, the oval window and round window (each covered with a membrane), and a ridge of bone called the promontory between these two membranes. The facial canal (holding the facial nerve) and horizontal semicircular canal are also contained within the medial wall of the tympanic cavity.

The tympanic cavity can be divided into three portions (Fig. 8.7). The **epitympanum**, or attic, is the superior portion of the tympanum. The head of the malleus and incus are located within the epitympanum. Crossing the epitympanum from the back of the tympanic cavity to the front, just beneath the head of the malleus and incus, is a branch of the facial nerve called the **chorda tympani**, which emerges from the posterior wall of the middle ear and exits via the anterior wall of the middle ear. The rest of the portions of the ossicular chain are located in the **mesotympanum**, the middle portion of the tympanic cavity. The **hypotympanum** is the crescent-shaped inferior portion of the middle ear cavity located below the inferior border of the annulus and below the eustachian tube (Spector & Ge, 1981).

The ossicles (Fig. 8.9) are suspended in the middle ear cavity by a series of muscles and ligaments. The **manubrium** of the malleus attaches to the cone of the tympanic membrane extending almost vertically from the tip of the cone. The anterior process of the malleus is attached to the anterior wall of the tympanic cavity by the **anterior ligament of the malleus.** The tendon of the tensor tympani muscle is also attached to the anterior surface of the malleus, close to the neck. The head of the malleus is firmly connected to the head of the incus. The posterior process of the incus is attached to the **posterior ligament of the incus,** which emerges from the posterior wall of the middle ear. The long process of the incus extends from the head of the incus in a downward direction to an L-shaped bend called the **lenticular process of the incus.** The lenticular process of the incus is attached to the head of the stapes at the **incudostapedial joint,** the smallest joint in the human body. The two crura (legs) of the stapes end at the stapes

*The internal carotid artery is one of the two paired arteries supplying blood to the brain. The other paired artery is the vertebral artery.

**The internal jugular vein is a vein that drains blood from the head and neck toward the heart.

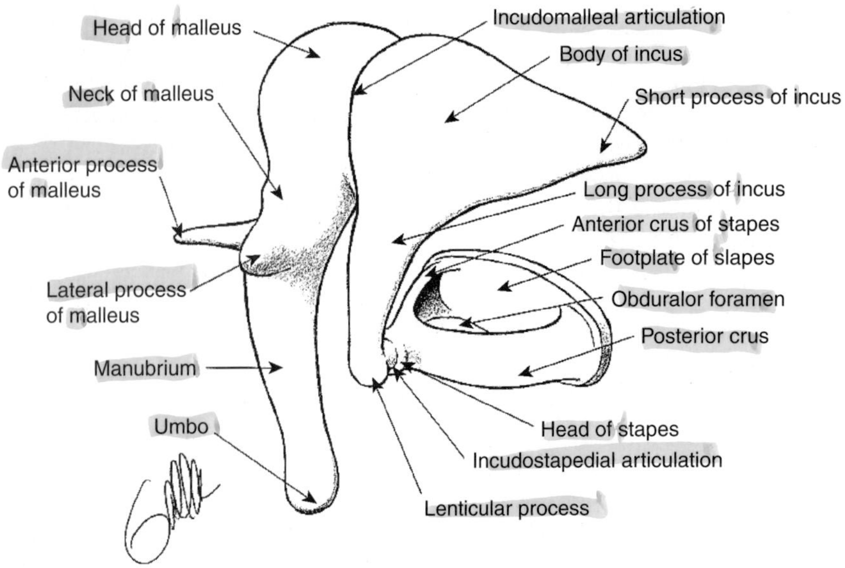

Figure 8.9. The ossicular chain with portions of the bones labeled. (From Janfaza P, Nadol JB, Galla Jr R, et al. Surgical Anatomy of the Head and Neck. Philadelphia: Lippincott Williams & Wilkins, 2001.)

footplate, which is held in the oval window by a ring-shaped ligament called the **annular ligament.** The hole between the crura of the stapes is called the **obturator foramen.** The tendon of the stapedius muscle attaches on one end to the posterior neck of the stapes and projects through the posterior wall of the middle ear to attach to the stapedius muscle. The malleus, incus, and stapes are not lined up in a straight line across the tympanum. The ossicular chain actually points backward (posterior) as it travels inward (medially).

The tympanic membrane is a thin, pearly gray, translucent (allowing light to pass through) membrane with an average thickness of about 100 μm (Donaldson & Duckert, 1991; Helmholtz, 1954). The thickness of the membrane varies both along the membrane's axes and among people. Kogo (1954) measured the thickness of the tympanic membrane at seven points in seven different ears and reported values ranging from 30 to 120 μm, and Lim (1970) reported a range of 30 to 90 μm. The weight of the tympanic membrane is approximately 14 mg (Zemlin, 1988). It has an oval shape with a vertical diameter of about 9 to 10 mm and a horizontal diameter of about 8 to 9 mm (Gelfand, 1990; Helmholtz, 1954). The cross-sectional area of the ear canal occupied by the tympanic membrane varies in humans from 55 to 90 mm^2 with an average value of 64 mm^2 (Harris, 1986; Zemlin, 1988); however, since the membrane is cone shaped, its surface area is slightly larger. The conical area of the tympanic membrane is not uniformly stretched and consists of two parts: the **pars tensa,** which is stretched (taut), and the **pars flaccida,** which is relatively loose (flaccid). The pars tensa is the only part of the tympanic membrane that effectively contributes to sound transmission. The other part (the pars flaccida) has a different function and much less effectively participates in the energy transfer between the air in the ear canal and the middle ear structures. Its function is to allow the tympanic membrane to work like a piston rather than a membrane fixed at its circumference. Thus, the average effective area of the tympanic membrane is only about 55 mm^2 (Zemlin, 1988).

The tympanic membrane can be examined by looking down the ear canal with an instrument called an **otoscope** that has a narrow tip, a light, and a magnifying lens. Figure 8.10 shows an illustration of the tympanic membrane as seen through the otoscope from the ear canal. The surface of the tympanic membrane can be divided into four quadrants: anterior superior, anterior inferior, posterior inferior, and posterior superior. The most prominent feature on the tympanic membrane during otoscopic examination is the **cone of light** or light reflex, located on the anterior inferior quadrant. The cone of light is caused by the reflection of the light from the otoscope off a section of the pars tensa. Sometimes, white, cloud-like patches called **tympanosclerosis** (scarring on the eardrum) can be seen on the tympanic membrane,

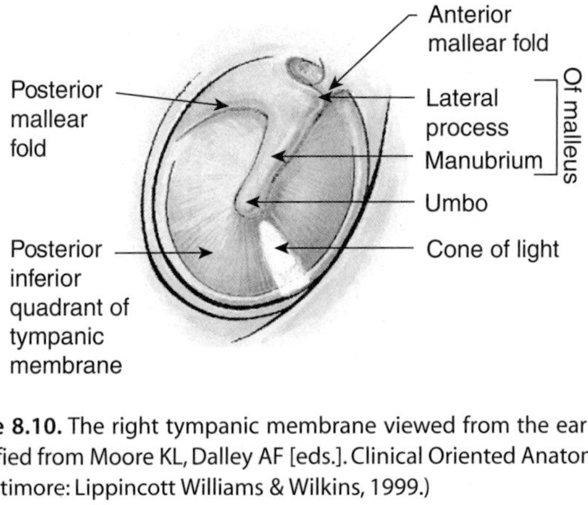

Figure 8.10. The right tympanic membrane viewed from the ear canal. (Modified from Moore KL, Dalley AF [eds.]. Clinical Oriented Anatomy. 4th Ed. Baltimore: Lippincott Williams & Wilkins, 1999.)

especially in people with a history of middle ear infections. The tympanic membrane is composed of three distinct layers. The outermost layer is continuous with the skin lining the ear canal. The innermost layer is continuous with the mucous membrane lining the middle ear. The middle layer is composed of two layers of fibrous tissue, one layer of radial fibers (fibers are lined up like spokes in a bicycle tire) and one layer of circular fibers (fibers lined up like the layers of a cinnamon bun). This membrane construction makes it relatively strong and resistant to changes in shape over years of use.

By looking at a normal tympanic membrane with an otoscope, several middle ear landmarks can be identified. The manubrium of the malleus and umbo can be seen clearly. The lenticular process of the incus can often be seen posterior to the manubrium of the malleus—in the left ear it appears like this: ᒪ, and in the right ear it appears like this: ᒧ see Fig. 8.11). Less often, the promontory and round window can be seen inferior to the long process of the incus.

When viewing a photograph of a tympanic membrane, it is usually easy to determine whether the tympanic membrane is from the right or left ear. Examine the relationship between the manubrium of the malleus and the cone of light in Figure 8.11. The most prominent feature for new ear canal explorers is the cone of light. If one can see the cone

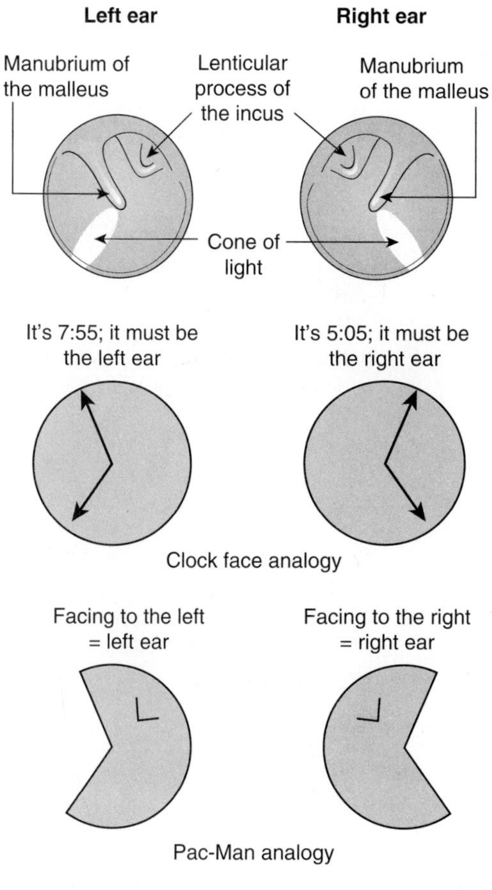

Figure 8.11. Ways to identify right and left tympanic membranes in otoscopic examination pictures.

of light, the otoscope can be pointed up and back from this point to explore the entire tympanic membrane. Two ways to remember the relative position of the manubrium of the malleus and cone of light in each ear are shown. The tympanic membrane is often compared to a clock face with the manubrium of the malleus and cone of light as the hands on the clock. We suggest another analogy, that of the Pac-Man in which the manubrium of the malleus and cone of light form the edges of the mouth of the Pac-Man and the lenticular process of the incus (when visible) forms the eye.

MIDDLE EAR PHYSIOLOGY

The middle ear, similar to the outer ear, has several functions including a sound transmission function, a pressure equalization function, and an inner ear protection function. Its main role is to act as a transducer to change the acoustic wave arriving at the tympanic membrane into the motion of fluids in the inner ear. A **transducer** is a device that changes energy from one form to another. The middle ear consists of transducers that convert sound to mechanical vibration (outer ear to middle ear) and then transmit the vibration from a solid (middle ear bones) to a fluid (inner ear fluid) medium. The ossicles function as a bridge that matches the impedance between the air in the outer ear and the fluid in the inner ear. This whole transmission system is located in the air cavity of the middle ear and the static air pressure in the cavity affects the stiffness of the tympanic membrane. If the air pressure is too low or too high compared with ambient (surrounding, environmental) pressure, the sound transmission function of the middle ear will be affected. Therefore, the middle ear must not only deliver sound to the inner ear, but also provide a pressure equalization function, maintaining the proper pressure on both sides of the tympanic membrane. The middle ear also provides some limited protection of the inner ear from excessively loud sounds via the stapedius muscle, which is connected to the ossicles.

Sound Transmission Function

Sound waves travel down the ear canal and reach the tympanic membrane causing it to vibrate in response to changes in sound pressure. Certain areas of the tympanic membrane, specifically the portions of the pars tensa between the outer rim of the tympanic membrane and its attachment at the manubrium, vibrate at greater amplitudes than others. Just like a trampoline will vibrate up and down with its greatest amplitude where a child is jumping and lesser amplitude at the attachment points around the edge, the tympanic membrane will vibrate best at certain locations based on its attachment points. For low-frequency sounds, the stretched part of the tympanic membrane moves up and down as one unit, like one child on a trampoline. For higher frequency sounds, the tympanic membrane has a multimodal vibration pattern that resembles a trampoline with several children jumping up and down in different locations. Due to the presence of the pars flaccida and the attachment points of the tympanic membrane, however, some parts of the pars tensa have a relatively larger freedom of movement than others and the multimodal vibration pattern is not uniform across the whole membrane.

When sound energy impinges on the tympanic membrane, the movements of the membrane are transferred through the ossicular chain to the oval window of the inner ear. This is the main transmission pathway for sounds through the middle ear. The role of the ossicles in the middle ear is to match the high impedance of the fluid filling the inner ear to the low impedance of the air in the ear canal and facilitate an effective transfer of energy to the inner ear. According to Lynch et al. (1982), the impedance of the inner ear fluid (Z_1) is approximately 160,000 rayls (acoustic ohms). For comparison, the impedance of water is about 144,000 rayls and the impedance of seawater is about 158,000 rayls. All of these values are very high in comparison to the impedance of the air (Z_2), which equals about 40 to 42 rayls depending on temperature and atmospheric pressure. The ratio of the inner ear fluid and air impedances (Z_1 to Z_2) is very high and equal to:

$$\frac{Z_1}{Z_2} = \frac{160{,}000}{40} = 4000$$

Since the impedance mismatch (ratio) is estimated to be about 4000, the middle ear must compensate for this inequality between the air and the fluid and increase the pressure at the oval window more than 63 times above the sound pressure acting at the tympanic membrane.* A ratio of 63 is equal to a 36-dB increase in sound pressure. Therefore, the middle ear can be thought of as a system that transforms the low acoustic pressure air that impinges on the tympanic membrane to the high pressure exerted by the oval window movements on the fluids of the inner ear. Without the middle ear system, 99.9% of the acoustic pressure acting on the tympanic membrane would be reflected back. In animals that live in a fluid environment, this conversion is not necessary, because there is no need to go from a low-impedance (air) to a high-impedance (fluid) environment. For example, fish do not have a middle ear because they live in a fluid environment and they do not need an impedance transformer.

Note that the movements of the tympanic membrane are transmitted not only to the ossicular chain, but also to the air filling the middle ear cavity. The changes in the air pressure in the middle ear cavity can also stimulate the membranes of the inner ear windows. This is, however, not the primary transmission pathway described in the previous paragraph; it is a shunt pathway. The effect of the shunt pathway is negligible due to the impedance mismatch between the impedances of the air and the inner ear fluid and the fact that the air pressure acts simultaneously on the oval and round windows of the inner ear (Chapter 9). The only way in which the shunt pathway becomes the primary pathway is if the ossicular chain is missing (or disconnected). In this case, the listener will have a moderate to severe hearing loss because his or her impedance transformer is missing.

The impedance transformer formed by the middle ear structures consists of three mechanisms: (1) the pressure transformer (area ratio transformer), (2) the ossicular lever, and (3) the catenary lever or buckling effect. There is by no means an agreement in the literature regarding the names of these three mechanisms or the exact contribution each one makes to the pressure transformer; however, these terms are commonly used.

The main of the three mechanisms is the **pressure transformer** resulting from the difference in the surface areas of the tympanic membrane and oval window. The concept of this pressure transformer is shown in Figure 8.12 (top).

If there is no loss of energy in the system shown in Figure 8.12, the force (F_2) acting on the fluids of the inner ear at the surface of the oval window membrane (S_2) should be equal to the force (F_1) acting on the surface of the tympanic membrane (S_1). Thus:

$$F_1 = F_2 \qquad (8.2)$$

Recall from earlier chapters that pressure is equal to force acting over an area.

$$Pressure = \frac{Force}{Area} \qquad (8.3)$$

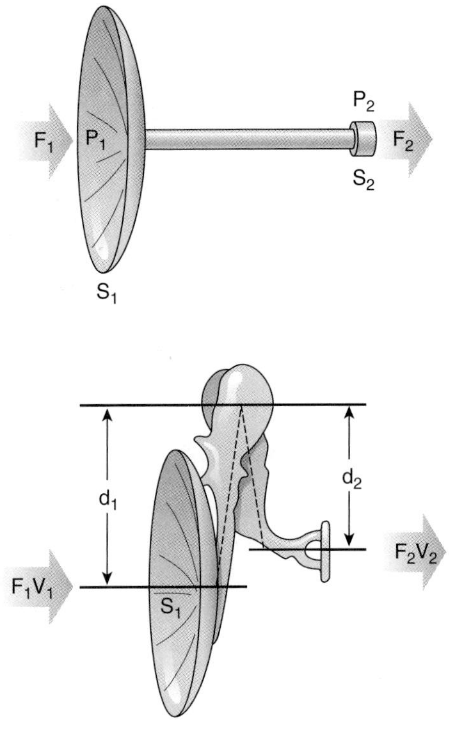

Figure 8.12. The concept of the pressure transformer. (Modified from Pickles JO. An Introduction to the Physiology of Hearing. 2nd Ed. New York: Academic Press, 1988. Used with permission from Elsevier.)

*For the power to be the same on both ends of the ossicular chain, the transmitted force needs to increase in proportion to the square root of the impedance ratio. See the discussion of transformer operation in Chapter 13.

If the force is held constant and the area varies, it is clear that the pressure will change.

$$\text{Tympanic membrane pressure} = \frac{\textit{Force}}{55\,\text{mm}^2}$$

$$\text{Oval window pressure} = \frac{\textit{Force}}{3.2\,\text{mm}^2}$$

Due to the fact that the active area of the tympanic membrane (S_1 = 55 mm^2) is approximately 17 times larger than the active area of the oval window (S_2 = 3.2 mm^2), this ratio works as a pressure amplifier. If the ossicles transmit a constant force from the manubrium of the malleus to the footplate of the stapes, then the pressure across the oval window should be about 17 times (about 25 dB) greater than the pressure across the tympanic membrane.

If you are having difficulty conceptualizing the increase in pressure in the middle ear system, consider a hiker walking through snow in normal boots and using snow shoes. The force of the hiker (his or her mass affected by the pull of gravity) is the same regardless of the type of shoes, but the pressure of the regular boots on the snow is much greater than the pressure offered by the snow shoes because of the difference in surface area. Therefore, hikers wearing snow shoes can walk on the surface of the snow although they would not be able to do this wearing just their normal boots.

The second transformer mechanism, the **ossicular lever,** results from the fact that the ossicular chain is firmly jointed at the junction between the malleus and the incus and the attachment of these two bones to the anterior ligament of the malleus and the posterior ligament of the incus, respectively, creates a rotational motion between the two, transferring energy from the relatively larger bone (malleus) to the smaller bone (stapes) (Fig. 8.12 bottom). If the middle ear were a perfect transmission system, the difference in the length between the malleus and the incus would result in a lever action that increases the force acting over the oval window by about a 1.15-to-1 ratio (1.2 dB)* (Pickles, 1988).

The third mechanism, the **catenary lever** or **buckling effect,** of the tympanic membrane is considered by several authors to be another type of lever action that may be operating in the middle ear. Helmholtz (1868) suggested that due to the conical shape of the tympanic membrane, the tip (the umbo) of the membrane is displaced less than the rest of the membrane surface. This smaller displacement (distance) of membrane movement at the umbo results in a smaller displacement of the manubrium of the malleus, which is attached at the umbo, as compared to the displacement of the rest of the membrane. Since the product of force and distance is constant in a lever mechanism, the relatively large displacement of the membrane due to the presence of a given external force (F_1) translated into a smaller movement at the umbo means a larger force (F_2) is acting on the malleus. Since the ossicular chain moves as one stiff system, changes at the beginning of the system (malleus) are transmitted to the end of the system (stapes) in the form of increased force at the stapes. The presence of this mechanism was questioned by several authors, including Békésy, but the results of holographic measurements of tympanic membrane vibrations conducted by Tonndorf and Khanna (1970, 1972) confirmed the presence of a small buckling effect. The catenary lever or buckling effect increases the impedance ratio of the system by about two times (6 dB) (Gelfand, 2001; Rosowski, 1996).

The combined effects of the three mechanisms results in a theoretical increase in the sound pressure at the footplate of the stapes by 17 × 1.15 × 2 = 40 times (approximately), which is about 32 dB. This value is quite close to the pressure loss in the air-to-fluid transmission taking place in human ears, which is considered to be about 36 dB. Thus, the middle ear is theoretically able to compensate for almost all of that energy loss.

Although the middle ear system provides an efficient impedance matching device, it is not a perfect transmission system. Even in a normally functioning middle ear, some of the sound energy reaching the tympanic membrane will be reflected back into the ear canal. The effectiveness of the middle ear transformer is also affected by pathologic changes in the middle ear. For example, a middle ear infection with fluid (otitis media with effusion) increases the input impedance of the ear and the amount of sound energy reflected back off the tympanic membrane.

Another limitation of the middle ear mechanism is that the impedance matching provided by the middle ear holds well for low and middle frequencies but fails at high frequencies. The typical mean middle ear gain is approximately 20 to 25 dB from 250 to 1000 Hz and then it decreases at about 6 to 8 dB per octave above that point (Puria et al., 1997; Battista & Esquivel, 2005). Above 1000 Hz several effects cause the middle ear function to become increasingly more inefficient at impedance matching. A complex pattern of vibration of the tympanic membrane at high frequencies reduces the area of the tympanic membrane that is contributing to sound transmission (Tonndorf & Khanna, 1972). In addition, the resonance properties of the middle ear cavities including the mastoid cavity and the aditus ad antrum affect the movement of the ossicular chain and cause a further decrease in the stapes motion in the 1500- to 3500-Hz range (Gyo et al., 1986; Killion, 1978; McElveen et al., 1982; Puria et al., 1997).

Brenkman et al. (1987) reported that the lever ratio contributing to the force amplification provided by the middle ear structures differs among individuals and may change as a function of frequency from about 1.0 at low frequencies to as much as 2.5 at 1000 Hz (0 to 8 dB). With increasing frequency, there is also a change in the way the ossicles vibrate, which decreases the efficiency of energy transfer along the ossicular chain (Battista & Esquivel, 2005). However, a large portion of the nonideal operation of the middle ear

*The difference in the length (d) increases the force at the footplate of the stapes by a factor of d_1/d_2 = 1.15; therefore $F_2 = F_1\,(d_1/d_2) = F_1 \times 1.15$. In other words, F_2 is 1.15 times the value of F_1.

transformer and the natural reduction in its efficiency at higher frequencies (above 2000 Hz) is compensated for by sound amplification by the outer ear system, which amplifies incoming sounds up to about 6000 Hz. Thus, all things considered, the outer and middle ear systems together compensate for most of the energy that would have been lost in a direct air-to-fluid transmission.

Note that the middle ear impedance seen at the tympanic membrane consists of both resistance (*R*) and reactance (*X*) components that are responsible for two different forms of energy loss (Chapter 4). The average middle ear resistance and reactance values (in rayls) measured by Zwislocki (1975) are shown in Figure 8.13. The top two lines represent resistance (*R*) as a function of frequency for males and females and the bottom two lines indicate reactance as a function of frequency (*X*) for males and females. Resistance is always a positive number, but the reactance is negative in the case of stiffness reactance and positive in the case of mass reactance (notice positive and negative numbers shown on the *y* axis). Notice from Figure 8.13 that at low frequencies (<1000 Hz) the impedance of the ear results mainly from stiffness reactance, which is primarily caused by the stiffness of the tympanic membrane. The size and tension of the tympanic membrane does not allow for the large displacements of the tympanic membrane needed for efficient reception of very-low-frequency sounds, thus limiting the amount of low-frequency energy that is transmitted to the ear. The stiffness reactance decreases as frequency increases and becomes negligible at about 600 to 800 Hz. At higher frequencies, the ear impedance results mainly from the mass reactance (inertia) of the middle ear structures. At high frequencies, the mass of the tympanic membrane is too large to accurately follow fast changes in sound pressure, and thus sound transmission becomes ineffective, as it is for very low frequencies. The total reactance of the ear is smallest in the 800- to 6000-Hz range, causing the energy transmission from the tympanic membrane to the inner ear to be at its maximum (most efficient) in this range (Gelfand, 1990). The resistance of the ear is relatively unaffected by frequency, and remains between 0 and 500 rayls from 200 to about 6000 Hz.

Dallos (1973) observed that the outer ear and middle ear transfer functions determine the shape of the threshold of hearing curve. Following these observations, Goode (1997) suggested that variations in the middle ear transfer function between individuals explained a significant part of the 25-dB range of hearing threshold variability observed in young people with normal ears. In other words, people with greater than normal middle ear resistance and reactance may have perfectly "normal" ears (no pathology or malformation), but have hearing thresholds poorer than the "average" ear as a result of this individual variability. Goode called the top 10% most sensitive ears "golden ears" and the 10% of individuals with the least sensitive ears "tin ears."

Pressure Equalization Function

The middle ear cavity is susceptible to damage from sudden ambient pressure changes. The middle ear pressure is governed by a classic gas law of physics known as the Boyle-Mariotte Law, which states that at a constant temperature, the volume (*V*) of a body of gas is inversely related to the pressure (*p*) to which it is subjected. A change in the external air pressure that is not compensated for by a change in the middle ear air pressure will result in a negative or positive pressure difference between the ear canal and the middle ear cavity. This difference may cause damage to the tympanic membrane or other ear structures by causing excessive bulging or retraction of the tympanic membrane and unusual stress applied to the middle ear structures.

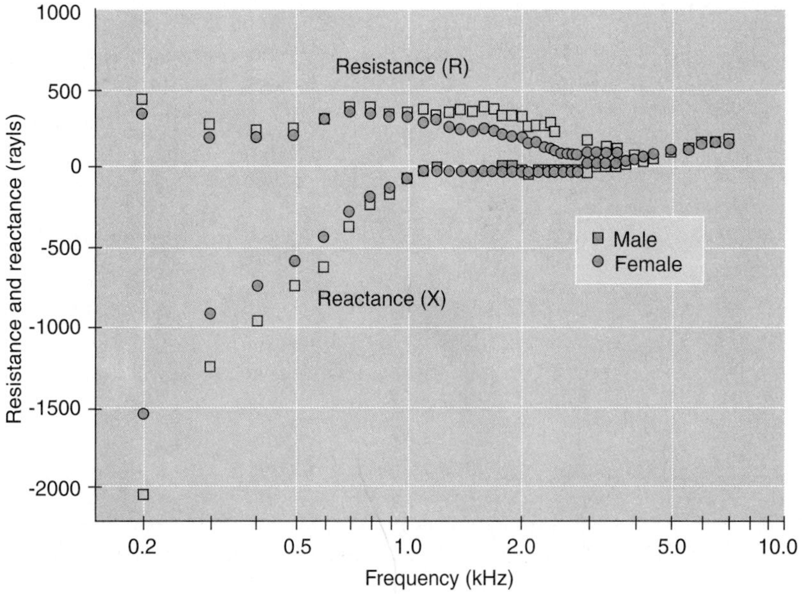

Figure 8.13. The average middle ear resistance and reactance. (Modified from Zwislocki J. The role of the external and middle ear in sound transmission. In: Tower DB (ed.). The Nervous System. Volume 3: Human Communication and Its Disorders. New York: Raven Press, 1975.)

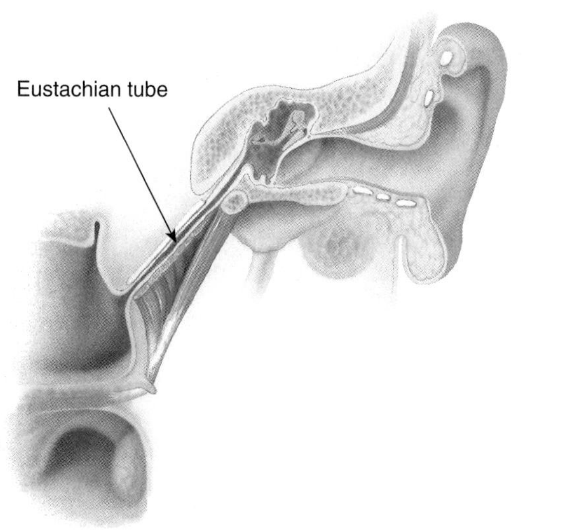

Figure 8.14. The eustachian tube. (Modified from an image created for the Anatomical Chart Co.)

In a healthy middle ear cavity, the pressure within the tympanic cavity is maintained at an air pressure similar to that of ambient air pressure by the eustachian tube (Fig. 8.14). For optimal listening, the middle ear cavity should be maintained at ambient pressure so that it functions efficiently. However, eustachian tube blockage or breathing unusually pressurized air (as in scuba diving or air travel) may cause an air pressure mismatch between the middle ear and the outside environment that needs to be corrected.

The cartilaginous portion of the eustachian tube (the portion closest to the throat) is normally closed but is opened intermittently during yawning, swallowing, and so forth by the contraction of the **tensor veli palatini muscle.** There is also evidence that the contraction of the **levator veli palatini muscle** assists in the opening of the eustachian tube (Ishijima et al., 2002). The air in the middle ear is constantly absorbed by the mucosal tissue surrounding the middle ear and must be replaced periodically or negative middle ear pressure will develop. The eustachian tube also provides drainage for fluid that has entered or is produced by the middle ear.

The opening of the eustachian tube causes a "popping" sound when a puff of air rushes into the middle ear to equalize the middle ear pressure with the ambient pressure. Although the eustachian tube opens normally during yawning, chewing, and swallowing, during activities that involve sudden or large changes in atmospheric pressure (air travel, scuba diving), it is sometimes necessary to force an opening of the eustachian tube to equalize the pressure. One way to do this is to hold the nose, close the mouth, and blow (not too hard!). This is called a **Valsalva maneuver.** When the opening of the eustachian tube is dysfunctional, due to a craniofacial anomaly or swollen tissue in the nasopharynx, it may not be possible to clear the ears by opening the eustachian tube. In some cases, small pressure equalization (PE) tubes are surgically inserted through the tympanic membrane to equalize the air pressure between the middle ear and the environment.

Ear Protection Function

Sometimes the impedance of the middle ear increases due to a pathologic state (e.g., fluid in the middle ear), which impedes the flow of energy through the middle ear system. The impedance of the middle ear may also be temporarily altered by the normal action of the middle ear in response to loud sounds. In response to loud sounds, the stapedius muscle will contract, pulling the stapes in an outward and downward direction away from the oval window. This is a bilateral (two-sided) reflex in which the right and left stapedius muscles will contract in response to a loud sound in either ear. This contraction increases the impedance of the middle ear system by increasing the stiffness of the ossicular chain. This effect is called the **acoustic reflex** (stapedius reflex, middle ear muscle reflex).

The acoustic reflex is normally triggered by sound exceeding about 85 to 95 dB SPL and it provides up to about 15 dB attenuation of the input signal (Borg, 1968; Brask, 1979). The latency (time delay between stimulus and response) of the acoustic reflex varies from about 25 to 100 ms depending on the frequency and intensity of the signal (Møller, 2000). Therefore, the protective function of the acoustic reflex is not effective for high-intensity impulse noise, which can enter and damage the cochlea in a time frame that is much quicker than the latency of the contraction. Furthermore, the contraction of the stapedius muscle will not continue indefinitely, but will quickly adapt to the loud sound and cease contracting. This is especially true for high-frequency sounds; thus, this protection function is only effective for low-frequency sounds (<2000 Hz) over a limited period of time. Most hearing loss due to noise is centered in the higher frequencies due to the lack of natural protective mechanisms in this frequency range and the enhancement in the sound provided by the resonance properties of the outer and middle ear.

Summary

The main functions of the outer and middle ear structures are to channel acoustic energy, convert acoustic energy into mechanical energy, and deliver it in the appropriate form to the inner ear. The pinna is the externally visible structure of the outer ear extending out from the side of the head. The external auditory canal (ear canal) begins at the external auditory meatus and forms an S-shaped curve ending at the tympanic membrane (eardrum). The outer ear performs several functions including frequency- and direction-dependent sound amplification and middle ear protection. The middle ear is an air-filled cavity called the tympanic cavity containing the three smallest bones in the body, the malleus, incus, and stapes, which are collectively called the ossicular chain. Sound waves travel down the ear canal and reach the tympanic membrane. The tympanic membrane will vibrate in response to these sounds. These vibrations are efficiently transmitted by a normal middle ear to fluid vibrations used by the cochlea, which is the location of the hearing organ.

Key Points

- Acoustic energy (sound waves in air) enters the outer ear and this energy is converted into mechanical motion in the middle ear.
- The outer ear consists of the pinna and the external auditory canal that is terminated by the tympanic membrane, which separates the outer ear from the middle ear.
- Localization is the ability to determine the location of a sound source in space and includes azimuth estimation and elevation estimation.
- The differentiation between sounds coming from left and right directions is primarily facilitated by binaural (two ear) cues, and differentiation between sounds of different elevation is primarily facilitated by monaural (one ear) cues.
- The ear canal is the primary resonator of the outer ear, amplifying sound around 3000 Hz in a relatively wide band from about 1500 Hz up to about 6000 Hz. In addition, sound reflections from the structures of the pinna (high frequencies) and torso (low frequencies) provide some amplification of sound entering the ear.
- The middle ear is an air-filled cavity containing a chain of three small bones: the malleus, incus, and stapes. The malleus is embedded in the tympanic membrane and is attached to the anterior ligament of the malleus and the tendon of the tensor tympani. The incus is attached to the malleus on one end, to the stapes at the other end, and to the posterior ligament of the incus. The stapes is embedded in the oval window and is also attached to the tendon of the stapedius muscle.
- The middle ear role is to change the acoustic energy arriving at the tympanic membrane into motions of the fluids in the inner ear and to provide a matching bridge to minimize energy loss between low-impedance (air) and high-impedance (fluid) environments.
- The tympanic membrane can be observed using an otoscope. The most prominent structures are the cone of light in the anterior inferior quadrant and the manubrium of the malleus in the anterior superior quadrant.
- The acoustic reflex offers some amount of protection of the ear at low and middle frequencies by contracting in response to loud sounds. This contraction increases the impedance of the middle ear.
- In a healthy middle ear cavity, the pressure within the tympanic cavity is maintained at an air pressure similar to that of ambient air pressure by the opening of the eustachian tube.

CHAPTER 9

The Inner Ear and Vestibulocochlear Nerve

Chapter Outline

Objectives

- To review the anatomy of the inner ear and vestibulocochlear nerve
- To review the physiology of the cochlea and the auditory nerve (the cochlear portion of the VIII nerve)
- To briefly review the anatomy and physiology of the vestibular system

Key Terms

Action potential (neural potential, nerve impulse)
Afferent neuron
Alternating current (AC) potential
Ampulla
Anastomosis of Oort (vestibulocochlear anastomosis)
Anion
Anterior (superior) semicircular canal
Auditory nerve (acoustic nerve, cochlear nerve)
Axon
Basilar membrane
Bioelectric potential
Boettcher cell
Bony labyrinth
Cation
Central nervous system
Characteristic frequency (CF)
Claudius cell
Cochlea
Cochlear amplifier
Cochlear microphonic
Collaterals
Compound (whole nerve) action potential
Contralateral
Cortex
Crista ampullaris
Cross-link
Cupula
Cuticular plate
Deiters cell
Dendrite
Depolarize
Direct current (DC) potential
Ductus reuniens
Dynamic range
Efferent neuron
Electric potential
Electromotility
Endocochlear potential
Endolymph
Endolymphatic duct
Endolymphatic sac
Exocytosis
Ganglion
Gap junction
Gray matter
Habenula perforata
Hair cell
Helicotrema
Hensen cell
Horizontal (lateral) semicircular canal
Inner hair cells (IHCs)
Inner phalangeal cell
Inner radial fiber
Inner sulcus cell
Internal auditory canal
Interneuron
Ion channel
Ion
Ipsilateral
Lateral olivocochlear neuron
Macula
Medial olivocochlear neuron

Membranous labyrinth
Modiolus
Nerve
Nerve fiber
Neural impulse (nerve impulse)
Neuron
Neurotransmitter
Nonlinear distortion
Nucleus
Olivocochlear bundle
Organ of Corti
Otoacoustic emissions
Otoconia
Otolithic membrane
Outer hair cell electromotility
Outer hair cell (OHC)
Outer spiral fibers
Outer spiral sulcus cell
Perilymph
Periodicity (temporal) theory
Peripheral nervous system
Phalangeal process
Phase locking
Place coding
Place theory
Posterior (inferior) semicircular canal
Prestin
Reissner's membrane
Resting potential
Reticular lamina
Rods (pillars) of Corti
Rosenthal's canal
Saccule
Saturation point
Scala media (cochlear duct, cochlear partition)
Scala tympani
Scala vestibuli
Semicircular canal
Shearing motion
Soma (cell body)
Space of Nuel
Spiral ganglia
Spiral lamina
Spiral ligament
Spiral limbus
Stereocilia
Stereocilia bundle
Stimulus-related potential
Stria vascularis
Striola
Summating potential
Synapse
Synaptic cleft
Tectorial membrane
Tip-to-side cross-link
Tonotopic organization (tonotopicity)
Traveling wave (transverse wave)
Tuning curve
Tunnel of Corti
Utricle
Vestibular ganglion
Vestibule
Volley theory

The inner ear contains the hearing and balance organs housed in an intricate bony labyrinth with an overall volume of about 200 mm^3 (Buckingham & Valvassori, 2001). This small space contains a sophisticated system of structures responsible for our ability to hear and to maintain our balance. To understand the anatomy and physiology of the inner ear is to marvel at what can be accomplished by nature in a very small space, as this volume is about the size of a peanut M&M.

The inner ear, as pictured in many textbooks, looks like the image in Figure 9.1., although one cannot dissect a human skull and find a freestanding bone in this shape. The familiar cochlea shape seen in many textbooks is actually the created image that is in the shape of a cavity (hole) called the **bony labyrinth** located within the petrous portion of the human temporal bone. If one were to make an impression of the bony labyrinth and then chip away the temporal bone, the resulting structure would look like Figure 9.1. This type of model makes a good introductory teaching model, but it must be understood that it is a negative image of the real structure; that is, it is a space of this shape located within a bone.

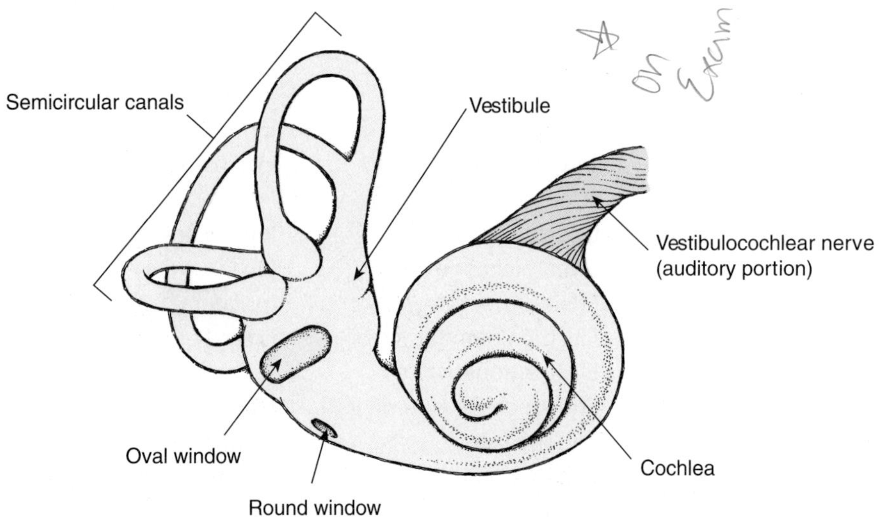

Figure 9.1. The shape of the bony labyrinth. (Modified from an image created by Neil O. Hardy, Westpoint, CT. Courtesy of Lippincott Williams & Wilkins. Used with permission.)

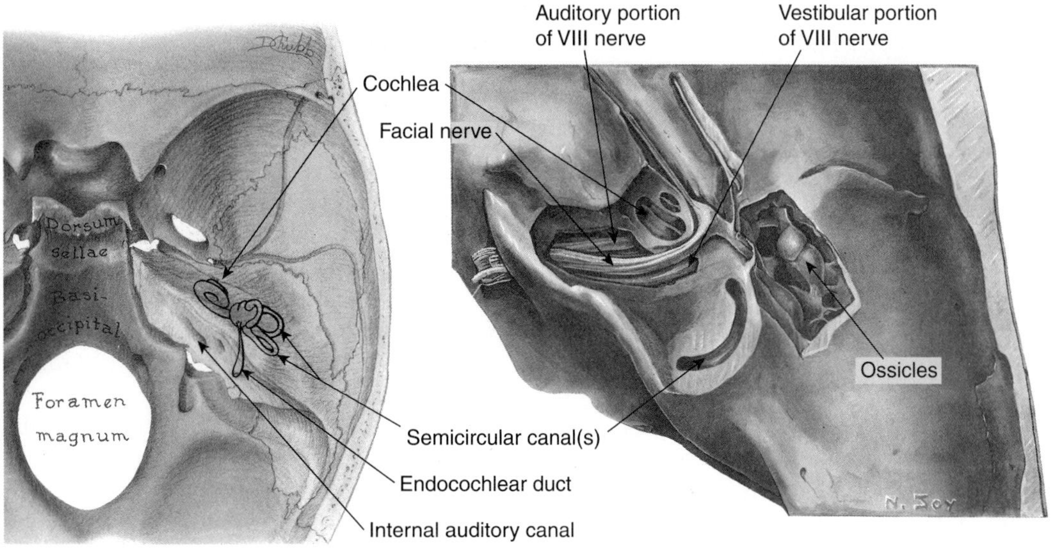

Figure 9.2. The inner ear seen in the superior view of the skull. An intact petrous portion **(A)** and dissected petrous portion **(B).** (Modified from Moore KL, Dalley AF. Clinical Oriented Anatomy. 4th Ed. Baltimore: Lippincott Williams & Wilkins, 1999. Used with permission.)

Figure 9.2 shows a superior view (view from above) of a human skull, with the petrous portion of the temporal bone visible. The view on the left shows the intact temporal bone with a superimposed line drawing indicating where the bony labyrinth is located within the bone. The view on the right shows the temporal bone as it would appear in a dissection. Notice in the second view that one of the three semicircular canals and two of the turns of the cochlea are shown. Within the cochlea, a central core of bone, the **modiolus,** can be seen. Also pictured is the **internal auditory canal,** which houses the vestibulocochlear (VIII) and facial (VII) nerves. The vestibulocochlear nerve will be discussed in more detail later in this chapter.

The bony labyrinth contains three main structures: the **cochlea,** which contains the organ of hearing, and the **semicircular canals** and **vestibule,** which contain the organs of balance. The cochlea is the most anterior (toward the front) of the three structures of the inner ear. The walls surrounding the base of the cochlea and a part of the vestibule together form the medial (middle) wall of the middle ear cavity.

A **membranous labyrinth** is located within the bony labyrinth and it follows all the curves and coils of the bony labyrinth. The shape of the membranous labyrinth is shown in Figure 9.3. The outside line seen in Figure 9.3 indicates the walls of the bony labyrinth. The membranous labyrinth is suspended within the bony labyrinth in a fluid called perilymph

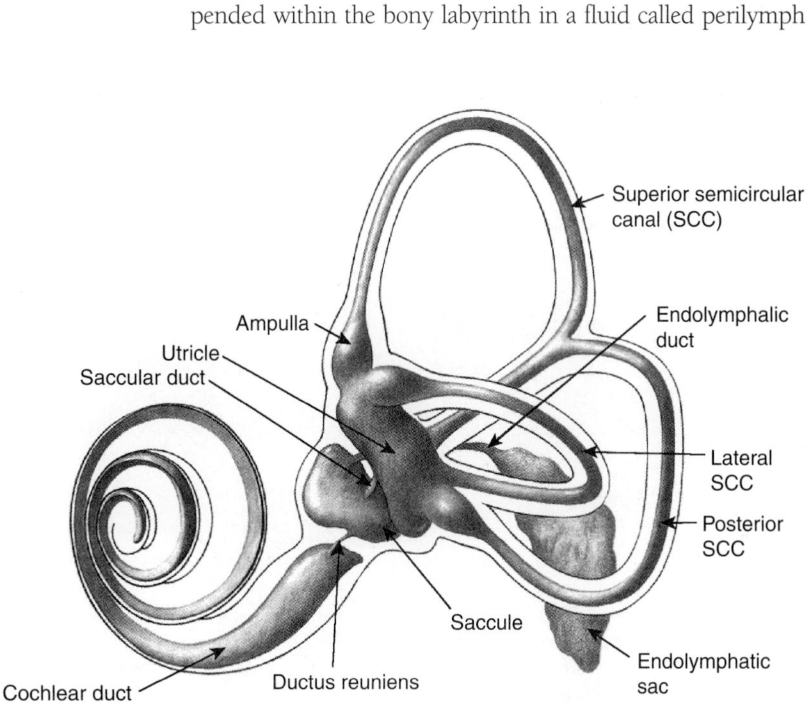

Figure 9.3. The membranous labyrinth shown within the bony labyrinth (outer line). (From Janfaza P, Nadol JB, Galla Jr R, et al. (eds.). Surgical Anatomy of the Head and Neck. Philadelphia: Lippincott Williams & Wilkins, 2001. Used with permission.)

and it is attached to the bony labyrinth along the edge of the cochlear spiral. The membranous labyrinth is filled with another fluid called endolymph and the chemical difference between these two fluids is important for the creation of electrochemical (neural) responses to sound entering the ear. This overall picture of the inner ear system provides the basis for discussing individual portions of the inner ear.

ANATOMY OF THE INNER EAR AND VESTIBULOCOCHLEAR NERVE

The Cochlea

The bony labyrinth of the cochlea forms a coiled tunnel about 35 mm long that turns 2¾ times through the petrous portion of the temporal bone (Polyak et al., 1948). The cochlea is about 6.8 mm high (Dimopoulos & Muren, 1990). The widest coil of the spiral is called the **base** of the cochlea. The narrowest end of the spiral, where the coils become tighter, is called the **apex.** Spiraling up through the center of the cochlea is a core of bone called the modiolus. The **spiral lamina** is a spiral, corkscrew-shaped bony shelf that projects from the side of the modiolus and partially divides the cochlear tunnel into smaller sections (Fig. 9.4).

The membranous labyrinth follows the cochlear spiral all the way from the base of the cochlea to just short of its end (the apex). Figure 9.4 shows a cross section of the entire bony spiral of the cochlea. The three separate channels seen in the cross section of the cochlea are the **scala vestibuli, scala tympani,** and **scala media.** The scala media is also known as the **cochlear duct** or **cochlear partition.** All three channels continue along the length of the cochlea, winding around as three parallel tunnels. The membranous part of the cochlea is the scala media and two other channels are bordered by the bony walls of the cochlea and are separated from each other by the scala media. Just prior to reaching the apex, the scala media channel ends and the scala tympani and scala vestibuli are connected together by a narrow passage called the **helicotrema.**

A detailed cross section of the cochlear tunnel is shown in Figure 9.5. Notice that the cross section of the cochlear duct forms a triangle shape. The short side of the triangle is attached to the wall of the bony labyrinth, whereas the two longer sides of the triangle are created by the **basilar membrane** and **Reissner's membrane** (after Ernst Reissner, 1824–1875), which stretch from the outside edge of the bony labyrinth to the inside (modiolus) edge. Located on the basilar membrane is the organ of hearing, called the **organ of Corti** (after Alfonso Corti, 1822–1876), which is the main structure responsible for converting mechanic vibrations that enter the cochlea into neural impulses.

On the outside edge of the scala media is the **stria vascularis.** *Stria* means "stripe" and *vascularis* refers to the vascular (blood) system. Reissner's membrane (vestibular membrane) forms the top edge of the scala media and the basilar membrane forms the bottom edge of the scala media. Reissner's membrane is attached on its inside edge to the **spiral limbus,** which sits on top of the spiral lamina. The basilar membrane is attached on its inside edge to the spiral lamina and on its outside edge to the **spiral ligament.**

The channel separated from the scala media by Reissner's membrane is the scala vestibuli and the channel separated from the scala media by the basilar membrane is the scala tympani. Notice that the orientation of the cross section in Figure 9.5 is different from the orientation of the cochlea shown in Figure 9.4. In Figure 9.4, the scala tympani is shown to be above the scala media, and in Figure 9.5, the scala tympani is shown to be below the scala media. The difference in the orientation of the cochlea in these two figures has been stressed to demonstrate that the same body part may be shown in different orientations on various diagrams and photographs. Even if the photograph or drawing of the cochlea is not clearly labeled, it is generally easy to differentiate Reissner's membrane from the

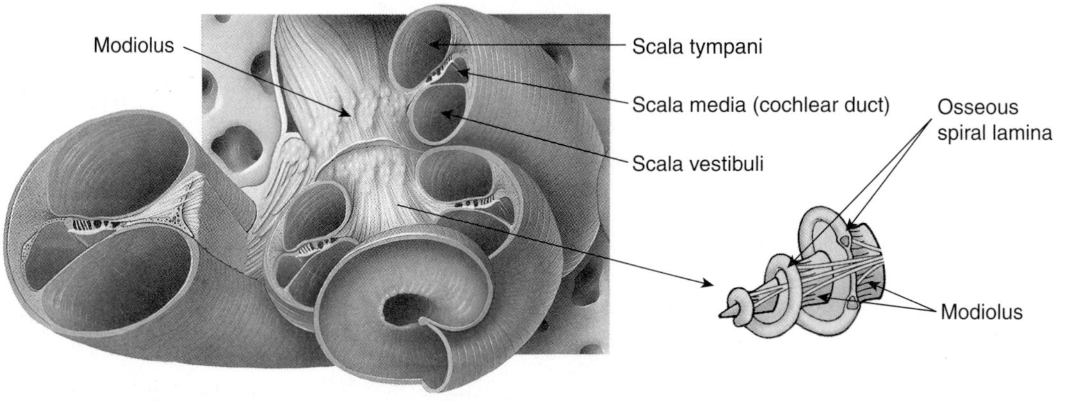

Figure 9.4. The turns of the cochlea. The corkscrew-shaped bone in the center of the cochlea is the modiolus with the spiral lamina (bony shelf) projecting in a spiral along the side. (A modified from an image created by the Anatomical Chart Co. B (modiolus core) modified from Moore KL, Dalley AF. Clinical Oriented Anatomy. 4th Ed. Baltimore: Lippincott Williams & Wilkins, 1999. Used with permission.)

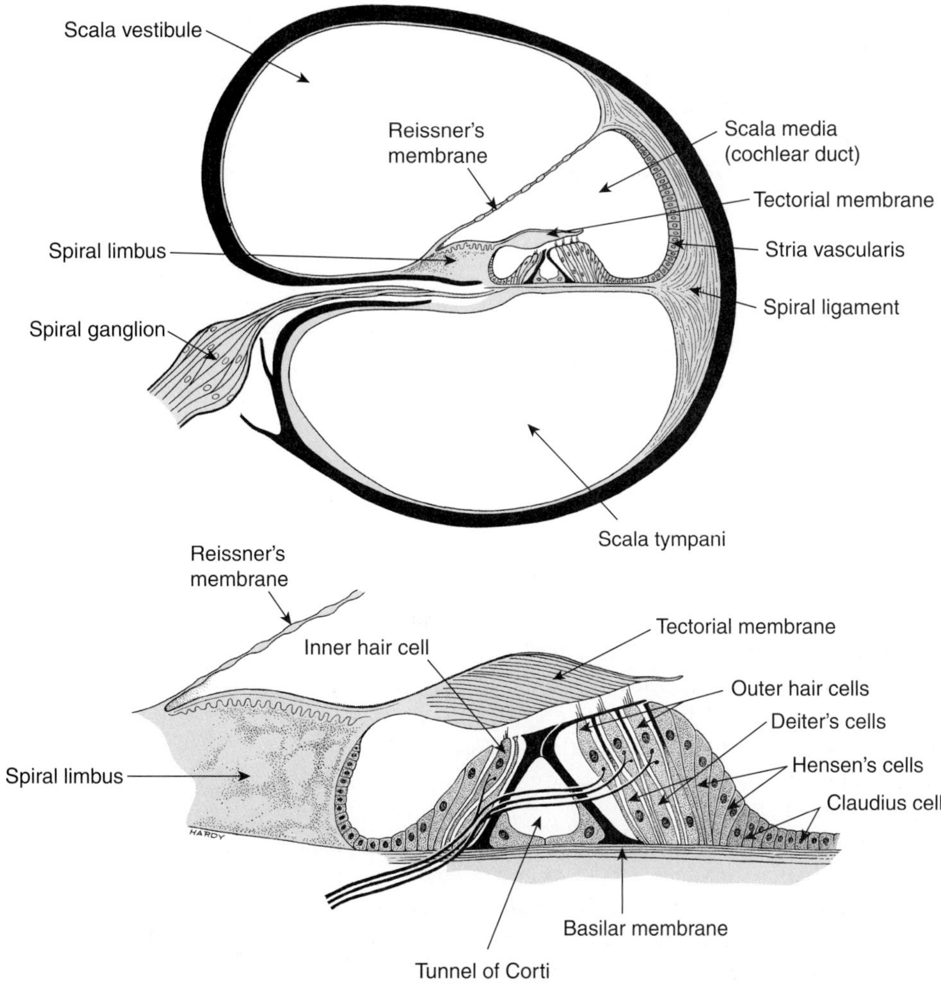

Figure 9.5. A cross section of the cochlea.

basilar membrane in a picture. The basilar membrane is thicker and it has an additional structure (the organ of Corti) spread across its width.

The three channels of the cochlea are filled with fluid. The scala vestibuli and scala tympani, together with the vestibule and semicircular canals, are filled with the **perilymph,** which is high in sodium (Na) and low in potassium (K). The membranous labyrinth, including the scala media, is filled with another fluid called **endolymph,** which is high in potassium and very low in sodium. Both of these fluids are almost incompressible; that is, they cannot be squeezed into smaller spaces (Cohen & Furst, 2004).

The relative positions of the three scalae compared with the location of the vestibule and middle ear wall are illustrated in Figure 9.6 in an uncoiled cochlea. Notice that at the base of the cochlea, the scala vestibuli is contiguous with the vestibule. During the process of sound transmission from the middle to inner ear, the inward motion of the stapes moves the membrane of the oval window, which is the entry point for the transmitted sound to the scala vestibuli. Farther into the cochlea, the scala vestibuli follows the cochlear spiral and connects to the scala tympani through the helicotrema passage located at the apex of the cochlea. The scala tympani winds down to the base of the cochlea and is terminated by the membrane of the round window, located in the middle ear wall.

The basilar membrane forms the border between the scala media and the scala tympani and it is the supporting structure for the organ of Corti. The up-and-down motions of the basilar membrane are crucial in the process of converting mechanic motions into electrochemical impulses. An important feature of the basilar membrane is that its mechanic properties gradually change along its length. The membrane is the thinnest and stiffest at the base of the cochlea (low mass and high stiffness) and thickest and most flaccid at the apex (large mass and low stiffness), and it can be considered like a mechanic system that consists of many segments having their own resonance frequencies, which decrease from the base toward the apex. Thus, different portions of the basilar membrane have a tendency to vibrate (resonate) at different frequencies. Low-frequency forces cause the membrane to vibrate most effectively at its apex and high-frequency forces cause the strongest vibration at the base of the cochlea.

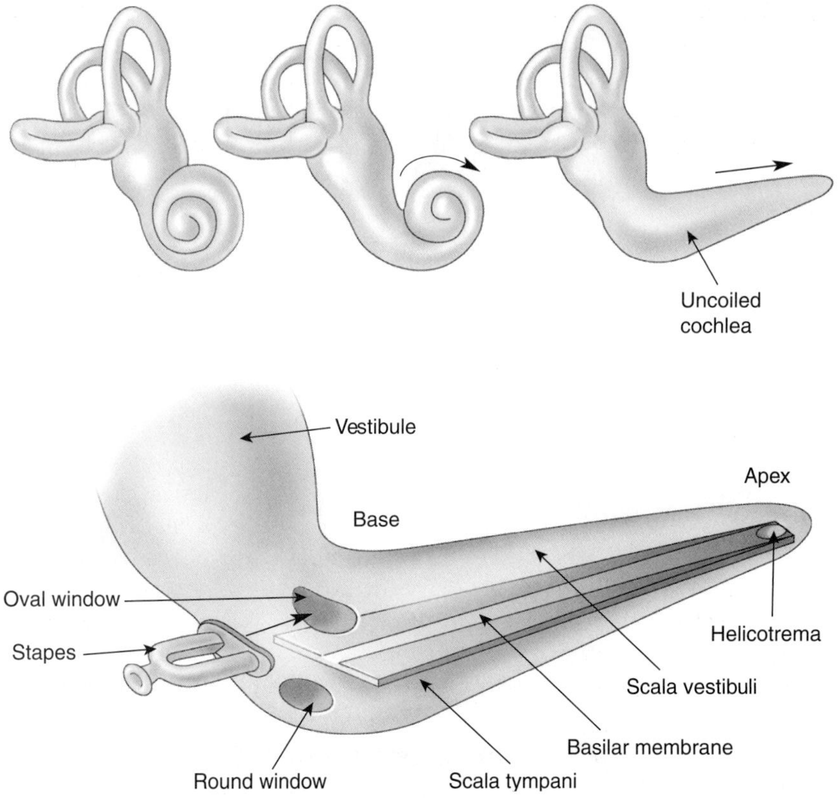

Figure 9.6. A view of the uncoiled cochlea. (Modified from Bear MF, Connors BW, Paradiso MA. Neuroscience: Exploring the Brain. Baltimore: Lippincott Williams & Wilkins, 2001. Used with permission.)

The sense organ of hearing, the organ of Corti, runs along the entire length of the basilar membrane, on the side of the scala media tunnel. The organ of Corti and surrounding structures are shown in Figure 9.5. Most of the organ of Corti sits on the basilar membrane, but a small portion extends onto the spiral lamina. The organ of Corti consists of hair cells and support cells. **Hair cells** are sensory (auditory) cells with stereocilia (tiny hairs) projecting from one end. These cells are responsible for changing mechanic motion into electrochemical impulses that can be transmitted by the nervous system.

The organ of Corti consists of one row of **inner hair cells** (IHCs) that are shaped like a flask and three rows of **outer hair cells** (OHCs) that are cylindrical in shape (Fig. 9.7). Approximately 3500 IHCs and 12,000 OHCs are in each cochlea. Between the IHC and the OHC is the **tunnel of Corti,** a triangular-shaped support structure created by the inner and outer **rods (pillars) of Corti.** The inner rod sits on the spiral lamina and the outer rod sits on the basilar membrane. The OHCs are further supported by narrow **Deiters cells** (after Otto Freidrich Deiters, 1834–1875). Deiters cells have a cup-shaped depression that holds the bottom end of each OHC and long **phalangeal processes** that project around the OHCs and extend up to the surface of the organ of Corti. The OHCs are held in place quite firmly at the top and bottom of the cell, but most of the length of the OHC is not firmly supported but is surrounded by a perilymph-filled space called the **space of Nuel** (Ulfendahl et al., 2000).

A number of supporting cells are located medially (modiolus side) and laterally (toward the spiral lamina) to the hair cells. Located medially to the IHCs are the **inner sulcus cells** (or inner spiral sulcus cells), which extend from the spiral limbus to the inside edge of the IHCs, and the **inner phalangeal cells** (or inner supporting cells), which provide support for the IHCs (Lim, 1986). Support cells that are

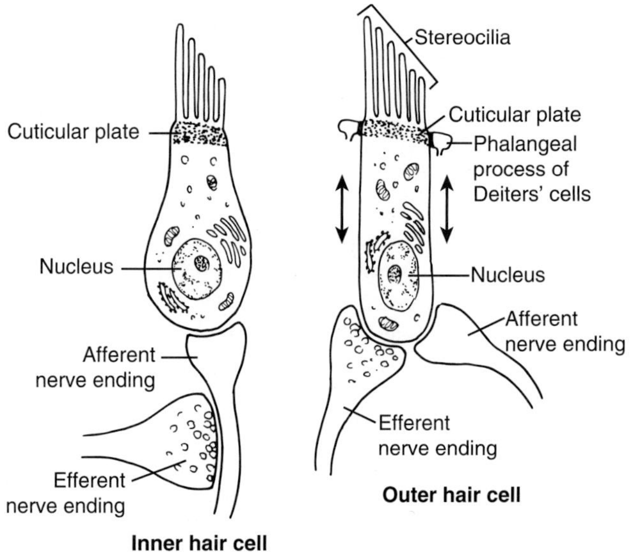

Figure 9.7. Inner hair cells **(A)** and outer hair cells **(B).**

located next to the OHCs are **Hensen cells** (after Viktor Hensen, 1835–1924). The other support cells include **Claudius cells** (after Matthias Claudius, 1821–1869), which are adjacent to the Hensen cells; **outer spiral sulcus cells,** which begin at the Claudius cells and continue along the spiral ligament; and **Boettcher cells** (after Arthur Boettcher, 1831–1889), which are found in the basal turn of the cochlea under the Claudius cells (Spicer & Schulte, 1994). Most of these cells are shown in Figure 9.5.

Projecting from the top of each hair cell are several rows of tiny hairs called **stereocilia.** There are 40 to 60 stereocilia on each IHC and 100 to 150 on each OHC. The group of stereocilia on the top of each hair cell is called a **stereocilia bundle.** The stereocilia are firmly anchored to the hair cell via a thickening at the top edge of the hair cell called the **cuticular plate.** The tops of the hair cells and supporting cells form the upper surface of the organ of Corti, called the **reticular lamina.** The reticular lamina isolates the organ of Corti from the endolymph of the scala media, with the exception of the stereocilia, which project through the reticular lamina into the endolymph. The length of the stereocilia bundle and the stiffness of the bundle vary from the base to the apex of the cochlea (Lim, 1986).

If the organ of Corti is viewed from the top, the stereocilia bundle projecting from the top of each IHC forms a shallow U shape and the stereocilia bundle projecting from each OHC forms a V or W shape (Fig. 9.8).

Attached to the superior surface of the spiral limbus is a fibrous membrane called the **tectorial membrane,** which extends out into the scala media over the entire organ of Corti, making contact with the tallest tips of the OHC stereocilia. The rows of stereocilia on each hair cell are arranged in gradually increasing height, like a set of steps with the tallest stereocilia located away from the modiolus. The tips of the largest stereocilia from the OHCs project into the tectorial membrane, but the stereocilia from the IHCs do not contact the tectorial membrane according to most sources (e.g., Steel, 1983), although it is possible that the IHC stereocilia in the basal turn of the cochlea may be loosely coupled to the tectorial membrane.

Individual stereocilia are connected to each other by thin fibers called **cross-links** (Pickles et al., 1984). The three types of cross-links are **side-to-side cross-links,** which form connections between the sides of adjacent stereocilia in the same row; **row-to-row cross-links,** which form connections between the sides of adjacent stereocilia across rows; and **tip-to-side cross-links** (often labeled "tip links"), which form connections between the top (smaller cilia) and the side (larger cilia) of adjacent stereocilia across rows (Gelfand, 1998). The tip-to-side cross-links control the state of mechanically gated ion channels. **Ion channels** are tiny openings in the hair cell membrane that allow potassium ions (K^+) to pass from the endolymph into the hair cells. It is believed that when the tip-to-side cross-links are pulled, they open the gates of the attached ion channels, and when the links return to their rest position, the gates close. This means that when the stereocilia are pushed away from the modiolus, the gates are pulled open (on the smaller cell), and when the stereocilia are pushed toward the modiolus, the gates are shut. The mechanical action of the basilar membrane (up and down) results in the movement of the stereocilia toward and away from the modiolus, and this causes the opening and closing of the ion channels, which begins the neurophysiologic process that leads to sound perception.

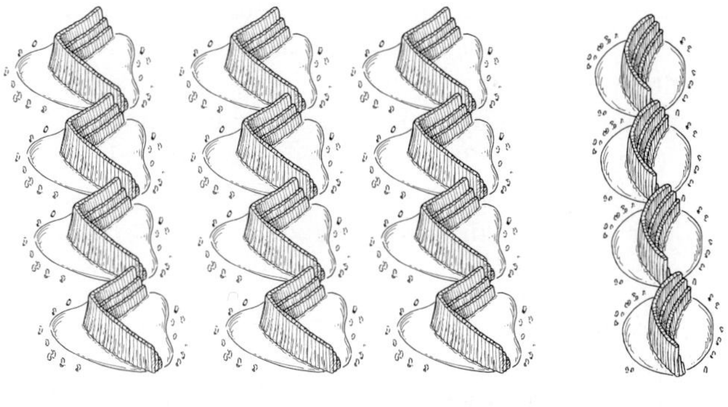

Figure 9.8. A top view of the hair cell stereocilia. The tectorial membrane has been removed.

The Vestibulocochlear Nerve

The vestibulocochlear nerve (the VIII cranial nerve) is the nerve that connects the systems of hearing and balance to the brain. The name of this nerve results from the fact that it has two portions: a vestibular portion and a cochlear portion. The vestibular portion begins at the sensory cells contained within the vestibule and semicircular canals and travels with the cochlear portion of the vestibulocochlear nerve to the entry point in the brainstem, where both parts take separate paths through the central nervous system. The cochlear portion of the vestibulocochlear nerve begins beneath the cochlear hair cells and joins the vestibular portion in the internal auditory canal (a channel in the temporal bone) on its way to the brain. The cochlear part of the vestibulocochlear nerve is called the **auditory nerve,** although in some books it is also referred to as the acoustic nerve or cochlear nerve.

Hair cells of the organ of Corti communicate with the brain via a network of cells called **neurons** (nerve cells). Neurons are cells that transmit electrochemical information within the nervous system of the body. The neuron has a **soma (cell body)** and two types of extensions, called axons and dendrites, which allow the nerve to communicate with other nerves at junctions called **synapses.** At the point where one neuron synapses with an adjacent neuron, information transfer (communication) occurs. The **dendrite** is the part of the cell that receives signals from other cells and the **axon** is the part of the cell that transmits signals to other cells. Axons extending from several neurons are bundled together, like wires in a telephone cable, forming communication pathways called **nerves.** If you would like to know more about neuron anatomy, consult the website. **Link 9-1**

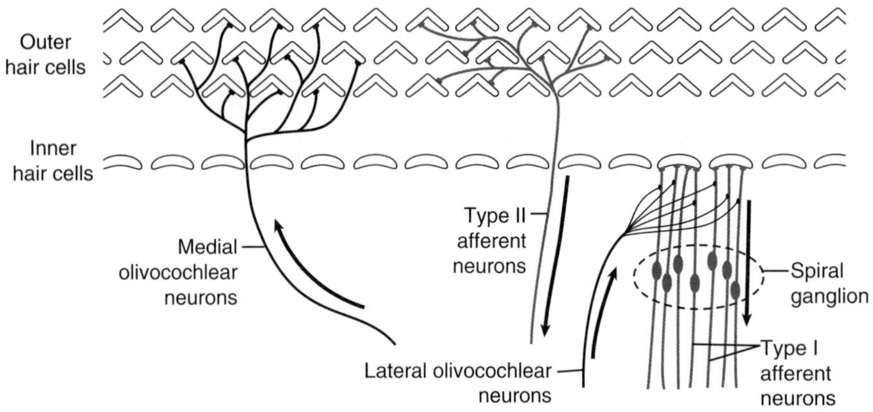

Figure 9.9. The innervation pattern of afferent and efferent neurons to the hair cells.

Within the nervous system, the cell bodies from many different neurons are grouped together. In the **central nervous system,** consisting of the brain and spinal cord, a group of cell bodies is called a **nucleus** except at the surface of the brain, where it is called a **cortex** or **gray matter.** In the **peripheral nervous system,** which includes the rest of the nervous system outside of the brain and spinal cord, a group of cell bodies is called a **ganglion**.*

Depending on the function of a neuron, all neurons can be divided into afferent neurons, efferent neurons, and interneurons. **Afferent neurons** (or sensory neurons) are the neurons that carry sensory information (touch, taste, smell, hearing, vision) from the peripheral nervous system to the central nervous system. **Efferent neurons** are neurons that carry information from the central nervous system to the peripheral nervous system (e.g., instructions to the leg muscles that allow us to walk). **Interneurons** provide communication between afferent and efferent neurons.

Within the auditory system, afferent neurons from the auditory nerve convey auditory information from the cochlea to the central nervous system and efferent neurons convey signals from the central nervous system back to the cochlea and other structures. The afferent system is by far the most well understood of the two systems. The afferent portion of the auditory nerve consists of two types of afferent neurons, type I afferent neurons and type II afferent neurons. Approximately 95% of the afferent neurons are type I and 5% are type II. Type I neurons (also called **inner radial fibers**) are the larger of the two types and they are covered with myelin. Type II neurons (also called **outer spiral fibers**) are thinner and not covered with myelin. A **nerve fiber** is a thread-like extension that comes out of a cell body. It is sometimes used synonymously with the term *axon*, which is usually a relatively long fiber; however, a dendrite is also referred to as a short fiber. The interface between the afferent auditory nerve and the cochlear hair cells is quite complex but it needs to be well understood to follow the basics of auditory perception.

The Auditory Nerve and Hair Cell Connection

Figure 9.9 illustrates the location of the auditory nerve endings relative to the IHCs and OHCs. The IHCs are connected to type I afferent auditory neurons and the OHCs are connected to type II afferent auditory neurons.* Approximately 20 type I afferent auditory neurons innervate each IHC. Each of these neurons is attached to only one hair cell. In contrast, type II afferent auditory neurons travel down the cochlea for a short distance and send multiple branches to several different OHCs. Auditory nerves enter the spiral lamina via holes in the bone called **habenula perforata** and project toward the center of the modiolus into a channel called **Rosenthal's canal** (after Friedrich Christof Rosenthal, 1780–1829), where the nerve cell bodies are located. Collectively, these cell bodies are called the **spiral ganglia.** The central processes of the spiral ganglion nerve cells exit the base of the modiolus, join with nerves from the vestibular portion of the vestibulocochlear nerve and the facial nerve, and travel via the internal auditory canal toward the brainstem. The neural pathway conveying auditory information beyond this point will be discussed in Chapter 10.

Similar to afferent auditory neurons, there are also two types of efferent auditory neurons in the cochlea. They are the **medial olivocochlear neurons** and the **lateral olivocochlear neurons** (Fig. 9.9). Together, these neurons make up the **olivocochlear bundle.** These neurons originate in the superior olivary complex in the brainstem (Chapter 10), travel with the vestibular nerve, and enter the cochlea via the **anastomosis of Oort** (also called the **vestibulocochlear anastomosis**). Each of the two types of efferent nerves is named by the location of the cell bodies in the brainstem. Medial olivocochlear neurons have cell bodies in the medial portion of the superior olivary complex and lateral olivocochlear neurons have cell bodies in

*One major exception to this rule is the misnamed "basal ganglia," which are cell bodies located deep in the brain. They are more correctly called the basal nuclei.

*The hair cells are not actually connected to the nerve fibers; they are separated by the small synaptic cleft. The term *connection* in this context refers to the communication connection between the hair cells and the nerves.

the lateral portion of the superior olivary complex. Medial olivocochlear neurons are large myelinated neurons that send collaterals (axon branches) to many OHCs, primarily to the **contralateral** (opposite side) ear. Lateral olivocochlear neurons are smaller unmyelinated neurons that send collaterals to the base of the IHCs, primarily on the **ipsilateral** side (same side). Lateral olivocochlear neurons terminate at the peripheral processes of the type I afferent neurons below the IHCs, rather than directly with the hair cells (Fig. 9.7).

PHYSIOLOGY OF THE INNER EAR AND VESTIBULOCOCHLEAR NERVE

The inner ear can be described as a transducer changing the mechanic energy of the ossicular chain of the middle ear into electrochemical impulses that can be transmitted by the nervous system to the brain. This is quite a complex task. Consider for a moment what is required for the translation of speech into nerve impulses. Speech is a dynamic sound consisting of rapid changes in frequency and intensity. The inner ear must take this highly dynamic signal and translate it virtually instantaneously into a series of pulses that can be carried through thousands of individual nerves to the brain where the signal is reconstructed into a meaningful message. If the frequency, intensity, and timing characteristics of the signal are distorted in the translation, speech will be unintelligible.

The process by which the cochlea breaks down complex sound and translates it into a series of nerve impulses has been investigated for many years and is not yet fully understood. Several basic mechanisms have been identified, however, that explain how the frequency, intensity, and timing characteristics of sound are coded by the cochlea and how the brain uses these neural codes to reconstruct messages.

Traveling Wave

The scala vestibuli and scala tympani of the cochlea are filled with perilymph, which is a virtually incompressible fluid. The oval window and the round window, located in the bony wall separating the inner ear from the middle ear, are two critical elements in the conversion of energy from the mechanic movement of the stapes to the wave motion inside the cochlea. These windows are covered with flexible elastic membranes, in contrast to the rest of the bony wall of the normal cochlea.* When the stapes (connected to the oval window) pushes in toward the cochlea, the excess fluid in the scala vestibuli tries to expand perpendicularly by pushing on the walls of the bony cochlea and the scala media. Since the scala media is filled with another incompressible fluid, endolymph, it cannot be compressed and the whole scala media is displaced perpendicularly, pushing the fluid in the scala vestibuli toward the scala tympani, which causes a bulging of the round window. The process is repeated in the opposite direction when the oval window moves outward, causing the scala media (including the basilar membrane and organ of Corti) to move toward the scala vestibuli. Thus, the scala media and the structures within it vibrate in response to the vibratory movement of the oval window. Since the mechanic properties of the basilar membrane vary along its length, the displacement of the basilar membrane is not uniform but varies along its longitudinal axis. The point of maximum displacement of the basilar membrane depends on the frequency of the oval window movement and it is located at the place where the resonance frequency of the basilar membrane segment is equal to the frequency of the stimulation. Thus, at high frequencies, the point of maximum vibration is located toward the base of the cochlea. For low frequencies, the point of maximum vibration occurs toward the apex of the cochlea; however, a large portion of the membrane vibrates because the energy travels along the cochlea from base to apex in the form of a traveling wave. A **traveling wave** (transverse wave) is a wave motion in which moving particles are displaced perpendicularly to the direction of the moving wave (Chapter 5). When the oval window is stimulated at a specific frequency, the traveling wave begins at the base of the cochlea and gradually increases in amplitude up to the point at which the resonance frequency of the vibrating segment of the membrane matches the stimulation frequency. Beyond this point the wave magnitude abruptly decays. Thus, the envelope of displacement of the basilar membrane is not symmetric; it rises gradually to the point of maximum displacement and then sharply decays. This specific characteristic of the basilar membrane motion is the reason that low frequencies mask higher frequencies more than the other way around; this phenomenon will be discussed in Chapter 12.

The correspondence between stimulation frequency and place along the cochlea is called **tonotopicity;** thus, the cochlea is said to be **tonotopically organized.** The traveling wave behavior and tonotopicity of the basilar membrane was first described by Georg von Békésy (1960), who won a Nobel Prize for his work. The pattern of the traveling wave propagating along the basilar membrane is shown in Figure 9.10.

If the signal entering the cochlea is a complex sound, various components of this sound will be represented by various points of vibration along the basilar membrane making the membrane behave as a biologic frequency analyzer where the distance along the membrane axis corresponds to signal frequency and the magnitude of the membrane displacement corresponds to the intensity of the spectral components. For example, if a tone with two components (e.g., 500 Hz and 3000 Hz) entered the cochlea, there would be separate areas of vibration for each of these components along the basilar membrane. The greater the spectral complexity of the input signal is, the more complex the vibration pattern will be across the basilar membrane.

*In some pathologic conditions, other "windows" or openings of the bony labyrinth wall are present. For example, superior semicircular canal dehiscence is an abnormal opening in the bony superior semicircular canal wall. Any abnormal opening in the bony wall of the cochlea can affect the normal function of the inner ear and can result in hearing loss and/or dizziness.

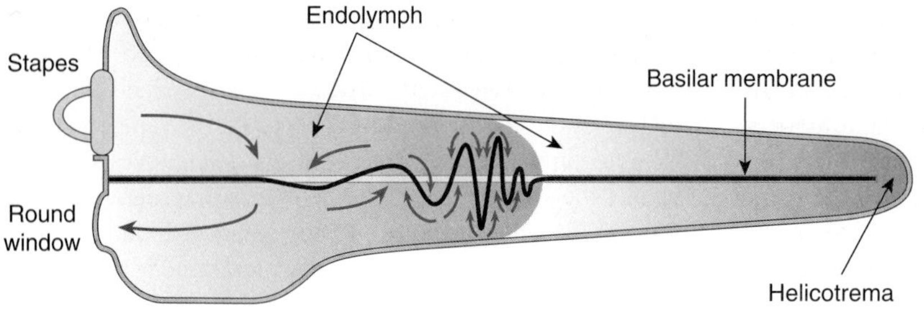

Figure 9.10. The traveling wave. (From Bear MF, Connors BW, Paradiso MA. Neuroscience: Exploring the Brain. Baltimore: Lippincott Williams & Wilkins, 2001. Used with permission.)

Electric Potentials in the Inner Ear

The mechanic movement of the basilar membrane does not create neural activity by itself. To generate neural signals, several other structures and mechanisms must exist. For example, the inner ear must contain a source of electricity. In general, electricity is created by separating charged particles, called **ions,** so that positively (+) charged particles (called **cations**) are stored in one location and negatively (−) charged particles (called **anions**) are stored in another location. These two opposing concentrations of particles constitute a source of electrical energy. When a system uses energy stored in the charged particles, the particles move from one area of the system to another in the form of a particle flow (electric current). The larger the differences in electric charge between the two areas are, the greater the force attracting the opposite charges. This force is called an **electric potential.** The basic elements of electric systems and their properties are discussed in Chapter 13.

In the inner ear, the electric potentials are created by various concentrations of positively and negatively charged ions in perilymph, endolymph, and hair cells. These ions include positive potassium ions (K^+), negative chloride ions (Cl^-), positive sodium ions (Na^+), and positive calcium ions (Ca^{2+}). Endolymph is rich in potassium (K^+) and is low in calcium (Ca^{2+}) and sodium (Na^+). Perilymph is low in potassium (K^+) and is rich in calcium (Ca^{2+}) and sodium (Na^+). The negative chloride ions (Cl^-) dominate the cell bodies of the hair cells. The various concentrations of these ions are separated by semipermeable membranes that surround the hair cells and separate the cochlear spaces. For this stored electricity to do work, some trigger mechanism must exist that causes the flow of charged particles from one place to another.

The electric potentials (i.e., differences in electrical charge) existing between various areas within the human body are called **bioelectric potentials.** Bioelectric potentials that normally exist in the human body without being affected by stimulation are called **resting potentials** and potentials generated by stimulation are called **stimulus-related potentials.** Stimulus-related potentials that are generated in individual neurons in response to external stimulation are called **action potentials, neural potentials, neural impulses,** or **nerve impulses.** When the action potentials from many different neurons occur at the same time, this is called a **compound (whole nerve) action potential** (CAP).

The endolymph in the scala media has a resting potential that is about +80 mV compared with the perilymph in the scala vestibuli and scala tympani. This resting potential is called the **endocochlear potential** (EP) and it is generated by the stria vascularis (Tasaki & Spyropoulos, 1959). The IHCs have a resting potential of about −40 mV and the OHCs have a resting potential of about −70 mV compared with the perilymph (Santos-Sacchi, 2001) (Fig. 9.11). Thus, the resting potential of the hair cells is approximately 120 mV (IHC) to 150 mV (OHC) lower than the resting potential of the endolymph.

When an acoustic stimulus excites the cochlea, three stimulus-related electric potentials appear and can be measured within the cochlea. They are the summating potential, the cochlear microphonic, and the CAP. The summating potential and the cochlear microphonic are generated within the inner ear by the hair cells and the CAP is the resulting electrical activity transmitted by the vestibulocochlear nerve caused by the activity of the whole cochlea.

The **summating potential** is a positive or negative change in the potential difference between the hair cells and

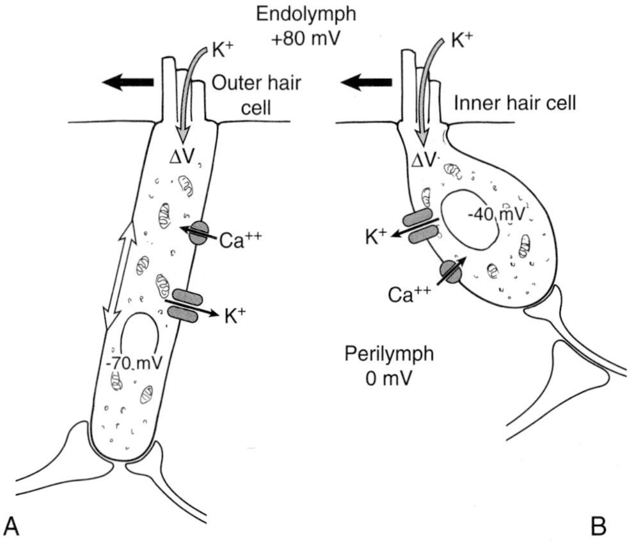

Figure 9.11. Electric potentials of inner **(A)** and outer **(B)** hair cells.

the endolymph. This potential begins when a signal begins and ends when a signal ends. The summating potential is a **direct current (DC) potential.** This means that the potential increases or decreases during the presence of stimulation but does not change its polarity; that is, it is either a sustained positive or a sustained negative change in the existing potential but the potential does not reverse itself.

The **cochlear microphonic** and **compound action potential** are both **alternating current (AC) potentials.** An AC potential is electrical activity in which both the magnitude and direction of the electrical flow vary periodically. The cochlear microphonic is a change in voltage produced at the reticular lamina that mimics the vibration pattern of the basilar membrane. As the basilar membrane moves up and down, the cochlear microphonic alternates between positive and negative polarity, mimicking the shape of the input signal. For example, if a 200-Hz pure tone enters the cochlea, the cochlear microphonic will mimic the signal and appear as a 200-Hz signal. A speech signal will create a cochlear microphonic that mimics the speech signal (Wever & Bray, 1930). The cochlear microphonic is not the neural response of the inner ear that results in our perception of sound, but is instead a byproduct of cochlear operation (e.g., an indication of the electromechanic feedback loop in the cochlea) (Causse, 1942; Furst & Cohen, 1994; Kellaway, 1944; Seymour & Tappin, 1951).

The CAP, also called the whole nerve action potential, is the summed AC potential generated by many neurons of the auditory nerve that are stimulated by a large number of IHCs. The magnitude of the CAP depends on the number of activated neurons.

Shearing of the Stereocilia

When the basilar membrane moves up and down, the hair cells that are located on the basilar membrane will also move up and down. Because the attachment point of the basilar membrane to the spiral lamina is farther away from the modiolus than the attachment point of the tectorial membrane to the spiral limbus, the up-and-down motion of the scala media will cause the basilar membrane and tectorial membrane to move back and forth relative to each other in a direction that is perpendicular to the motion of the basilar membrane (Fig. 9.12). This is called a **shearing motion** and it results in a shearing force acting on the stereocilia, which makes them bend.

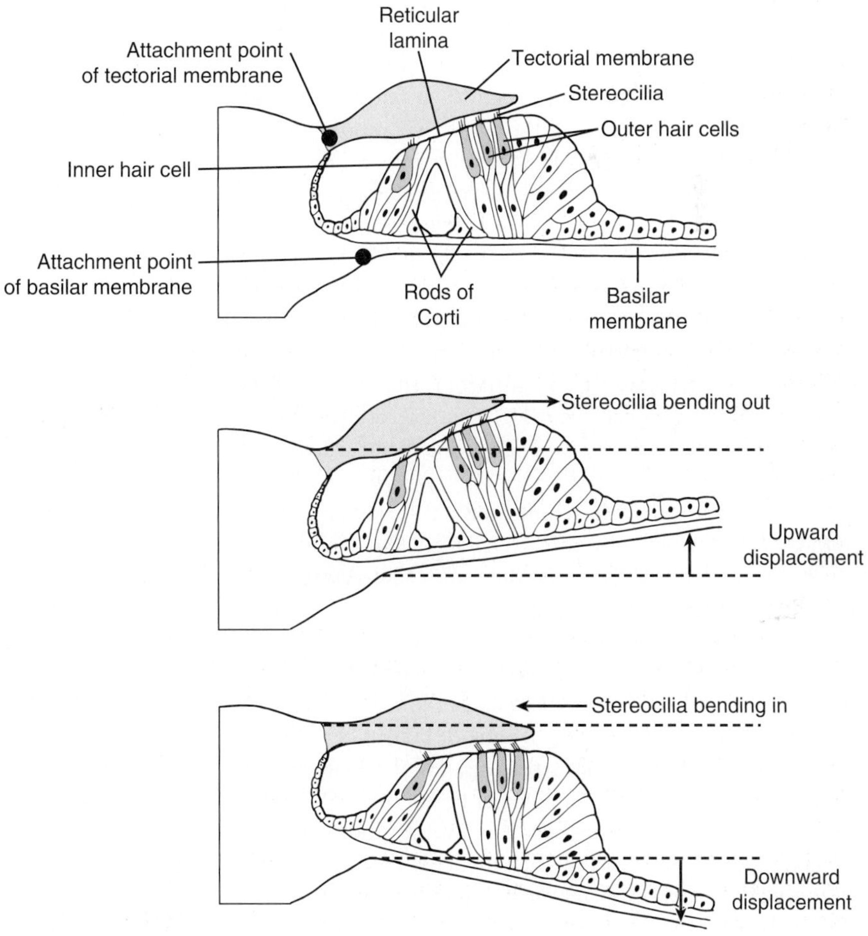

Figure 9.12. Shearing of the hair cell stereocilia. (Modified from Bear MF, Connors BW, Paradiso MA. Neuroscience: Exploring the Brain. Baltimore: Lippincott Williams & Wilkins, 2001. Used with permission.)

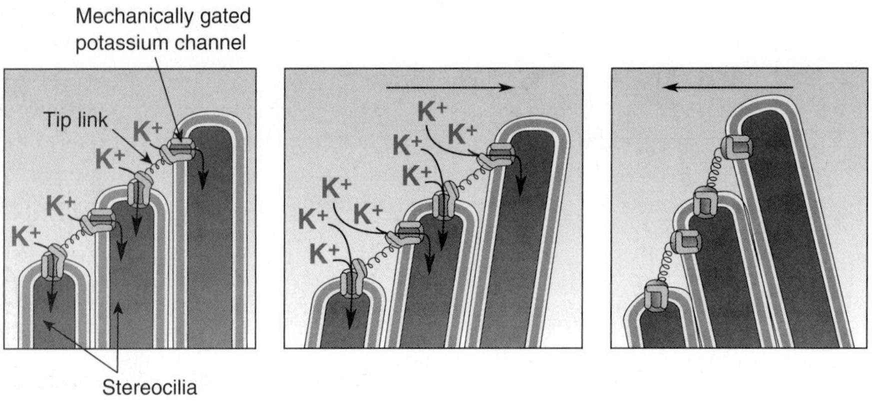

Figure 9.13. Mechanical gating of ion channels by tip links. Potassium (K^+) enters the cell when the gates are open. (Modified from Bear MF, Connors BW, Paradiso MA. Neuroscience: Exploring the Brain. Baltimore: Lippincott Williams & Wilkins, 2001. Used with permission.)

Recall that the largest of the stereocilia from the OHCs are embedded in the tectorial membrane. Thus, the largest stereocilia will be pulled back and forth with the tectorial membrane following the shearing motion between the basilar membrane and the tectorial membrane. The stereocilia of the IHCs are not embedded in the tectorial membrane, but they will also move back and forth in response to the fluid motion across the stereocilia (Dallos et al., 1972).

When the stereocilia bundle is bent toward the largest stereocilia, the mechanic action of the tip-to-side links results in the opening of the ion channels in the stereocilia, allowing positively charged potassium ions (K^+), which are the main cations in the endolymph, to rush into the negatively charged hair cell (Fig. 9.13) and depolarize its content. The word **depolarization** means a change in the electrical potential existing between the inside and outside of a cell, away from its resting state toward zero. During this change the cell is excited, and if the change exceeds a certain threshold value, it generates a nerve impulse. When the stereocilia bundle is deflected away from the largest stereocilia, the ion channels are closed and the negative resting potential of the hair cell is restored. Thus, the back-and-forth motion of the stereocilia causes the hair cells to change the electrical potentials of the cells.

The OHCs and IHCs have different and specific reactions to the chemical influx of K^+ ions. OHCs react to this change in electrical potential by expanding and contracting, and IHCs react by releasing a special substance called a **neurotransmitter** (chemical messenger) from the base of the cell into the synapse with the afferent auditory nerve fibers. The release of the neurotransmitter initiates the transmission of information to a neuron. The actions of both types of hair cells require that the K^+ ions be in plentiful supply in the endolymph. Therefore, K^+ ions must be continuously recycled and reused in the inner ear. The source producing and recycling the K^+ ions in the scala media is the stria vascularis, which is responsible for maintaining the positive endocochlear potential. In a normal ear, K^+ travels from the base of the cell through a series of channels known as **gap junctions** back to the stria vascularis, which sends it back to the endolymph.*

The Action of the Outer Hair Cells

The OHCs can be considered automatic gain control (AGC) cells that affect the mechanic motion of basilar membrane. In response to a change in the cell potential (when K^+ rushes into the cell and is then pumped out of the cell), the OHC is alternately compressed and expanded in length. The mechanic changes in the length of the OHCs are referred to as the OHC electromotility (motor action, motility function). **Electromotility** is the ability of the OHCs to act as small motors in responses to changes in the electrical potential of the cell. The motion of the OHCs changes the shape of the traveling wave, increasing its displacement in the narrow area at the location of the vibrating OHCs. The greater displacement of the traveling wave increases the mechanic input to the IHCs, which are located next to the vibrating OHCs. This increase in the mechanic stimulation of the IHCs increases their activity level. Therefore, the OHC motility that results in the increase in the IHC response is called the **cochlear amplifier.** The amplification of the incoming sound by the OHC movement varies as a function of the intensity of the sound and is the greatest at low intensities. If the OHCs are substantially missing, the missing cochlear amplifier results in a hearing loss of approximately 50 dB.

Outer hair cell motility is attributed to a protein called **prestin** located in the OHC wall (Dallos & Fakler, 2002; Zheng et al., 2000). Recent evidence suggests that the stereocilia bundle, which appears to be "tuned" to respond best at specific frequencies, also contributes to the active process (Kennedy et al., 2005; Ricci, 2003; Withnell et al., 2002). In addition, the coil-like shape of the cochlea appears to contribute to increased vibrations at the outside edge of the

*A number of genetic forms of hearing loss are associated with the malformation of proteins that create gap junctions (e.g., the connexin 26 gene mutation) (Steel, 1999).

spiral and the transmission of low frequencies that are mapped at the end of the cochlea (Manoussaki et al., 2006).

The motility of the OHC was first observed by Brownell and colleagues (1985), who described changes in the length of the OHC in vitro (in an artificial environment) in response to changes in an applied external voltage; however, the existence of an active process in the cochlea that acts as a mechanic amplifier within the cochlea was hypothesized long before by Gold (1948). Gold stated that a cochlear amplifier would be necessary to overcome the large degree of damping offered by the cochlea and to explain humans' exquisite ability to differentiate very small differences in frequency (e.g., to perceive the difference between 1000 and 1004 Hz), something that is not adequately explained by the behavior of the broad traveling wave observed and described by von Békésy.

In 1978, David Kemp reported a phenomenon he had recorded from the human ear canal. In response to a sound introduced into the ear canal, he was able to record "cochlear echoes," which are sound waves reflected from the inner ear back out to the ear canal. This echo was hypothesized to be a byproduct of the cochlear amplifier and it provided evidence that energy is generated within the cochlea. This energy is sent through the middle ear to the outer ear, with the tympanic membrane acting as a speaker cone creating acoustic waves in the external ear canal. The very-low-intensity echo can be observed in a normal ear, but it is absent in an ear with a hearing loss caused by OHC damage. These echoes are now called **otoacoustic emissions** (OAEs). Kemp's research led to a revolutionary new clinical testing procedure that is now common practice for hearing screening and diagnosis in hospitals and clinics around the world.

Little is known about the afferent neural connections of the OHCs, although some limited evidence demonstrates that they are functional (Engel et al., 2006). Several OHCs synapse with each single, unmyelinated, type II, slow-reacting neuron, which connects directly to nuclei in the superior olivary complex. The fact that the OHCs connect to slow-reacting neurons indicates that they may respond to average levels of cochlear excitation. Their function may be informing the olivary nuclei centers about the state of vibration of the basilar membrane or the coding of the overall intensity of the cochlea stimulation.

The Action of the Inner Hair Cells

The response of the IHCs to the influx of potassium ions (K^+) is the release of neurotransmitter substance from the base of the hair cell into the **synaptic cleft** (space between neurons) via a process called **exocytosis** (Fig. 9.14). The neurotransmitter travels across the synaptic cleft to bind to receptor sites on the auditory nerve endings. The auditory nerve will respond to this chemical message by firing (sending) an electrical signal down the nerve. If you would like to learn more about neuron physiology, please consult the website. **Link 9-2**

The neurotransmitter substance released by the IHC at the synaptic junctions with the afferent neuron appears to be glutamate (Nordang et al., 2000). Since 95% of the afferent fibers from the auditory branch of the vestibulocochlear nerve innervate IHCs, the IHC is the primary mechanism for sending the signal to the nervous system. The translation of the excitation of the IHC into the neural code (impulses) is the focus of various theories of hearing.

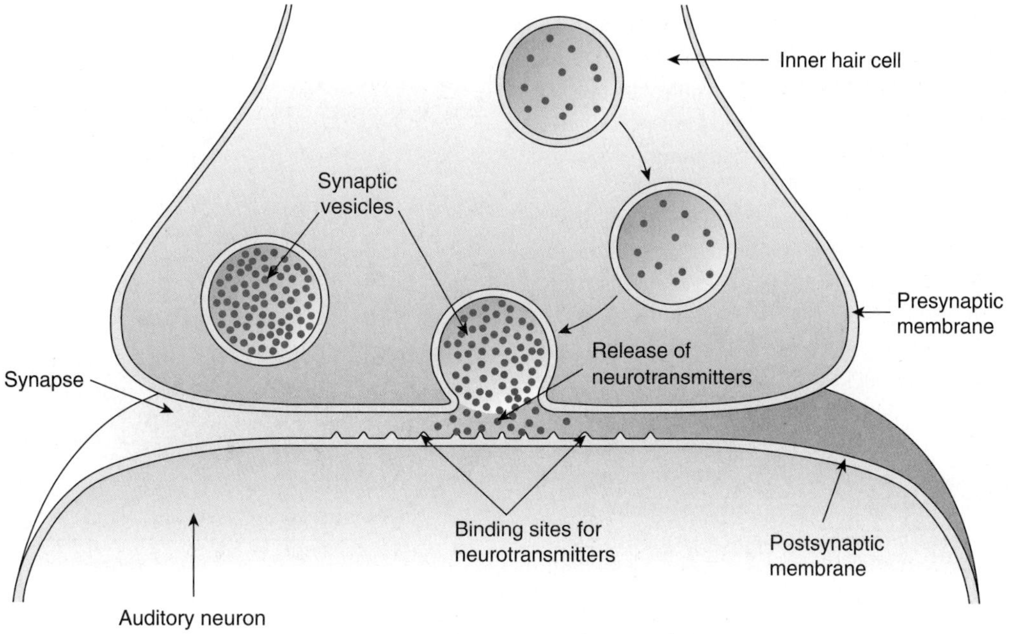

Figure 9.14. Neurotransmitter release in the synaptic junction.

THEORIES OF HEARING

The cochlea is the organ responsible for analyzing the incoming sound and translating it into nerve impulses that are carried by thousands of neurons to the brain for assembly into a sound perception. Two types of neural codes are observed in the neural output of the cochlea that convey information from the cochlea to the auditory centers in the brain: place code and temporal code. Their roles and the relative importance of these two codes remain unclear. The theories explaining how the inner ear translates arriving vibrations into neural code are called theories of hearing. To date, a number of theories explaining how the inner ear converts the frequency of the incoming signal into a series of electrochemical signals have been proposed, but all of them are variants of two main theories: place theory and periodicity (temporal) theory. The **place theory** states that frequency information is represented by place coding, and the **periodicity theory** states that frequency information is represented by temporal coding. The anatomic and physiologic function of the cochlea and auditory nerve is the same regardless of which theory is considered; however, these theories differ in how much importance is placed on the place of stimulation along the cochlea versus the frequency at which the basilar membrane vibrates.

Place Theory of Hearing

As previously discussed, frequency is represented in the cochlea by the tonotopic mapping of the signal frequency along the length of the basilar membrane. The maximum displacements of the basilar membrane caused by sounds of different frequency are physically distributed along the membrane due to the progressively changing mechanic properties of the basilar membrane (width and stiffness). The mapping of stimulus frequencies to *place* (on the basilar membrane) is frequently referred to as **place coding** and the theory attempting to explain the process of hearing based on place coding is called the place theory of hearing. According to the place theory, two sounds are perceived as being different because they cause two different groups of neurons to respond.

The first place theory can be attributed to Helmholtz (1862). Helmholtz assumed that the basilar membrane was composed of a series of small resonators. Thus, this theory is frequently called the resonance theory. The basis for the more current place theory of hearing is the traveling wave theory proposed by von Békésy (1960). This theory states that the stimulation of hair cells along the basilar membrane occurs at the place of greatest displacement of the basilar membrane. The main weaknesses of place theories are their inability to explain the phenomenon of hearing the missing fundamental of a complex sound (Chapter 4) and to account for perceptual differences in low-frequency stimulation where the tuning curves are rather wide (Mann, 2002).

In support of place theories is the fact that the tonotopic mapping of the cochlea is preserved in the auditory nerve. Each type I afferent auditory neuron connects to only one IHC. Therefore, the IHC excitations, caused by a specific frequency component in a signal, are relayed to spatially separate auditory neurons. The spatial separation of nerve fibers also continues along the auditory nerve (low-frequency fibers in the middle, high-frequency fibers around the edge) and the mapping of frequency to different places continues throughout the entire central auditory nervous system including the brain (Chapter 10).

Tuning Curves

The main support for the place theory comes from the fact that each hair cell and nerve cell is sharply tuned to respond best to one specific frequency, called the **characteristic frequency** (CF). This property is needed to effectively translate place-coded stimulus frequencies into neural responses. Individual hair cells and their associated nerve cells fire (generate nerve impulses) in response to sounds of various frequency, but they are most effective in responding to frequencies equal to their CF. The specific value of the CF of a hair cell depends on the cell's location along the length of the cochlea. A curve representing the effectiveness of the cell firing as a function of the stimulus frequency is called a **tuning curve.** In other words, the tuning curve graphically illustrates the intensity required to stimulate a specific hair cell or nerve cell as a function of sound frequency. An example of the tuning curve for an auditory neuron with a CF of 5000 Hz is shown in Figure 9.15. The frequency of the sound is represented along the *x* axis and the intensity of the sound is on the *y* axis. The tuning curve represents the lowest intensity of a sound of a specific frequency needed for a neuron (or hair cell) to fire. Although the shape of the tuning curve varies depending on its CF, a typical curve looks like a letter V with a tail on the low-frequency side. The CF of the neuron corresponds to the tip of the V. The white area represents the response area of the hair cell or auditory neuron.

The hair cell shown in Figure 9.15 has a CF of 5000 Hz and it responds at this frequency to a very low stimulation

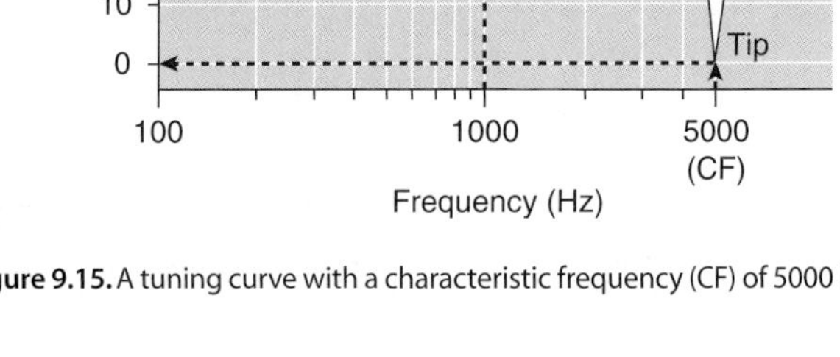

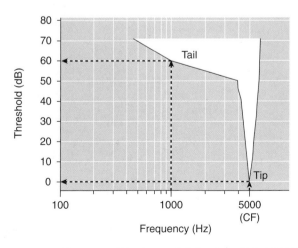

Figure 9.15. A tuning curve with a characteristic frequency (CF) of 5000 Hz.

level, denoted in this figure by a value of 0 dB. The same cell will also respond to a stimulus with a frequency of about 1000 Hz, but only if the sound intensity of the stimulating tone is 60 dB higher (dashed line) than that of the 5000-Hz tone. In other words, a 1000-Hz sound must be 60 dB greater than a 5000-Hz sound to activate a cell that has a CF of 5000 Hz. The farther the stimulus frequency is from the CF, the greater the intensity required to activate the cell.* The threshold difference between the tip (CF) of the curve and the start of the tail of the curve is generally about 40 to 50 dB; that is, a stimulus with a frequency in the tail region must be 40 to 50 dB more intense to cause that cell to fire.

Periodicity (Temporal) Theory of Hearing

Place coding and place theories of hearing explain several auditory phenomena, but they cannot account for all of them. The inability of place theories to explain some auditory phenomena gave rise to another set of hearing theories based on periodicity (temporal, frequency) coding. Periodicity coding theories state that the cochlea transmits frequency information based on the period of the waveform arriving at the cochlea; thus, the rate or *frequency* of neural impulses is the mechanism for coding frequency.

All nerve fibers fire spontaneously (without stimulus) a certain number of times per second. This is called the resting firing rate of the nerve and it is considered to be neural noise. The basis for the periodicity theory of hearing is the fact that the resting firing rate of auditory neurons is increased when IHCs are excited and decreased when IHCs are inhibited (Fig. 9.16).

Imagine a 200-Hz tone traveling through the air. This 200-Hz tone consists of alternating compression and rarefaction portions (pressure changes) that vary 200 times per second. When the signal reaches the middle ear, the tympanic membrane and the ossicular chain will vibrate at a frequency of 200 Hz. The stapes will move in and out of the oval window at a frequency of 200 Hz also. Subsequently, the basilar membrane will vibrate up and down 200 times per second. The movement of the basilar membrane up and down 200 times per second will cause the stereocilia of the OHC to bend back and forth 200 times per second. Whenever the stereocilia bend with sufficient force, the hair cell releases neurotransmitters and the auditory nerve fires. Assuming the auditory nerve fires every time neurotransmitters are released, the 200-Hz frequency would be translated into 200 pulses per second by the nerve fiber. The number of pulses per second of the nerve firing will vary with the frequency of the sound wave; thus, the signal frequency could be coded by the impulse rate. In other words, according to the periodicity theory, two sounds are perceived as being different because they cause the same neurons to respond at different rates; that is, their responses differ in the duration of the time interval between firing spikes.

Historically, the best known periodicity theory is the telephone theory proposed by Rutherford* (1886). This theory states that all the hair cells in the cochlea are simultaneously stimulated by sound of any frequency and the complete sound analysis is performed in the brain. One early argument against the periodicity theory was the fact that individual neurons cannot fire more frequently than about 1000 times per

*This is similar to the concept of the resonance curve presented in Chapter 3 where we discussed mechanic systems. Recall that a mechanic system can be made to vibrate at frequencies other than the resonance frequency, but with much less efficiency.

*Lord Ernest Rutherford (1871–1937) was a New Zealand physicist who received a Nobel Prize in Chemistry (1908) for his investigations into the disintegration of the atom and the chemistry of radioactive substances.

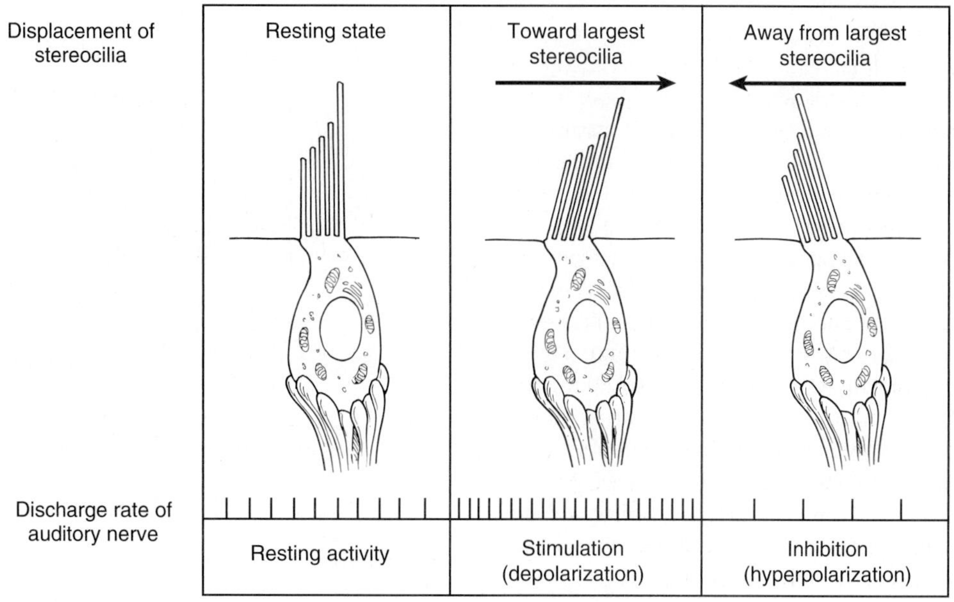

Figure 9.16. Discharge rate of auditory nerve fibers at rest and during excitation and inhibition.

second; therefore, individual neurons cannot provide temporal coding (phase locking) for frequencies higher than 1000 Hz. **Phase locking** means that the firing pattern of the nerve is synchronized with the phase of the incoming auditory signal; thus, the nerve will only fire at certain phases of the periodic signal, or at integer multiples of the period of stimulation. This argument was addressed by Wever (1949) in his version of the periodicity theory called the volley theory.

The **volley theory** states that the firing limit of a single neuron can be overcome if the CAP is a sum of multiple neurons firing within a volley (think volleyball, where multiple team members work together to get the ball from one side of the court to the other; here multiple neurons work together to get the auditory signal from the cochlea to the nerve). This theory is supported by mammal research that has shown that groups of neurons working together can phase lock to auditory stimuli with frequencies of up to 4000 to 5000 Hz by having individual neurons fire to every *n*th cycle of the sound (Kiang et al., 1965; Rose et al., 1967). For frequencies higher than about 5000 Hz, however, place cues appear to be the only cues that are available for the brain to determine frequency. Periodicity theory is useful in explaining several auditory phenomena that cannot be explained by the place theory, such as the perception of the missing fundamental and the reason a single electrode in a cochlear implant can result in some degree of auditory perception. Therefore, it is likely that both the place code and the temporal code are used together to convey information about the signal frequency and their synergy results in our auditory sensations.

Coding of Intensity

Both the place and frequency theories of hearing are in reality two different theories describing how humans perceive sound frequency. They do not provide any elaborate schemes regarding intensity coding. Both place coding and temporal coding, however, can be used to convey information about signal intensity.

To understand how the auditory system codes sound intensity, let us realize that the greater the sound intensity is, the greater the number of neural spikes included in the CAP. Low-intensity sounds create a fairly small and narrow traveling wave on the basilar membrane and create a relatively small back-and-forth movement of the hair cell stereocilia in a limited region. Large-intensity sounds create a much larger and broader traveling wave and thus a much larger back-and-forth motion of the hair cell stereocilia across a much larger area. The broader traveling wave results in a greater number of hair cells that fire, and the greater stereocilia deflection results in an increase in the amount of neurotransmitter released from the IHCs into the synaptic cleft, thus increasing the likelihood that an afferent auditory nerve fiber will fire. Thus, sound intensity is most likely coded via the type and number of auditory neurons that are activated.

Recall that a neuron at rest fires spontaneously from time to time. When a sound enters the ear and reaches an auditory nerve, the firing rate of the nerve will increase above its spontaneous firing rate. As the intensity of the sound increases, the firing rate will increase, up to a point called the **saturation point.** Once the firing rate has reached the saturation point, the firing rate will stay the same regardless of an increase in intensity. The intensity range between the threshold of the neuron (the lowest intensity that will cause a neuron to fire) and the saturation point is called the **dynamic range.** The dynamic range of a single neuron varies from about 25 to 40 dB for most auditory neurons. Thus, to transmit a larger dynamic range for acoustic signals, other neural mechanisms must account for this range. The two mechanisms appear to be (1) group firing of several neurons at the same time and (2) different sensitivities of various neurons responding to the specific stimulation.

As we have already discussed, a more intense sound creates a broader traveling wave, which excites a larger number of hair cells and auditory neurons. Evidence for this, for example, is in the widening of the tuning curves seen at high intensity levels. In addition, there appears to be three different types of auditory neurons, with overlapping but not identical dynamic ranges. These three types of neurons were identified by Lieberman (1978) on the basis of the differences in their resting (spontaneous) firing rate and were labeled high-, medium-, and low-spontaneous activity neurons. Figure 9.17 illustrates the change in the firing rate of these three types of neurons as a function of the intensity of a sound. Notice that the discharge rate for all three types of neurons increases as intensity increases and that all of the neurons reach saturation (seen as a relatively flat line) at some point. Notice also that the dynamic ranges of the three neurons are across different intensity regions. The firing rate of the high-spontaneous fibers increases between about −10 and 30 dB, medium-spontaneous fibers increase between about 5 and 35 dB, and low-spontaneous fibers increase between about 25 and 40 dB. This means that the

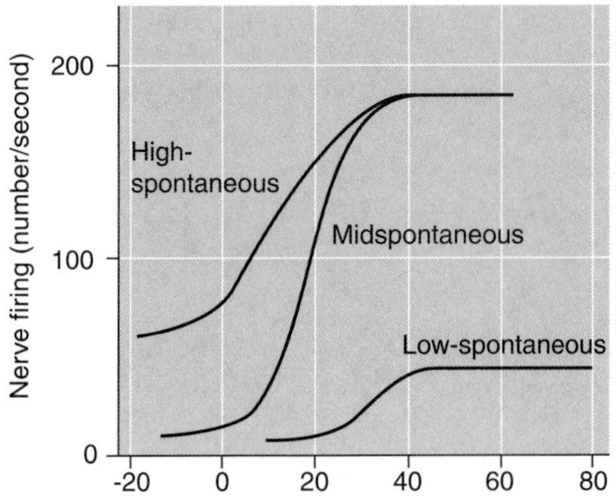

Figure 9.17. Firing rates of the three types of auditory neurons as a function of sound pressure. (Based on the work of Liberman MC. Auditory nerve response from cats raised in a low-noise chamber. *J Acoust Soc Am* 1978;63:442–455.)

range of intensities that can be coded by the number of activated neurons and the overall rate of firing of auditory nerve is much larger than would be possible if only one type of neuron was in the auditory nerve.

NONLINEAR BEHAVIOR OF THE INNER EAR

The auditory system is a nonlinear system. Nonlinear systems, and more specifically nonlinear amplifiers, are described in detail in Chapter 14; however, the basic concept of a nonlinear system is that the processing of the input signal depends on the magnitude of that signal and the shape of the output waveform is different from the shape of the input waveform. This difference in shape is called **nonlinear distortion.** The main source of the nonlinear distortion in the auditory system is the electromotility of the OHCs and the resulting level-dependent cochlear amplification. Some nonlinear distortions are produced in the middle ear, but they only occur at very high stimulation levels.

The presence of nonlinear distortions in the auditory system means that the output signal from the cochlea that is sent to the auditory nerve is not a direct replica of the input signal that enters the ear canal. The characteristic feature of nonlinear distortions is that they create some frequency components that may not exist in the input signal. We never hear or are bothered by these distortions because they are the result of the normal operations of the ear and we have never heard the world without them.

The original studies of the cochlea assumed that its behavior was linear, that is, that the signals converted in the neural impulses were direct replicas of the sound waves impinging on the tympanic membrane. Linear processing in the cochlea, however, did not explain several experimental findings. For example, the broad and crude vibrations of the basilar membrane observed originally by von Békésy in the 1940s (von Békésy, 1960) could not explain the highly precise and selective response of the auditory system to small changes in signal frequency or the high acuity of the auditory system. It was clear that some kind of additional nonlinear mechanism was needed to describe how basilar membrane movements worked to create the high-resolution responses of the auditory system. In the late 1970s, through the works of Rhode (1978), Kemp (1978), Brownell et al. (1985), and others, nonlinear behavior was experimentally observed and formally accepted. This nonlinear mechanism results primarily from the compression and expansion of the OHCs, that is, OHC motility, previously discussed in this chapter. The OHC motility operates only at low to moderate intensity levels; thus, the nonlinear behavior of the cochlea causes low-intensity sounds to be amplified more than high-intensity sounds.

The specific experimental observations indicating that the cochlea is a nonlinear system include both physiologic and psychoacoustic data. Some of the observations that have indicated nonlinear behavior in the inner ear are nonlinear distortions of the input signal (e.g., difference tones), spontaneous otoacoustic emissions, two-tone suppression (in which a greater intensity tone can mask a lower intensity tone), the upward spread of masking (Chapter 12), and nonlinear loudness growth (loudness recruitment). The last three phenomena are psychoacoustic observations, whereas the first two are physiologic observations. For example, the nonlinear products that are produced as a result of the normal function of the hair cells can propagate back toward the middle ear and tympanic membrane and be recorded as otoacoustic emissions. OAEs are useful in clinical audiology for diagnostic purposes. If distortion products are present at normal levels, the cochlea is probably functioning normally. If the distortion products are absent, then an abnormality exists in the system.

VESTIBULAR SYSTEM: THE ORGANS OF BALANCE

The primary focus of this textbook is hearing science, and a discussion of the vestibular (balance) system is outside the scope of most hearing science courses. The balance system, however, is closely associated with the auditory system and located in the same part of the human body. Several pathologic states of the inner ear involve both the cochlea and the vestibular system. For completeness of the inner ear discussion, a brief description of the anatomy and physiology of the vestibular system is included in this chapter.

ANATOMY OF THE ORGANS OF BALANCE

The vestibular system is a complex balance system that together with the cochlea occupies the bony labyrinth in the temporal bone. The vestibular system consists of the vestibule and three semicircular canals (Fig. 9.1). The main function of the vestibule is to inform the brain about the direction of the force of gravity in reference to the position of the head, and the main function of the semicircular canals is to inform the brain about angular changes in body velocity.

Anatomy of the Vestibule

The vestibule is the bony cavity between the semicircular canals and the cochlea. With the bony vestibule, the membranous labyrinth forms two elements of the balance system: the **utricle** and the **saccule** (Fig. 9.3). Narrow ducts projecting from the utricle and the saccule join together to form the **endolymphatic duct**, which projects to the **endolymphatic sac** located in the dura mater (one of the three brain coverings, collectively called the meninges). The saccule is connected to the cochlear duct via a narrow channel called the **ductus reuniens.** The utricle is connected to all three semicircular canals.

The utricle and saccule each contain a sense organ called a **macula**; thus, there is a utricular macula and a saccular macula (i.e., there are two maculae). These sense organs are the source of internal information about head position relative to the earth and about the linear acceleration of the body. Each macula consists of hair cells, support cells, and a gelatinous membrane called the **otolithic membrane** (Greek, *oto-*, meaning ear, and *lithos*, meaning stone). The otolithic membrane contains **otoconia** (singular: otoconium), which are calcium carbonate crystals. Stereocilia and one kinocilium (a large cilium) project from the top of each hair cell into the otolithic membrane. The macula of the utricle is located on the anterior wall of the utricle in somewhat of a horizontal plane and the macula of the saccule is located on the medial wall of the saccule in somewhat of a vertical (up and down) plane. The maculae are not perfectly vertical (saccule) or horizontal (utricle); they are actually somewhat curved in orientation. The curved central line down the middle of each macula is called the **striola.** The stereocilia are oriented such that the kinocilium from each hair cell in the utricle faces the striola and the kinocilium from each hair cell in the saccule faces away from the striola.

Anatomy of the Semicircular Canals

The semicircular canals (Fig. 9.1) are a group of three canals—the **anterior** (or **superior**), **posterior** (or **inferior**), and **horizontal** (or **lateral**) **semicircular canals**—that are oriented in an almost orthogonal (right angle) manner to each other. Their function is to detect acceleration of the body in the three perpendicular planes. The anterior semicircular canal is at a 90° degree angle in comparison with the posterior canal, and both the anterior and posterior canals are at a right angle to the horizon. The horizontal (lateral) canal is not parallel with the horizon, however, and is about 30° off the true horizontal plane.

Each semicircular canal contains a semicircular duct, which has the same name as the canal in which it is housed, and a bulge at one end called an **ampulla,** which contains a sense organ called the **crista ampullaris** (plural: cristae ampullares), which blocks the canal at that point. The ampullae are located at the anterior opening of the horizontal canal, the anterior opening of the anterior canal, and the inferior opening of the posterior canal. The crista ampullaris is composed of a gelatinous mass called a **cupula,** support cells, and hair cells. Unlike the gelatinous mass that makes up the macula of the utricle, the cupula does not contain calcium carbonate in its healthy state.* Stereocilia and kinocilium project from the top of the hair cells and their tips are embedded in the cupula. The crista ampullaris is oriented so that it is perpendicular to the long axis of each semicircular canal. The stereocilia from each hair cell are oriented so that all the kinocilia from each crista are in the same direction. In the anterior and posterior canals, the kinocilia are on the canal side of the ampulla (away from the utricle) and in the horizontal canal, the kinocilia are on the utricle side of the ampulla (away from the canal).

*In a pathology known as benign paroxysmal positional vertigo (BPPV), otoconia from the otolithic membrane enter the canal and affect the normal operation of the semicircular canals. In this pathology, the semicircular canals become sensitive to gravity and the sensation of spinning will result in response to angular acceleration.

At the bottom of each hair cell in the vestibular system are the peripheral projections of the vestibular portion of the vestibulocochlear nerve. The cell bodies for the vestibular portion of the vestibulocochlear nerve, called the **vestibular ganglion** (or Scarpa's ganglion), are located within the internal auditory canal, where the auditory and vestibular nerve fibers travel together from the inner ear to the brainstem.

PHYSIOLOGY OF THE VESTIBULAR SYSTEM

The ability of humans and other species to move in a specific direction and to maintain a specific body position depends on the ability of the central nervous system to coordinate sensory input from three sensory systems: the vestibular system, the visual system, and the somatosensory (sensors for tissues within the body, e.g., sensors in joints and muscles) system. Signals from these three systems are integrated by the central nervous system. Some of the connections between the vestibular system and the visual system result in coordinated eye movements in response to changes in head position. In fact, the connection between the eyes and the ears is the basis for diagnostic tests that identify vestibular pathology on the basis of eye movement.

Physiology of the Utricle and Saccule

The maculae of the utricle and saccule are responsible for sending information to the central nervous system about head position relative to the earth and about linear (straight line) acceleration of the body. The otolithic membrane is denser than the surrounding endolymph. Therefore, when the head is tilted, the otolithic membrane is pulled by gravity toward the earth. In addition, when the body accelerates in a straight line, the otolithic membrane lags behind the movement of the rest of the vestibule because of inertia. This lag means that the otolithic membrane will move in the opposite direction to the direction of movement. When the otolithic membrane is shifted in position relative to the position of the hair cells, the stereocilia bend. If the stereocilia are bent toward the kinocilium, the cell is excited and will send signals to the central nervous system. If the stereocilia are bent away from the kinocilium, the cell is inhibited from sending signals. The movement of the stereocilia is very small, on the order of tenths of a micron even at the greatest displacement. Because of the unique orientation of the kinocilium relative to the striola, each head position results in a unique combination of hair cell bending. For each head position, some hair cells will be excited (depolarized) and some will be inhibited to various degrees, coding neural information about head position and linear acceleration of the body.

Physiology of the Semicircular Canals

The semicircular canals are responsible for sending information to the central nervous system about angular acceleration. When the head makes an angular movement, the fluid (endolymph) and the cupula in the semicircular canal that is in the same plane as the head motion will move in the opposite direction. For example, as the head turns right, the fluid in the horizontal semicircular canals lags behind the movement of the head due to inertia. Therefore, a head turn to the right will result in a fluid movement to the left relative to the canal position. Because the bottom of the hair cells in the crista ampullaris is fixed and moves with the canal and the stereocilia of the hair cell move with the fluid, the leftward movement of the fluid will cause the stereocilia to bend to the left. If the stereocilia are bent toward the kinocilium, the cell will be excited, and if the stereocilia are bent away from the kinocilium, the cell will be inhibited. Because of the orientation of the kinocilium in the horizontal canals, a head turn to the right causes the hair cells in the right horizontal canal to be excited and the hair cells in the left horizontal canal to be inhibited. The horizontal semicircular canals act as polar opposites, one excited while the other is inhibited. The anterior and posterior canals work similarly, but the anterior canal on each side is paired with the posterior canal on the opposite side. Depending on the direction the head turns, a unique pattern of excitation and inhibition will be transmitted to the central nervous system.

Summary

The inner ear is located in a bony labyrinth (cavity) in the petrous portion of the temporal bone. It consists of the cochlea, which contains the organ of hearing, and the vestibule, which contains the organs of balance: the maculae (in the utricle and saccule) and the cristae ampullares (in the semicircular canals). The organ of Corti is the sense organ responsible for responding to sound, the maculae are the sense organs that respond to gravity and linear acceleration, and the cristae ampullares are the sense organs that respond to angular acceleration. The bony labyrinth contains a fluid called perilymph. The membranous labyrinth that is located within the bony labyrinth is filled with another fluid called endolymph.

The organ of Corti is located along the basilar membrane on the side of the scala media. The organ of Corti contains support cells and hair cells. Hair cells are sensory cells with a bundle of stereocilia (hairs) projecting from the top of each cell. The stereocilia are responsible for changing the mechanical motion of the basilar membrane into electrochemical impulses used by the nervous system. The auditory nerve (the cochlear portion of the vestibulocochlear nerve) begins beneath the organ of Corti. Approximately 95% of the afferent auditory nerve fibers innervate IHCs. The majority of efferent auditory nerve fibers innervate OHCs. Efferent auditory nerve fibers are either medial olivocochlear fibers or lateral olivocochlear fibers, depending on the cell bodies' location within the superior olivary complex of the brainstem.

The physical properties (width and stiffness) of the basilar membrane change gradually along its length. This property is the basis for the direct mapping of sound frequencies to vibrations in specific locations of the basilar membrane. This relationship is called tonotopicity or tonotopic organization. The place coding theory of hearing states that the coding of stimulus frequency is based on the place of stimulation along the basilar membrane. The base of the cochlea is responsible for coding high-frequency sounds and the apex of the cochlea is responsible for coding low-frequency sounds. An alternate theory of hearing, called the periodicity (temporal, frequency) theory of hearing, states that the cochlea transmits frequency information in the form of the number of pulses per second in response to the period (frequency) of the sound wave. Some phenomena cannot be explained by either theory alone; thus, it is likely that both place coding and periodicity coding work together. Intensity is coded via two mechanisms, the number of auditory neurons that are activated and the rate at which they fire.

Key Points

- The bony labyrinth of the cochlea is about 35 mm long and twists about $2\frac{3}{4}$ times from its base to its apex.
- The cell bodies (spiral ganglion) of afferent auditory nerve fibers are located within a central core of bone called the modiolus.
- A cross section of the cochlea shows the three divisions of the cochlea: the scala vestibuli, the scala tympani, and the scala media (cochlear duct).
- The organ of Corti is located within the scala media and runs along the entire length of the basilar membrane. The organ of Corti consists of

one row of inner hair cells and three rows of outer hair cells.

- A traveling (or transverse) wave of the basilar membrane causes the bending (shearing) of the stereocilia of the hair cells.
- The bending of the stereocilia of inner hair cells results in electrochemical impulses along the afferent auditory nerve fibers.
- The bending of the stereocilia of outer hair cells results in an electromotility function of the outer hair cells. The outer hair cells change in length along their long axis in response to changes in voltage.
- Most of the afferent auditory nerve fibers innervate the inner hair cells and most of the efferent auditory nerve fibers innervate the outer hair cells. This supports the function of the inner hair cells as the sensory transduction mechanism and the outer hair cells as the provider of a motor action.
- The traveling wave of the basilar membrane is amplified by an active process in a living cochlea. The active process has been attributed to outer hair cell electromotility. The reason for outer hair cell electromotility is attributed to a protein called prestin in the outer hair cell wall. Other possible mechanisms are still under investigation.
- The stria vascularis is responsible for generating the cochlear resting potential (of about +80 mV) called the endocochlear potential. Stimulus-related potentials, generated by sound entering the ear, include the cochlear microphonic, summating potential, and compound action potential.
- Each hair cell and nerve cell is tuned to respond best to one specific frequency, called the characteristic frequency, but cells will also respond to sounds close in frequency to the characteristic frequency. A tuning curve graphically illustrates the intensity required to stimulate a specific hair cell or nerve cell as a function of sound frequency.

Chapter Outline

CHAPTER 10

Central Auditory Nervous System

Diana C. Emanuel, Laurie Williams-Hogarth, and Tomasz Letowski

Objectives

- To review basic terminology necessary to study the central nervous system
- To review the organization of the brain including structures in the forebrain, midbrain, and hindbrain
- To review the central nervous system with emphasis on integrating the location of auditory nuclei and pathways
- To list and briefly describe the function of the cranial nerves
- To review the primary afferent pathway that transmits signals from the vestibulocochlear nerve to the brain, including the major nuclei and fiber tracts
- To introduce the anatomy and function of the olivocochlear system

Key Terms

Abducens nerve
Afferent
Angular gyrus
Anterior
Anterior commissure
Anterior ventral cochlear nucleus (AVCN)
Arbor vitae
Arcuate fasciculus
Area triangularis
Brachium of the inferior colliculus
Brainstem
Broca's area
Bushy cell
Central auditory nervous system (CANS)
Central nervous system (CNS)
Central sulcus
Cerebellar cortex
Cerebellopontine angle
Cerebellum
Cerebral aqueduct (mesencephalic aqueduct, aqueduct of Sylvius)
Cerebral cortex
Cerebral hemisphere
Cerebral peduncle
Cerebrospinal fluid (CSF)
Chopper pattern
Chorda tympani
Choroid plexus
Cochlear nucleus
Coincidence detector
Commissure of the inferior colliculus
Corpora quadrigemina
Corpus callosum
Decussate
Diencephalon
Dorsal
Dorsal acoustic stria (stria of Monaco)
Dorsal cochlear nucleus
Dorsal commissure of the lemniscus (commissure of Probst)
Efferent

Epithalamus
Facial nerve
Fiber tract
Fissure
Folia
Foramen magnum
Forebrain
Fornix
Frontal lobe
Frontal/coronal
Gyri
Heschl's gyrus (transverse temporal gyrus)
Hindbrain
Horizontal
Hypothalamus
Inferior
Inferior colliculus
Insular lobe
Interaural intensity difference (IID)
Interaural time difference (ITD)
Intermediate acoustic stria (stria of Held)
Internal capsule
Lateral
Lateral lemniscus
Lateral olivocochlear bundle (LOCB)
Lateral sulcus (sylvian fissure)
Lateral superior olivary (LSO) nucleus
Limbic system
Longitudinal fissure
Medial
Medial geniculate nucleus (or medial geniculate body)
Medial olivocochlear bundle (MOCB)
Medial superior olivary (MSO) nucleus
Medulla (medulla oblongata)
Midbrain
Nuclei
Nucleus of the trapezoid body
Occipital lobe
Octopus cell
Oculomotor nerve
Olive
Olivocochlear bundle
Onset pattern
Parietal lobe
Pauser pattern
Periolivary nuclei
Plane
Planum temporale
Plasticity
Pons
Pontomedullary junction
Postcentral gyrus (primary somatosensory cortex)
Posterior
Posterior ventral cochlear nucleus (PVCN)
Precentral gyrus (primary motor cortex)
Primary (afferent) ascending pathway
Primary auditory area (A1)
Primary auditory cortex
Primary-like pattern
Pyramids
Right ear advantage
Sagittal
Section
Signal processing
Subthalamus
Sulci
Superior
Superior olivary complex (SOC)
Superior temporal gyrus
Supramarginal gyrus
Tectum
Telencephalon
Temporal lobe
Thalamus
Third ventricle
Transverse
Transverse fissure
Trapezoid body
Trigeminal nerve
Trochlear nerve
Vagus nerve
Ventral
Ventral acoustic stria
Ventricle
Vermis
Vestibular-ocular reflex (VOR)
Vestibulocochlear anastomosis (anastomosis of Oort)
Vestibulocochlear nerve
Wernicke's area

The **central auditory nervous system (CANS)** is a sound-processing network of **afferent** (ascending) and **efferent** (descending) auditory **fiber tracts*** and **nuclei** (groups of cell bodies) that connect the ear with the brain. Note that the central auditory nervous system is abbreviated *CANS* (note the "A") and it is a part of the overall central nervous system, which is abbreviated *CNS*. By far the best understood auditory pathway is the **primary afferent (ascending) pathway**, which is responsible for taking a coded auditory signal from the vestibulocochlear nerve *upward* through the brainstem to the cortex.* The primary afferent pathway is much better understood than the **efferent (descending) pathway**, which travels from the cortex and various nuclei in the brainstem *downward* to modify the operating characteristics of lower levels of afferent neurons in the brainstem and the hair cells in the cochlea. Quite a few different efferent auditory fiber projections have been identified in the CANS, but the main efferent auditory system affecting sound processing in the cochlea is the olivocochlear system, which will be described

*Within the central nervous system, a group of axons is no longer referred to as the nerve but by using a variety of terms including tract, white matter, fasciculus, column, lemniscus, funiculus, and bundle.

*Other ascending pathways (e.g., polysensory) branch off the auditory pathway into nonauditory areas, as well as from other systems (e.g., somatosensory) to the auditory system, allowing for the integration of information from other sensory systems and connections with the limbic system; this chapter will not discuss these pathways.

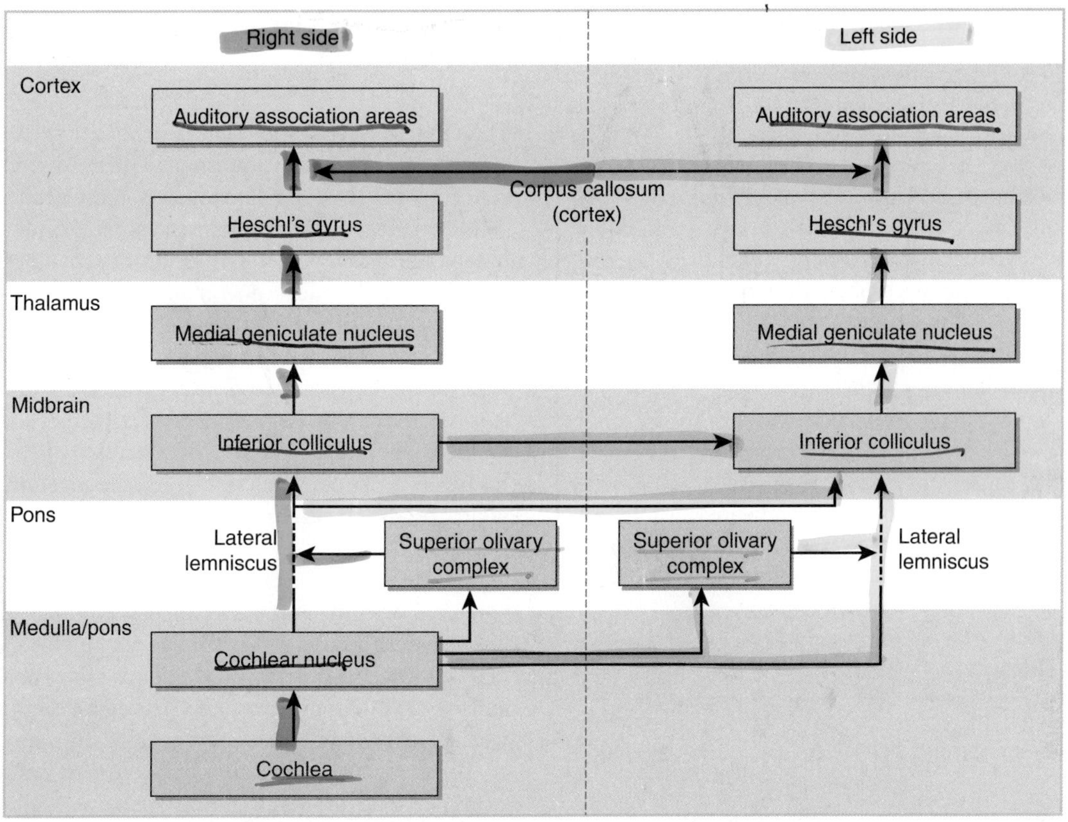

Figure 10.1. A diagram of the major nuclei in the ascending central auditory nervous system. Projections are from one cochlea. The opposite ear auditory pathway mirrors this.

later in this chapter. A diagram showing the ascending auditory pathway from one ear is shown in Figure 10.1. A similar diagram can be made for the opposite ear.

Notice in Figure 10.1 that in several locations, fibers **decussate** (cross from one side to the other), allowing the CANS to process information from both ears at the same time. In Figure 10.1 the fibers are crossing from the right side to the left side, but for the opposite ear the fibers will be crossing over from the left to the right pathway. The main elements of the CANS, listed in ascending order from the most peripheral (bottom of Fig. 10.1) to the most central (top of Fig. 10.1), are listed below:

- Cochlear nucleus
- Superior olivary complex
- Lateral lemniscus
- Inferior colliculus
- Medial geniculate nucleus or medial geniculate body
- Heschl's gyrus (primary auditory cortex)
- Auditory association areas

The CANS is one of the many parts of the CNS. To understand the CANS, one must first be familiar with and understand the general anatomic structure of the CNS. Therefore, this chapter is divided into two primary sections: (1) the anatomy of the CNS with an emphasis on the parts of CNS anatomy that are specifically involved in auditory processing and (2) the physiology of the CANS with an emphasis on binaural and sequential processing of information. This chapter is very terminology intensive. To make reading easier, please review the Anatomy Terminology box so you are familiar with the common anatomic terms that are used throughout this chapter.

Box 10.1 Anatomy Terminology

Anatomists use specific terms to describe the spatial orientation of two- and three-dimensional models and specimens (see figure). The main terms used to describe the location of anatomic structures within the body are:

- **Anterior**—toward the front
- **Posterior**—toward the back
- **Inferior**—toward the bottom
- **Superior**—toward the top
- **Medial**—toward the middle
- **Lateral**—toward the side
- **Ventral**—anterior (below the midbrain) or inferior (above the midbrain)
- **Dorsal**—posterior (below the midbrain) or superior (above the midbrain)

Notice that the terms *ventral* and *dorsal* change meaning depending on the location of the structure. In reference to the central nervous system (CNS), these terms are used assuming the CNS pathway is a straight vertical line. In reality, the brain has a curve along the vertical axis much like a candy cane, with the bend of the candy cane beginning at the midbrain. The terms *ventral* and *dorsal* disregard this curve; therefore, ventral is synonymous with anterior in the spinal cord and brainstem and ventral is synonymous with inferior above the brainstem.

A **plane** view (two-dimensional surface) or **section** (cut or slice in a specimen) is described based on the orientation of this plane or cross section relative to the body. The most common terms used to describe planes and cross sections are:

- **Sagittal**—divides the body into right and left parts. If exactly on the midline, it is called a median sagittal cut. If to one side of midline, it is described as parallel to median sagittal (or parasagittal).
- **Frontal/coronal**—divides the body into front and back. On a 90° angle compared with the sagittal plane.
- **Transverse**—divides the body into top and bottom parts.
- **Horizontal**—parallel with the horizon in reference to a standing person.

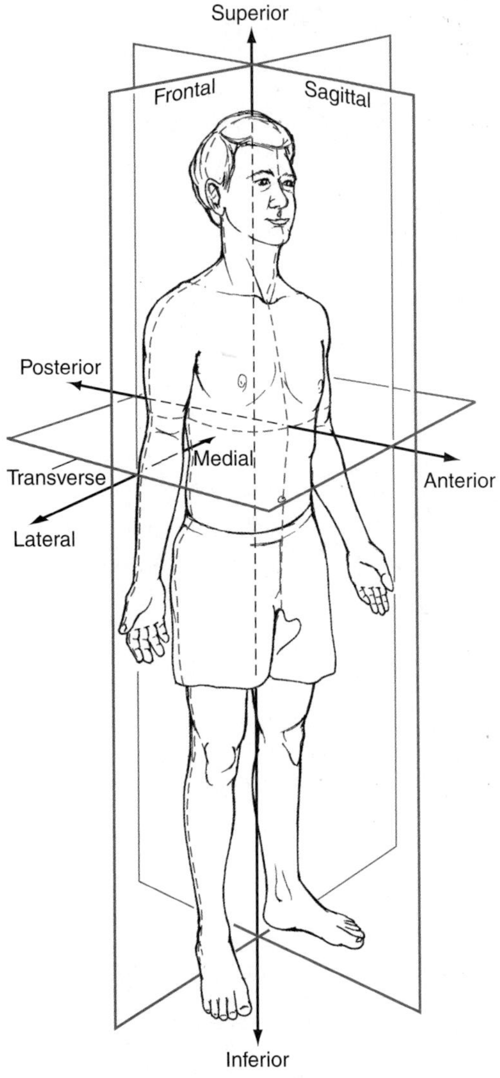

ANATOMY OF THE CENTRAL NERVOUS SYSTEM

The **central nervous system** is divided into the brain and spinal cord, but only the brain will be discussed in this chapter since the spinal cord is not involved in auditory signal processing. The brain is the control center for all voluntary, conscious actions of living organisms. Brain tissue consists of cell bodies (gray matter) that make up the outer layer of the brain and various nuclei deep within the brain. Brain tissue also includes myelinated axons (white matter), which connect various structures within the brain and outside of the brain. In addition, the center of the brain includes four fluid-filled cavities called brain **ventricles.** Each ventricle contains a structure called a **choroid plexus,** which produces **cerebrospinal fluid** (CSF), which protects the brain.

The human brain is customarily divided into three primary regions: the forebrain, the midbrain, and the hindbrain, based on the embryonic development of the human nervous system. If you would like to know more about the embryonic development of the nervous system, consult the website. **Link 10-1**

The three basic regions of the human brain and their main parts are shown in Figure 10.2. Each of these regions has a very distinct function and structure, which will be discussed in the next few sections.

Forebrain

The **forebrain** is the largest region of the brain. It consists of two portions:

1. Telencephalon
2. Diencephalon

Telencephalon

The **telencephalon** undertakes the processing of conscious thoughts and intellectual functions, controls the initiation of body movement, and perceives sensations. The telencephalon consists of two **cerebral hemispheres:** right and left. The internal portion of the cerebral hemispheres contains the basal nuclei, the ventricular system, and a number of other supporting structures. For more information on the basal nuclei and the ventricular system, consult the website. **Link 10-2**

The cellular surface of each cerebral hemisphere is called the **cerebral cortex** and it includes six neural layers numbered from I to VI. The cortex structure is a pleated series of peaks and valleys that function to increase the surface area of the cortex. The peaks are called **gyri** (singular: gyrus) and the valleys are called **sulci** (singular: sulcus). Extremely deep sulci are called **fissures.** The main sulci and fissures that divide the cerebrum into two hemispheres and eight lobes (four on each side) are shown in Figure 10.3. These include:

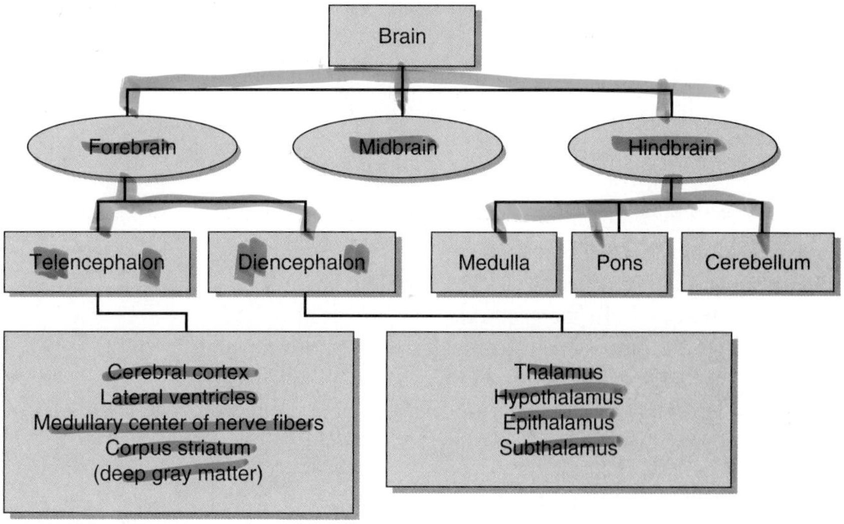

Figure 10.2. The major divisions of the brain.

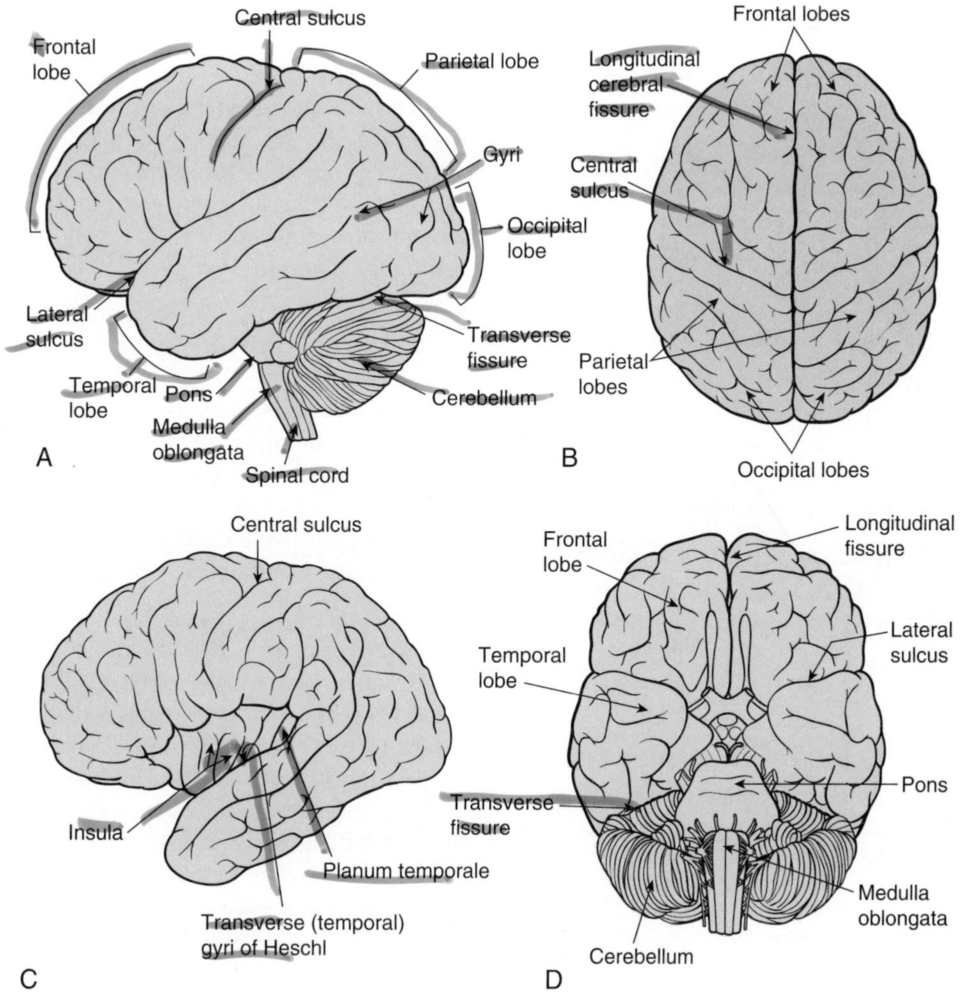

Figure 10.3. Four views of the brain including **(A)** lateral, **(B)** superior, **(C)** lateral with the lateral fissure pulled out and down to expose the insula and the planum temporale, and **(D)** ventral. (A modified from Cohen BJ. Medical Terminology. 4th Ed. Philadelphia: Lippincott Williams & Wilkins, 2003. B from Stedman's Medical Dictionary. 27th Ed. Baltimore: Lippincott Williams & Wilkins, 2000. D from Bear M, Conner B, Paradiso M. Neuroscience, Exploring the Brain. 2nd Ed. Baltimore: Lippincott Williams & Wilkins, 2000. Used with permission.)

- **Longitudinal fissure**—separates the right and left hemispheres
- **Central sulcus**—separates the frontal and parietal lobes
- **Lateral sulcus** (sylvian fissure)—separates the frontal lobe (and part of the parietal lobe) from the temporal lobe
- **Transverse fissure**—separates the cerebral hemispheres from the cerebellum

The two cerebral hemispheres are generally symmetric and are connected by a neural bridge called the **corpus callosum.** Although both hemispheres are involved in all human activities, one of them has a tendency to dominate when processing specific information. In most people, the left hemisphere is more active in processing sequential information and logical reasoning for tasks such as language processing (understanding speech, reading, and writing) and sequential arithmetic calculations. In contrast, the right hemisphere is more active in processing emotions, intuitive decisions, spatial processing, and perception of music and pictures. The amount of dominance of one hemisphere over the other is person dependent and may change over our lifetime as a result of pathology, medical intervention, or specific training.

Each hemisphere is divided into four principal lobes and two additional "lobes" or systems. The four principal lobes of the cerebrum and their primary functions are listed below:

- **Frontal lobe**—voluntary skilled movements
- **Parietal lobe**—tactile and proprioceptive (body position) perception, spatial orientation, conscious taste perception, and the integration of auditory information with other sensory information (e.g., visual, tactile)
- **Occipital lobe**—visual processing
- **Temporal lobe**—auditory processing, comprehension of language, higher order processing of visual information (e.g., recognizing faces or facial expression), and aspects of learning and memory (in combination with other brain centers including the hippocampus)

The two additional "lobes" are not technically lobes in the anatomic sense. However, they have specific physiologic functions that are different from the primary lobes. These are:

- **Limbic system** (from the Latin *limbus*, meaning border*)—processing of drive-related (e.g., sex drive, eating and drinking behavior) and emotional behaviors
- **Insular lobe** (also known as the insula or island of Reil)—autonomic processes including activities that are not consciously controlled, such as regulating the internal environment of the human body

Several areas of the cerebral cortex are specialized for processing specific types of information (Fig. 10.4). These

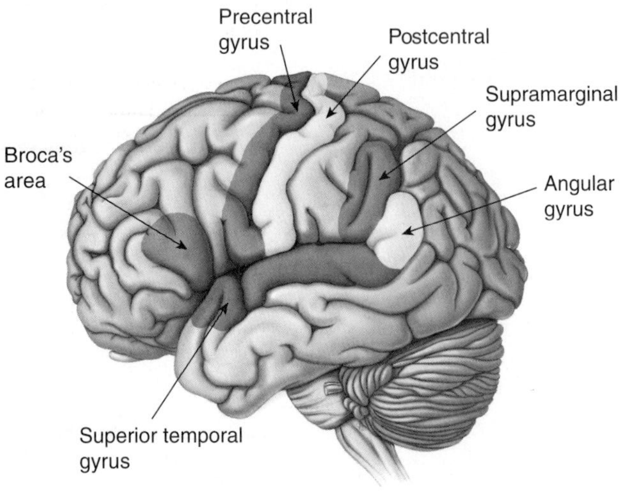

Figure 10.4. Specialized areas of the cerebral cortex. (Modified from Bear M, Conner B, Paradiso M. Neuroscience, Exploring the Brain. 2nd Ed. Baltimore: Lippincott Williams & Wilkins, 2000. Used with permission.)

cortical areas form several principle gyri, which are labeled by name as well as by Brodmann area number* (based on the work of anatomist Koribian Brodmann, 1909). The specific processing areas that are of interest in this book are listed below. The Brodmann area numbers are indicated in the text by the number in parentheses following the name.

- Precentral gyrus or primary motor cortex (area 4)
- Postcentral gyrus or primary somatosensory cortex (areas 3, 1, 2)
- Heschl's gyrus or transverse temporal gyrus (areas 41, 42)
- Superior temporal gyrus or Wernicke's area (area 22)
- Area triangularis or Broca's area (area 44)
- Angular gyrus (area 39) within the parietal-occipital-temporal junction (i.e., region where the three lobes meet)
- Supramarginal gyrus (area 40)

The gyrus that is most important from an auditory-processing point of view is the **transverse temporal gyrus** or **Heschl's gyrus** (after Richard Heschl, 1824–1881). Heschl's gyrus contains the primary auditory cortex, which is the first part of the cortex to receive auditory information.

Heschl's gyrus can be seen by pulling down the temporal lobe and peering into the lateral (sylvian) fissure and looking for a gyrus that is perpendicular to the superior temporal gyrus (Fig. 10.3C). Sometimes there is only one Heschl's gyrus and sometimes there are as many as three gyri; however, we will use the singular term gyrus when

*The name *limbic system* has a dual connotation because the limbic lobe anatomically *borders* the telencephalon and the diencephalon while it also functionally *borders* conscious and unconscious neurologic processing.

*Brodmann areas are 52 areas of the brain identified and numbered by German anatomist and neurologist Koribian Brodmann (1868–1918) on the basis of their physiologic activities determined by staining brain cells.

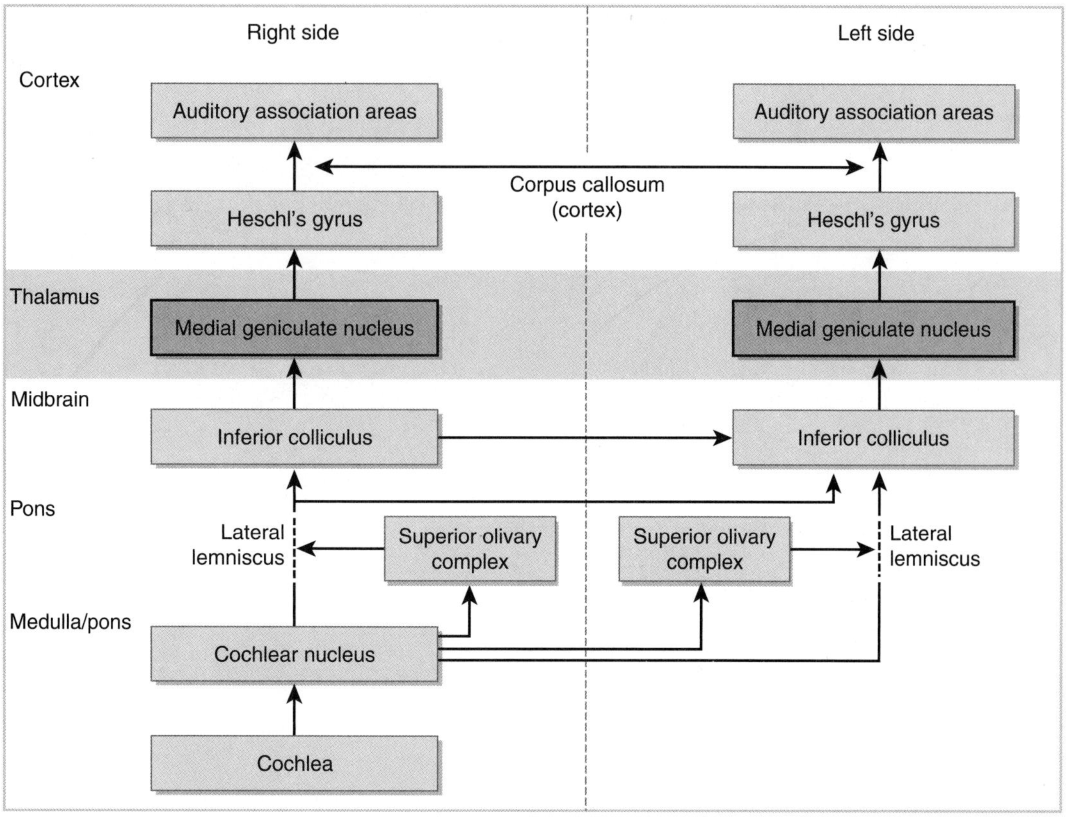

The medial geniculate body is divided into three parts, listed below:

- Ventral portion
- Dorsal portion
- Medial portion

Nerve fibers from the primary ascending pathway project from the ventral portion of the **medial geniculate nucleus** to Heschl's gyrus via a large bundle of fibers called the **internal capsule.** The medial and dorsal nuclei are part of the nonprimary ascending pathway and their projections connect the medial geniculate body to other areas of the brain, including the limbic system.

Box 10.3 The Diencephalon: Key Concepts

Developmentally speaking, the diencephalon is the inferior part of the embryologic forebrain. It is situated between the cerebrum and the midbrain. It has four major subdivisions: the thalamus, hypothalamus, epithalamus, and subthalamus. Within the thalamus is the medial geniculate body (nucleus), a relay region in the auditory pathway. Afferent fibers project from the ventral portion of the medial geniculate nucleus to Heschl's gyrus, forming part of the internal capsule.

Midbrain

The **midbrain** (mesencephalon) is the superior portion of the brainstem. The **brainstem** is the lowest part of the brain and it is structurally continuous with the spinal cord. It constitutes a major communication route between the forebrain, the spinal cord, and the peripheral nervous system. In addition to the midbrain, the brainstem includes the pons and the medulla oblongata, which belong to the hindbrain and will be discussed in the next section. Structures in the midbrain include:

- **Cerebral peduncles**—two large fiber tracts connecting the brainstem with the brain; they look like pillars in an anterior view (Fig. 10.6A)
- **Corpora quadrigemina** ("four twin bodies")—four round bumps on the dorsal surface of the midbrain, containing the superior colliculi (part of the visual system) and inferior colliculi (part of the auditory system) (Fig. 10.6B)
- **Cerebral aqueduct** (mesencephalic aqueduct, aqueduct of Sylvius)—aqueduct that runs through the midbrain, connecting the third ventricle to the fourth ventricle. *Cerebral aqueduct* is the traditional term for this passageway, although it may be considered "old fashioned"; the *mesencephalic aqueduct* is the most current term, and the *aqueduct of Sylvius* is very commonly used in many health care fields.

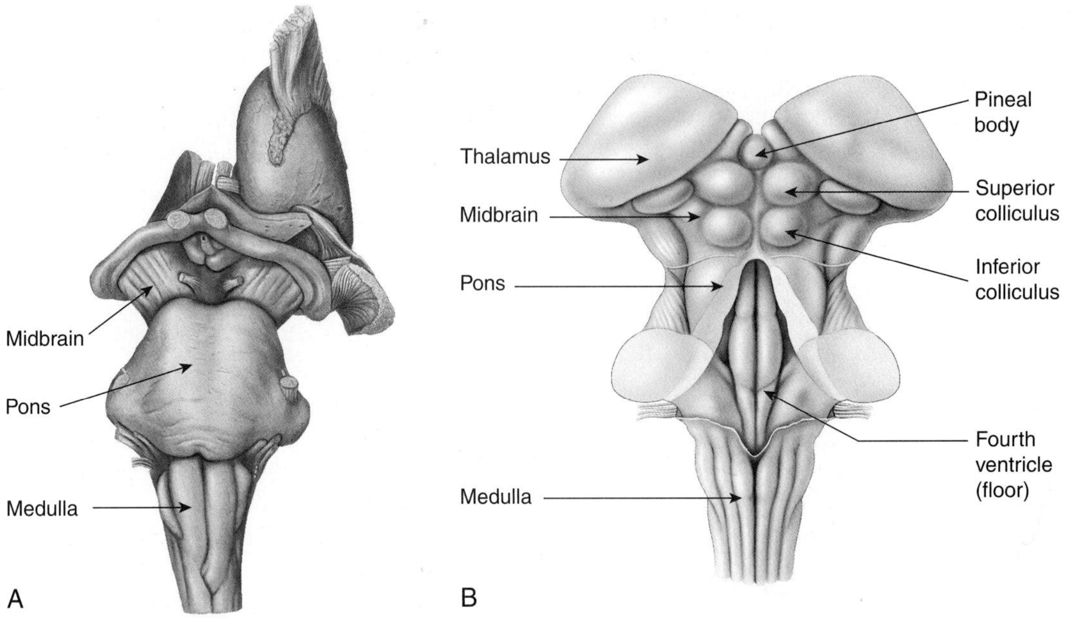

Figure 10.6. The brainstem in an **(A)** anterior and a **(B)** posterior view. (A from Grants Atlas of Anatomy. B from Bear M, Conner B, Paradiso M. Neuroscience, Exploring the Brain. 2nd Ed. Baltimore: Lippincott Williams & Wilkins, 2000. Used with permission.)

The main parts of the midbrain involved in auditory processing are the inferior colliculi (right and left), which appear as the bottom two of the four round projections on the **tectum** (roof) of the midbrain. The inferior colliculi are a major connection point in the auditory pathway, receiving projections via the lateral lemniscus from all primary ascending fiber tracts and processing and transmitting this information to the thalamus.

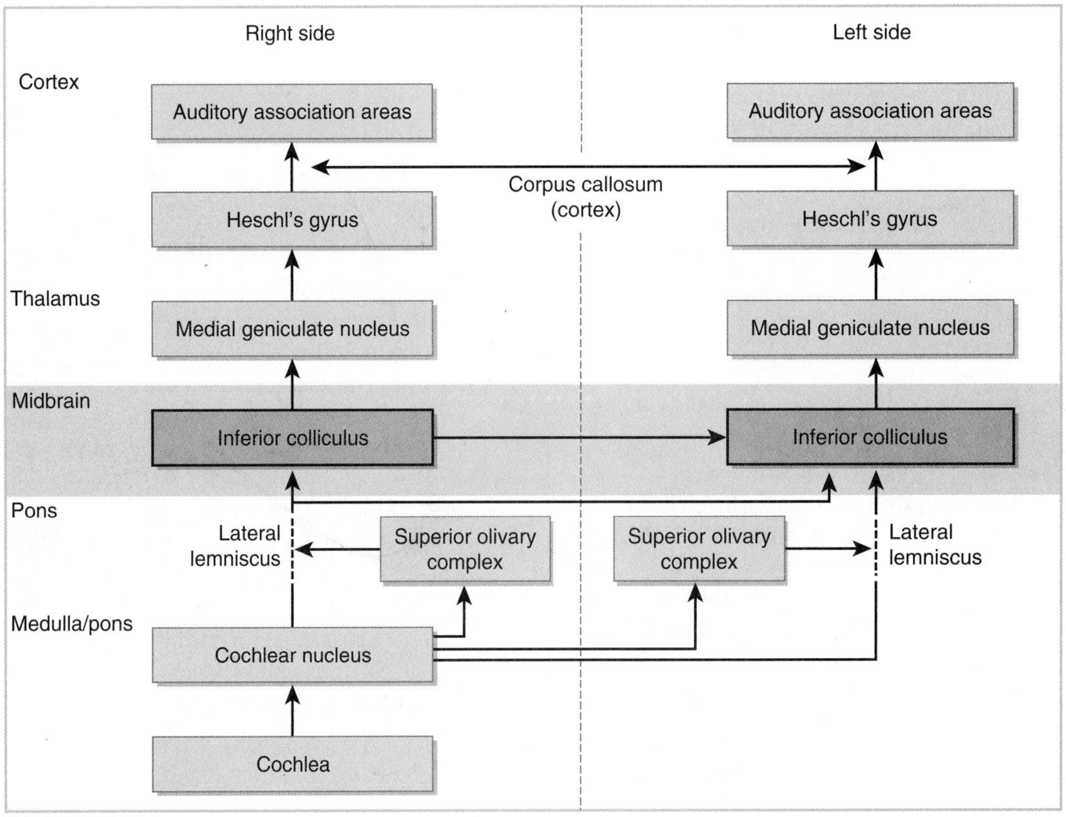

A fiber tract called the **commissure of the inferior colliculus** connects the two inferior colliculi to allow information to cross between the two sides. From the inferior colliculus, nerve fibers travel via a tract called the **brachium of the inferior colliculus** to the medial geniculate nucleus in the thalamus.

Box 10.4 The Midbrain: Key Concepts

The midbrain, also known as the mesencephalon, develops from the middle of the embryonic brain vesicles. Many auditory and vestibular fiber tracts travel through the midbrain en route to and from higher brain centers. The inferior colliculus is an auditory center on the dorsal aspect of the midbrain. Afferent fibers from the inferior colliculus form the brachium of the inferior colliculus and project to the medial geniculate nucleus of the thalamus before reaching the cerebral cortex.

Hindbrain

The **hindbrain** (rhombencephalon) is the most posterior (toward the back) part of the embryo, which develops into three brain structures:

- Medulla (medulla oblongata)
- Pons
- Cerebellum

Medulla Oblongata and Pons

The **medulla** (Fig. 10.6A) connects with the spinal cord through a large opening at the base of the skull called the **foramen magnum.** The ventral surface of the medulla contains prominent fiber bundles called the **pyramids,** which are made up of motor neuron tracks connecting the spinal cord to the cortex. Dorsolateral (dorsal and lateral) to each pyramid is the **olive,** which is a bulge containing the inferior olivary nucleus.

The medulla oblongata is connected with the **pons.** The ventral surface of the pons looks like an apple (Fig. 10.6A), whereas the dorsal surface of the pons has a diamond-shaped depression, which is the location of the fourth ventricle (Fig. 10.6B). Together, the pons and medulla make up an important area for the processing of auditory information. The vestibulocochlear nerve enters the brainstem between the pons and medulla (the **pontomedullary junction**) close to the angle created by the cerebellum and the pons (the **cerebellopontine angle**), and the right and left auditory nerves end at the **cochlear nuclei** on each side of the brainstem in this area.

The ventral and dorsal cochlear nuclei on each side of the brainstem form a continuous curved band of cells spanning dorsal and lateral portions of the brainstem surface at the pontomedullary junction. As the auditory nerve enters the brainstem, it splits into two branches; one branch enters the **anterior ventral cochlear nucleus** (AVCN) and the other enters the **posterior ventral cochlear nucleus** (PVCN). Fibers projecting to the PVCN branch split again, with fibers

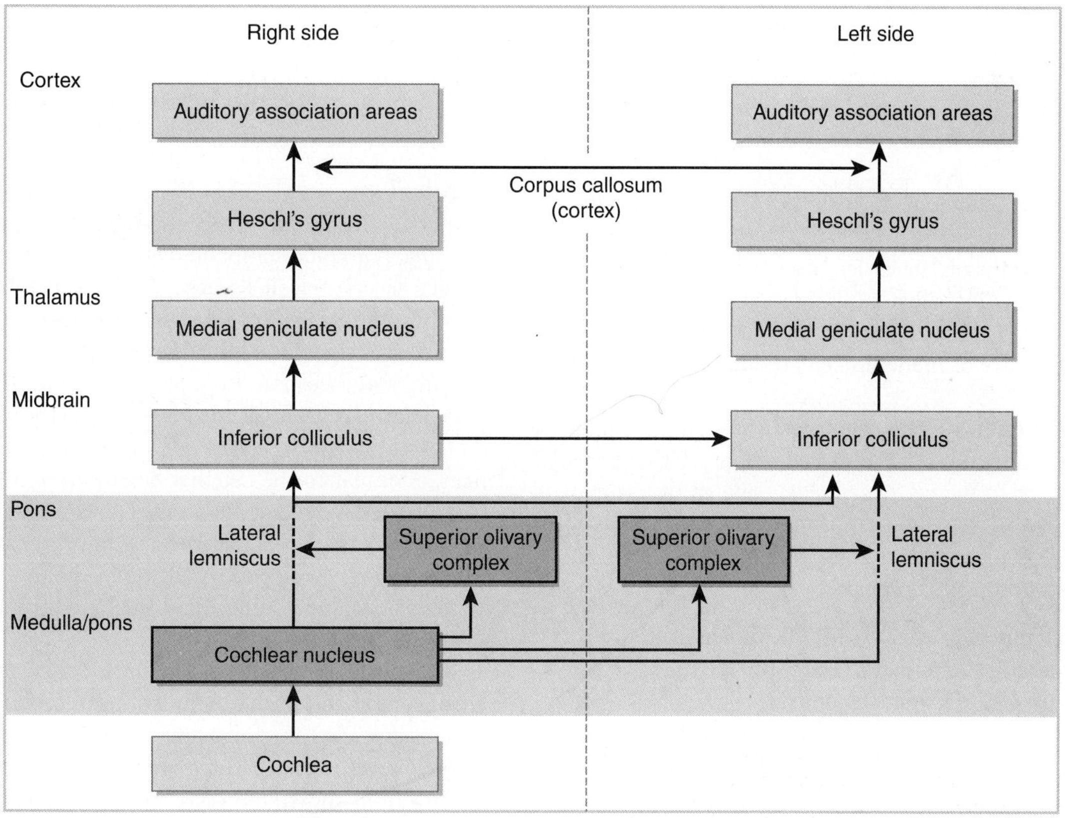

projecting further, into the **dorsal cochlear nucleus** (DCN). Thus, each nerve fiber sends projections to all three divisions of the cochlear nucleus.

Each of the three divisions of the cochlear nucleus is connected via separate fiber tracts to one large fiber tract called the lateral lemniscus. Most of the fibers from these tracts project to the lateral lemniscus located on the contralateral (opposite) side of the brainstem; thus, the tracts from the right cochlear nucleus project to the left lateral lemniscus and vice versa. A much smaller number of axons project to the ipsilateral (same side) lateral lemniscus. Because of this bilateral (two side) projection pattern, information from both ears is projected to each lateral lemniscus. The three fiber tracts traveling away from the cochlear nucleus are:

- **Dorsal acoustic stria** (stria of Monaco) from the PVCN
- **Intermediate acoustic stria** (stria of Held) from the DCN
- **Ventral acoustic stria (trapezoid body*)** from the AVCN

Whereas the majority of the fibers from each stria project directly to the contralateral lateral lemniscus, some of the fibers, including a majority of fibers from the ventral acoustic stria (trapezoid body), project first to the contralateral superior olivary nucleus (discussed in the next section). The superior olivary nucleus projections then travel up to the lateral lemniscus (Adams, 1986; Møller, 2000). The ventral acoustic stria fibers also project to nuclei associated with the **facial nerve** (which innervates the stapedius muscle in the middle ear) and the **trigeminal nerve** (which innervates the tensor tympani muscle in the middle ear) (Møller, 2000).

The **lateral lemniscus** (from the Greek *lemniskos*, meaning "ribbon") is a flat band of fibers that begins in the pons and travels to the posterior surface of the midbrain. Although most fibers travel straight through the lateral lemniscus, some synapse with nuclei within the lemniscus. Within the lateral lemniscus are two nuclei:

- Dorsal nuclei of the lateral lemniscus (DNLL)
- Ventral nucleus of the lateral lemniscus (VNLL)

The majority of lateral lemniscus fibers project to the ipsilateral inferior colliculus; some axons, however, travel from the DNLL to the opposite side of the brain in the **dorsal commissure of the lemniscus (commissure of Probst)** (Moore, 1987).

The **superior olivary complex (SOC)** is a group of nuclei located within the pons just a short distance medial and superior to the cochlear nuclei. The entire complex is surrounded by ascending axons traveling from the cochlear nucleus to the lateral lemniscus (Moore, 1987). The SOC is composed of three main nuclei:

- **Medial superior olivary (MSO) nucleus**
- **Lateral superior olivary (LSO) nucleus**
- **Nucleus of the trapezoid body**

*The trapezoid body appears in cross section as a trapezoid shape.

The MSO nucleus and LSO nucleus are relatively large nuclei. In contrast, the nucleus of the trapezoid body is smaller and has been described as not really a nucleus at all in humans, but just "scattered" neurons (Moore, 1987). The MSO and LSO nuclei are surrounded by various small nuclei called **periolivary nuclei.**

The main efferent system of the CANS, the olivocochlear system, begins at the periolivary nuclei of the superior olivary complex and extends to the cochlea. The descending motor fibers from the periolivary nuclei are called the **olivocochlear bundle** (OCB), also known as Rasmussen's bundle (Rasmussen, 1942).

The efferent system is divided into two main parts:

- **Medial efferent system** or **medial olivocochlear bundle** (MOCB)
- **Lateral efferent system** or **lateral olivocochlear bundle** (LOCB)

As their names imply, the medial efferent fibers project from periolivary nuclei that are more medial in location, close to the MSO nucleus, and the lateral efferent fibers project from periolivary nuclei that are more lateral in location, close to the LSO nucleus. The medial efferent neurons have large myelinated axons and project primarily (approximately 70%) to the contralateral cochlea, where they synapse directly with the outer hair cells (Sahley et al., 1997). The lateral efferent nerve fibers have smaller, unmyelinated axons that project primarily (approximately 90%) to the ipsilateral cochlea, where they synapse with the type I afferent auditory nerve fibers at the base of the inner hair cells (Sahley et al., 1997). Both fiber types travel out of the brainstem with the vestibular branch of the vestibulocochlear nerve, through the internal auditory meatus, and via the **vestibulocochlear anastomosis (anastomosis of Oort)** of the internal auditory meatus to the cochlea (Arnesen & Osen, 1984). (An anastomosis is a merging together of two structures).

Cerebellum

The **cerebellum** (Latin for "little brain") is connected to the medulla, pons, and midbrain by three fiber tracts. It includes surface layers of cell bodies called the **cerebellar cortex,** which form folds called **folia,** and the fiber tracts projecting to and from the cortex called **arbor vitae** (meaning "tree of life" in Latin, because of the resemblance to the branches of a tree). Similar to the deep gray matter in the cerebrum (i.e., the basal nuclei), the cerebellum also contains deep gray matter. Similar to the cerebral hemispheres, the cerebellum (Fig. 10.7) is divided into two hemispheres by a central structure called the **vermis** (which means "worm"). Alternately, it can be structurally divided into three lobes and several lobules including the flocculonodular lobe, anterior lobe, and posterior lobe.

The cerebellum is associated with the vestibular (balance) system and primarily functions to produce changes in skeletal muscle tone for maintaining equilibrium, posture, and coordination of voluntary movements. It receives information from the spinal cord and various sensory systems

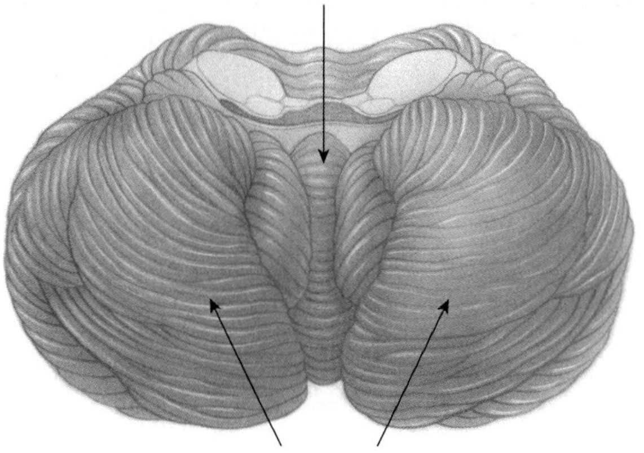

Figure 10.7. The cerebellum. (Image from Grants Atlas of Anatomy. Used with permission.)

and coordinates operations of the muscular skeletal system. The cerebellum is also involved in the control and **plasticity** (ability of the brain to reorganize itself) of the vestibular-ocular reflex (VOR), which is described later in this chapter.

Box 10.5 The Hindbrain: Key Concepts

The hindbrain develops from the most inferior end of the embryonic brain vesicles. It is composed of several structures including the medulla oblongata, pons, and cerebellum. The ventral surface of the medulla contains motor fiber bundles called pyramids. Dorsolateral to the pyramids is a structure called the olive, which is formed by the underlying inferior olivary nucleus. The ventral surface of the pons contains the rootlets of several cranial nerves including the vestibulocochlear nerve (CN VIII). The dorsal pontine surface (along with the dorsal medulla) contributes to the formation of the fourth ventricle. Several fiber bundles, including the trapezoid body, course beneath the dorsal surface of the pons (tegmentum). The cerebellum is attached to the brainstem via three fiber bundles called cerebellar peduncles, which contain projections between the cerebellum and the olivary and vestibular nuclei.

CRANIAL NERVES

Information to and from the CNS and peripheral nervous system (PNS) is carried by 12 pairs of cranial nerves (12 on the left, 12 on the right). Each pair of the cranial nerves is labeled with Roman numerals, from I to XII. All of the cranial nerves, except the first two, which connect directly with the brain, attach to structures of the brainstem (Fig. 10.8).

To memorize the names of the 12 cranial nerves in the right order, anatomy students for generations have used a mnemonic rhyme to help them to remember the nerves: "On old Olympus' towering top, a Finn **and** German viewed a hop." The first letter of each word in the rhyme corresponds to the initial letter of each pair of cranial nerves. Note, however, that the eighth cranial nerve is represented by the word

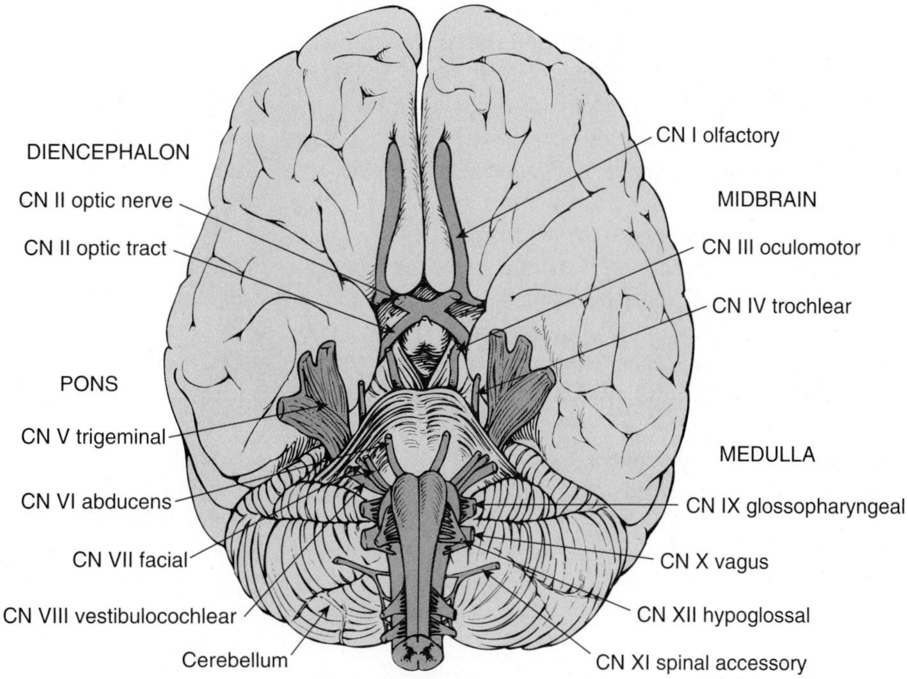

Figure 10.8. The entrance points for the 12 cranial nerves. (Modified from Weber J, Kelley J. Health Assessment in Nursing. 2nd Ed. Philadelphia: Lippincott Williams & Wilkins, 2003. Used with permission.)

"**and**" because the old name for that nerve is the auditory nerve (or acoustic nerve). The term vestibulocochlear nerve is more widely used today, although the cochlear portion of the vestibulo*cochlear* nerve is still called the auditory nerve today (as we discussed in Chapter 9). The 12 cranial nerves, in order of their connection with the brain, are:

- I Olfactory
- II Optic
- III Oculomotor
- IV Trochlear
- V Trigeminal
- VI Abducens
- VII Facial
- VIII Vestibulocochlear
- IX Glossopharyngeal
- X Vagus
- XI Accessory spinal
- XII Hypoglossal

The most important cranial nerve to the operation of the auditory and vestibular systems is the **vestibulocochlear nerve,** which was described in Chapter 9. This nerve is responsible for conveying hearing and balance information from the inner ear to the central nervous system. Several other cranial nerves are also involved with the auditory and vestibular systems.

The **oculomotor, trochlear,** and **abducens** nerves control the movement of the eyeball. These nerves are of interest because the movement of the eyes is connected to the vestibular system. Specifically, the **vestibular-ocular reflex** is a reflex that allows the eyes to stay focused on an object, even when the body is moving. When the head moves, a signal is sent from the vestibular part of the inner ear to the vestibular nuclei in the brainstem and then to the nuclei that control eyeball movement. As a result of this neural feedback, a head turn in one direction results in the same amount of eye movement in the opposite direction maintaining a stable image on the retina.

The **trigeminal nerve** provides sensory innervation to the tympanic membrane and motor innervation to the tensor tympani muscle in the middle ear and to the tensor palatini muscle, which opens the eustachian tube. Similarly, the auricular branch of the **vagus nerve** (Arnold's nerve) and the **facial nerve** provide sensory innervation to the outer ear and tympanic membrane, so both these nerves convey information about air pressure in the outer ear and operational conditions of the tympanic membrane to the brain. A branch of the facial nerve called the **chorda tympani** travels through the middle ear from the posterior wall to the anterior wall where it joins the lingual nerve, transmitting taste sensations from the anterior two thirds of the tongue. Another branch of the facial nerve provides motor innervation to the stapedius muscle (attached to the stapedius bone in the middle ear). More general information about the anatomic properties and functions of individual cranial nerves is provided on the website. **Link 10-3**

PHYSIOLOGY OF THE CENTRAL AUDITORY NERVOUS SYSTEM

The anatomy of the CANS has been studied extensively in both humans and animals via postmortem dissection. The physiology of the CANS is studied on living creatures; therefore, much of the basic physiology research has been conducted on animals by using microelectrodes inserted directly into neurons. In regard to the auditory system, the activity in specific neurons is observed after stimulating them either by an acoustic stimulus delivered to the ear or by an electrical stimulus delivered to the neuron. Although some microelectrode research has been conducted on humans, human physiology is generally inferred from animal research or studied by noninvasive imaging procedures that examine metabolic activity using the evaluation of blood flow in the brain (functional magnetic resonance imaging, positron emission tomography) or create pictures of bone and/or soft tissue within the head (radiographs, computed tomography scans, magnetic resonance imaging). Auditory physiology is also studied indirectly by monitoring the electrical activity in the CANS via electrodes placed on the head (evoked potential testing) and via the use of behavioral testing (i.e., human responses to various auditory stimuli).

Primary Afferent (Ascending) Central Auditory Nervous System

The major nuclei of the auditory pathway are shown in Figure 10.1. The auditory nerves leaving the right and left cochleae (Chapter 9) synapse with the right and left cochlear nuclei on the same side of the brainstem. After passing the cochlear nuclei, most of the nerve fibers cross to the opposite side of the brainstem to a large fiber tract called the lateral lemniscus. Some auditory fibers make this connection directly, whereas others connect first at the superior olivary complex before entering the lateral lemniscus. From the lateral lemniscus, nerve fibers project to the inferior colliculus, continue to the medial geniculate nucleus (body), and then enter the cortex. The major nuclei listed above are the main processing centers of auditory information where neural coding and recoding take place.

It is important to remember that whenever a nerve fiber reaches a nucleus, the individual nerve fiber ends there and the transmitted information is sent further via the next nerve in the chain. It is also important to realize that the CANS is not a direct transmission line that delivers auditory nerve impulses straight from the cochlea to the cortex. The nuclei of the CANS perform various **signal-processing** functions along the pathways between the vestibulocochlear nerve and the cortex and they gradually produce a much more refined signal to the brain than that originally encoded in the auditory neurons. Each nucleus in the CANS appears to use both place and temporal coding, indicating that the original time, frequency, and intensity information generated in the cochlea is used across all stages of signal processing. Recall from

Chapter 9 that place coding means that the signal frequency is coded by the place of activity within the cochlea or group of neurons and temporal coding means that signal frequency is coded by the rate of nerve firing.

Tonotopic organization of frequency information initiated at the basilar membrane of the cochlea has been found within every nucleus of the CANS. The specific orientation of the frequency maps (i.e., the place in the nucleus that corresponds to high- and low-frequency sounds), varies widely among the nuclei. The organization of the tonotopic map depends on the type of nucleus and the type of species. The degree to which the CANS needs the tonotopic organization for decoding of frequency is not entirely understood. The brain likely uses both place and temporal coding to determine sound frequency because neither coding strategy can account for the high resolution of human hearing across the whole audible frequency range.

The temporal coding of sound is processed differently both *between* and *within* the various nuclei. The relatively simple phase-locking pattern seen at the level of the auditory nerve changes as the signal travels through the central nervous system. Some central auditory neurons seem to provide a modified relay function. In other words, the signal preserves all its main characteristics but is "fine-tuned" (reduced in its ambiguity) in the transmission from one neuron to the next. Some neurons respond to specific differences between incoming signals, some neurons respond to the beginning and end of the signal (edge detectors), and some neurons are only active when a signal is present or when the signal changes. Thus, the CANS works like a large array of processors, each extracting different aspects of the signal from the initial code to create new codes. These new codes are then sent to the brain for further processing and then for conversion into sensation and perception. The CANS also includes interaural (between ear) connections and various feedback loops where the ongoing signal coming up the chain can be modified by signals coming down or across the chain.

Cochlear Nucleus and Acoustic Stria

The majority (about 95%) of auditory nerve fibers are type I, meaning they have large myelinated axons, and they begin at the base of the inner hair cells. These nerve fibers transfer electrochemical signals to the second-order neurons, which have their cell bodies in the cochlear nuclei. In contrast to the type I fibers, little is known about the function of the smaller and unmyelinated type II fibers, which make up about 5% of the fibers in the auditory nerve and begin at the base of the outer hair cells.

The complex place and temporal coding created at the cochlea travels along the auditory nerve and is delivered to the cochlear nucleus. The place coding is preserved at the level of the auditory nerve by the tonotopic arrangement of nerve fibers, with low-frequency fibers from the apex of the cochlea traveling in the center of the auditory nerve and high-frequency fibers from the base of the cochlea traveling along the periphery of the auditory nerve (Spoendlin & Schrott, 1989).

The size of a nerve fiber and the presence of myelin are the two primary factors affecting the nerve conduction velocity (the speed at which a signal travels down the nerve). The temporal coding that originated at the cochlea most likely arrives intact at the cochlear nucleus because the auditory nerve fibers do not vary considerably in size. Since the fibers are similar in size, it is hypothesized that all the signals reach the cochlear nucleus in the same temporal (time) order in which they were sent by the hair cells of the inner ear. Timing patterns in children may be more synchronized than in adults, since the variability in fiber size appears to increase with age (Spoendlin & Schrott, 1989).

A number of different firing patterns have been recorded from various cells within the cochlear nuclei. The same patterns have also been identified in other nuclei all the way up the CANS (Kiang et al., 1965; Pfeiffer, 1966). These patterns include:

- **Primary-like patterns**—firing patterns that are similar to the signal in the auditory nerve in which the repetition rate of the firing matches the frequency of the stimulus
- **Chopper patterns**—firing patterns produced by cells that fire periodically, but the period of their response does not match the period of the stimulus
- **Pauser patterns**—patterns produced by cells that fire in response to the onset of a stimulus and then take a break for a short time and resume firing at a lower level
- **Onset patterns**—patterns produced by cells that fire only at the onset of the stimulus

The nerve firing patterns that are commonly seen in the cochlear nucleus are illustrated in Figure 10.9 using post-stimulus time (PST) histograms. A PST histogram shows the amount of neural activity (number of nerves firing, *y* axis) as a function of time (*x* axis). Time $t = 0$ indicates the presence of a specific event that triggered the response. The higher the lines in the PST histogram, the greater the neural activity is at a specific point in time. The response of a neuron with a primary-like response pattern stimulated by a tone with a frequency of 3500 Hz is shown in Figure 10.9A. Note that the primary-like neurons are firing throughout the stimulus, similar to the pattern seen in the auditory nerve for a high-frequency sound. The firing pattern of a neuron with a chopper response pattern is shown in Figure 10.9B. This is also a periodic pattern of firing (it appears *choppy* but periodic), but the period of the firing does not correspond to the period of the acoustic stimulus that entered the ear.

A neuron with a pauser-type firing pattern is shown in Figure 10.9C. Note that the pauser neurons fire when the signal starts, then there is a short period with no nerve activity, and this period is followed by a lower level of neural activity. Figure 10.9D shows the firing pattern of the onset neuron in which neurons fire only at the onset of the stimulus.

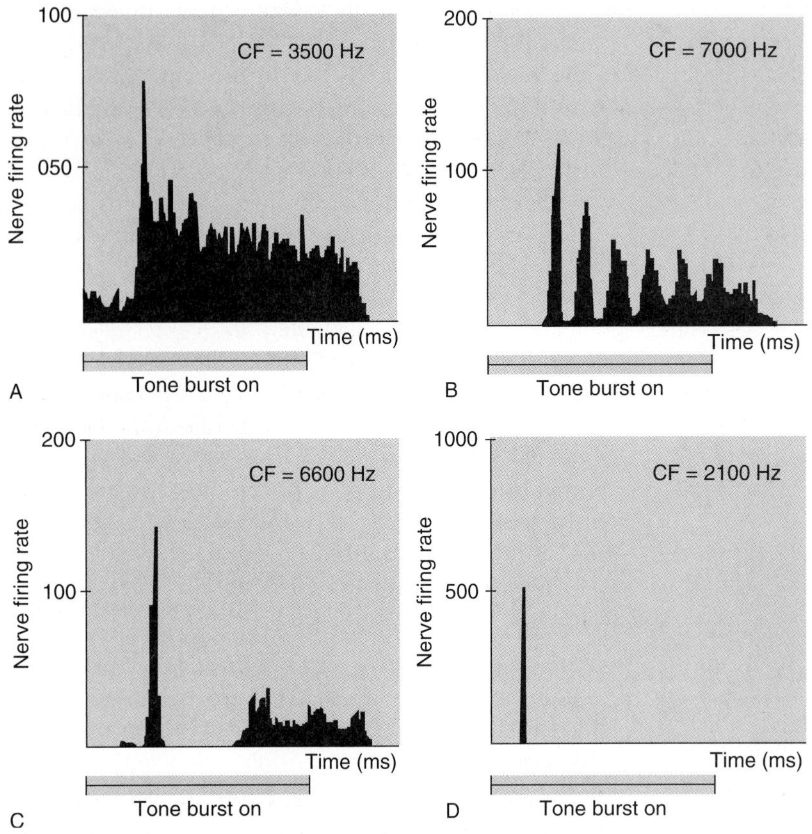

Figure 10.9. Poststimulus time (PST) histograms illustrating commonly reported firing patterns in the cochlear nucleus including **(A)** primary-like, **(B)** chopper, **(C)** pauser, and **(D)** on. (From Pfeiffer RR. Classification of response patterns of spike discharges for units in the cochlear nucleus: tone-burst stimulation. Exper Brain Res 1966;1:220–235. With kind permission of Springer Science and Business Media.)

In addition to the relatively simple general patterns of neural response discussed above, several subcategories of response pattern exist within each category, including at least three types of onset response and at least three categories of chopper response (e.g., Rhode & Smith, 1986). They may be generated by different types of cells or the same cell may have different polarization conditions resulting in different output patterns. Furthermore, these response patterns vary depending on the intensity, duration, and complexity of the signal entering the ear (Pfeiffer, 1966). In other words, the well-documented primary-like, chopper, pauser, and onset firing patterns seem to be observed only in response to simple tonal stimuli, and they most likely do not provide a good picture of the way neurons respond to complex signals, such as speech. The different response patterns seen for tone bursts, however, do provide convincing evidence that a number of different coding processes take place in the cochlear nucleus.

The firing pattern of a neural cell appears to be determined by a variety of factors including the type of axon terminal on the presynaptic neuron, the number of signals received by the cell during a specific time period, the presence of signals from other nuclei that can inhibit or excite the cell (Cant, 1982; Ostapoff et al., 1994; Rhode & Smith, 1986), and the type of cell that is receiving the signal.

In the AVCN, the auditory neurons synapse on a relatively large part of the dendrite of a **bushy cell** (cell that resembles a bush) with only a few auditory neurons connected to each bushy cell. The cells that synapse on each bushy cell are from adjacent places on the cochlea, which means that each AVCN bushy cell processes information from only a narrow range of frequencies processed by the cochlea. Therefore, it is likely that the firing pattern of the bushy cell is responsible for the primary-like pattern of nerve firing. The temporal coding (phase locking) seen at the auditory nerve level is not just duplicated by the bushy cell, but is also enhanced (Joris, Carney, et al., 1994; Joris, Smith, et al., 1994; Louage et al., 2005). Joris, Carney, et al. (1994) reported that the firing pattern of a bushy cell has better phase locking to the original signal than the firing pattern of the auditory nerve. They suggested that the bushy cell is an excitatory-excitatory (EE) cell that acts as a **coincidence detector;** that is, it only responds to stimulation when it receives coincident (concurrent) signals from several neurons. Thus, random firing of the auditory nerve fiber does not cause excitation of the bushy cell. Other researchers have suggested that the fine-tuned firing of the bushy cell also involves an inhibitory input from other neurons (Kopp-Scheinpflug et al., 2002). This means that under certain processing conditions, the bushy cells are prevented from firing by inhibitory signals received from other neurons.

In the PVCN, the predominant cell type is the **octopus cell** (cell that resembles an octopus with tentacle-like dendrites). Small nerve endings from a larger number (about 50) of different auditory nerve fibers synapse with each octopus cell along its dendrites and soma. Therefore, octopus cells are more broadly tuned than bushy cells and respond to signals across a wider range of frequencies as compared with a narrowly tuned neuron such as the bushy cell (Golding et al., 1995).

The octopus cell will only fire if a group of auditory nerve fibers, originating from various locations in the cochlea, fire at about the same time, so the octopus cell appears also to be a coincidence detector responding to synchronous firing from many different frequency fibers (Ferragamo & Oertel, 2002; Oertel et al., 2000). Octopus cells have been reported to respond well to very brief stimuli (e.g., clicks) and to tones that are modulated (periodically altered) in amplitude (Oertel et al., 2000), but they have been found to basically turn off in response to a continuous stationary wideband noise (Levy & Kipke, 1998). Therefore, octopus cells appear to behave as multi-input onset cells. The bushy cells and octopus cells are only two of the many types of cells seen in the CANS, but their different responses serve to illustrate the different types of responses that contribute to the multifaceted signal processing that occurs in the CANS.

Superior Olivary Complex

The SOC is the lowest level place in the CANS pathways where the neurons receive input from both ears. Therefore, it is the first stage of coding binaural (two ear) information in the CANS. It receives stimulation primarily from the ipsilateral and contralateral AVCN with most neurons arriving at the ipsilateral LSO nucleus and contralateral MSO nucleus. Both the MSO and LSO nuclei are predominantly made of two-input neuron cells: EE (excitatory-excitatory) coincidence detector cells and EI (excitatory-inhibitory) difference detector cells that respond to binaural input.

Binaural listening is critical for auditory spatial orientation including sound source localization and auditory distance estimation. The ability to localize sound in a three-dimensional space allows people to hear speech messages in the presence of background noise, since signals and noise sources are spatially separated. Listening with two ears also has an impact on sound loudness, the detection of signals in noise, and sound quality (timbre). All of these perceptual effects will be discussed in Chapter 12.

Recall from Chapter 8 that sound localization in the horizontal plane depends primarily on:

- **Interaural timing difference** (ITD)—a difference in time of sound arrival at two ears
- **Interaural intensity difference** (IID)—a difference in sound intensity at two ears

The ITDs are used by the CANS to determine the horizontal location of low-frequency sound sources and IIDs are used by the CANS to determine the horizontal location of high-frequency sound sources; both mechanisms are based on differences between contralateral and ipsilateral signals. The MSO nucleus is made up predominantly of neurons that respond to low- to midfrequency sounds, with high-frequency cells making up a much smaller part of the nucleus (Moore, 1987). Studies have shown that the MSO is the primary nucleus for detecting temporal differences between ipsilateral and contralateral signals and these differences are the basis for localization of low-frequency sounds (Masterton et al., 1967; Masterton et al., 1975). Therefore, most MSO neurons are EE neurons, but the MSO nucleus also includes some EI neurons (Mannell, 2002). The coincidence detectors (EE neurons) respond when signals arrive at the same time from both ears and difference detectors (EI neurons) respond to ipsilateral input and are inhibited by contralateral input (Seikel et al., 2000). If you would like to know more how coincidence detectors operate, consult the website. **Link 10-4**

The LSO nucleus has a frequency map quite different to that of the MSO nucleus. The majority of the LSO nucleus is dedicated to high-frequency stimuli (Moore, 1987). The LSO neurons are mainly the EI neurons that respond to the difference in intensity of stimulation of the ipsilateral and contralateral ear. The LSO nucleus, however, also houses a small group of EE neurons (Mannell, 2002). The LSO nucleus most likely works with nuclei in the lateral lemniscus and inferior colliculus to code IIDs needed to localize high-frequency sounds.

Lateral Lemniscus and Inferior Colliculus

The **lateral lemniscus** is the largest fiber tract in the auditory brainstem. It includes projections from a number of different nuclei within the cochlear nucleus and from the superior olivary complex on both sides of the brainstem and it contains various nuclei within this bundle of ascending tracts.

The **inferior colliculus** is another brainstem center that plays a role in coding binaural information based on intensity and timing differences between ears. The coding created in the SOC nucleus along with coding created in the inferior colliculus and decoding in the auditory cortex are the three processing stages that are required for sound perception in a three-dimensional space (Masterton et al., 1967; Møller, 2002). Damage to the central auditory pathway above the SOC nucleus, preventing the coded localization signals from both sides from reaching the cerebral hemispheres, affects localization ability. The lateral lemniscus may also be a place where directional information is recombined with the primary coding of signal frequency and intensity to create a complex sound image (Seikel et al., 2000).

Medial Geniculate Body, Heschl's Gyrus, and Auditory Association Areas

The medical geniculate body (MGB) is the final precortical processing nucleus of the ascending auditory pathway. It includes both monaural and binaural (EE and EI) neurons of the same kind that can be found in the inferior colliculus (Ehret, 1997). The nerve fibers of the MGB project to various parts of the cortex and cerebrum, most importantly to the primary auditory cortex (Heschl's gyrus) and auditory association areas. The primary auditory cortex "appears to perform sound analysis by synthesis, i.e., by combining spatially distributed coincident or time-coordinated neural responses" (Ehret, 1997).

The auditory centers in the brain receive their inputs from the ipsilateral MGB and thus respond primarily to signals received by the contralateral ear. Recall that the majority of auditory fibers leaving the cochlear nucleus cross from one side of the brainstem to the other. This means that ear-specific information is carried up by a relatively small number of ipsilateral fibers and a much greater number of contralateral fibers. In other words, most of the processing of signals arriving at the right ear is performed in the left hemisphere and most of the processing of signals arriving at the left ear is performed in the right hemisphere. For most people, the left hemisphere is the language-dominant hemisphere, so speech information directed to the left ear must be transported from the right hemisphere (where it arrives first) to the left hemisphere for decoding. Similarly, for most people, decoding of complex sounds with tonal quality (e.g., music) appears to occur primarily in the right hemisphere, so tonal signals that enter the right ear and arrive at the left hemisphere must be delivered to the right hemisphere for decoding. The information transferred between hemispheres occurs primarily across the corpus callosum.

Hemispheric specialization is probably the reason that most people process speech better when it is directed toward the right ear. For example, a telephone conversation is slightly easier to understand for most people when listening with the right ear. This difference is more pronounced in young children, and it becomes much smaller in adulthood. This is due to the fact that most of the speech processing is done in the left (language dominant) hemisphere. This slight difference in interpreting the auditory signal is called the **right ear advantage.**

The primary auditory cortex maintains a representation of the tonotopic organization (frequency map) of the basilar membrane that was preserved at all successive nuclei (Aitkin, 1990; Ehret, 1997). The map is repeated several times involving neurons of different selectivity and response (i.e., some neurons are uniquely sensitive to specific temporal patterns such as up-and-down glides in frequency and intensity that are important for speech recognition and the perception of music). Each hemispheric cortex also contains a spatiotopic (body centric) map of acoustic space with prioritized contralateral input (Ehret, 1997; Rayes, 2006). It seems like the acoustic coding stages appear to end at the primary auditory cortex and from this point on decoding for identification and classification is performed.

In addition to connections from the MGB to the primary auditory areas, there are also complex connections between the MGB and the limbic system. Consider the fact that some sounds make you happy and some make you sad or anxious. Did you ever wonder why? A number of connections exist between the auditory system and the limbic system, including a connection between the medial geniculate body and the amygdala. The amygdala plays a key role in perception and expression of emotional responses. Specifically, it appears that the amygdala receives sensory information (visual, auditory, etc.), processes the information, and sends signals to centers that control behavior, memory, endocrine (hormone), and autonomic nervous system functions. These connections appear to be responsible for "emotional memory," which is a conditioned response of the body caused by specific sensations. For example, if you were to hear a sound that always occurred together with something unpleasant, then, after a period of time, this sound would automatically be linked with a specific physical response. The sound might trigger a reaction by the autonomic nervous system response, causing an increase in heart rate or pupil dilation, or it might cause a general feeling of anxiety, and so forth.

Processing in the cortex is actually far more complex than the rather simple process described in this chapter, but more detailed analysis of cerebral processing is outside the scope of an introductory hearing science textbook.

Efferent Central Auditory Nervous System Pathway

The function of the olivocochlear bundle, especially the MOCB, appears to be to control the electromotility of the outer hair cells and to decrease the amplification of the auditory signal at the level of the cochlea (Chapter 9). The function of the MOCB has been investigated experimentally using two types of procedures. First, the MOCB in animals has been stimulated using an electrical stimulus applied to the neurons, and this stimulation affects the way in which the hair cells function. Second, the MOCB has been stimulated indirectly by introducing noise or other acoustic stimuli into the ear. The noise is carried by the ear via the regular primary afferent pathway, but it also causes the activation of the MOCB neurons, which connect with the outer hair cells. Stimulation of the MOCB via direct electrical stimulation and via noise presented to the ears also decreases the magnitude of otoacoustic emissions normally recorded in the ear canal as well as the magnitude of the electric activity in the auditory nerve as measured via evoked potential. Thus, it appears that the MOCB controls outer hair cell motility and that this action affects our ability to hear signals in three-dimensional space under adverse listening conditions. A number of studies have shown that the action of the MOCB improves our ability to understand speech in a background of noise (Giraud et al., 1997; Kumar & Vanaja, 2004). Far less is known about the function of the unmyelinated fibers of the LOCB compared to the MOCB.

Summary

A familiarity with basic neuroscience is essential for the study of the central auditory nervous system. The brain is customarily divided into three regions: the forebrain, the midbrain, and the hindbrain. The forebrain includes the telencephalon and the diencephalon, the midbrain is the superior portion of the brainstem, and the hindbrain includes the pons, cerebellum, and medulla oblongata. Specialized cortical areas in the brain include the primary auditory cortex, also known as Heschl's gyrus, and the primary auditory association area, also known as Wernicke's area. Information between the central nervous system and peripheral nervous system is carried by the 12 cranial nerves. The auditory portion of the vestibulocochlear nerve is responsible for conveying auditory signals to the CANS.

The CANS has afferent and efferent pathways. The primary afferent (ascending) pathway is responsible for conveying the auditory signal from the peripheral nervous system through the brainstem to the cortex. The afferent auditory system does not just relay a copy of auditory nerve impulses straight from the cochlea to the cortex, but also provides complex signal processing. Each nucleus along the CANS is tonotopically organized and each nucleus is responsible for relaying and enhancing temporal cues. Central auditory nuclei appear to be able to modify frequency, intensity, and timing cues via a variety of mechanisms including coincidence detection and inhibition. The efferent pathway travels downward via various nuclei and modifies signals that are on their way to the auditory center in the brain. The best understood efferent pathway is the olivocochlear bundle, which projects from the superior olivary complex to the outer hair cells of the cochlea, modifying the function of these cells by controlling their electromotility.

Key Points

- Each hemisphere is divided into four principal lobes and two additional lobes. The principal lobes are the frontal lobe, the parietal lobe, the occipital lobe, and the temporal lobe. The two additional lobes are the limbic lobe and the insular lobe.
- The cortex of each cerebral hemisphere is a series of peaks called gyri and valleys called sulci or fissures. Large sulci visible on the brain's surface include the longitudinal fissure, the central sulcus, the transverse fissure, and the lateral sulcus (sylvian fissure).
- The brainstem consists of three structures: the midbrain, the pons, and the medulla oblongata.
- The 12 cranial nerves, in order, are the olfactory, optic, oculomotor, trochlear, trigeminal, abducens, facial, vestibulocochlear, glossopharyngeal, vagus, accessory spinal, and hypoglossal.
- The oculomotor, trochlear, and abducens nerves connect the balance system of the ear to the muscles that move the eyeballs, an important connection that is responsible for the vestibular-ocular reflex.
- The major connection points along the central auditory nervous system are the cochlear nucleus, superior olivary complex, lateral lemniscus, inferior colliculus, medial geniculate nucleus (medial geniculate body), and Heschl's gyrus, which is also called the primary auditory cortex.
- The degree to which the CANS uses tonotopic and temporal organization for decoding of frequency is not entirely understood. It is likely that the brain uses both coding schemes to receive precise information about auditory stimulation across a wide frequency and intensity range.
- Well-documented cell firing patterns seen in the CANS including primary-like, chopper, pauser, and on patterns. These patterns have been recorded in response to simple tonal stimuli but most likely do not provide a good representation of the way neurons respond to complex signals, although they do provide evidence that different neurons process sound in different ways.
- The medial and lateral superior olivary nuclei are the first place where auditory signals from both ears come together. These nuclei provide an important first step in our perception of the location of a sound source.
- Most of the CANS fibers cross to the opposite side of the brainstem between the cochlear nucleus and the lateral lemniscus. The number of contralateral fibers is larger than the number of ipsilateral fibers, indicating that the primary processing of acoustic signals is performed within the contralateral hemisphere (i.e., signals from the right ear are processed primarily in the left hemisphere and vice versa).
- Language and speech processing is mostly performed in the left cerebral hemisphere and perception of music and spatial orientation depend primarily on the right cerebral hemisphere.
- The olivocochlear bundle (specifically the medial OCB) appears to improve the ability of human listeners to understand speech in a background of noise via the control of the mechanic action of the outer hair cells.

CHAPTER 11

Bone Conduction

Chapter Outline

Objectives

- To define bone conduction and to describe how sound is conducted to the cochlea via vibrations of the skull
- To discuss how the outer, middle, and inner ear are involved in the processing of bone-conducted sound
- To describe the differences in skull vibration based on the frequency and location of a bone vibrator
- To introduce the concept of bone conduction communication

Key Terms

Air conduction
Bone conduction
Bone conduction hearing aid
Bone vibrator (clinical bone vibrator, communication bone vibrator)
Compressional vibration
Contact microphone
Distortional mechanism
Inertial middle ear mechanism (ossicular-inertial mechanism)
Inertial vibration
Inner ear mechanism
Middle ear mechanism
Occlusion effect
Osteotympanic mechanism
Outer ear mechanism

Bone conduction is the process of receiving auditory signals through vibrations of the skull and associated soft tissue. This chapter covers the mechanics of bone conduction and describes how various parts of the ear contribute to bone conduction hearing. This description is followed by a discussion of the conditions under which bone conduction contributes to the perception of a sound. Since the head is a complex mechanical system, the effect of bone conduction depends on the location of the applied force, the type of coupling between the force and the head, and the impedance mismatch between the source of force and the head structures. In addition to these topics, bone conduction transmission will be discussed as a method of two-way communication.

BONE CONDUCTION HEARING

There are two basic mechanisms by which physical stimuli can stimulate the hearing receptors of the inner ear: air conduction and bone conduction (Békésy, 1932).

- **Air conduction** is the process by which an acoustic signal travels through the structures of the outer and middle ear and arrives at the cochlea.
- **Bone conduction** is the process by which an acoustic signal vibrates the bones of the skull to stimulate the cochlea. Vibrations of the skull bones can result from either acoustic or mechanical stimulation of the skull.

Sounds existing in the environment are usually heard via air conduction because the outer and middle ear systems are designed to provide an effective impedance transformer (i.e., a "bridge") between the impedance of the air in the environment and the impedance of the fluid of the cochlea (Chapter 8). Sounds in the air that reach other parts of the head are not transmitted efficiently to the cochlea because of the impedance mismatch between the low impedance of the air and the high impedance of the skull, skin, and other tissues. However, bone conduction plays an important role in sound reception in three circumstances:

- The reception of high-intensity sounds
- The reception of direct vibrations
- The reception of one's own voice

Reception of High-Intensity Sounds

Intense environmental sounds can evoke vibrations of the skull that are strong enough to create an auditory sensation. If the outer and middle ear systems are working normally, the contribution of vibrations transmitted through the head to the cochlea will be minimal compared to the contribution of the vibrations arriving at the cochlea via the air conduction pathway. If sounds are prevented from entering the air conduction pathway, however, then the bone conduction pathway will become an important or even the primary pathway. Barriers preventing sounds from traveling via the air conduction pathway include pathology of the outer and/or middle ear (conductive pathology) and hearing protection systems (e.g., earplugs and/or earmuffs). The fact that high-intensity sounds can be received via direct bone conduction pathways sets an upper limit on the effectiveness of individual hearing protection devices. In other words, if a sound is intense enough, it will get to the cochlea, even with the most effective earplugs and earmuffs. The difference in the sensitivity of human hearing to air conduction and bone conduction stimulation does not exceed 50 to 60 dB and it is frequency dependent. Some civilian and military noises have peak pressure levels as large as 180 to 190 dB and continuous pressure levels of 140 to 150 dB. Since the hearing protection offered by the best hearing protection devices cannot exceed the difference between air conduction and bone conduction sensitivity (i.e., 50 to 60 dB), the bone conduction transmitted sound can still be as intense as 130 dB (peak) and 90 dB (continuous). These sounds are still quite loud and detrimental to human hearing.

Reception of Direct Vibrations

Vibrations of the skull can be caused by sound waves propagating in the air as well as by mechanic vibrations applied directly to the skull through contact with the teeth, skin, or bones. When a mechanic force is applied directly to the structures of the head, the difference in impedance between the vibrating object and the head is relatively small and the transfer of energy to the skull is much more efficient than when the head vibrations are caused by sound waves. This type of mechanic stimulation occurs when a listener's head is placed in direct contact with a vibrating object, such as a piano or a loudspeaker box, or when a mechanic vibrator is applied to the head and held in place. Common mechanic vibrators include a **clinical bone vibrator**, which is a calibrated device used for hearing testing; a **communication bone vibrator**, which is used for speech communication in various commercial systems; and a **bone conduction hearing aid**, which is a hearing aid that directly vibrates the bones of the skull for patients with outer and/or middle ear pathology.

Reception of Own Voice

Vibrations of the skull can be produced not only by external stimulation, but also by a high acoustic pressure buildup in the upper throat during speech production, which is transferred to the surrounding structures. This bone conduction pathway, together with the air conduction pathway from the mouth and around the head to the ear, provides feedback to the talker that allows the talker to control voice level and monitor speech production. The fact that we hear ourselves differently when we speak compared to when we listen to our recorded voice is due primarily to the lack of bone conduction transmission when we listen to our recorded voice (and to a smaller extent, by the frequency response of the recording equipment). You can easily hear the difference in your voice when you record a phrase and play it back and then hear yourself saying it live. Consult the website for instructions on how to record and play back your voice on your PC. **Link 11-1**

Sounds generated within the vocal tract during speaking, chewing, and crunching food are not optimally transmitted to the ear via bone conduction, and this is a good thing.

Vowel sounds generated at the back of the pharyngeal cavity can be quite intense and reach 140 dB (Killion et al., 1988). If these sounds could effectively be transmitted to the cochlea, they would be a permanent source of hearing loss. In addition to the poor transmission of sound through the tissues, the middle ear acoustic reflex is activated prior to speaking, further protecting us from our own voices.

BONE CONDUCTION VIBRATION PATTERNS

The manner and the intensity with which the skull vibrates in response to a mechanic vibrator placed against the skull varies based on the frequency of the vibration and the placement of the vibrator (Békésy, 1932). Figure 11.1 illustrates the vibration pattern of the skull in response to a vibrator placed against the forehead.

As you can see in Figure 11.1A, at low frequencies around 200 Hz the entire skull vibrates back and forth as a unit. This type of vibration is called **inertial vibration.** At 800 Hz the direction of the motion is still the same but the vibration pattern changes and the back and the front of the skull move 180° out-of-phase. When different elements of a vibrating system move against each other, this type of vibration is called **compressional vibration.** This motion is shown in Figure 11.1B. At even higher frequencies the vibration mode of the skull changes again and around 1600 Hz the skull begins to vibrate as a combination of two perpendicular compressional vibrations (Fig. 11.1C). Similar vibration patterns can also be observed in the vertical direction (Békésy, 1932).

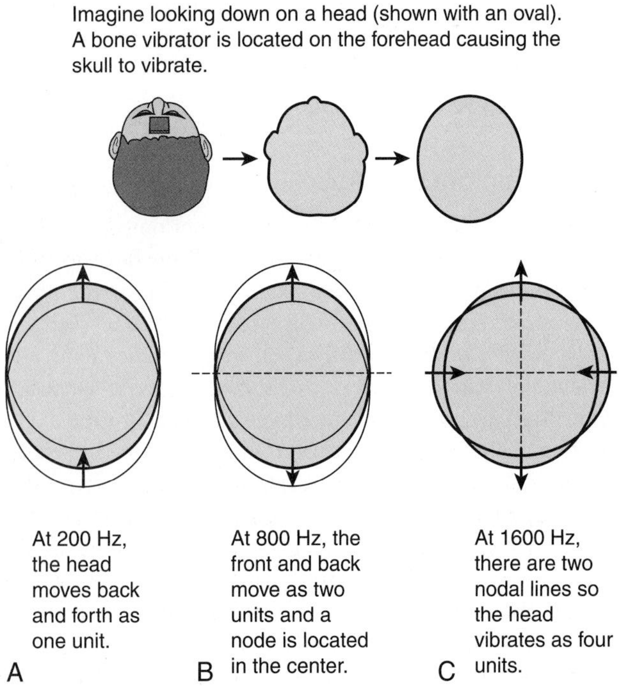
Imagine looking down on a head (shown with an oval). A bone vibrator is located on the forehead causing the skull to vibrate.
At 200 Hz, the head moves back and forth as one unit.
A
At 800 Hz, the front and back move as two units and a node is located in the center.
B
At 1600 Hz, there are two nodal lines so the head vibrates as four units.
C

Figure 11.1. Modes of bone conduction vibration for three different frequencies observed. (Based on von Békésy G. Zur theorie des hörens bei der schallaufnahme durch knochenleitung. *Ann Phys* 1932;13:111–136.)

The patterns of skull vibration shown in Figure 11.1 for 800 Hz and 1600 Hz are called the first compressional mode and the second compressional mode of skull vibration, respectively. The modal character of skull vibration is even more complex at very high frequencies, but the magnitude of these vibrations is very small and is effectively damped by the soft tissue surrounding the bones (Håkansson et al., 1994, 1986).

The main axes and magnitudes of both horizontal and vertical vibration depend on the location of the vibrator exciting the skull. In some cases, direct vibration of the head may also cause forced antiresonances of the skull. For example, for the mastoid placement of the vibrator, strong ipsilateral antiresonances can be observed around 400 Hz and 2000 Hz that may result in a stronger perception of the sound in the contralateral ear than in the ipsilateral ear (Stenfelt, 1999; Stenfelt et al., 1999; Tonndorf & Jahn, 1981; Zwislocki, 1953).

BONE CONDUCTION TRANSMISSION

Both the air-conducted signals and the bone-conducted signals ultimately arrive at the cochlea and produce vibrations of the basilar membrane, but the pathways taken by a bone-conducted signal are different from those taken by an air-conducted signal. Air-conducted signals travel along a single pathway extending from the pinna of the outer ear to the fluids of the inner ear. Bone-conducted signals vibrate multiple cranial and facial bones, cartilages, and soft tissue structures and through them excite the fluids of the inner ear. The skull vibrations and the sound waves propagating through the skull transfer some energy to the outer and middle ears, which additionally contribute to bone conduction hearing. Such complex and multifaceted vibrations of the head result in several mechanisms that contribute to the transmission of vibrations from the skull to the cochlea. In fact, Tonndorf (1966) described seven different ways by which the vibrations of the skull affect the cochlea, and Stenfelt and Goode (2005) indicated that five pathways were potential contributors to bone conduction. In general, all of the pathways of bone conduction can be grouped into three main mechanisms:

- The **inner ear mechanisms**
- The **middle ear mechanism**
- The **outer ear mechanism**

The primary pathway of bone conduction transmission is from the bones of the skull directly to the cochlea, without the involvement of the outer and middle ear; however, both the outer and the inner ear can contribute to the perception of bone-conducted sounds under some transmission conditions.

The Inner Ear Mechanism

Recall from Chapter 9 that the cochlea is housed in the bony labyrinth of the temporal bone. Vibrations of the skull cause the bony portions of the cochlea (including the walls of the labyrinth and the spiral lamina) to vibrate, moving the cochlear fluids and changing the size and shape of the cochlear cavity. This inner ear pathway consists of three mutually supportive mechanisms:

- Compressional cochlear mechanisms
  - First compressional cochlear mechanism
  - Second compressional cochlear mechanism
- Inertial cochlear mechanism

The Compressional Cochlear Mechanisms

The **first compressional cochlear mechanism,** also called the **distortional mechanism,** results from alternating compressions and expansions of the bony labyrinth, which cause changes in the shape and size of the cochlear cavity. The vibrations of the temporal bone cause the bony labyrinth to change its shape and volume, shown in Figure 11.2A. Because the scala vestibuli is larger than the scala tympani, the change in shape of the bony labyrinth results in an alternating upward and downward displacement of the basilar membrane (Tonndorf, 1962). The resulting upward and downward motion of the basilar membrane is similar to that created by the air conduction mechanism and it leads to the activation of the electrochemical processes in the hair cells and subsequently to auditory perception.

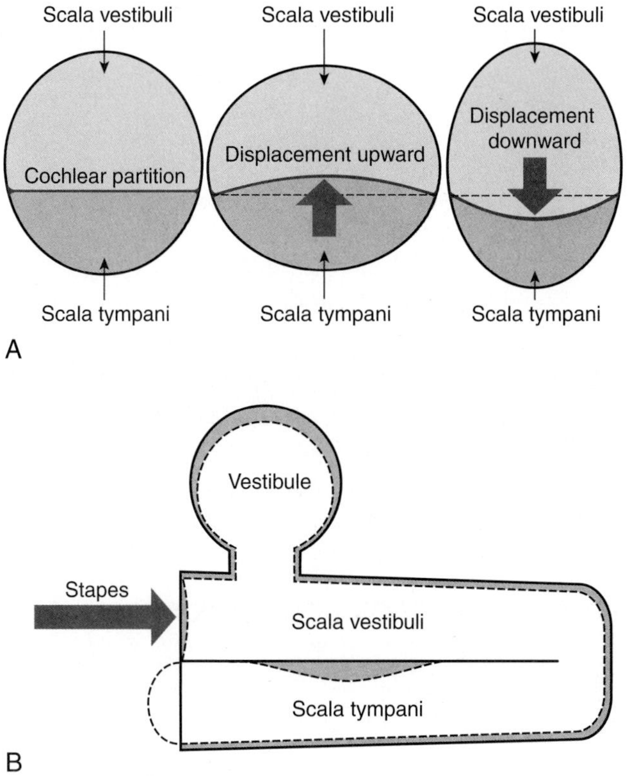

Figure 11.2. Bone conduction transmission based on the distortional mode **(A)** and the compressional mechanism **(B).** (From Gelfand SA. Essentials of Audiology. 2nd Ed. New York: Thieme, 2001. **(A)** Based on the work of Tonndorf J. Compressional bone conduction in cochlear models. *J Acoust Soc Am* 1962;34:1127–1131. **(B)** Based on the work of Bekesy von Békésy G. Zur theorie des hörens bei der schallaufnahme durch knochenleitung. *Ann Phys* 1932;13:111–136. Used with permission.)

The above behavior is supplemented by the difference in stiffness between the oval window and the round window that results in the second compressional cochlear mechanism. If the air conduction pathway is not activated, the stapes is fixed in the oval window. The membrane in the oval window membrane is not as mobile as the membrane of the round window. Recall that the bony labyrinth is filled with virtually incompressible fluid; to accommodate the changes in the size of the cochlear cavity due to temporal bone vibration, the oval and round windows must accommodate some amount of fluid. The difference in stiffness between both windows will cause the round window to bulge in and out more than the oval window (Fig. 11.2B), resulting in an additional mechanism forcing a displacement of the basilar membrane.

The compressional cochlear mechanisms are the oldest theoretical explanations of how vibrations of the skull conduct vibrations that are perceived as sound; however, recent research on temporal bones indicates that this mechanism may not play as significant a role in bone conduction transmission as previously thought and the inertial cochlear mechanism is most likely the primary bone conduction mode (Stenfelt & Goode, 2005).

The Inertial Cochlear Mechanism

The inertial cochlear mechanism is the result of the inertial lag between the movement of the walls of the bony labyrinth and the motion of the fluid and membranes within the bony labyrinth. Tonndorf (1966) observed that the cochlear fluids, oval window, and round window were only loosely coupled to the temporal bone and therefore lagged behind the motion of the bony walls. In addition, Stenfelt et al. (2003a) reported bone conduction hearing due to the inertial movement of the osseous spiral lamina. Therefore, the inertial mechanism of the cochlea can be considered as the sum of several separate inertial mechanisms associated with the fluids, the spiral lamina, and both windows. These mechanisms work in synergy with the compressional mechanisms of the cochlea resulting in the movements of the basilar membrane. The concept of inertia as it affects bone conduction is explained in more detail in the next section.

The Middle Ear Mechanism

The middle ear mechanism, also called the **inertial middle ear mechanism** or **ossicular-inertial mechanism,** is the result of bone vibration on the relative position and movement of the ossicular chain. Recall from Chapter 2 that inertia is the tendency of an object at rest to stay at rest and an object in motion to stay in motion until acted on by an outside force. Recall also (Chapter 8) that the ossicles are not rigidly attached to the skull but are suspended in the middle ear by a series of ligaments and muscles. The suspended nature of the ossicles results in their delayed movement in response to the vibrations of the surrounding temporal bone and constitutes the ossicular-inertial mechanism of bone conduction.

To understand the ossicular-inertial mode of bone conduction (and the cochlear fluid inertia from the previous section), imagine a car coming to a sudden stop. The car stops quickly but the driver does not stop as quickly and will lurch forward. This is due to the loose connection between the driver and the car. The effect of the stopping force on the driver's body is delayed and therefore the driver continues to travel for a short time due to the force of inertia. Now imagine a bone vibrator placed on the mastoid portion of the temporal bone that is forcing the skull to vibrate back and forth. When the skull moves back and forth, the ossicles also move back and forth, but with a slight time lag due to the relatively loose connection to the bones of the skull (temporal bone). This slight lag means that instead of the stapes moving in-phase with the bony wall that separates the middle and inner ears, it moves out-of-phase with the bony wall. This out-of-phase movement of the stapes and the surrounding bones makes the stapes move in and out of the oval window in the same way it does during sound transmission via the air conduction pathway (Chapters 8 and 9). Therefore, the inertia of the ossicular chain contributes to the perception of sound received through bone conduction stimulation.

The magnitude of the bone conduction effect caused by the ossicular-inertial mechanism of the middle ear is quite small compared to the inner ear component and it depends on the frequency of vibration and the location of the mechanic vibrator. A larger ossicular-inertial component is seen for a mastoid placement of a bone vibrator (i.e., on the side of the head) as opposed to a forehead placement. Common explanations for this include the fact that a bone vibrator placed on the side of the skull will result in more of a side-to-side vibration pattern of the skull compared to a greater front-to-back vibration pattern for a forehead placement of the vibrator. Since the normal motion of the ossicular chain is a side-to-side motion, this explains why a bone vibrator placed on the side of the head results in much more efficient bone conduction stimulation than the placement of the vibrator on the front of the head. The front-to-back vibration is perpendicular to the normal motion of the ossicles, creating almost no vibration due to the ossicular-inertial mechanism.

If a pathology in the middle ear (e.g., otosclerosis) causes the stapes to be more firmly fixed in the oval window niche than normal, then the ossicular-inertial mechanism of the middle ear may be decreased or absent (especially across the frequency range of resonance for the ossicles) and the overall bone conduction vibration reaching the cochlea will be decreased in intensity (Stenfelt et al., 2002). This change is indicated during hearing tests and it is used to help in the diagnosis of middle ear pathology.*

*The diagnostic pattern seen on a hearing test for a patient with otosclerosis is called a "Carhart Notch." A Carhart Notch is a decrease in bone conduction hearing ability around 2000 Hz because of the reduction of vibration of the ossicles near their resonance frequency.

The Outer Ear Mechanism

The outer ear contribution to bone conduction transmission is another bone conduction compressional mechanism. This mechanism has also been called the **osteotympanic mechanism,** although this name may be somewhat misleading, since "osteo" means bone and some researchers have indicated that it is actually the cartilaginous portion of the ear canal that is the primary cause of this component (Stenfelt & Goode, 2005). The outer ear mechanism only plays a role in bone conduction when the outer ear is closed, for example, by an earphone or a hearing aid. Békésy (1932), Stenfelt et al. (2003b), and others observed that when the ear canal is closed, the sound caused by bone vibration becomes louder. The increase in the perceived intensity of bone-conducted sounds caused by the occlusion (covering) of the external ear is called the **occlusion effect.** The occlusion effect is primarily a low-frequency phenomenon and it depends on the volume of the occluded space. The sound pressure increase in the ear canal due to the occlusion effect may be as large as 20 to 25 dB (Berger & Kerivan, 1983; Watson & Gales, 1943).

To experience the occlusion effect, hum with both of your ears open. Keep humming and occlude one ear by pushing your ear lobe over your ear canal or sticking a finger in your ear canal. You should hear the sound of your voice become louder in the covered (plugged) ear. This is due to the fact that during bone conduction (and humming is conducted to the ear primarily by bone conduction), the vibrations of the head cause vibrations of the walls of the ear canals. When ears are unoccluded, most of the energy created from these vibrations will leave the ear canal via the external auditory meatus because sound waves always take the "path of least resistance." Since the tympanic membrane offers greater resistance to the flow of energy than the open meatus, the opening of the ear canal provides a natural outlet for sound energy to exit the ear canal. When the ears are occluded, however, the acoustic energy from the vibrations of the ear canal walls is transmitted via the tympanic membrane to the middle and then inner ear. This additional energy arriving at the cochlea is part of the bone conduction signal, adding to the magnitude of vibration at the cochlea.

BONE CONDUCTION COMMUNICATION

It is important to recall that vibrations of the skull bones can be produced by both external stimulation and by the person's own speech or other vocal production. Therefore, it is possible to record the bone vibrations of a talker and use them as a communication signal. These signals can be delivered to another person through a bone vibrator, creating a bone conduction communication system. The system can operate in a two-way mode; that is, a person can wear both a vibrator and a **contact microphone** and be able to both receive and transmit speech signals.

Bone conduction recordings are made using a special microphone that is sensitive to vibration. This type of microphone is called a contact microphone. Contact microphones can be placed on the surface of the human head to record skull vibration or they can be placed on any vibrating object to capture its vibrations. For example, musicians attach contact microphones to various elements of musical instruments to obtain special music effects or just to enhance the volume of sound produced by the instrument. Transducers based on the same principle (i.e., converting vibration to electrical and then acoustic signals) are also used to convert vibrations from the old-fashioned gramophone (record player) needle into an electrical signal. More information about various types of transducers and their characteristics is included in Chapter 14.

One important advantage of contact microphones over traditional air microphones is that they are much less sensitive to external noise and can be used effectively in noisy environments. A view of a commercial bone conduction communication system is shown in Figure 11.3.

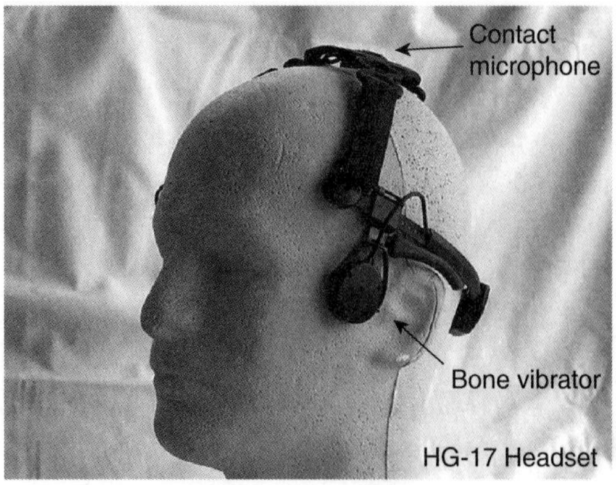

Figure 11.3. Bone conduction communication system. (Photograph courtesy of Canadian Wireless Technologies, www.canadianwireless.ca.)

When a contact microphone is placed on the head of the talker to record the talker's voice, the preferred location for a bone conduction microphone is on the jaw or on the top of the head rather than on the side of the head, which is the preferred location for a clinical bone vibrator. This is due to the fact that the air flow in the vocal tract and the movements of the jaw bone during speech production cause the strongest skull vibration in up-and-down and front-to-back (midsagittal plane) directions rather than a side-to-side direction. All other rules regarding impedance matching and the need for good contact with the head apply equally to bone vibrators and contact microphones. In addition, both require the device to be in a stable position and placed in a manner comfortable for the user.

Summary

Bone conduction is the process of receiving auditory signals through vibrations of the skull and associated soft tissue. Bone conduction plays an important role in sound reception in three circumstances: when high-intensity acoustic waves cause skull vibrations strong enough to be heard, when vibrations of the skull are made by direct contact with mechanical vibrations, and when vibrations of the skull are caused by the talker's own speech production. In bone conduction, low frequencies cause the entire skull to vibrate back and forth as a unit (inertial vibration) and higher frequencies cause portions of the skull to vibrate out-of-phase with each other (compressional vibration). Transmission of bone vibrations involves inner ear, middle ear, and outer ear structures.

The inner ear mechanisms consist of two compressional mechanisms, by which the size and shape of the cochlea change, and an inertial mechanism, which results from the inertial lag between the movement of the walls of the bony labyrinth and the motion of the fluid and membranes within the bony labyrinth. The middle ear mechanism is due to the inertial lag between the ossicles and the skull. The outer ear mechanism results from the vibrations of the ear canal walls, which vibrate the air in the ear canal. When the ear canal is open, the sound energy created in the ear canal exits the ear and the mechanism is not as effective. When the ear canal is occluded, however, the sound energy in the canal is entrapped and forced to enter the middle ear through tympanic membrane vibrations. The primary component of bone conduction is the inner ear component.

Bone conduction can be used as a means of speech communication. Bone-conducted signals can be received through contact microphones (talker) and delivered through bone vibrators to another person (listener). Such communication systems are mainly used by the military and people working in high noise conditions since they are not sensitive to environmental noise.

Key Points

- Air-conducted signals travel from the pinna to the middle ear to the inner ear, whereas bone-conducted signals vibrate multiple structures in the head and through them transfer energy to the inner ear.
- The effect of bone conduction depends on the location of the applied force, the type of coupling between the force and the head, and the impedance matching between the source of force and the head structures.
- High-intensity environmental sounds can cause skull vibrations strong enough to cause an auditory sensation, but bone conduction is not the primary pathway of sound reception by a person with normal hearing.
- Bone conduction and air conduction are involved in the feedback system used by a talker to monitor speech production.
- At low frequencies, the entire skull vibrates back and forth as a unit (inertial vibration). At higher frequencies, portions of the skull vibrate out-of-phase with each other (compressional vibration).
- The occlusion effect is an increase in intensity of the bone-conducted sound when the ear canal is closed (occluded) compared with an unoccluded ear canal.

CHAPTER 12

Psychoacoustics

Chapter Outline

Objectives

- To describe the relationship between the acoustic characteristics of intensity, frequency, duration, and spectral complexity and the perceptual characteristics of loudness, pitch, perceived duration, and timbre
- To introduce the concept of threshold and discuss methods of determining absolute and difference thresholds
- To review signal detection theory and how listener bias affects the hit rate and false alarm rate in a detection task
- To discuss psychophysical scales used in psychoacoustics and hearing science
- To review the concept of masking
- To define the critical band and discuss how the critical band influences auditory perception
- To discuss various aspects of binaural perception and spatial hearing

Key Terms

Absolute threshold
Auditory response area
Backward masking
Bark
Bark scale
Bias
Binaural advantage
Critical band
Cone of confusion
Detection threshold
Difference limen (DL)
Difference threshold
Discriminability index (d-prime, d′)
Equal-loudness curve
Fechner's Law
Forward masking
Hearing area
Judgment
Just noticeable difference (jnd)
Listener
Lateralization
Loudness
Loudness level
Loudness scale
Masking
Mel scale
Metathetic continuum
Method of Adjustment
Method of Constant Stimuli
Method of Limits
Minimum audible angle (MAA)
Minimum audible movement angle (MAMA)
N-Alternative Forced Choice (nAFC) technique
Ogive curve
Paired comparison
Perception
Periodicity pitch
Phon
Pitch
Probability (p)
Prothetic continuum
Psychoacoustics
Psychophysical function
Psychophysics
Recognition threshold

Receiver operating characteristic (ROC)
Response bias
Response criterion (β)
Scale
Sensation
Sensation magnitude
Simultaneous masking
Sone scale
Sound Quality
Spatial orientation
Speech range
Stevens' Power Law
Stimulus magnitude
Temporal masking
Terminal threshold
Test stimuli
Threshold
Threshold of hearing
Timbre
Trained listener
Upward spread of masking
Weber's fraction
Weber's Law
YN (yes–no) technique

Psychoacoustics is the study of the relationship between the acoustic world and our auditory image of this world. It is a branch of **psychophysics**, which is the study of the relationship between the physical world and the perceptual world across all of the senses: hearing, taste, vision, smell, and touch. The term *psychophysics* was originally introduced by Gustav Theodore Fechner (1801–1887), a German psychologist, in his book *Elemente der Psychophysik* (1869). The perceptual world includes our sensations and perceptions. **Sensation** is the awareness of an external stimulus or some change in the internal state of the body caused by an external stimulus. **Perception** is the act of recognition and interpretation of a stimulus based on previous experiences. The result of a perception is a new experience that is added to our knowledge base as part of the cognitive process involving learning by experience. Examples of auditory sensations are loudness, pitch, and the sensation of a sound source moving from the left to the right. Examples of perceptual processes are speech recognition, voice identification, and recognition of a tune based on two or more sounds.

The measurement of sensation is called **psychophysical measurement** or psychophysical testing. Physical stimuli used in psychophysical measurement are called **test stimuli** and human responses to these stimuli are called **judgments.** Psychophysical measurement is a far more complex task than the measurement of the physical characteristics of a stimulus. Human responses are highly variable and are greatly influenced by instructions, listener bias, fatigue, anticipation, external and internal noise, attention, motivation, and so forth. In addition, the perceptual reaction of a listener involves complex probabilities that are affected by the stimulus itself and by all the factors listed above. Thus, each perceptual reaction has some degree of uncertainty and the same stimulus may be heard or missed if the probabilities change.

An acoustic stimulus may be expected or not. It also may be heard or not. If a person expects to hear an auditory stimulus, we call this person a **listener.** The fact that the person could actually miss the stimulus is irrelevant. This person is still a listener. Thus, the acts of hearing and listening are not the same process. We are physically able to hear many sounds in our everyday environment, but our central auditory nervous system "tunes out" most of them to protect us from the overwhelming onslaught of sounds that enter the ears all day long. To actually listen to a sound involves a conscious effort—we must focus on the sound of interest. The more people actively listen to sound, the better they become at detecting subtle changes in sounds. The listening experience and familiarity with both the sounds of interest and the surrounding acoustic environment greatly affect human ability to detect and recognize sound sources. People who know how to listen are referred to in the psychoacoustics literature as **trained listeners.** A trained listener is simply a listener who is able to detect subtle changes in a sound better than other listeners having the same physiologic capabilities. One may become a trained listener by specialized training, by experience gained from participation in psychoacoustic experiments, or by customarily performing listening-related tasks, such as those performed by car mechanics or speech-language pathologists. You may actually have had listening training in the past without being aware of it. If you are a musician or if you have studied a foreign language, you have received some listening training. Over the course of your training, you probably noticed that you were able to more easily detect subtle changes in sounds than before your training began.

In the acoustics portion of this book we discussed the main physical characteristics of acoustic stimuli: intensity, frequency, duration, and spectral complexity. When these stimuli act on human hearing, they become auditory stimuli and the physical characteristics of sound are reflected in an auditory image (i.e., as a sensation of sound). The sensations generally associated with intensity, frequency, duration, and spectral complexity are loudness, pitch, perceived duration, and timbre. As a general rule, when intensity increases, loudness increases; when frequency increases, pitch increases; when duration increases, perceived duration increases; and when spectral complexity changes, the perception is a change in timbre. The relationship between the physical and the perceptual worlds, however, is far from simple, and changes in each category of perception can be caused by changes in more than one acoustic parameter. For example, an increase in intensity usually causes an increase in loudness, but it also may be perceived as a change in pitch, even if the frequency does not change. This chapter will examine the connection between physical stimuli and the psychological impressions that these stimuli evoke.

THRESHOLDS AND SCALES

Psychophysical testing involves the determination of perceptual thresholds and the development of psychophysical scales. Perceptual **threshold** is the point at which the intensity level of a stimulus is just large enough to cause a change in the mental response of a person affected by the stimulus. For example, a hearing threshold is the lowest sound intensity level at which a listener can barely detect the presence of a sound. A psychophysical **scale** is a graded measure of a specific sensation in which a faint sensation is located on one end of the scale and an increase in the degree of stimulation is associated with a point farther along the scale. An example of a *physical* scale is the sound intensity scale, which is a tool for comparing the acoustic energy of various sounds using sound measurement equipment. An example of a *psychophysical* scale is a loudness scale, which is a tool for comparing the perceived strength of various sounds based on human responses.

Perceptual Thresholds

To step across the threshold of a doorway is to pass from the outside to the inside of a house. To pass through a perceptual threshold is to pass from one mental state to another. There are three types of psychological thresholds: absolute thresholds, terminal thresholds, and difference thresholds. An **absolute threshold** is the minimum value of a stimulus that elicits a specific reaction. Examples of absolute thresholds are the threshold of hearing or the threshold of touch. Absolute perceptual thresholds can be either sensory thresholds ("I hear speech") or cognitive thresholds ("I understand speech").

A **terminal threshold** is the maximum value of a stimulus that elicits a given response. A terminal threshold separates stimuli that produce a specific perceptual response from those that do not because their magnitudes are too large. An example of a terminal threshold is the intensity at which the sensation caused by a sound changes from an auditory sensation to a pain sensation.

A **difference threshold** is the smallest physical difference between two stimuli in which a listener can determine that the two stimuli are perceptually different. Examples of difference thresholds are the smallest noticeable difference in the pitch of a sound and the smallest noticeable difference in the perception of the direction of an incoming sound.

Absolute Threshold

Unlike a threshold across a doorway, an absolute perceptual threshold is not a narrow, well-defined border between two types of sensation. When a stimulus is at about the threshold level, it will be noticed sometimes and not noticed at other times, depending on the plethora of factors mentioned at the beginning of this chapter. This situation is shown in Figure 12.1. The less intense (e.g., quieter) the stimulus, the smaller the percentage of times the stimulus will be detected. The more intense the stimulus, the greater percentage of times it

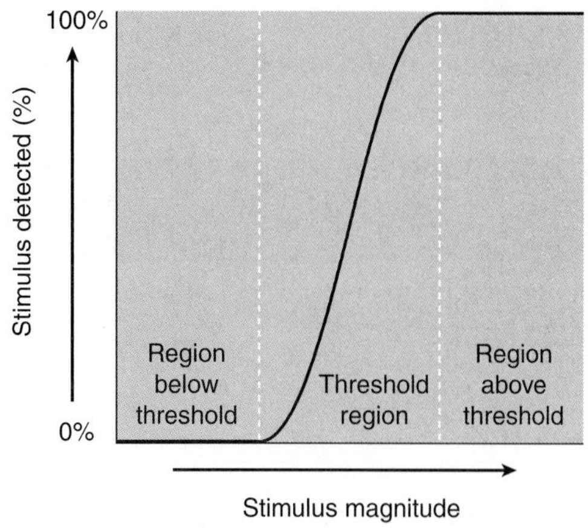

Figure 12.1. Threshold is not a quick step between always not noticeable and always noticeable stimuli or events.

will be detected. Thus, an absolute threshold is a value on a continuum somewhere between the points at which a sound will never be detected (0%) and will always be detected (100%). The percentage value that represents threshold can be chosen arbitrarily; for most applications, however, the absolute threshold is defined as the magnitude of a stimulus that elicits a specific response 50% of the time.

The curve shown in Figure 12.1 is a generic growth curve showing changes in a living organism's response due to changes in environmental conditions. These changes may be applicable to sensation, population growth, and progress of training. The *x* axis can be stimulus intensity. The curve shown in Figure 12.1 is referred to in literature as an **ogive curve** (logistic curve, logistic function, sigmoid curve, S-curve).

An absolute threshold can be either a detection threshold (sensory threshold) or a recognition threshold (cognitive threshold). **Detection threshold** is the lowest intensity of a stimulus that can be detected a specific percentage of times, usually 50%. **Recognition threshold** is the lowest intensity of a stimulus at which the stimulus can be recognized a specific percentage of time, usually 50%. Two common techniques used to determine detection thresholds are:

1. **YN (yes–no) technique:** The listener is given a number of trials with some of them containing a signal and some of them not containing a signal. The listener is asked to respond *yes* or *no* at each trial.
2. **N-Alternative Forced Choice (nAFC) technique:** The listener is presented with a number (*n*) of observation intervals. The signal is present during only one of the intervals and the listener must indicate which of the intervals contained the signal.

There are many different experimental procedures that utilize the above techniques, which can be fixed or adaptive. In a fixed procedure, subsequent trials are not dependent on each other and each trial contains a signal that was predetermined by the experimenter. In an adaptive procedure, the stimulus presented during each trial is dependent on the previous responses of the person responding to the stimuli.

PRACTICE PROBLEMS: ABSOLUTE THRESHOLD

Examine the graph below and answer questions 1 through 4.

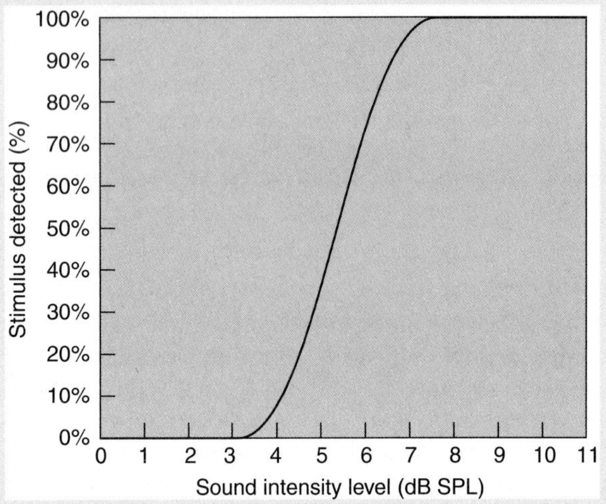

1. What percentage of the time would you expect a listener to respond to a signal presented at 4 dB SPL?
2. If the percentage criterion for determining the detection threshold is 50%, what is the detection threshold based on this figure?
3. If the percentage criterion for determining the detection threshold is 75%, what is the detection threshold based on this figure?
4. Based on the above figure, you notice that a listener can detect a 5-dB SPL signal a specific percentage of the time. How large does the signal intensity need to be for a listener to detect it twice as often as a 5-dB SPL signal?

Answers (If you need help with these problems, consult the website.) **Link 12-1**

1. Approximately 8% of the time
2. Approximately 5.6 dB SPL
3. Approximately 6.4 dB SPL
4. Approximately 6.1 dB

Signal Detection Theory

The main reason that the threshold of detection fluctuates in time even when the stimuli remain the same is that even under optimal operational conditions, some amount of time-varying noise is generated both outside and within the person's body, forcing the person to make a decision regarding whether the specific signal is embedded in noise or if he or she is just hearing the noise alone. In addition, each person responding to stimulation develops an internal criterion that dictates how the person responds to a specific task under the condition of uncertainty. These criteria are called **response bias (response criteria)**. The effects of noise and human bias on the detection of signals in noise are the focus of signal detection theory.

Signal detection theory (SDT) is a method of examining (1) the difficulty of the decision-making process in which people must differentiate between two classes of items (e.g., signal or noise, day or night, friend or foe) and (2) the **bias** favoring a particular type of response (e.g., the probability that you are more likely to identify someone as a friend or as a foe if you are not sure). As applied to sound detection, SDT assesses the probability that a listener will respond to a sound when the specific intensities of the stimulus and the noise are known. **Probability** is the likelihood that an event will occur under specific circumstances. For example, if you roll a six-sided die, the probability that you will roll a one is one sixth. The probability can be written as a decimal or a fraction ($1/6 = 0.17$) or it can be multiplied by 100 and reported as a percentage ($0.17 \times 100 = 17\%$). So the probability of rolling a 1 on a six-sided die is 0.17 or 17% for each roll of the die. Similarly, the probability of not rolling a 1 is five sixths or 83%. A coin toss is also governed by the rules of probability. A coin toss can result in a "head" or "tail"; thus, there are two possible outcomes and the probability of each of them occurring is 0.50 (or 50%) assuming that the coin is equally balanced. The probabilities associated with human response to acoustic signals are a bit more complex because they depend on three elements: the stimulus, the noise, and listener bias.

If an experimenter presents a tone to a listener and asks whether the tone is present or not, the listener usually has two* possible responses. The listener could indicate that a tone was heard (*yes*) or the listener could indicate that a tone was not heard (*no*) or could do nothing, which is generally equated with a *no* response. When the intensity of a tone is close to the threshold of detection, the decision may be difficult. Imagine a listener who is taking a hearing test, and she needs to do well on the test to keep her job. Under these conditions, she may decide to respond that she heard a tone even if she is not really sure. With this type of bias, she will most likely indicate that she heard a tone even when a tone is not actually presented. Conversely, imagine a listener who does not want to make a mistake by saying he heard a tone that was not there. With this type of bias, he will most likely wait to respond until he is absolutely sure that a tone is present, so he will most likely miss several low-intensity sounds.

There are four outcomes (possibilities) associated with a detection task. These outcomes are often reported in a 2 × 2 decision table shown in Figure 12.2. The names in each box in Figure 12.2 indicate the type of outcome. If a sound is

*In some cases the listener is allowed to select one out of three possible responses: "Yes," "No," and "I do not know."

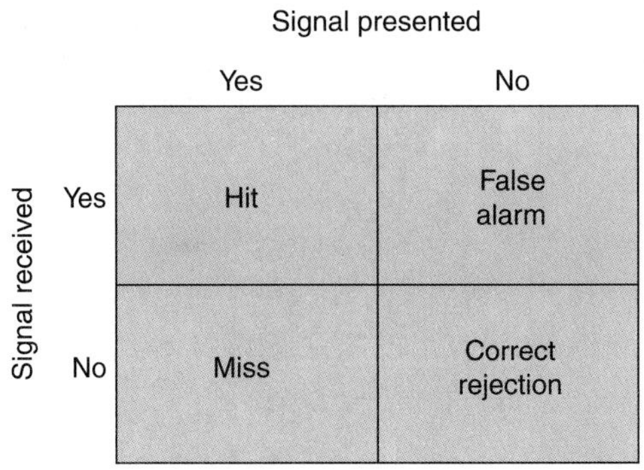

Figure 12.2. The four possible outcomes of a yes–no detection task shown as a 2 × 2 decision table.

presented and a listener responds to it, this outcome is called a "hit." If a sound is presented and the listener fails to respond to it, this outcome is called a "miss." If no sound is presented but the listener responds that the sound is present, this outcome is called a "false alarm," and, finally, if no sound is presented and the listener does not respond, this outcome is called a "correct rejection." Like a coin toss, if a signal is actually presented, the response can only result in two types of outcome: either a hit or a miss. Therefore, the probability of a hit added to the probability of a miss must equal one; that is, H + M = 1. Similarly, if a signal is NOT presented, the response must be either a false alarm or a correct rejection. Therefore, the combined probability of a false alarm and correct rejection is equal to one; that is, FA + CR = 1. If detection tasks were easy and responses were perfect, all of the responses would fall into either hit or correct rejection categories. Human responses are not perfect, however, and there is uncertainty in every decision task.

Data analysis used by signal detection theory is based on the relationship shown in Figure 12.3. The *x* axis represents the magnitude of some internal response to a specific physical variable. The internal response could be the perceived intensity of sound expressed in some arbitrary units (psychological response) or it could be the rate of nerve firing in the auditory system (physiologic response). The two curves in Figure 12.3 represent changes in the probability of generating a certain internal response when either noise alone or noise and signal are present. The probability of the response "I hear only noise" varies with the magnitude of the internal response according to a bell curve representing a Gaussian distribution,* and this shape is represented in Figure 12.3. This is the probability distribution function of the noise level that may exist at a given moment in time. The height and the width of this curve will vary depending on the specific processes affecting the internal response.

When no signal is present, only the random fluctuating activity (noise) of the external and internal environments of the listener affects the listener's decision. This situation is

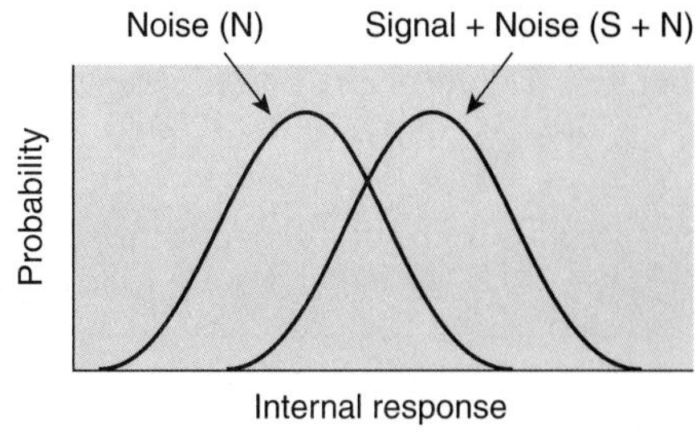

Figure 12.3. The probability functions for internal responses generated by noise (*N*) and signal plus noise (*S* + *N*).

represented by the left noise (*N*) curve. The curve to the right represents the presence of both the signal and the noise (*S* + *N*). The noise never goes away in a detection task (i.e., there is always the perception of some amount of noise), so it will always affect the decision process. Notice in Figure 12.3 that the *N* and *S* + *N* curves overlap, so sometimes the same internal signal can be generated by either the *N* or the *S* + *N* curve.

The probability distribution functions shown in Figure 12.3 are shown again in a different manner in Figure 12.4. The new element of Figure 12.4 is the response criterion (β) (listener response bias) shown by an additional vertical line. This line indicates the point on the internal response scale that the listener has chosen as the response criterion, that is, as the minimal value on the internal response scale indicating that the signal is present. If the internal response is lower than the response criterion, then the listener responds that the signal is not present. If the internal response is higher than the response criterion, then the listener responds that the signal is present. The four categories of response from the 2 × 2 decision table shown in Figure 12.2 are superimposed on Figure 12.4 and indicated by different shading patterns. If the *S* + *N* creates an internal response greater than the response criterion, the listener will respond with "yes" and this will be classified as a hit. If the *S* + *N* creates an internal response less than the criterion, the listener will respond with "no" and this will be classified as a miss.

If the vertical line indicating the response criterion passes through the point where the *N* and *S* + *N* distributions intersect (cross each other), this response criterion is called

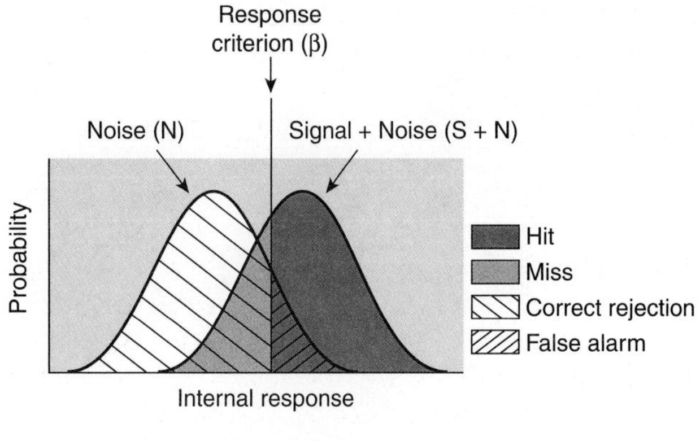

Figure 12.4. The four possible response categories based on a specific response criterion (β) of the listener.

*The Gaussian distribution is frequently referred to as a normal distribution because it is the most common distribution of natural events.

the ideal criterion ($\beta = 1$) since it does not favor either of the distributions. The ideal criterion represents the concept of an ideal observer (listener). If the response criterion of a listener is to the left of the ideal criterion, then $\beta < 1$ and this listener is called a liberal listener. If the response criterion of a listener is located to the right of the ideal criterion, then $\beta > 1$ and this listener is called a conservative listener. Recall from the previous discussion the woman who did not want to miss any tones because she would lose her job. Her response criterion (β) would be located to the left compared to the response criterion of the man who was waiting to respond "yes" until he was pretty sure he heard a signal. If the response criterion moves to the left, the hit rate increases but so does the false alarm rate. If the response criterion moves to the right, the false alarm rate decreases but so does the hit rate. In this type of response task, there will always be errors (e.g., misses and false alarms) if the noise and noise and signal distributions overlap.

In the situation shown in Figure 12.4, the only way to increase the hit rate and decrease the false response rate at the same time is to separate the *N* and *S* + *N* distributions on the internal response scale. This may be achieved by decreasing the average noise level, which is rarely possible, or by increasing the signal intensity level, which may not always be possible. The separation between the *N* and *S* + *N* distributions is typically measured with a statistic called the **discriminability index** or **d-prime** (d') shown in Figure 12.5A. D-prime varies from 0 (completely overlapping distributions) to 4 (almost no overlap between distributions) or more.

The relationship between the hit rate and the false response rate as a function of d' is shown in Figure 12.5B. This relationship is commonly called a **receiver operating characteristic (ROC).**

The *x* axis in Figure 12.5B indicates the false alarm rate and the *y* axis indicates the hit rate. Each curve in the figure corresponds to a specific value of d'. Optimally, a test result will have a high hit rate and a low false alarm rate, which requires a large d'. In addition, moving from the left to the right side of the ROC graph along any specific d' curve corresponds to a change in the response criterion (β) of the listener from more strict (right side of the curve) to more lax (left side of the curve). Knowing the hit and false alarm rates of a specific listener and knowing the ROC curves for the specific test, we are able to determine the difficulty level (d') of the test for the listener as well as the response bias (β) of the listener.

PRACTICE PROBLEMS: USING SIGNAL DETECTION THEORY

1. If d' is equal to zero and the probability of a hit is 0.5, what is the probability of a false alarm?
2. If d' is equal to 2 and the false alarm rate is 0.25, what is the probability of a hit?
3. What would the hit rate be if the false alarm rate is 0.75 and d' is equal to 2?
4. What would the miss rate be if the false alarm rate is 0.5 and d' is equal 1?

Answers (If you need help with these problems, consult the website.) **Link 12-2**

1. 0.5
2. Approximately 0.88
3. 1
4. About 0.2

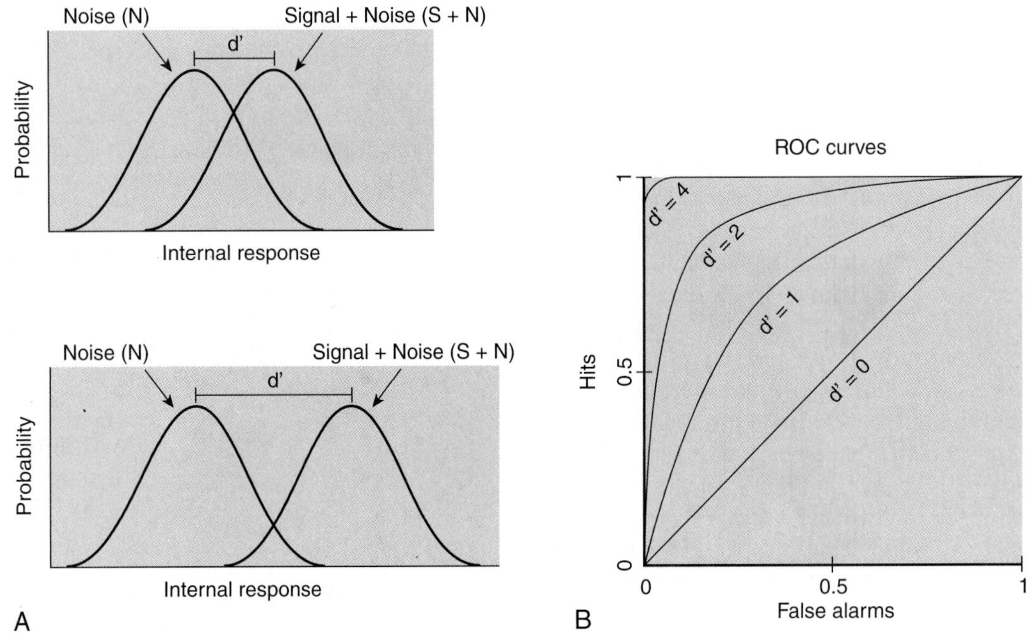

Figure 12.5. (A) Two distributions that differ in the amount of overlap and therefore in their d' value. **(B)** Receiver operating characteristic (ROC) indicating the relationship between the hit rate and false alarm rate for four values of d-prime.

Difference Threshold

The difference threshold, also called the **difference limen (DL)** or **just noticeable difference (jnd)**, is the smallest change in a stimulus that can produce a change in sensation. Similar to the absolute threshold, the DL is a statistical measure and it is calculated as a percent of specific responses (usually 75%). The reason that the DL value is set at 75% and not at 50% is because the outcome of simple same–different comparisons is greatly affected by guessing. The effect of guessing is discussed further in the Psychophysical Methods section.

One way to determine the DL is to listen to and compare several test sounds, which change gradually on a specific characteristic, against a reference sound that is fixed on that characteristic. The DL is the smallest difference that is just barely audible between the test sound and the reference sound. Depending on the type of DL that is measured, the test sounds can differ in intensity, frequency, duration, and so forth. The same two psychophysical techniques (yes–no and forced choice) that are used to determine absolute thresholds are also used to determine difference thresholds, but their specific technical forms are obviously slightly different.

The result of a DL measurement can be expressed in absolute or relative form. Let us assume, for example, that we use a 1000-Hz tone at 40 dB SPL as the reference tone and vary the frequency of the test tone until we find the frequency that is just noticeably different. If we find that the smallest noticeable difference between both tones is 4 Hz, the DL expressed in absolute form would be 4 Hz. Using a relative scale, we can also express the same DL for frequency as a fraction or percentage. Such a fraction can be written as:

$$DL(f) = \frac{\Delta f}{f} \qquad (12.1)$$

where $DL(f)$ is the difference limen for frequency, Δf is the absolute change in the signal frequency that corresponds to DL sensation, and f is the magnitude of the reference tone. In the case described above:

$$DL(f) = \frac{4\text{ Hz}}{1000\text{ Hz}} = 0.004$$

or

$$DL(f) = \frac{4\text{ Hz}}{1000\text{ Hz}} \times 100\% = 0.4\%$$

In Chapter 7 we discussed the fact that a human's reactions to stimuli are based on relative changes in stimulus magnitude and not on absolute changes. It is easier to notice a 1-kg change in a mass if the mass changes from 1 to 2 kg (a 100% change) than when it changes from 101 to 102 kg (a 1% change). This is a manifestation of the general property of human perception that the smallest perceived change in stimulus intensity is proportional to the stimulus magnitude. This general functional relationship was originally developed by Ernst Heinrich Weber (1795–1878), a German physiologist who is considered, together with Gustav Fechner and Hermann Helmholtz, as one of the three fathers of psychophysics. This general functional relationship is known as

Weber's Law. Weber's Law states that the stimulus needs to be changed by a constant percentage of its initial value for this change to be perceived. Weber's Law can be expressed mathematically as:

$$\frac{\Delta I}{I} = K \qquad (12.2)$$

where ΔI is the smallest perceived increment, I is the original magnitude of the stimulus, and K is a constant called the **Weber fraction.** The Weber fraction is dependent on the type of stimulus and its specific characteristics.

Although Weber's Law is a good general approximation of human reaction to changes in a stimulus, it does not hold at the absolute thresholds of perception for sound intensity. To compensate for the baseline magnitude of the stimulation that must be surpassed to establish a linear relationship between the magnitude and the perceived increment, the equation representing Weber's Law can be modified as follows:

$$\frac{\Delta I}{I + I_0} = K \qquad (12.3)$$

where I_0 is the sound intensity corresponding to the absolute threshold of perception and depends on the specific stimulus and its characteristics. This modified Weber fraction is useful when stimuli are presented at a sound intensity close to the threshold of sensation (0 dB SL to about 20 dB SL).

PRACTICE PROBLEMS: CALCULATING DIFFERENCE THRESHOLD

1. Determine the DL in relative terms if the absolute change in the signal frequency is 35 Hz and the magnitude of the reference tone is 5000 Hz.
2. What is the DL in absolute terms if the relative change in the signal frequency is 10% and the magnitude of the reference tone is 3000 Hz?
3. Using Equation 12.3, determine the value of ΔI if a listener's threshold is 2×10^{-4} Pa, the reference stimulus is 4×10^{-4} Pa, and the modified Weber fraction is equal to 10%.
4. Two studies reported DL values for sound intensity as 15% and 1.5 dB. Which of these two values is higher and by how much?

Answers (If you need help with these problems, consult the website.) **Link 12-3**

1. 0.007
2. 300 Hz
3. 0.000042 Pa or 4.2×10^{-5} Pa
4. The first value (15% or 0.6 dB) is lower than the second value (1.5 dB) by 0.9 dB.

Psychophysical Methods

Psychophysical measurements of absolute and differential thresholds can be made using various variants of YN and nAFC measurement techniques, but all of these variants have their origin in three classical psychophysical methods:

1. **Method of Limits,** in which the stimulus is gradually increased and decreased until the threshold has been reached
2. **Method of Constant (Random) Stimuli,** in which the value of the stimulus in individual trials is determined at random
3. **Method of Adjustment,** in which a listener manually adjusts the stimuli presented in the subsequent trials until the stimuli meet a predetermined threshold criterion

The Method of Constant Stimuli results in the most precise threshold values, but it is also the most time consuming of the three methods and it is generally reserved for research studies. It also requires a preliminary prediction of the threshold value to make the threshold determination feasible in a realistic time. In other words, it requires the selection of a "ballpark" intensity that the examiner expects to be close to the threshold value and the placement of all the presentation levels around this value. The Method of Adjustment helps the listener to focus on the required task and is well suited for tests that require long listening sessions; this method is both time efficient and attractive to listeners because of their direct involvement in the stimulus manipulation. The Method of Limits is the easiest of the three methods and relatively quick. It offers an optimal combination of time effectiveness and test reliability so it is the most common clinical procedure used for hearing testing. All three methods were first formally described by Fechner in his book *Elemente der Psychophysik* (1869, 1966).

The Method of Limits uses a series of stimuli with gradually increasing (ascending) and decreasing (descending) magnitudes and defines the threshold as a *change* in the listener's response. An example of this procedure is shown in Figure 12.6A. If the series is ascending, the change is from no (−) to yes (+). If the series is descending, the change is from yes (+) to no (−).

Hearing testing in the field of audiology is generally conducted using a modified Method of Limits such as the one recommended by the American Speech-Language-Hearing Association (ASHA) (1978). An example of an application of the ASHA method is shown in Figure 12.6B. The ASHA method (which is based on the up 5, down 10 procedure first described by Hughson & Westlake, 1944) begins with either an ascending trial (shown in Fig. 12.6B) or a descending trial (not pictured) to locate the approximate threshold region. When the listener's response changes from "no" to "yes," the actual threshold search begins. The intensity of the signal is decreased in 10-dB steps in response to a "yes" and increased in 5-dB steps in response to a "no." Threshold is determined as the lowest intensity level at which the response is at least 50%, with a minimum of three responses at that level.

To measure absolute threshold using the Method of Constant Stimuli, both the YN and the nAFC techniques can be used. The YN technique calls for the experimenter to select several signals of different intensity and present them in a random order. All of the selected signals (e.g., 2, 4, 6, 8, 10, and 12 dB SPL) are presented the same number of times and threshold is determined as the intensity at which a signal is detected 50% of the time.

A serious limitation of the YN procedure is that the obtained data depend on the guessing strategies used by the listener. For example, the listener may choose to answer "yes" on each and every trial regardless of the signal audibility. Therefore, to minimize the effect of guessing on the results of the test, several no-stimulus trials are added to the test and the ratio of incorrect responses during these trials is used in threshold calculations as an indicator of the guessing rate of the listener. If the guessing rate is found to be k (%), then the absolute threshold is calculated as the percent of correct responses:

$$p(\%) = 50 + \frac{k}{2} \tag{12.4}$$

The value of the stimulus resulting in a probability $p(\%)$ of correct responses is the value that would be selected (heard) 50% of the time if the listener was an ideal listener. For example, imagine $k = 50\%$; that is, 50% of the time the

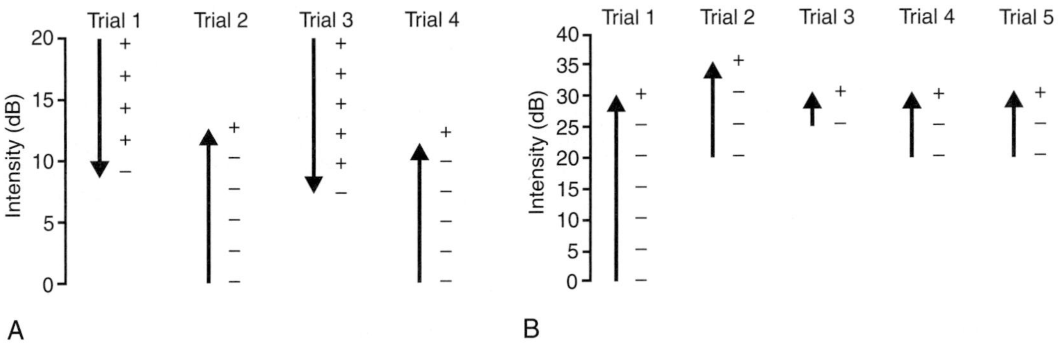

Figure 12.6. (A) The descending (trials 1 and 3) and ascending (trials 2 and 4) series of the Method of Limits. The "−" indicates lack of listener response and the "+" indicates the presence of a listener response. **(B)** An example of a modified Method of Limits.

listener indicates (guesses) that there is a signal present during an interval when there is no signal. Using Equation 12.4, we can determine that with a 50% guessing rate, the actual 50% probability of detecting the signal would correspond to a listener response rate of 75% correct responses (i.e., $p = 75\%$ from Equation 12.4). This means that to determine the hearing threshold for this person, we would need to use a criterion of 75% (i.e., the intensity at which the listener responds 75% of the time).

Another absolute threshold variation of the Method of Constant Stimuli uses the nAFC technique. In this case, the same stimuli are used as before but the listener is presented with *n* observation intervals and needs to indicate which of the presented intervals contains the stimulus. Both the magnitude of the stimulus and the interval number in which the stimulus is presented change from trial to trial. The order of presentations may be counterbalanced or random. A combination of the Method of Constant Stimuli and the nAFC technique can also be used to measure DLs. In this case, the listener is presented with a sequence of *n* stimuli and must determine which one, if any, is different. As before, from trial to trial, the stimuli vary both in magnitude and in the place they fall in the sequence of choices. The order of presentations may be counterbalanced or random.

The most common variant of the nAFC technique applied to the Method of Constant Stimuli is the 2AFC technique, known more widely as the **paired comparison** procedure. Two stimuli, or two observation intervals, are presented in one trial and the listener's task is to select one of them on the basis of a specific criterion. For example, the listener may be asked to select the stimulus that is louder, to indicate whether the stimuli were identical or not, or to report whether the first or the second observation interval contained a stimulus. A similar form of the 2AFC technique may also be applied to measure DL with the Method of Limits if the first stimulus in all pairs is identical and the second stimulus changes gradually (in an ascending or descending direction) from one presentation to another.

Similarly, as in the case of YN techniques, the results of all nAFC tests need to be corrected for guessing. For example, if the test is presented using the 2AFC technique and the listener is randomly selecting "1" or "2," on average 50% of these guesses will be correct. Therefore, to determine the detection threshold that results in a 50% probability of detection using the described technique, the interval between 50% and 100% needs to be divided in half and the value of 75% is used for threshold determination. The larger the *n* in the nAFC technique, the smaller the effect of listener guessing and the closer the real threshold point is to 50%. The percent of responses that indicate threshold (taking into account guessing) can be calculated for any *n* using the formula:

$$p(n) = \frac{1}{2}\left(1 + \frac{1}{n}\right) \times 100\% \qquad \textbf{(12.5)}$$

where $p(n)$ is the percent of responses that need to be obtained using an nAFC procedure to determine the value of the stimulus resulting in 50% detectability by an ideal observer and *n* is the number of stimuli or observation intervals in a single trial, where $n > 1$. For example, if there are six internals ($n = 6$) in the trial, then $p = 58\%$, and this is the percent correct that corresponds in this test to a 50% detection rate. Note that if $n = 1$, this equation does not apply because the test does not involve a comparison task.

In the Method of Adjustment, also called the Method of Average Errors, the listener adjusts the intensity of the stimulus in each trial according to given instructions. The control device can be a knob, slider, or control switch. Examples of tasks required of the listener include adjusting the sound to be barely audible, adjusting one sound to be equally loud as another, and adjusting the frequency of one sound to be an octave higher than the frequency of another sound. The absolute threshold is calculated as the mean value of several adjustments (Cardozo, 1965). The differential threshold is calculated as the standard deviation of the adjustments. The standard and test (adjustable) stimuli may be presented sequentially or simultaneously.

One automated variant of the Method of Adjustment procedure is the Bekesy tracking procedure. This procedure uses a sweep-frequency stimulus (although the same procedure can also be applied to a single-frequency signal). In the Bekesy tracking procedure, the sound is on continuously and the frequency increases gradually to determine the shape of the threshold of hearing. The listener responds by pressing or releasing a control button. The listener presses a button when a sound is heard and the automated system makes the sound gradually quieter. If the listener does not press the button, the sound gets gradually louder. The speed at which the sound changes is typically around 2 to 3 dB/s. The listener's task is to keep the sound oscillating around the threshold of hearing by repeatedly pressing and releasing the button. The threshold value is calculated as the average value of the deviations of the resulting zigzag curve.

Psychophysical Scales

A scale is a system of rules by which numbers or categories (labels) are assigned to various objects. Scales can be physical, when physical objects (e.g., distances) are assigned numbers based on a physical measure (e.g., number of meters), and psychological, when human reactions (e.g., preference) are assigned labels based on psychological measures (e.g., very bad, bad, average, good, very good). A psychophysical scale is the relationship between human reactions and the physical stimuli causing these reactions. If the differences between physical stimuli can be specified in terms of the magnitudes of a specific physical property, the relationship between the psychophysical scale and the physical stimuli may be represented in the form of a psychophysical function; the process of constructing or using such a function is called psychophysical measurement. The concept of a function was introduced in Chapter 1 and the concept of psychophysical measurement was discussed earlier in this chapter. Thus, a **psychophysical function** is a function relating the strength of a sensation, called the **sensation**

magnitude, to the strength of the physical stimulus, called the **stimulus magnitude,** which caused the sensation. In other words, a psychophysical function relates changes in human perception to changes in stimulation. The relationship between the stimulus magnitude and the sensation magnitude varies depending on the basic category of the sensation (e.g., hearing, vision), the specific sensation that is evoked (e.g., loudness and pitch for hearing, light intensity and color for vision), and the type of stimulus. Psychophysical measurement is not always as simple and straightforward as physical measurement because humans do not all respond to physical characteristics in the same way. In addition, a person may respond differently to the same set of stimuli at different times, depending on a number of internal and external factors including the order of stimuli presentation. It is also important to realize that most physical scales have a natural zero point, whereas some psychological scales have it (e.g., loudness) and some do not (e.g., pitch). To systematize some of the possible relationships among variables in both physical and psychological scales, Stevens (1946, 1951) introduced a hierarchy of four types (levels) of psychophysical scales together with their permissible mathematical operations. These four levels of measurement scales are nominal, ordinal, interval, and ratio scales. For more information on these levels of measurement, see the website. **Link 12-4**

Psychophysical Continua

Each sensation underlining a psychophysical scale exists along a continuum. In other words, sensations vary from a low (minimum) point to a high (maximum) point on a scale assigned to this sensation. For example, a cup of tea may be examined for sweetness. If the tea has no sugar, it may be judged as having a low sweetness; if the tea has one spoon of sugar, it may be judged as having moderate sweetness; and if the tea has two spoons of sugar, it may be judged as having high sweetness (depending on the individual). The sensation of warmth may also be assessed for this cup of tea along a continuum of cold to hot. The strength of tea flavoring (weak to strong) may also be evaluated.

There are two basic types of continua underlying sensations. They are called **prothetic continua** and **metathetic continua** (Stevens, 1975). Prothetic continua are *quantitative sensations* that vary in the quantity or magnitude of the sensation in response to the change in the stimulus. Metathetic continua are *qualitative sensations* for which a change in the stimulus elicits a change in the similarity (or dissimilarity) between two sensations rather than a change in the magnitude of sensation. Prothetic continua have a natural zero point (lack of property), whereas metathetic continua do not. A common example of a prothetic continuum is the loudness of sound. It is relatively easy for a listener to assign a numeric value to a stimulus indicating when a sound is quiet or loud and how much one sound is louder than another. Perceived duration is another quantitative continuum. It is rather easy to determine that one sound is shorter than another and how much one sound is longer than another. Pitch, on the other hand, is an example of a metathetic continuum (Stevens, 1975). While it is relatively easy to make a judgment about a difference in pitch between two sounds, it is far less intuitive to determine if one sound is two or three times the pitch of another sound, although it can be done.

Fechner's Law

The concept of the psychophysical scale was developed by Gustav Fechner, who based this scale on Weber's Law assuming that (1) the DL is defined by the Weber fraction and (2) the DL is the same perceptual entity across the whole range of stimulation and it can be used as a psychological unit of measurement. These two assumptions led to the formulation of a functional relationship know as **Fechner's Law.** Fechner's Law states that the magnitude of a sensation (R) increases proportionally with the logarithm of the stimulus intensity (I); that is:

$$R = k \times \log_a(I) \qquad (12.6)$$

where k is a constant and a is the base of the logarithm. Fechner's Law can be plotted as a function assuming that DLs are equal units of response (y axis) resulting from specific changes in stimulus intensity (x axis). An example of a logarithmic function illustrating Fechner's Law is shown in Figure 12.7A.

Fechner's Law is the foundation of many psychophysical scales used in acoustics and hearing science, which demonstrate a logarithmic-like relationship between sensation magnitudes and stimulus magnitudes. These scales are good representations of some qualitative (metathetic) scales such as the pitch scale, but they are less appropriate approximations of quantitative (prothetic) scales, such as the loudness

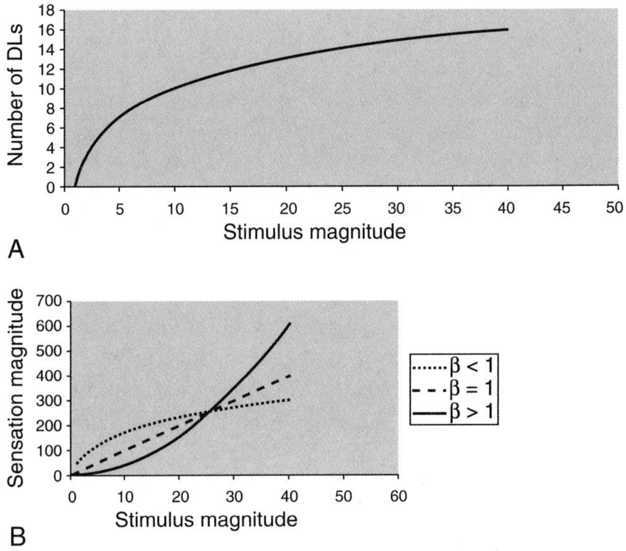

Figure 12.7. (A) A logarithmic function illustrating Fechner's Law showing the relationship between the number of difference limens (DLs) and the stimulus magnitude. **(B)** Three examples of power functions based on Steven's Power Law with various β and k values.

scale, which have a natural zero point. Most quantitative scales (e.g., loudness scale) do not exactly follow Fechner's Law and are better represented by Stevens' Power Law.

Stevens' Power Law

The results of many experimental studies have demonstrated that the relationship between some sensations and the physical stimuli that elicit these sensations is not always well represented by Fechner's Law and logarithmic function. Research has shown that psychophysical relationships involving prothetic continuum and a physical stimulus usually have an exponential form (expressed by a power function). The concept of using a power function to describe the relationship between physical stimuli and prothetic sensations was originally proposed by American psychologist Stanley Smith Stevens (1906–1973), and this relationship is known as **Stevens' Power Law.** Stevens' Power Law states that prothetic sensations follow power functions of the physical stimuli. According to Stevens, "The power function tells us that there exists a beautifully simple relationship between stimulus and sensory response" (Stevens, 1975, p. 16). Stevens' Power Law can be written as:

$$R = k \times I^{\beta} \qquad (12.7)$$

where R is the magnitude of the sensation, I is the magnitude of stimulation, β is an exponent that is based on the specific perceptual continuum under consideration, and k is a constant that depends on the type of stimulus. Several examples of hypothetical power functions, with varying β and k values, are illustrated in Figure 12.7B. The exact shape of the power function will vary considerably depending on the specific sensation that is studied. For example, for the loudness of sound, the brightness of light, and the intensity of smell and taste, $\beta < 1$. For the perceived length of an object and the magnitude of coldness, $\beta \approx 1$, and for weight, warmth, and electric shock sensations, $\beta > 1$. Thus, a graph of the relationship between the loudness and intensity of sound will look quite different than the relationship between the warmth of a metal object pressed against the skin compared to the temperature of the object. Within psychoacoustics, quite a lot of scaling research has been conducted to explore how changes in sensation are related to changes in physical characteristics.

HEARING AREA

The **threshold of hearing,** also called the threshold of audibility, is the lowest sound intensity that can be heard under specific listening conditions. The specific magnitude of an acoustic signal that corresponds to the threshold of hearing is dependent on many attributes of sound such as frequency, duration, spectrum, and temporal envelope. Because the intensity and frequency of sound are the two most important factors associated with the audibility of sound, the threshold of sound is most often illustrated as a function of frequency (i.e., with frequency along the x axis and intensity along the y axis) (Fig. 12.8).

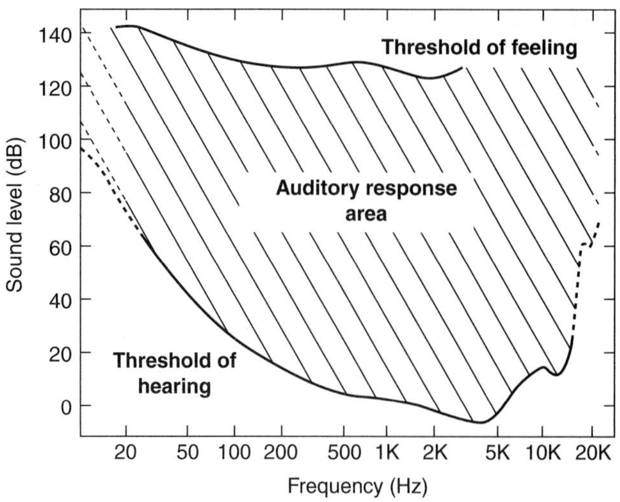

Figure 12.8. The area of hearing. (From Durrant J, Lovrinic J. Bases of Hearing Science. Baltimore, MD: Lippincott Williams & Wilkins, 1995. Used with permission.)

The range of intensities that are perceived as sounds is limited at its upper level by the threshold of pain, also called the threshold of feeling, since the sensation of pain is associated with an impression that something is touching the ear. The range of perceived intensities across frequency from the lowest intensity sound a human can perceive to the threshold of pain and from the lowest to highest frequency humans can hear is called the **hearing area** or **auditory response area.** The extent and shape of the auditory response area are shown in Figure 12.8.

As you can see in Figure 12.8, the normal auditory system of humans is capable of perceiving sounds across a wide range of frequencies and intensities. This area extends from about 20 Hz to 20,000 Hz along the frequency scale and from about 0 dB SPL to 120 dB SPL along the sound intensity scale. However, as shown in Figure 12.8, the human ear is not equally sensitive across the entire frequency range. Human hearing is the most sensitive in the range around 1000 to 5000 Hz and quite sensitive for tones in the 300- to 5000-Hz range, which is also called the **speech range** since energy in this range is critical to differentiating between various speech sounds. Beyond this range the threshold of hearing quite abruptly increases at both low and high frequencies. Thus, the human ear is naturally tuned to receive speech sounds. Notice also in Figure 12.8 that the line indicating the threshold of feeling is quite a bit flatter than the minimum audibility curve. This means that sounds of various frequencies become painful at about the same sound pressure level in contrast to the threshold of hearing, where they need to differ more to be heard.

In addition to frequency, hearing threshold is quite dependent on the duration of a signal. The threshold is higher for very short signals and increases with duration at a rate of about 3 dB per doubling of duration until the duration reaches about 200 ms (Zwislocki, 1960). Beyond 200 ms, the effect of duration on signal audibility is practically negligible.

LOUDNESS

Loudness is the property of sound that allows sounds to be ordered on a scale extending from quiet (soft) to loud. The loudness of sound depends primarily on sound intensity, but, to a lesser degree, it also depends on sound duration, frequency, and spectral complexity. In general, when an increase in sound intensity exceeds a certain minimum value (DL), any further increase in sound intensity results in a change in the loudness of the sound. However, two sounds of the same intensity but of different frequency or spectral complexity may also differ in their loudness. Similarly, two sounds of the same intensity but with different durations may be perceived as not being equally loud if one sound is shorter than 200 ms. Most perceptual phenomena need a stimulus of a certain minimal duration to develop a full sensation, and this minimal duration is about 200 ms for loudness.

Difference Limen for Intensity

The difference limen for intensity [DL(I)] refers to the smallest perceivable change in sound intensity. The value of the DL(I) depends on the frequency and intensity of the sound. This relationship is illustrated in Figure 12.9. In the graph shown in Figure 12.9, the frequency of a sound is shown on the *x* axis, the sound intensity of a given sound is on the *z* axis, and the difference threshold for intensity, expressed as the Weber fraction ($\Delta I/I$), is on the *y* axis. Note that the intensity of the reference tone is expressed in sensation level (dB SL). Sensation level is the intensity of a sound expressed in decibels above the threshold of hearing for an individual listener.* Note also that this graph shows that the classic Weber's Law does not hold for low sensation levels and needs a correction factor (see Equation 12.3). If the classic Weber's Law were true, all of the lines would be flat (parallel with the *z* axis), regardless of the intensity of the sound.

The DL(I) varies from about 0.5 dB to 1 dB for tones and music sounds heard in laboratory conditions to about 3 dB for everyday sounds heard by an average listener. The DL(I) is high for very short sounds, decreases with signal duration, and above about 200 ms becomes independent of duration. If you would like to hear pairs of sound that differ in their intensity by specific amounts, see the website. **Audio clip 12-1**

*One other commonly used measurement scale in psychoacoustics is hearing level (dB HL). Hearing level is the intensity of a sound expressed in decibels above the average normal hearing threshold at each frequency. For the ideal average listener the values in dB HL and dB SL would be identical. For more information on the hearing level scale, consult any audiology textbook.

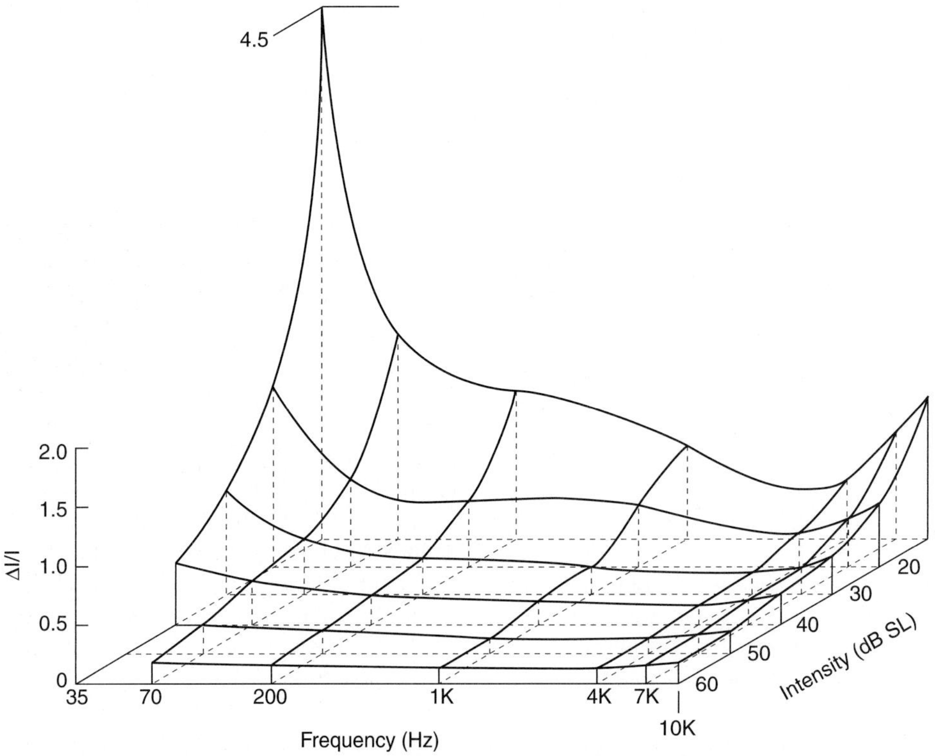

Figure 12.9. The relationship between frequency, intensity, and difference limen for intensity. (From Gulick WL. Hearing: Physiology and Psychophysics. New York: Oxford University Press, 1971. Based on data from Riesz RR. Differential intensity sensitivity of the ear for pure tones. *Phys Rev* 1928;31:867–875. Copyright 1971 Oxford University Press, Inc. Used with permission.)

Loudness Level

Loudness depends primarily on sound intensity, but it is also affected by sound frequency. If we present two pure tones with different frequencies and adjust their intensity so that they sound equally loud, they are said to have the same **loudness level.** In psychoacoustics, the reference point for equal loudness levels is a 1000-Hz tone at various sound pressure levels (i.e., a 1000-Hz tone at 20 dB SPL, 40 dB SPL, 60 dB SPL, and so forth). The unit of loudness level is the **phon.** The name *phon* was proposed by German physicist Heinrich Georg Barkhausen (1881–1956) and adopted as a unit of loudness level in 1937 at the First International Acoustic Conference in Paris. A sound is said to have a loudness level of 40 phons if it has the same loudness as a 1000-Hz tone having an intensity level of 40 dB SPL. So, a 1000-Hz tone with an intensity of 20, 40, and 60 dB SPL would have phon levels of 20, 40, and 60 phons, respectively. Loudness level is a broad concept that applies to all sounds independent of their complexity and frequency content. The loudness level of sounds other than a 1000-Hz tone is determined by adjusting the intensity level of a 1000-Hz tone to a value that sounds equally loud with the other sound. The intensity level of this adjusted 1000-Hz tone, expressed in phons, is the loudness level of the other sound.

The dependence of loudness level on both the sound intensity and sound frequency for tones can be shown in an intensity-frequency graph as a line connecting the sound intensities having the same loudness level. This line is called an **equal-loudness curve** or **equal-loudness contour,** isoloudness curve, or phon curve. A family of the equal-loudness curves for pure tone sounds is shown in Figure 12.10.

The phon level of the equal-loudness curves in Figure 12.10 is indicated by the intensity level of a 1000-Hz tone. Examine, for example, the 40-phon line. Notice that the intensity of the 40-phon line is 40 dB SPL at 1000 Hz. This is because 40 dB SPL at 1000 Hz is the reference point with the intensity scale. Note also that a 100-Hz tone with an intensity level of about 52 dB SPL has the same loudness level (40 phons) as a 1000-Hz tone at 40 dB SPL. A 10,000-Hz tone with an intensity level of about 48 dB SPL has the same loudness level (40 phons) as a 1000-Hz tone at 40 dB SPL. The equal-loudness contours at low-intensity levels are almost parallel to the minimum audibility curve, but the contours flatten out somewhat at higher intensity levels as the stimuli reach the threshold of pain.

Loudness Scale

Loudness level expressed in phons indicates how intense a sound must be to sound just as loud as a 1000-Hz tone. Loudness level, however, does not indicate how much louder (how many times) one sound is as compared with another. To determine the relative loudness of two or more sounds, we need to use the concept of loudness and of a **loudness scale.** The most common loudness scale is the **sone scale*** introduced by S.S. Stevens. One **sone** has been defined as the loudness of a 1000-Hz tone with an intensity level of 40 dB SPL. Since such a tone has a loudness level of 40 phons, a sound with a loudness level of 40 phons has a loudness of 1 sone. A sound that is twice as loud as 1 sone is assigned a loudness of 2 sones, a sound that is 10 times as loud is assigned a loudness of 10 sones, and so forth.

Figure 12.11 illustrates the loudness growth function in which the loudness in sones, displayed using both a linear (A) and logarithmic (B) *y* axis, is graphed as a function of the

*A Fechner scale (Fig. 12.7A) built by adding DLs is another example of a loudness scale.

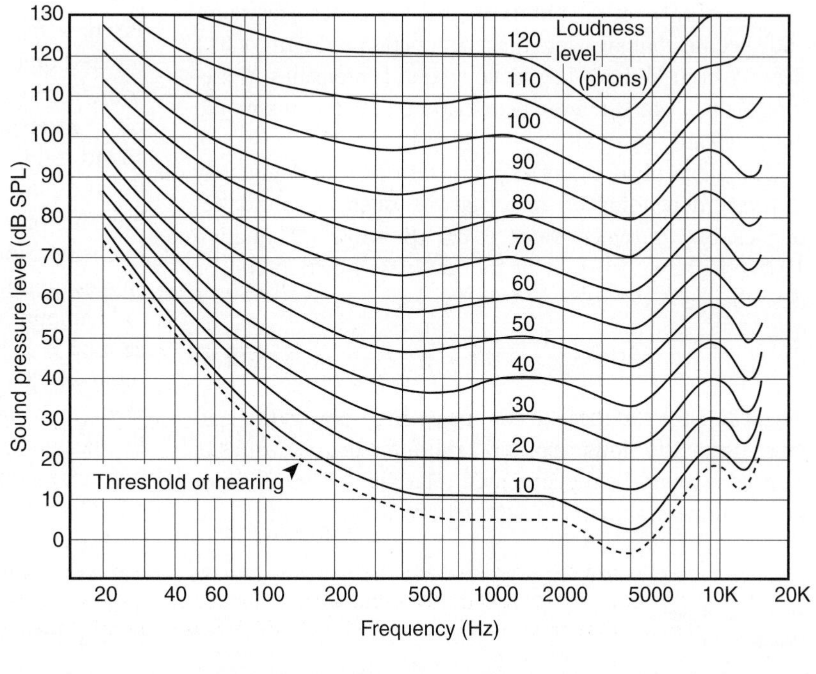

Figure 12.10. Equal loudness curves.

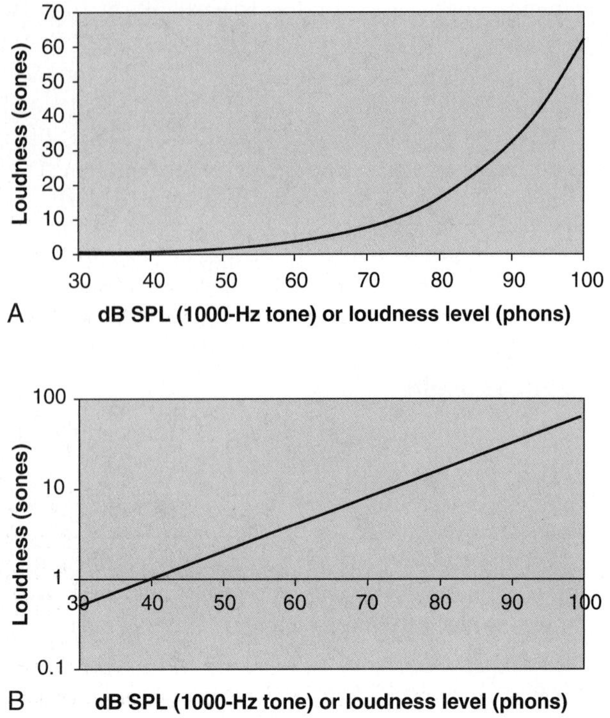

Figure 12.11. Loudness in sones as a function of dB SPL for a 1000-Hz tone shown with **(A)** a linear *y* axis and **(B)** a logarithmic *y* axis. Note that since the sound pressure levels of a 1000-Hz tone are numerically equal to the loudness levels of a 1000-Hz tone, the *x* axis can also be expressed as loudness level in phons.

sound pressure level (dB SPL) of a 1000-Hz tone. Since the sound pressure levels of a 1000-Hz tone are numerically equal to the loudness levels of a 1000-Hz tone, the *x* axis of the graph in Figure 12.11 can also be expressed as loudness level in phons. Further, since various sounds that are equally loud are expressed by the same number of phons, the graph shown in Figure 12.11, *with the x axis in phons but not dB SPL,* can apply to all sounds regardless of their frequency and spectral content. Note that the function in Figure 12.11 departs from Weber's Law at low sound intensities; therefore, if the *x* axis extended below 30 dB SPL, the line would curve toward the *x* axis.

The slope of loudness as a function of sound intensity can vary depending on many factors, such as sound frequency, but its typical value is 0.3 ($\beta = 0.3$ in Equation 12.8); therefore, in general, the loudness function can be described as*:

$$L = \frac{1}{15.85} \times \left(\frac{I}{I_0}\right)^{0.3} \qquad (12.8)$$

where L is the loudness of sound in sones, $\frac{1}{15.85}$ is the specific constant for loudness, and I and I_0 are the intensities of a specific sound being compared (Hartmann, 1997). Since both loudness and loudness level are functions of sound intensity, it is possible to determine a direct relationship between these two functions such that:

$$L = 10^{(-1.2 + 0.03LL)} \qquad (12.9)$$

where L is loudness in sones and LL is loudness level in phons.

PRACTICE PROBLEMS: LOUDNESS CALCULATIONS (USING FIGS. 12.10 AND 12.11)

1. What is the loudness of a 2000-Hz tone played at a loudness level of 80 phons?
2. What is the sound intensity level of a 300-Hz tone having a loudness of 1 sone?
3. How much louder would a 1000-Hz tone be if its loudness level increased from 60 phons to 90 phons?
4. How much louder would a 2000-Hz tone be if its loudness level increased from 50 phons to 60 phons?

Answers (If you need help with these problems, consult the website.) **Link 12-5**

1. About 16 sones
2. 38 dB SPL
3. 7.5 times as loud
4. 2.0 times as loud

PITCH

Pitch is the property of sound that allows sounds to be ordered on a scale extending from low to high. The pitch of sound changes primarily with sound frequency, where low pitch corresponds to low frequency and high pitch correspond to high frequency. Pitch and frequency, however, are not the same thing—pitch depends not only on frequency, but also on other characteristics of sound such as sound intensity, duration, and spectral complexity. Similar to intensity and loudness, if sound frequency changes by a perceptible amount (equal to the DL for frequency), then the perception is a change in pitch. It is also possible, however, for pitch to change when frequency does not change (e.g., a change in intensity may sound like a pitch change). Furthermore, it is also possible to perceive pitches that do not correspond to any frequency contained in the physical stimulus (i.e., we hear something that is not actually there, such as the missing fundamental, described later). Last but not least, sounds can differ in the strength of pitch sensation and there are some complex sounds that do not appear to have a perceptible pitch at all.

*If the sound loudness is expressed as a function of sound pressure, the coefficient $\beta = 2 \times 0.3 = 0.6$.

Difference Limen for Frequency

The difference limen for frequency [DL(f)] refers to the smallest change in the frequency that can be perceived. The DL(f) differs enormously among people and becomes smaller with extended practice. Some people can notice changes in frequency that are less than 0.01%, whereas others are "tone deaf" and have great difficulty hearing a change in frequency and identifying the direction of frequency change. The amount of perceived change is also dependent on the methodology used in determining DL(f) value. Typical DL(f) values for pure tones of middle and high frequencies are on the order of 0.1% to 1% and they become larger at low frequencies (i.e., below 500 Hz) (Shower & Biddulph, 1931). The relationship between the frequency (*x* axis) of the reference tone, the intensity of the reference tone (*z* axis), and the DL for frequency expressed in relative units ($\Delta f/f$) is shown in Figure 12.12.

Figure 12.12 illustrates that the lines are fairly flat from about 500 to 8000 Hz and from 10 to 60 dB SL (i.e., $\frac{\Delta f}{f}$ is constant). Below 500 Hz the DL(f) is independent of frequency and equal to about 5 Hz. If you would like to hear pairs of sounds that differ by specific amounts in their frequency, consult the website. **Audio clip 12-2**

Pitch Scale

An increase in pitch is generally associated with an increase in frequency. The amount of change in frequency, however, does not correspond to the same amount of change in pitch. In other words, when frequency doubles, the perception is not a doubling of pitch. The scale relating frequency and pitch is the **mel scale** developed by S.S. Stevens (Stevens & Volkmann, 1940; Stevens et al., 1937). The mel scale is a scale of pitches judged by listeners to be equal in distance from one another. The mel scale was created by presenting to a listener a reference tone (1000 Hz at 40 dB SL) and then asking the listener to create a scale of tones from this reference

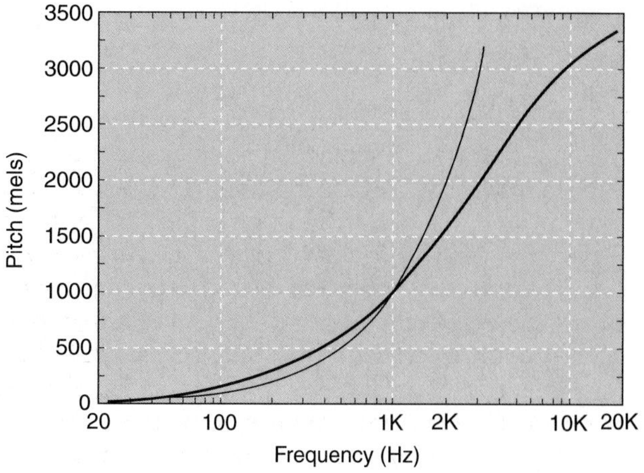

Figure 12.13. The mel scale (*thick line*) and the hypothetical octave scale drawn assuming that each octave represents a doubling in pitch (*thin line*). (From Stevens SS, Volkmann J. The relation of pitch to frequency: a revised scale. *Am J Psychol LIII* 1940;3:329–353. Copyright 1940 by the Board of Trustees of the University of Illinois. Used with permission of the University of Illinois Press.)

tone by doubling and halving the pitch of the sound. The reference tone of 1000 Hz at 40 dB SL is assigned a value of 1000 mels. The tone that has twice the pitch of a 1000-mel tone is assigned the value of 2000 mels, the tone that is perceived to have half the pitch of a 1000-mel tone is assigned the value of 500 mels, and so forth across the entire pitch range. Similar to all logarithmic functions, the pitch scale in mels does not have a natural zero point.

The relationship between the frequency scale in Hz and the pitch scale in mels is illustrated in Figure 12.13. The mel scale is shown by the thicker line and the octave scale (music interval scale) is represented by the thinner line. The octave scale drawn in Figure 12.13 assumes that each octave represents a doubling in pitch. Notice that the pitch scale is very closely related to the octave scale at low and middle frequencies up to about 1500 Hz but diverges from it at higher frequencies. Notice also that pitch increases as

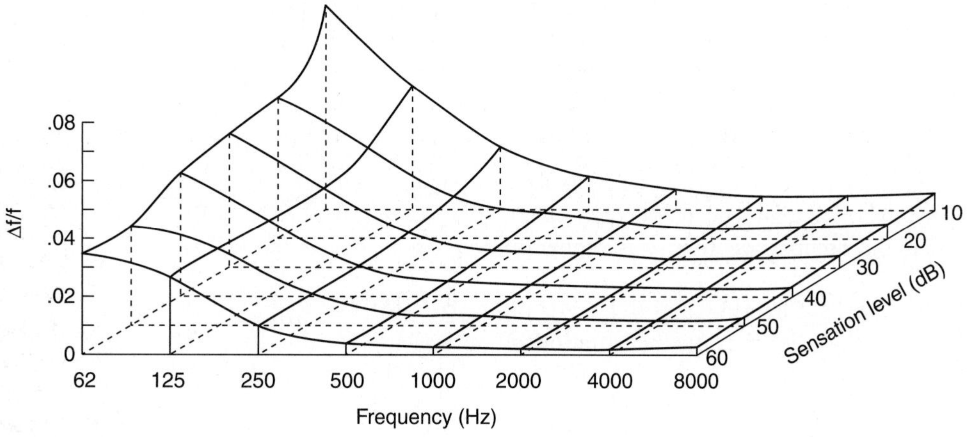

Figure 12.12. Difference limen for frequency as a function of frequency and intensity. (From Gulick WL. Hearing: Physiology and Psychophysics. New York: Oxford University Press, 1971. Based upon data by Shower EG, Biddulph R. Differential pitch sensitivity of the ear. *J Acoust Soc Am* 1931;3:275–287. Copyright 1971 Oxford University Press, Inc. Used with permission.)

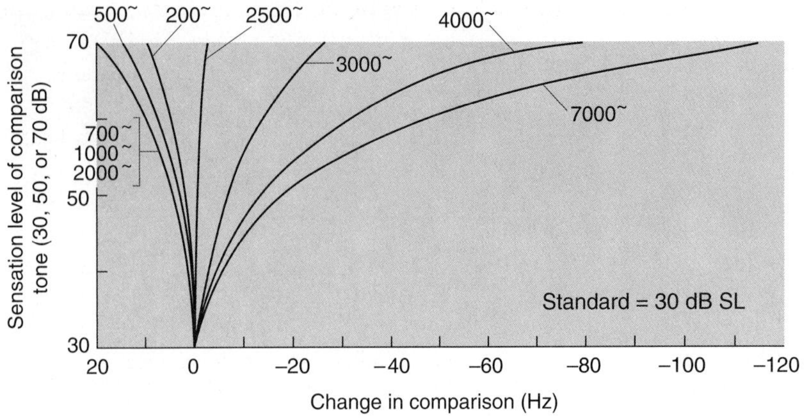

Figure 12.14. Intensity influences on pitch perception. (From Gulick WL. Hearing: Physiology and Psychophysics. New York: Oxford University Press, 1971. Copyright 1971 Oxford University Press, Inc. Used with permission.)

frequency increases but the relatively large frequency range from 20 Hz to 20,000 Hz is contained within a relatively small pitch range extending only to 3400 mels.

Although pitch is mainly dependent on frequency, changes in other physical characteristics of sound also can influence pitch perception. For example, changes in the intensity of a sound may cause both positive and negative changes in pitch. Stevens (1935) has shown that when a pure tone above 2500 Hz is increased in intensity, listeners perceive that the tone increases in pitch, and when a pure tone below 2500 Hz is increased in intensity, listeners perceive the tone decreases in pitch.

The effects of sound intensity on sound pitch reported by Gulick (1971) are shown in Figure 12.14. In this study, listeners were presented with a series of reference tones that varied in frequency from 70 to 7000 Hz (each frequency is shown in the figure with a separate line). The reference tone was always set to an intensity of 30 dB SL. Each reference tone was then presented with a second (comparison) tone, first at 30 dB SL, then at 50 dB SL, then at 70 dB SL. The frequency of the second tone was adjusted until the listener indicated that both tones had the same pitch. Look at the line marked 4000 Hz in the figure. When the comparison tone was 50 dB SL (indicated on the *y* axis), the comparison tone had to be decreased by about 12 Hz (indicated on the *x* axis) for both tones to have the same pitch. In other words, when the comparison tone was more intense, the pitch increased and it had to be decreased in frequency to have the same pitch as the reference tone. The differences become more marked when the comparison tone was higher in intensity (70 dB SL).

In addition to the effects of intensity and frequency on pitch, the sensation of pitch depends on the duration of sound. Tones with an extremely short duration are perceived as clicks that do not seem to elicit any sensation of pitch. Once the duration reaches a certain length (about six cycles for frequencies below 1000 Hz and about 10 ms for frequencies above 1000 Hz), the clicks become more tonal but their pitch is different from the pitch of a continuous tone. Finally, when the tone duration reaches about 250 ms, the tone reaches its natural pitch (Gulick, 1971).

The auditory system can also create the perception of a pitch that does not correspond to any specific frequency component of the signal entering the ear. This pitch sensation is called **periodicity pitch** or residual pitch. Consider, for example, a complex tone with a missing fundamental, as previously mentioned in Chapter 4. Imagine a complex wave consisting of a series of harmonics in which the greatest common factor of the harmonics is missing. For example, a tone consisting of 1000, 1500, 2000, and 2500 Hz **Audio clip 12-3** has four components that are all related harmonically to the number 500, which is the greatest common factor of all four numbers. Thus, the 500-Hz tone is the fundamental frequency of the complex tone. Since 500 Hz is not actually a component of this complex wave, it is called a "missing" fundamental. If a listener hears the 1000-, 1500-, 2000-, and 2500-Hz tones played together, a 500 Hz tone can be perceived, even though there is no energy present at 500 Hz. The perception of the missing fundamental is most likely created either at the level of the cochlea by timing cues or farther along in the auditory system based on pattern recognition detectors, which look for relationships among signals. Investigation of activity within the cortex had indicated that the tonotopic organization of the auditory cortex is based on the pitch of the sound and not the frequency, so the missing fundamental, which has no energy when the sound enters the ear, creates a sensation by the time the signal reaches the brain (Pantev et al., 1989).

MASKING

Masking is the ability of one sound (the masker) to completely block out or to decrease the audibility of another sound (the maskee). There are two basic forms of masking: simultaneous masking and temporal masking. Simultaneous masking takes place when two sounds arrive at the listener together and the stronger one masks the other one. As a matter of fact, both sounds mask each other but one of them has a bigger effect on the other than the other way around. Temporal masking takes place when two sounds arrive in succession closely enough in time that they influence each other.

An example of masking in everyday life is a conversation that takes place in a crowd of people talking. The signal that you are trying to hear is masked by the background noise of other voices. The term *noise* in this context is any background sound that is unwanted. Using masking terminology, the signal is the maskee and the noise is the masker. When signal and noise arrive at the ear together (or in quick succession), both of them excite the basilar membrane at the same time and their vibration patterns often overlap. Whether or not the signal can be heard above the noise depends on their difference in intensity and similarity in frequency, spectrum, and temporal pattern.

Simultaneous Masking

Simultaneous masking is the masking resulting from the presence of two or more sounds at the same time. Much of our basic understanding of simultaneous masking is based on research that began in the early part of the 1900s. A classic masking study conducted by Wegel and Lane (1924) described the masking of pure tones by other pure tones. The authors used pure tones for both the signal and the noise (tone-on-tone masking), varied the relationship between their frequencies, and measured the threshold of hearing for the signal tone. Some of the results of their work are shown in Figure 12.15. The graph shows the changes in the threshold of hearing for the tone signal at various frequencies (indicated by the *x* axis) when a 1200-Hz pure tone masker was delivered to the same ear. The masker was presented at three different intensities, 44, 60, and 80 dB. The three lines on the graph show the changes in hearing threshold that occurred for each of these three maskers.

The masking curves shown in Figure 12.15 can be used to highlight a few basic facts about masking. First, the greater the intensity of the masker, the greater the upward shift in the hearing threshold is. The 44-dB masker resulted in the smallest threshold shift (lowest line on the graph), whereas the 80-dB masker resulted in the greatest shift (top line in the graph). This finding is not surprising since we intuitively know that a loud background noise masks a signal to a greater degree than a quiet background noise. The amount of threshold shift represents the amount of masking, which is the increase in the signal level that must be added to the signal to restore its audibility.

Second, the amount of masking is greatest when the frequency of the masker is close to the frequency of the signal. Notice that when the frequency of the signal was close to the frequency of the noise (i.e., 1200 Hz), the masking was greatest. The dashed lines in Figure 12.15 indicate the level where the peak would be predicted if this rule was the only masking rule that applies to these data. The solid lines represent the actual shift in threshold. Notice some dips in the amount of masking right at the frequency of the masker or its harmonics. They occur because when the signal and the masker are very close in frequency, their interaction creates beats (see Chapter 6) that improve the detection of the tone.

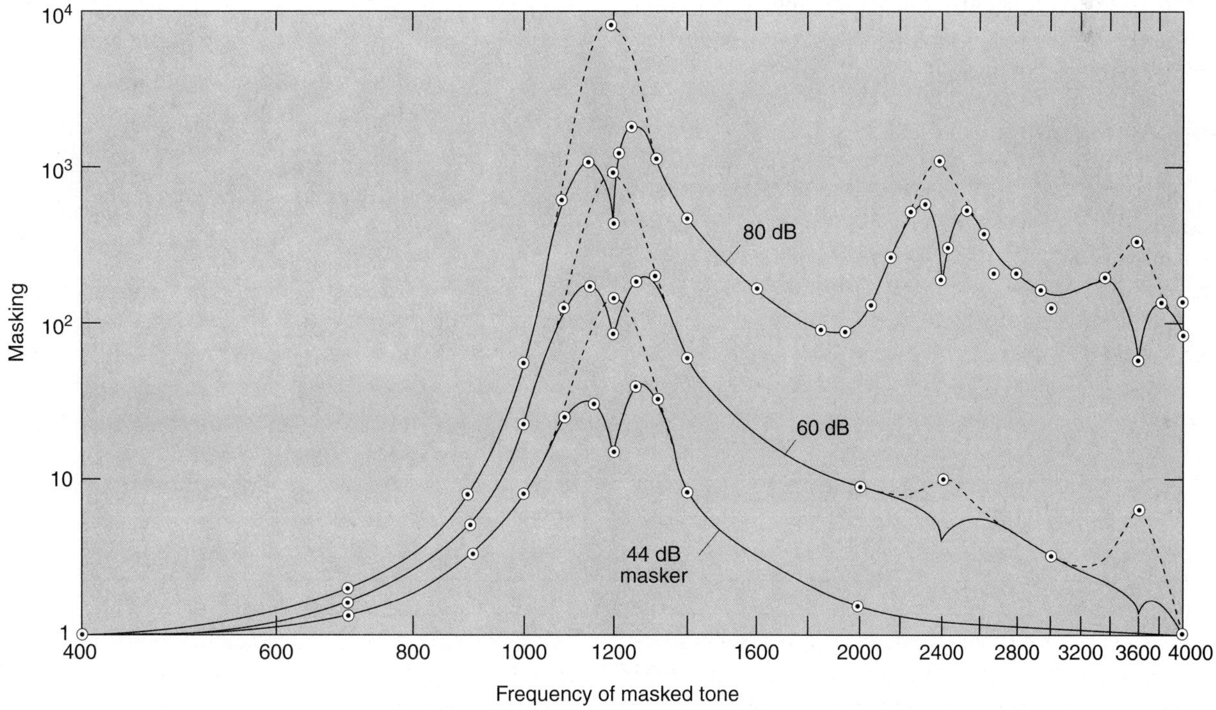

Figure 12.15. Tone-on-tone masking. (Reprinted figure from Wegel RL, Lane CE. The auditory masking of pure tone by another and its probable relation to the dynamics of the inner ear. *Physiol Rev* 1924;23:266–285. Copyright 1924 American Physical Society. Used with permission.)

During beats the two tones move in and out of phase, alternately reinforcing and canceling each other and creating an amplitude-modulated signal that is easy to hear.

Third, low-frequency signals mask high-frequency signals better than high-frequency signals mask low-frequency signals and this effect is most pronounced at high-intensity levels. Notice that the lowest curve is fairly symmetric, indicating that when the masker was relatively low in intensity (44 dB), the masking was very similar for tones lower and higher than 1200 Hz. When the intensity of the masker increased, however, the masking curves became asymmetric with an increased amount of masking at high frequencies. This phenomenon is called an **upward spread of masking** and it is especially pronounced with very intense maskers. The upward spread of masking means that a masker is able to mask signals of higher frequency to a greater degree than those of lower frequency. This effect is caused by the asymmetry of the excitation pattern along the basilar membrane.

Fourth, notice that for the moderate (60 dB) and most markedly for the high (80 dB) intensity masker, the masking level increases around the harmonics of the masking tone. This suggests that at high-intensity levels, the ear generates nonlinear distortions in the form of additional harmonics. Since 2400 Hz and 3600 Hz are harmonics of 1200 Hz, these distortions increased the effective noise masking for tones near 2400 and 3600 Hz.

The discussion presented above was limited to the effects of narrow band maskers such as tones. Typically, however, real-world sounds and the maskers used in hearing science applications are wideband stationary noises such as white noise or pink noise. The masking curves produced by such noises are much less frequency dependent and free from local disturbances caused by beats. If you would like to hear the effects of various signal-to-noise ratios on the audibility of the signal, consult the website. **Audio clip 12-4**

Temporal Masking

When two sounds arrive at a listener in a quick succession, the listener may only hear one of them. This phenomenon is called **temporal masking.** There are two basic forms of temporal masking: **forward masking,** where the masker is presented slightly before the signal, and **backward masking,** where the masker is presented slightly after the signal. The effects of forward and backward masking are illustrated in Figure 12.16. The left panel shows the effect of backward masking and the right panel shows the effect of forward masking. The time difference between the arrival of the signal and the masker (*x* axis) varies from 0 to 100 ms (notice that the 0 point for backward masking begins at the far right of the graph). When the time difference between the arrival of both sounds is close to 0 ms, the amount of masking is the greatest, and the masking decreases fairly rapidly as the time difference between the two sounds increases. In other words, the farther apart the masker and the signal are, the less efficient the masker is. Temporal masking plays a very large role in speech perception and room acoustics. For example, the strong reflection of a sound from a nearby wall arriving shortly after the direct sound can mask speech arriving from a direct route. If you would like to hear the effects of the temporal separation of sounds on their temporal resolution and integration, consult the website. **Audio clip 12-5**

CRITICAL BANDS

There is a large body of research supporting the theory that the cochlea processes information in frequency bands. The basilar membrane and hair cells can be theorized to act like an overlapping row of filters, breaking down auditory signals into different spectral (frequency) bands so that various frequencies of the auditory signal can be transmitted, via a series of time-coded impulses, along the central auditory nervous system for decoding at the brain. One of the largest bodies of literature showing that bands of hair cells and nerve fibers appear to act together to process auditory information concerns the concept of the **critical band.**

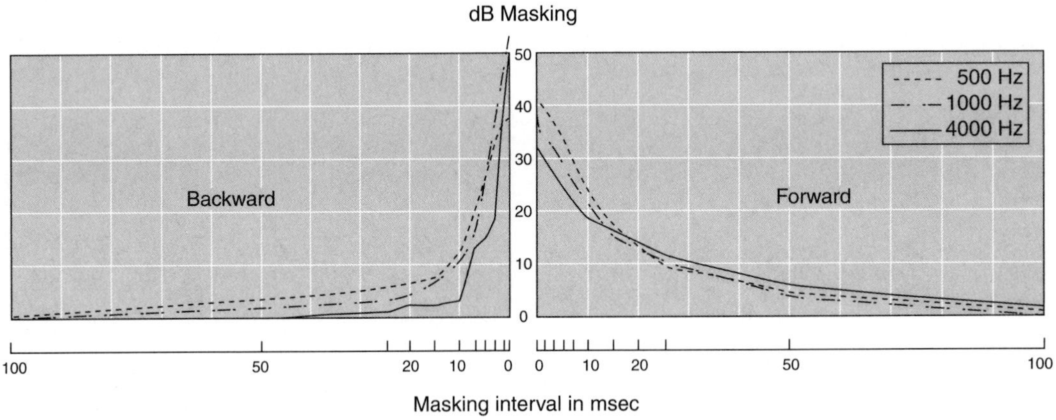

Figure 12.16. The amount of masking created by backward (*left panel*) and forward (*right panel*) maskers as a function of time between the masker and the signal. (From Elliott LL. Backward and forward masking of probe tones of different frequencies. *J Acoust Soc Am* 1962;34(8):1116–1117. Used with permission of the American Institute of Physics.)

The **critical band** is a range of frequencies that is integrated (summed together) by the auditory nervous system and affects the perception of various aspects of sound. The ear can be said to be a series of overlapping critical bands, each responding to a narrow range of frequencies. This concept was introduced by Fletcher (1940) to explain the masking of a pure tone by wideband noise. Fletcher masked a pure tone with a band of noise, keeping the spectrum level (the amount of noise energy per 1-Hz band) constant but changing the noise bandwidth (i.e., changing the overall power of the masking noise by increasing the width of the spectrum). When the width of the noise band increased, the threshold of hearing for the masked tone also increased, but only until the noise band reached a certain width. Any further increase in the noise band beyond this point did not affect the masked threshold. To account for this finding, Fletcher introduced the concept of an auditory filter and referred to its bandwidth as a critical band. Thus, a critical band is the bandwidth within which changes in noise energy affect the detectability of a tone centered within the band and outside which masker energy has very limited effect on the tone detectability.

Following Fletcher's study many listening experiments, including loudness judgment, masking, and quality judgment studies, have shown that the hearing system integrates the sounds within the critical band differently than the sounds outside of the critical band (e.g., Scharf, 1970). For example, imagine a narrow-band noise that expands its bandwidth while decreasing the spectrum level (energy level in each 1-Hz band) so as to maintain the same overall power. As long as the bandwidth of the noise is less than the critical band, the loudness of the noise is practically constant. Once the bandwidth exceeds the size of the critical band, the loudness of the wideband noise gradually increases despite the fact that the overall power of the noise is kept constant (Zwicker & Fastl, 1999). This relationship is shown in Figure 12.17. The critical band concept is also important for understanding masking, pitch perception, and timbre resolution.

In developing the concept of the critical band, Fletcher made assumptions that the auditory filter has a rectangular shape and that the noise energy needed to mask a tone is equal to the energy of the tone. Both of these assumptions were not correct and had to be modified based on the results of subsequent research. Several studies have demonstrated that the auditory filter has certain slopes that affect the contribution of various frequency components at both sides of the filter in response to the energy passing through the filter. In addition, the noise energy needed to mask a tone has been determined to be about 2.5 times larger than the energy of the tone and to vary with the center frequency of the tone (Scharf, 1970). Therefore, both the shapes and the widths of the critical band had to be revised and the actual critical bands are about 2.5 times wider than the bands proposed by Fletcher. For example, the revised critical band shown in Figure 12.18 is about 160 Hz wide at 1,000 Hz. To differentiate the new critical bands from the old critical bands proposed by Fletcher, the old bands are currently referred to as *critical ratios*.

The width of the critical band changes with signal frequency. Zwicker et al. (1957), Zwicker and Fastl (1972, 1990), and several other authors reported that at low frequencies, up to about 500 Hz, all critical bands have approximately the same bandwidth of about 100 Hz. Above 500 Hz, however, the bandwidth increases with frequency at a ratio of about 0.2, which means that $\Delta f = 0.2f$, where f is the central frequency of the band. The general relationship between the size of the critical band and the frequency is shown in Figure 12.18.

The full frequency range of audible frequencies spans across 24 side-by-side critical bands in which the edges and crossing points between the bands are located at frequencies of 0, 100, 200, 300, 400, 510, 630, 770, 920, 1080, 1270, 1480, 1720, 2000, 2320, 2700, 3150, 3700, 4400, 5300, 6400, 7700, 9500, 12,000, and 15,500 Hz. These 24 bands create a special frequency scale called the **critical band scale** extending from 0 to 24. The unit of this scale is called the **bark** and the scale itself is called the **bark scale** (in honor of

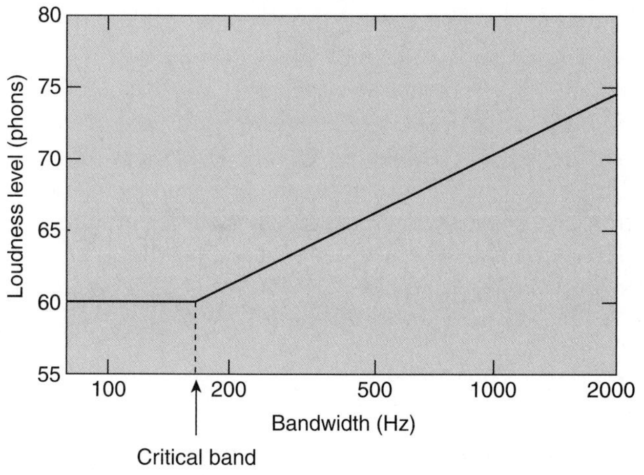

Figure 12.17. The effect of critical band on loudness.

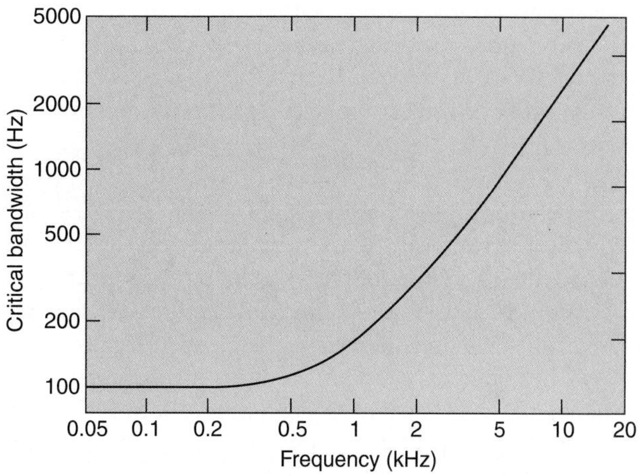

Figure 12.18. The width of critical band as a function of frequency.

Heinrich Georg Barkhauses, who introduced the term *phon*). When the bark scale is plotted along the length of the basilar membrane, each critical band occupies about 1.3 mm of the basilar membrane and extends across about 150 inner hair cells (Zwicker & Fastl, 1990). This scale can be considered another form of the Stevens' mel scale and each bark corresponds to about 100 mels (Zwicker & Fastl, 1990). Other studies have revealed that the actual auditory filters do not have a constant bandwidth below 500 Hz and the critical bands continue to decrease at about the same rate below 500 Hz (Moore & Glasberg, 1983; Glasberg & Moore, 1990; Moore et al., 1990). Based on these data, Glasberg and Moore (1990) introduced the concept of the equivalent rectangular band (ERB) of an auditory filter that changes with frequency such that:

$$ERB = 24.7 \times [(4.37 \times f) + 1] \qquad \textbf{(12.10)}$$

If you would like to hear the effects of sound bandwidth, including critical bandwidth, on sound loudness, consult the website. **Audio clip 12-6**

TIMBRE AND SOUND QUALITY

Pure tones form perceptual images based on their loudness, pitch, and perceived duration. Most real-world sounds, however, are not pure tones but sounds with much more complex spectra and temporal patterns. People are able to differentiate easily between two complex sounds that have identical loudness, pitch, and perceived duration, but different spectra. For example, it is easy to differentiate between the sound of a violin and the sound of a flute. The perceived characteristic that facilitates this differentiation is called the timbre. **Timbre** is formally defined as the attribute of auditory sensation by which a listener can judge that two sounds having the same loudness and pitch are different (American National Standards Institute, 1994). This definition does not indicate what timbre is but rather what timbre is not. Therefore, for practical reasons, it is more intuitive to equate timbre with sound character that allows for the recognition of a sound source and for perception of sound complexity.

A stationary sound needs to last at least 50 to 100 ms to have the recognizable timbre (sound character) of a sound. Timbre also depends on the rise time and, to a smaller degree, the decay time of the sound. For example, the rise time and fall time of music sounds are different, so if you play a music sound in reverse, it may sound like it was played by a different music instrument. If you would like to hear sounds with different rise and decay times, consult the website. **Audio clip 12-7** If you would like to hear the effects of signal duration on sound loudness, pitch, and timbre, consult the website. **Audio clip 12-8**

Timbre is a multidimensional phenomenon with many underlining scales that are used to describe sound. Some examples of scales of timbre are sharpness (sharp–dull), roughness (rough–smooth), and brightness (dark–bright). All of these terms describe some specific properties of sound, but they do not carry any emotional content. In other words, one sound may be more sharp (less dull) than another, but it does not mean that one of these sounds is better. The property of sound that allows us to scale sounds along emotional scales is called **sound quality.** Sound quality can be measured on various quality scales such as pleasantness, clarity, annoyance, or, in the case of speech perception, speech intelligibility. Both timbre and sound quality have an important role in hearing science since they are used to describe the sound source, its complexity, and its esthetic effect on the listener.

BINAURAL HEARING

All of the discussions of auditory sensations thus far assumed listening only with one ear. Under normal listening conditions, listeners use both ears, which makes the process of listening much more efficient. As a general rule, binaural hearing is superior to monaural hearing because binaural hearing increases signal loudness, and improves sound quality, speech intelligibility in noise, and localization ability, compared to monaural hearing.

The improvement in auditory perception when a person is listening with two ears is called the **binaural advantage** or binaural summation. For example, an improvement in hearing sensitivity is usually about 2 to 3 dB near threshold. At suprathreshold levels, the summation of sound received by two ears results in a doubling of sound loudness, which is comparable to an increase in sound intensity of 3 to 10 dB (Hawkins et al., 1987). Binaural listening also affects signal detection in noise, speech intelligibility, and sound quality judgments since it allows a listener to separate the various directions of incoming sounds and to attend to a specific sound source. Therefore, spatial separation of sound sources facilitated by binaural hearing is frequently referred to as spatial unmasking.

The binaural advantage is especially important for speech intelligibility when the talker and the source of the masking noise (or other unwanted talkers) are spatially separated. For one or more maskers that are spatially distinct from the talker's location, the binaural advantage can be as large as 4 to 7 dB (Bergault & Erbe, 1994; Hawley et al., 2004). This means that by spatially separating the signal from the noise, the increase in talker intelligibility is comparable with that achieved by increasing the level of the talker voice by 4 to 7 dB.

SPATIAL HEARING

The discussion of binaural hearing in the previous section addressed several situations in which binaural listening outperforms monaural listening. However, it did not address the most important effect of binaural hearing, which is a greatly improved spatial orientation. **Spatial orientation** is the act of determining the position of a sound source in space and the relationship between this position and the position of the listener. To identify both relative positions, the listener needs to determine the direction from which the sound is coming and the distance to the sound source. These two activities are auditory localization and auditory distance estimation.

Auditory localization is the process of judging the direction of an incoming sound. This process depends on binaural cues and monaural cues (mentioned in Chapters 8 and 10), head movements, and familiarity with the sound source. Judging the distance to a sound source depends on the intensity of the sound and properties of the sound that result from sound reflection, absorption by the air, etc., and familiarity with the sound.

Binaural cues are the interaural differences in intensity and time (phase) of sounds arriving to both ears. The interaural intensity difference (IID), also called the interaural level difference (ILD), results from different intensities of sounds arriving to the left and the right ear. It is mainly caused by direction- and frequency-dependent diffraction of sound around the listener's head. The IID cue is most effective at high frequencies where the dimensions of the human head are larger than the wavelengths of the traveling sounds. For example, if a sound source is located exactly in front of a listener, the sound arriving to each ear will have approximately the same intensity. However, if a sound source is located on one side of the listener's head, one ear will receive a direct sound whereas the other one will be located in the acoustic shadow of the human head and receive a much reduced sound intensity compared to the first ear.

The other binaural cue, the interaural time difference (ITD), results from the difference in the time of arrival of the sound to each ear. If the sound source is located off the median (midline), the sound takes longer to get to the farther ear than to the nearer ear. In the extreme situation when the sound source is located exactly on the side of the listener's head (in front of one ear), the time delay of sound reaching the opposite ear is about 600 to 800 μs, depending on the size of the listener's head. The ITD cue operates most efficiently at low frequencies, where the time difference is unambiguously converted into a phase difference between sounds arriving at the ears of the listener. Since the difference in timing can be expressed as the difference in the phase of the signal, the ITD is sometimes called the interaural phase difference (IPD). At higher frequencies, where the wavelength of the sound is smaller than the size of the listener's head, the phase cues will be ambiguous. For example, the phase at each ear may be identical if the difference in phase exceeds 360° and both ears receive the same phase of the wave in different cycles.

Both binaural cues, IID and ITD, are schematically shown in Figure 12.19. Binaural cues aid sound localization mainly along the left–right axis of the listener in the horizontal plane. The timing and intensity of sound arriving at both ears is practically identical for sound sources located at various elevations and along the median axis of the listener (equidistant between ears). In addition, sounds that are close together in location can result in sounds that are identical at both ears. For example, imagine a hypothetical cone extending outward from the ear of the listener. All points on the surface of this cone result in identical binaural cues and

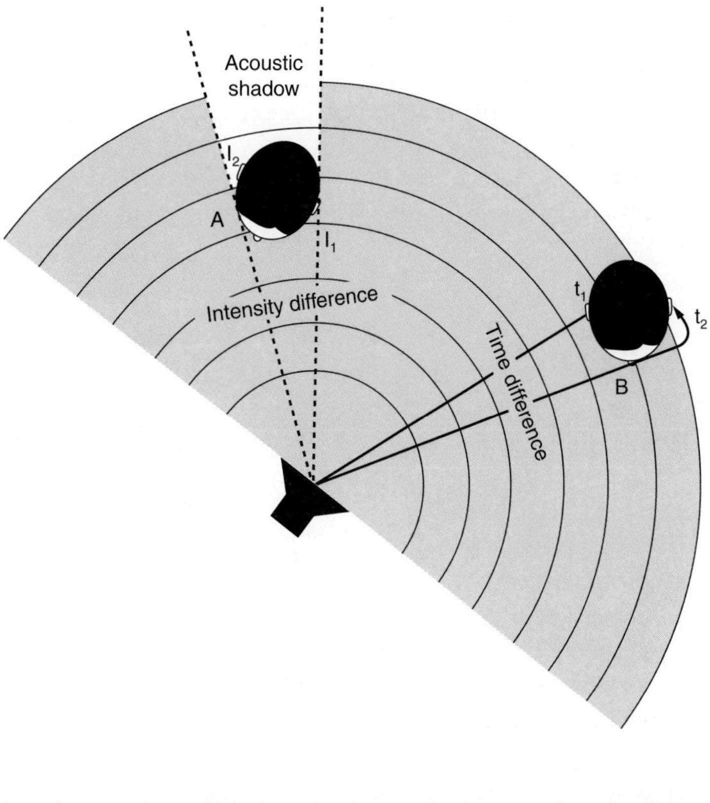

Figure 12.19. Localization of sound sources using the binaural cues: **(A)** interaural intensity difference and **(B)** interaural time difference.

the listener relying exclusively on the binaural cues is not able to distinguish between the directions of sound arriving from any two of these points. This cone is called the **cone of confusion** and it defines the limits of human ability to detect the location of a sound using binaural cues.

Monaural cues are the directional cues resulting from sound reflections and diffractions around the ridges of the pinnae and upper torso. They modify (filter) the sounds entering the ear and depend on the direction of the incoming sound. Monaural cues are very sensitive to the elevation of the sound source and to a large degree to the front or back position of the source.

The other class of localization cues includes head movements (involuntary and voluntary) and familiarity with the sound source (auditory memory). Head movements are important aids in sound localization for longer sounds. When listening to longer sounds, the listener can scan the space by slightly shifting or rotating the head. In addition, familiarity with both the sound source and the environment surrounding the listener significantly aids the listener in sound source localization. For example, a person who is familiar with the voice of another person can more easily determine the direction of an incoming sound compared with listening to an unknown voice.

Sound localization ability can be measured similarly to other perceptual phenomena, such as the absolute or difference threshold. Absolute localization is expressed as the absolute localization error in the horizontal or vertical plane. The absolute localization error depends on the type of sound source and its location and varies from about 5° to about 180° depending on the listening conditions.

Differential localization ability is the ability to notice a change in the sound source location. It is usually referred to as the **minimum audible angle** (**MAA**) for stationary sources and the **minimum audible movement angle** (**MAMA**) for moving sound sources. The MAA measured at a 0° horizontal angle (in front of the listener) is fairly frequency independent and varies from about 1° to 3°. At other elevations, MAAs are larger and can be as large as 10°. MAAs are relatively independent of sound frequency up to about 1000 Hz but increase with frequency above 1000 Hz (Mills, 1972).

The MAMA is a measure of our ability to detect sound source movement. It is defined as the smallest detectable change in an angular location of a moving sound source. It depends on the type of sound source, its speed, and the direction of movement. In general, MAMAs are about twice as large as MAAs, although for slowly moving sound sources MAMAs can be as small as 2° to 5° (Chandler & Grantham, 1992; Grantham, 1986, 1997; Middlebrook & Green, 1992).

In addition to listening to sound sources in a sound field, the listener may listen to sounds through earphones. In this case, the recorded ("phantom") sound sources are usually localized inside the head. By changing the IID or ITD between signals arriving to the left and right ear, the phantom sound source can be moved within the head on an imaginary arc connecting both ears. The act of identifying the location of a phantom sound source within the head is called **lateralization.**

None of the localization cues discussed above, except for the familiarity with the sound source and environment, is an effective cue for auditory distance estimation. The perceived distance of a sound source depends primarily on sound intensity (dominating factor in an open space) and the reverberation properties of the space (dominating factor in a closed space). The sound intensity cue is not a very reliable one when the listener is not familiar with the sound source or is placed in an unfamiliar environment. It is only an effective cue if the listener knows how loud the sound source is at various distances. Reflections from space boundaries such as the ground (open space) or the floor and walls (closed space) provide more reliable cues than sound intensity, but they are very limited in an open space. Furthermore, these cues are better utilized if the listener has some familiarity with the environment and the sound source. In addition, both auditory and visual estimates of large distances are affected by the relatively poor human ability to convert distance perceptions into distance estimates in physical units. People usually have great difficulties in reporting the distance to a specific source of sound or even a specific visual object in physical units; however, this ability can be improved with training.

Summary

Psychoacoustics is the study of the perception of sound by a listener. The acoustic characteristics of sound—intensity, frequency, duration, and spectral complexity—are generally associated with the perceptual characteristics of loudness, pitch, perceived duration, and timbre. The relationship between the stimulus magnitude and the sensation magnitude is complex. Loudness is the property of sound that allows sounds to be ordered on a scale extending from quiet (soft) to loud. Pitch is the property of sound that allows sounds to be ordered on a scale extending from low to high. Timbre can be defined as the sound property that allows for the recognition of a specific sound source and the perception of sound complexity.

Threshold is the level of a signal at which a specific sensory response is obtained a specific percentage of the time. Perceptual thresholds and the detection of sound sources are the focus of signal detection theory, which is a method of assessing the decision-making process under conditions of uncertainty.

A scale indicates the relative magnitude of an object or event in comparison to another object or event. The two most common psychophysical scales are the loudness scale and the pitch scale.

Masking is the ability of one sound to completely block out or to decrease the audibility of another sound. Masking usually results from the simultaneous reception of two or more sounds. Masking can also result when two sounds are received sequentially but very close together in time. The greatest amount of masking is produced by a high-intensity sound (masker) that is close in frequency and time to the signal (maskee).

Hair cells and nerve fibers appear to act together to process auditory information in frequency bands called critical bands. For this reason, if two sounds enter the cochlea at the same time and their frequencies are close enough to belong to the same critical band, their integration within the auditory system will be different than when the frequencies of the two sounds are farther apart than the critical band.

Spatial orientation is a listener's ability to identify the position of a sound source in space. It includes the acts of auditory localization (judging direction) on the horizontal (azimuth estimation) and vertical (elevation estimation) planes and auditory distance estimation (judging distance). Auditory localization cues include binaural cues (interaural time and intensity differences), monaural cues (filtering), and behavioral cues (head movement and sound familiarity). Auditory distance estimation is a more difficult task than sound source localization and it is dependent on the sound intensity and reverberant properties of a space.

Key Points

- There are two basic techniques used in hearing science to determine the threshold of sensation. They are the YN (yes–no) technique and the n-Alternative Forced Choice (nAFC) technique. They can be used with any of the three basic psychophysical methods of threshold determination: the Method of Limits, the Method of Constant Stimuli, and the Method of Adjustment.
- The dynamic range of hearing for a normal human ear extends from about 20 Hz to 20,000 Hz and from about 0 dB SPL to 120 dB SPL. However, the human ear is not equally sensitive across the entire frequency range.
- The improvement in auditory perception when a person is listening with two ears is called the binaural advantage.
- In a signal detection task there are four possible outcomes. If a sound is presented and the listener indicates that he or she heard it, the response is classified as a "hit." If a sound is presented and the listener fails to respond, the response is classified as a "miss." If no sound is presented but the listener indicates that he or she heard a sound, the response is classified as a "false alarm." If no sound is presented and the listener fails to respond, that is classified as a "correct rejection."
- The difference threshold is the smallest perceptible change in the magnitude of stimulation. The difference threshold is also known as the difference limen or just noticeable difference. The DL for intensity, or DL(I), refers to the smallest perceivable difference in sound intensity between two sounds. The DL for frequency, or DL(f), refers to the smallest change in the frequency that can be perceived.
- Weber's Law is based on the assumption that the DL corresponds to a constant relative change in the value of a stimulus regardless of the actual magnitude of the stimulus. This law does not hold for very low magnitudes of a stimulus that are close to the threshold of hearing.
- The most common scale of loudness is the sone scale. One sone is defined as the loudness produced by a 1000-Hz tone having an intensity of 40 dB SPL. The scale allows a listener to determine in sones how much one sound is louder than another.
- Equal-loudness contours (phon curves) indicate equal loudness levels of sounds of different frequencies. The reference is the loudness of a 1000-Hz tone.
- The scale relating frequency and pitch is called the mel scale.
- Masking phenomena, observed via tone-on-tone masking, include the following: (1) high-intensity sounds are more effective at masking than low-intensity sounds, (2) masking is most effective when the frequency of the masker is close to the frequency of the maskee, (3) low-frequency signals mask high-frequency signals better than high-frequency signals mask low-frequency signals (upward spread of masking), and (4) harmonics of a masking signal, created by the cochlea, can also act as maskers.

PART IV

Audio Systems

CHAPTER 13

Electricity and Electric Circuits

Tomasz Letowski, Diana C. Emanuel, and Stephen Pallett

Chapter Outline

Objectives

- To review the basics of electricity including the movement of electrons, voltage, current, resistance, and Ohm's Law
- To introduce the concepts of electric, magnetic, and electromagnetic fields
- To list and describe the common components of electric circuits including resistors, capacitors, inductors, and semiconductors (diodes, transistors)
- To describe the two types of circuits, parallel and series, and some basic concepts associated with electric circuits
- To describe the concept of electric impedance and how it relates to power transmission
- To describe the importance of grounding and shielding in electric circuits

Key Terms

Active component
Actuator
Alternating current (AC)
Ampere (A)
Amplifier
Atom
Audio signal
Battery drain
Capacitance
Capacitive reactance (X_c)
Capacitor
Chip
Conductor
Coulomb (*C*)
Crosstalk
Diode
Direct current (DC)
Electric charge (*Q*)
Electric circuit
Electric component
Electric current (*I*)
Electric field
Electric flux
Electric impedance
Electric installation
Electric load
Electric source
Electric switch
Electricity
Electromagnet
Electromagnetic field
Electromotive force (*E*)
Electron
Force field
Free electron
Ground
Grounding
Ground wire
Henry (H)
Hot wire
Inductance
Inductive reactance (X_L)
Inductor
Insulator
Interference noise
Ion
Ionized
Isotopes

Magnetic field	Permanent magnet	Series circuit
Magnetism	Permeability (μ)	Shielding
Magnetomotive force (*M*)	Permittivity (ε)	Thermal noise
Negative pole	Positive pole	Transformer
Network	Potential difference (*E*)	Transformer ratio (*r*)
Neutron	Potentiometer	Transistor
Ohm (Ω)	Proton	Transmitted noise
Ohm's Law	Resistance	Valence shell
Parallel circuit	Resistor	Volt (V)
Passive component	Safety ground	Voltage (*E*)
	Semiconductor	Voltage drop

ELECTRICITY

The study of electricity and electric circuits is critical for the study of hearing science. In almost every application, sound is measured, recorded, transmitted, and manipulated in its electric form, not in its acoustic or mechanic form. This electric signal is called an **audio signal** and the equipment used for recording, transmitting, and reproducing audio signals is called audio equipment. A good grasp of the concept of electricity and the principles of operation of basic electric circuits is needed for the proper use of audio equipment and effective sound manipulation. For example, an understanding of batteries and the concept of current drain is needed to determine how long a battery-operated device, such as a hearing aid or battery-operated audiometer, will function properly on one charge or one set of batteries. The selection of proper microphones and loudspeakers for sound recording and reproduction requires a good familiarity with electric specifications on these devices. A solid understanding of electric signals and circuits is needed to troubleshoot electric devices that are malfunctioning. A familiarity with the concept of electric impedance is needed for the effective use of electrodes in such audiology tests as the Auditory Brainstem Response (ABR) test. The list of applications of electricity is endless. Electricity is everywhere and it powers almost all of our technology. Most notably it powers our nervous system. Without a good understanding of what electricity can do and what is required for its proper use, we cannot do much in the modern world.

Atoms and Charges

Electricity is a form of energy resulting from an uneven distribution (potential energy) and directional flow (kinetic energy) of electrons. A change in the distribution of electrons results in the transfer of energy from one place to another as electrons move across a long chain of atoms. Thus, to study electricity, it is necessary to briefly review the atomic structure of matter. Matter is anything that occupies space and has mass. All matter (solids, liquids, and gasses) is composed of tiny building blocks called **atoms** with an average diameter of 10^{-8} cm. Atoms are made up of three types of particles: **protons** (which carry a positive charge), **electrons** (which carry a negative charge), and **neutrons** (which are neutral). The charges carried by protons and electrons are numerically identical; therefore, a proton–electron pair is electrically neutral. Protons are located in the nucleus of an atom and the number of protons in an atom is called the atomic number. For example, an atom with one proton (hydrogen) has an atomic number of 1, an atom with two protons (helium) has an atomic number of 2, and so forth. All of the elements (matter composed of one type of atom) are listed in order of their atomic number in the Periodic Table of the Elements, which can be found in any basic chemistry book. Neutrons also reside in the nucleus of atoms. They have a mass similar to that of a proton but do not have any electric charge. The number of neutrons plus the number of protons indicates the atomic mass of an element. Electrons do not practically contribute to the atomic mass of an atom since an electron's mass is about 1/1838 of the mass of a proton. The number of neutrons (but not the number of protons) in an element can vary and these variations are called **isotopes.** For example, the element carbon generally has six neutrons and six protons, so it has an atomic mass of 12 (called carbon 12 or C12). But in another isotope of carbon with eight neutrons, the atomic mass would be 14 (called carbon 14 or C14).

The electrons of an atom orbit the nucleus and are located at some distance away from it, creating multilayered electron "shells." If the number of electrons in an atom is the same as the number of protons, the atom is neutral. If the number of electrons is higher than the number of protons, the atom will have a negative (−) charge. If the number of electrons is lower than the number of protons, the atom will have a positive (+) charge. An atom that carries a charge is called an **ion.** A substance containing a lot of charged particles is said to be **ionized.** Understanding the concepts of electrons and ions is the key element to understanding electricity and electric systems.

Electric Current

An electric current is the organized flow of electrons. For current to flow, one must have a source of electrons that are free to move. Recall that each basic element (type of atom) has a specific number of protons that distinguishes one element from another. In all basic elements, the number of electrons spinning around the nucleus is equal to the number of protons in the nucleus. Individual electrons are organized in several shells located at different distances from the nucleus. The spinning path of electrons within a shell is called an orbit. The shells differ in the energy level of the electrons spinning within a shell. The first shell, closest to the nucleus, can only have two electrons. All other shells may have eight or more electrons located at various subshells and orbits. The farther away the shell is from the nucleus, the weaker the force of attraction is between the nucleus and the electron. This force of attraction is another form of the force of gravity discussed in Chapter 2.

The outer shell of an atom is called the **valence shell** and the electrons located on this shell are called valence electrons. If an electron on the valence shell is attracted by another atom more than it is attracted by its own nucleus, it can break away and become what is called a **free electron.** In some elements, such as copper, the electrons located on the valence shell are so weakly attracted by their own nucleus and at the same time they are so close to the nuclei of other atoms that the valence electrons start to drift randomly from one atom to another. The same phenomenon also takes place in more complex forms of matter that consist of several different elements. If some external force is applied to this type of matter, the randomly drifting electrons can be organized and start flowing in one specific direction. This flow of free electrons is called electric current. Since electrons are negatively charged particles, they move away from a negative (−) charge and toward a positive (+) charge. It is conventional, however, to draw current as flowing from the higher (+) to the lower (−) charge. This convention is in agreement with the natural flow observed in other areas of physics such as the flow of water that always moves from a higher level toward a lower one. It is a confusing concept that the current flows in the opposite direction than the electrons flow, but this convention is accepted in most scientific texts.

The intensity (strength) of **electric current (*I*)** is determined by the number of electrons passing through a point of observation in 1 second. In other words, the intensity of electric current is defined as the amount of electricity, called the **electric charge (Q),** passing through a specific point in 1 second. This number of electrons is usually astronomically high, so the number of electrons would not be a convenient unit of electric charge. Therefore, electricity is usually measured in a more practical unit called the **coulomb (C)** after the French physicist Charles de Coulomb (1736–1806), who is best known for his work on electricity and magnetism and is the author of Coulomb's Law. Coulomb's Law states that the force between two electric charges is proportional to the product of those charges and inversely proportional to the square of the distance between them. This law is an electric version of the Law of Gravitation (Chapter 2) and it determines the force of attraction between the nucleus and electrons spinning in various shells. A charge of 1 coulomb is equal to the amount of electricity contained in 6.24×10^{18} (6.24 quintillion) electrons. Subsequently, electric current is measured in the number of coulombs passing through a point of observation in 1 second. The current resulting from 1 coulomb of electricity passing through a point of observation in 1 second is called 1 **ampere** (A). The ampere was named after another French physicist, André Ampère (1775–1836), who developed the foundations of electromagnetism.

Electromotive Force

For free electrons to flow in an organized manner, they need an external force pushing them from one place to another. This force is called an **electromotive force (E), potential difference,** or **voltage** and it is measured in **volts (V)*.** Electromotive force is the force needed to pass an electric charge between two points in space. One volt is the force that generates 1 joule (J) of work when pushing an electric charge of 1 coulomb (C) across a certain distance. Thus, $V = J/C$.

The terms *electromotive force, potential difference,* and *voltage* represent the same physical phenomenon but are used in different contexts depending on the source of energy and whether they represent energy (the ability to do work) or work (e.g., electromotive force is the ability to deliver a voltage). All three quantities are denoted in this book by the letter *E*; however, in other books, they may be referred to as *U* or *V* or different letters may be assigned to each of these terms. The names *voltage* and *volt* were established in honor of Italian physicist Alessandro Volta (1745−1827), who invented the first chemical battery.

The source of electromotive force is an electric charge that has no place to go and that has accumulated at one specific location. This charge is called static electricity. For more information or static electricity, see the website. **Link 13-1** The presence of static electricity creates another opposite and equal charge in space, resulting in the presence of two groups of oppositely charged ions that are accumulated at different locations. The positively charged ions are called cations and the negatively charged ions are called anions. These groups are said to have a positive (+) and negative (−) potential and to constitute the **positive pole** and **negative pole** of the force field created by their presence. The force field created by two opposite poles is called an **electric field.** An electric field is a form of potential energy. In mechanics, potential energy is related to mass and the force of gravity or elasticity. In electricity, potential energy is related to charge and electromotive force. The total amount of electric field passing across a certain surface is called an electric flux. The **electric flux** is the amount of electric charge acting over a specific area. An electric flux of

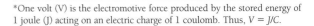

*One volt (V) is the electromotive force produced by the stored energy of 1 joule (J) acting on an electric charge of 1 coulomb. Thus, $V = J/C$.

1 coulomb per second creates an electric current of 1 ampere. If the accumulated electric charge finds a place to go and flows from one place to another (due to an attraction by an opposite charge), the result is electric current flow. The change from stored electric energy to a flow of current is a change from potential energy to kinetic energy. The electric current flow causes a decrease in the original voltage along the current pathway and this decrease in charge is called a **voltage drop.**

A natural phenomenon or device that causes the flux to flow and that generates an electromotive force is called an **electric source** or a source of electricity. A practical example of a source of electricity is a battery. A battery is an electrochemical device that can be charged and stores electricity. A battery is a system of two electrodes (poles, terminals) that carry opposite charges (+ and −) that are the source of the static electricity. If the poles of the battery are connected together by a conductor or other electric circuitry, the electrons are "pushed" through this external pathway by the voltage of the battery from its negative pole to its positive pole, forming a current. The current that is drawn from the battery is called a **battery drain** and it depends on the type of battery and properties of the circuitry connected to the terminals of the battery. The magnitude of the available electromotive force depends on the difference in charge between the two poles of the battery. Most common household batteries, including AA, AAA, C, and D, are intended to deliver a voltage of 1.5 V when connected to a load. Another common battery is the rectangular 9-V battery, which, as its name implies, delivers a voltage of 9 V.

If the voltage of a battery that is creating a flow of electrons is not sustained by an external source of energy, the flow of electrons gradually decreases and the electromotive force ceases to exist. Once the charge between the two poles of the battery is gone, there is no voltage at the output of the battery and the battery is dead. Some batteries (e.g., lead-acid batteries used in cars, lithium ion batteries used in computers) can be recharged and used again, whereas some others (e.g., alkaline batteries, zinc-air batteries, and mercury batteries) are not rechargeable.

Direct and Alternating Current

The source of electricity may be a static potential difference (voltage), which causes the current to flow in only one specific direction, or it may be an oscillating potential difference (voltage), which periodically changes its direction across time and causes the current to reverse its direction periodically. A current produced by a static potential difference is called a **direct current (DC),** which means that electrons are always flowing in only one direction. A common example of a DC source of electricity is a battery, such as a car battery or a hearing aid battery. An oscillating potential difference results in an oscillating current, which changes direction periodically. This oscillating voltage will result when an acoustic signal is converted into an electric signal. It may also be produced by special bidirectional electricity generators or converters, such as those used in power plants for supplying electricity to our homes and businesses.* A current produced by an oscillating voltage is called an **alternating current (AC).** Alternating current means that the current flow periodically changes its value and direction, usually following a sinusoidal pattern. Any device that is plugged into a standard wall outlet draws AC from the wall (although it may be converted to DC, as we will explain later in the chapter). Figure 13.1 shows examples of both types of current with the magnitude of the voltage shown on the *y* axis and time shown on the *x* axis. Notice that the alternating current shown in Figure 13.1A has the familiar sinusoidal form discussed in Chapter 3.

During the first half of the cycle in Figure 13.1A, the voltage is positive, and during the second half of the cycle, the voltage is negative. The duration of the wave period is 17 ms, which corresponds to a waveform frequency of 60 Hz. This specific frequency is used in the United States and some other countries (mainly South America) to transmit electric

*Electric power production and transmission that is commonly used for commercial and domestic use has the form of AC rather than DC due to its lower energy losses over large distances of transmission and easier ways to change voltage values.

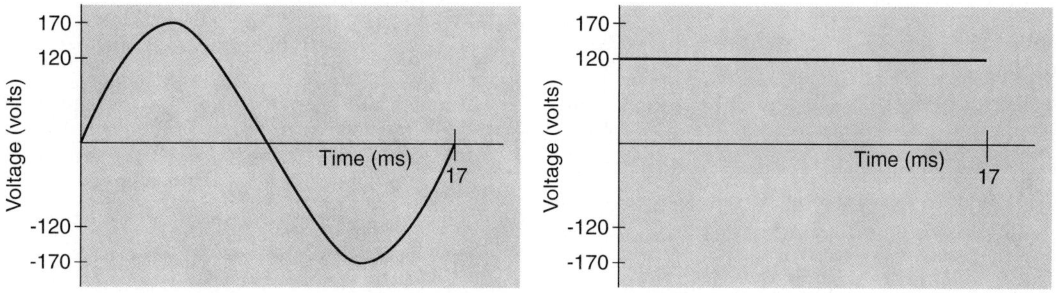

A **Alternating current**

B **Direct current**

Figure 13.1. Electromotive force (voltage) in volts as a function of time for one cycle of alternating current **(A)** and direct current **(B)** occurring over the same time period.

power from power plants to all energy users (60 Hz, 110 to 120 V). In Europe and in the rest of the world, 50 Hz (50 Hz, 220 to 240 V) is used for electricity production and transmission.*

Most electric devices that provide heat or move mechanic objects, such as electric stoves, refrigerators, fans, and shavers, use AC power for their operation. However, another large group of electric devices that transmit and process information, such as computers, audiometers, and audio equipment, require DC power for their proper operation. In many cases, when only AC power is available but DC power is required to operate a device, the AC power must be converted to DC power. This can be accomplished by an AC/DC converter that may appear as a big black box attached to the power cord of a computer or other device. Devices powered by batteries do not need an AC/DC converter, because batteries already supply DC.

Electric Power

In the section above we discussed electric power. Recall from Chapter 2 that mechanic power is defined as the product of force and velocity ($P = F \times v$). Similarly, electric power (P) is defined as the product of voltage (E) and electric current (I), because voltage is the electric counterpart to force and electric current is the electric counterpart to velocity.

$$P = E \times I \qquad (13.1)$$

The unit of electric power, just as in mechanic and acoustic power, is the watt (W). The watt is the unit for all forms of power since power is the ability to do work and it is not concerned with the physical means that contribute to this work. In the case of electric power, if a 12-V battery results in 1 A of current flowing through the electric system of a car, the power drawn from the battery is equal to 12 V × 1 A = 12 W. The power is subsequently related to the work that can be performed by an electric system. Recall that work (W) is equal to the product of power (P) and time (t). A source of electricity delivering 12 W of power for an hour has performed 12 Wh (watt-hours) or 43.3 kJ of work. Since the number of watt-hours is much easier to calculate than the number of joules, the watt-hour is the most commonly used unit of work in the domain of electricity. Consider now a 100-W light bulb. This type of bulb is rated for a specific number of hours of operation, such as 1000 hours, which is specified on the bulb package. This means that this bulb was designed to perform work equal to 100 W × 1000 hr = 100,000 Wh = 100 kWh, after which it will most likely fail.

According to Equation 13.1, power is the product of voltage and current. This equation describes the very straightforward relationship between power, voltage, and current in DC systems. To determine power consumption in AC systems, one needs to recall from Chapter 3 that there are a number of ways to indicate the magnitude of a periodic waveform. The specific magnitudes include the amplitude, average magnitude, root mean square (RMS) magnitude, and so forth. The magnitudes of an alternating electric signal can be described in the same way. Most commonly, the magnitude of an AC is indicated using the RMS magnitude, because when an AC source has an RMS magnitude equal to the value of a DC source, both sources provide the same amount of power. To illustrate this statement, consider the sinusoidal voltage provided by a standard electric outlet in your home. This voltage in the United States is rated as 120 V, 60 Hz. The value 120 V is not the amplitude of the waveform but is its RMS magnitude and it is frequently written as Vrms (for RMS voltage). The *amplitude* of the voltage delivered by the power plant in the United States is actually 170 V (Fig. 13.1A). Recall that RMS magnitude = amplitude × 0.707 (Chapter 3). Thus, a DC power source with a voltage value of 120 V produces the same power as an AC power source with an RMS magnitude of 120 V, which would occur when the amplitude of the AC power source is 170 V (170 × 0.707 = 120 V).

*Devices designed to operate with power sources having a 60-Hz frequency may not operate properly when used with power sources operating with a 50-Hz power frequency and vice versa. The use of the proper power frequency is especially important in the case of television systems since most countries choose their TV picture refresh rate to be equal to their power frequency. It is also important to realize that the speed of AC motors is proportional to the frequency of the supplied power.

PRACTICE PROBLEMS: POWER, VOLTAGE, AND CURRENT

1. What is the power drawn from a 9-V battery if the attached electric system draws 2 A of current?
2. What is the voltage of a battery that delivers 100 W of power while supplying 25 A of current?
3. What is the current intensity drawn from a 12-V battery supplying 50 W of power to its load?
4. What is the RMS magnitude of an AC power source that supplies the same amount of power as a DC source with a voltage of 320 V?
5. What is the voltage amplitude of an AC power source that supplies the same amount of power as a DC power source with a voltage of 320 V?
6. What is the voltage of a DC power source that supplies the same amount of power as an AC (sinusoidal) power source with a voltage amplitude of 200 V?

Answers (If you need help with these problems, consult the website.) **Link 13-2**

1. 18 W
2. 4 V
3. 4.17 A
4. 320 V
5. 452.62 V
6. 141.4 V

MAGNETISM AND ELECTROMAGNETIC FIELD

Magnetism is the property of matter that results from the movement of charged particles, such as electrons, through the matter. Similar to electricity, this is a phenomenon by which charged (magnetized) objects attract or repel other objects. An electromotive force results from the *presence* of opposing stationary charges. The opposing charges produce an electric flux and cause electric current to flow. A **magnetomotive force (*M*)** (magnetic force) results from the *movement* of charges, that is, the flow of electric current. The flow of current creates a magnetic flux (analogous to the electric flux introduced earlier in this chapter) that affects other currents flowing in the area and/or creates new currents. Magnetomotive force may also result from the natural spin of electrons (like Earth spinning around its axis) or the orbital motion of electrons around their atoms (like Earth orbiting around the sun). When the motions of electrons in neighboring atoms interact in such a way that the orbital motion of all the electrons of the group is aligned along the same axis, they form materials that have magnetic capabilities and are called **permanent magnets.** A permanent magnet can be natural (e.g., magnetite) or it can be created by an external process. In addition, passing a current through a coil of wire wound around a metal core can create a temporary magnetic force. This source of magnetic field is called an **electromagnet.**

Recall that according to Newton's Law of Gravitation (Chapter 2), two bodies (masses) separated in space attract each other with a force (*G*) called the force of gravitation. The presence of such a force in a certain area is referred to as a gravitational field. A gravitational field is an example of a force field, within which the particles of matter are acted upon by a specific force created by some form of potential energy. An electric field (electrostatic field) and a **magnetic field** are two other examples of force fields. Although a force field may conjure up images of science fiction movies, keep in mind that a **force field** is simply an area in which a force such as gravity, electricity, or magnetism is causing objects to be affected in certain ways. In electric and magnetic fields, respective electric and magnetic charges can attract or repel each other, causing currents to flow and charged objects to move. A magnetic field can be created by electrons spinning around the nucleus of an atom and by Earth spinning around its axis. Figure 13.2 illustrates this basic concept of attraction that occurs between two opposite charges and repulsion that occurs between two like charges, which repel each other.

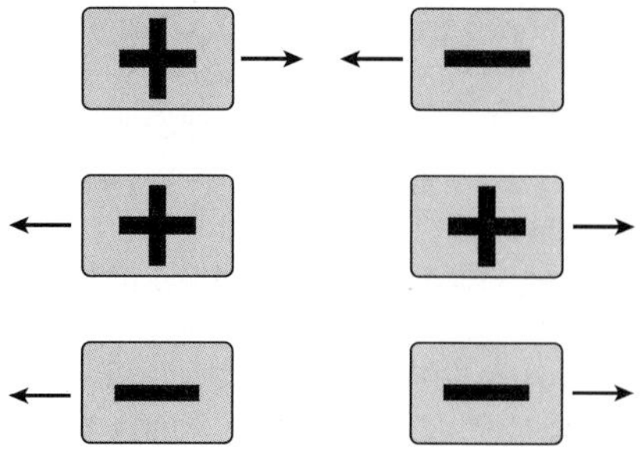

Figure 13.2. Opposite charges attract and like charges repel.

Both electric and magnetic fields are characterized by their respective flux and flux density. Electric flux was defined earlier in this chapter as the amount of electric charge acting over a specific surface. Similarly, magnetic flux is the amount of magnetism acting over a specific surface. The unit of magnetic flux is the weber (Wb). The name *weber* was established in honor of German physicist and acoustician Wilhelm Weber (1804–1891), who considerably advanced our understanding of electric and magnetic fields. A change in flux of 1 Wb per second creates an electromotive force of 1 V. Therefore, 1 Wb = V × sec. A mechanic analogy of the flux* is the quantity of fluid pushed through a pipe of a certain cross section during a specific time. It is important to realize that fluids of different viscosities, that is, different resistance to flowing, will result in different amounts of fluid pushed through the pipe in a specific amount of time, assuming that the same power is acting on the fluid. The same is true for electric and magnetic fields. Different materials have different properties that affect the transmission of flux; that is, they determine the amount of the field that can enter the material. These properties are called **permittivity (ε)** for an electric field and **permeability (μ)** for a magnetic field. They can be considered the electric and magnetic analogs of mechanic friction (fluid viscosity).

The most common measure of field intensity is flux density. The electric flux density (*D*), also called the electric displacement, is the density of electric flux per unit of area, that is, the rate at which electric current would flow through a certain area if the current could flow. The unit of electric flux density is coulomb over meter squared. The magnetic flux density (*B*), also called magnetic induction, is the density of magnetic flux per unit of area. The unit of magnetic flux density is the telsa (T), which is equal to weber per meter squared. Both *D* and *B* refer to a flux of energy through a specific material. The absolute (highest) flux density is produced if the material is a perfect insulator, that is, a dielectric material (electric field) or a nonferromagnetic material (magnetic field). To understand this concept, remember the concept of the "force field" from science fiction movies mentioned at the beginning of the chapter. When a magnetic field is present between two poles, but the poles are not connected, there is nothing flowing between the poles but there exists a force between them. Consider, for example, two huge magnets fixed to the floor so they

*The same analogy applies to both flux and electric current. The difference is that flux represents the intensity of the field with no conductor present in this area and the current represents the intensity of the resulting electron flow when the conductor is placed in this area.

cannot move and separated by a certain distance with opposing poles turned toward each other. Nothing is flowing between them, but if you put a paper clip somewhere between them it will not stay there but will "fly" toward the N pole. If both these magnets were connected by a piece of ferromagnetic metal (good conductor of the magnetic field) and you put a paper clip next to it, it would not move because there would be very little magnetic field to act on it.

The absolute electric flux density that results from given electric charges is called the electric field strength (K), and $D = \varepsilon K$. The absolute magnetic flux density that results from a given amount of magnetism is called magnetic field strength (H), and $B = \mu H$. If the material is a perfect electric insulator, then $\varepsilon = 1$ and $D = K$. If the material is a perfect magnetic insulator, then $\mu = 1$ and $B = H$. Thus, if one measures very low biologic potentials, these measurements need to be conducted in a well electrically and magnetically insulated booth to prevent the induction of external interferences in the measurement circuits. This means that the booth should be surrounded by well-conducting electric and magnetic material to minimize the flux density passing inside the booth.

Both electric and magnetic fields can be thought of as families of invisible lines of force connecting the two opposing poles of the source of the field and organizing particles of matter along theses lines. Actually, most of the formal definitions of flux refer to it as a group of "lines of force" passing through a specific surface. These lines provide an easy way to visualize the direction and extent of a specific field. An example of a magnetic field caused by a natural magnet and the lines of force representing the magnetic field are shown in Figure 13.3. An electric field created by the presence of positive and negative charges would have a very similar pattern.

According to common terminology, the two opposite poles of a magnetic field are called the North Pole (N) and the South Pole (S). This convention reflects the fact that the most widely known magnetic field, Earth's magnetic field, is created by a magnetic dipole with the poles located close to the geographical poles of Earth. This magnetic field extends thousands of kilometers into space and is caused by the rotational movement of Earth and the presence of both magnetic materials

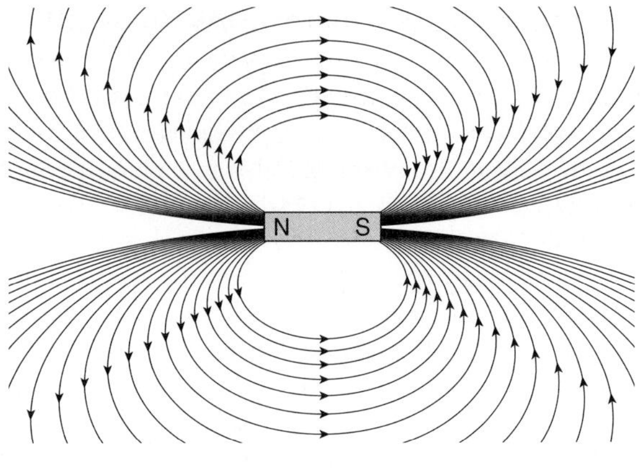

Figure 13.3. Magnetic lines of force of a bar magnet.

and electrically conductive fluids (such as fluid iron and nickel) in Earth's outer core.*

Unfortunately, the terminology related to magnetic poles is a bit confusing. Let us consider Earth to be a big magnet. In this magnet, the North Pole is denoted as N and the South Pole is denoted as S and the lines of force have a direction from south to north. However, in the case of all other magnets, N denotes the end of magnet being pulled toward Earth's N pole and S denotes the end of magnet being pulled toward Earth's S pole. Therefore, N seeks N and N repulses S, which is the opposite of the way positive (+) and negative (−) symbols are used in electricity. The origin of this magnetic convention is the labeling used in a magnetic compass. The end of the magnetic needle showing the direction toward N is historically labeled N although as a matter of fact it is the S pole of the small magnet used in the compass.

Figure 13.4A illustrates an example of a magnetic field created by the flow of a current. The current (I) passing through a wire creates a magnetic field (B) (shown by the

*The earth can be divided into the inner core, the outer core, and the surface (crust, shell). Due to the high temperature inside the earth, its inner core is still fluid. Fluids such as volcanic lava are also present in the outer core. The magnetic materials of the rotating earth will generate electric currents in the moving conductive fluids of the earth's core. However, only fluids located off center, in the outer core, move and therefore create the earth's magnetic field. This is the so-called dynamo theory of the earth's magnetic field.

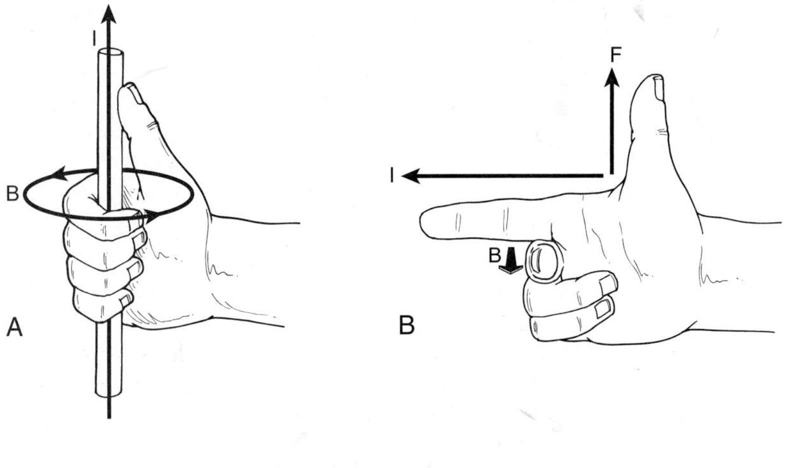

Figure 13.4. The right-hand rule used to demonstrate **(A)** the relationship between the direction of the current (*I*) flowing through a wire and the direction of the magnetic field (B) around the wire and **(B)** the directions of the current (*I*) flowing through a wire, the direction of the magnetic field (B) around the wire, and the direction of the force (*F*) that can move a wire.

circular line on the figure) that is perpendicular to the current flow. One way to picture the direction of the magnetic field is to use the "right-hand rule." The right-hand rule is a way to predict the direction of the magnetic field (B) produced by a current (I) passing through a wire. If you curl your right hand around a wire and stick your thumb out in the direction of the current flow (using the conventional notation that current flows from "+" to "−"), the direction of the fingers shows the direction of the magnetic field.

Imagine now a situation in which a wire passing a current (I) is placed in an external static (i.e., not alternating) magnetic field (B). The magnetic field produced by the electric current interacts with the external magnetic field (B), creating an electrodynamic force (F), which is trying to change the intensity of the electric current. If the wire has the ability to move, such as the coil in a dynamic loudspeaker (Chapter 14), it will move in the direction of the force (F). The direction of the force (F) and the direction of movement of the loudspeaker can be determined by another form of the "right-hand rule" shown in Figure 13.4B.

In Figure 13.4B, the right-hand rule uses the relative orientation of three fingers: the thumb, index finger, and middle finger (which are all at right angles to each other) to indicate the direction of the force (F), current (I), and magnetic field (B). If the index finger points in the direction of the current (I) and the middle finger points toward the magnetic field (B), then the thumb position indicates the direction of the force (F), which would be the expected direction of wire movement if the wire could move. The opposite is also true; moving a wire in the presence of a magnetic field results in the creation (induction) of an electric current in the wire. This opposite phenomenon is the principle of a dynamic microphone (Chapter 14).

The discussion presented above indicates that electric and magnetic fields are related and actually create each other, resulting in a complex **electromagnetic field.** Electric charges produce an electric field and cause the flow of a current. The flow of a current produces a magnetic field. When the velocity of the charged particles changes, the magnetic field changes and results in the creation of new electric currents. The new electric currents create changes in the electric field and new electromagnetic fields are created. In other words, an electromagnetic field is the interaction between the electric field generated by the presence of particles possessing an electric charge and the magnetic field generated by the relative movement of these particles in space. If we have a changing electric or magnetic field the other field is automatically created. Please note that an electric field and a magnetic field are the same force field created by stationary charges or by moving charges.

ELECTRIC COMPONENTS AND CIRCUITS

An **electric component** is a physical object that conducts current. The source of electricity and various electric components connected together are called an **electric circuit.** The final components of an electric circuit, that is, the component that uses electricity for a specific work, is called the **electric load** or simply the load. An electric circuit consisting of a source of electricity and a load is called a closed circuit. A circuit without a load connected to the source of electricity is called an open circuit. The main components of electric circuits include resistors, capacitors, inductors, switches, transformers, and active semiconductive elements.

Conductors and Insulators

Electricity travels through matter because of the movement of electrons along a chain of atoms like a long line of people passing a series of balls (Gibilisco, 2005). Electrons move very easily through some materials and not quite so easily through other materials. Their flow is dependent on the strength of the atomic forces (fields), the number of electrons on the valence shell of individual atoms, and the density of atoms in the matter (composition of the matter). These electrochemical properties of the matter are reflected in the resistance, capacitance, and inductance of the matter and will be described later. Together they represent the total opposition of the matter to electron flow, called the **electric impedance** (Z). Electric impedance is the electric analog of mechanic impedance that was discussed earlier in this book. Matter that has low electric impedance and conducts electricity easily is called a **conductor.** Matter that has high electric impedance and allows very few electrons to flow through it is called an **insulator** (e.g., dielectric). The matter forming an electric circuit can be lumped (concentrated) at specific locations or distributed across a circuit. The lumped electric components that represent resistance, capacitance, and inductance in an electric circuit are called resistors, capacitors, and inductors, respectively. A wire (conductor) connecting two components is an example of a component with resistance, capacitance, and inductance continuously distributed along its length.

Matter that can conduct electricity under some conditions but not others is called a semiconductor. Semiconductors are good materials for controlling the flow of electric current and are used in various electronic devices such as amplifiers and electronic switches. Both conductors and semiconductors operate by passing electric current. For an electric current to flow through a component, however, the atoms within the component must be willing to give and take electrons. Good conductors, like copper, easily accept and give away electrons, whereas good insulators, like silicon and glass, do not.

For an electric current to flow, it needs an electric circuit, that is, a pathway that allows the flow of an electric current from one pole of an energy source to another. A basic electric circuit is a loop created by wires connecting a series of various electric components. Depending on the type of voltage source attached to the circuit, all circuits can be divided into DC circuits and AC circuits. The basic difference between these circuits is that resistance affects current flow in both DC and AC circuits, whereas capacitance and inductance affect the current flow only in AC circuits, since their opposition to current flow is a function of frequency. If a DC source is connected to a circuit including capacitive or inductive components, their opposition to DC is either infinite (capacitance) or none (inductance).

As discussed above, the main electric components of DC circuits are resistors, whereas AC circuits include resistors, capacitors, and inductors. Both types of circuits can also employ various auxiliary components such as switches, electric light devices, and fuses. All these components are called **passive components** (passive elements). They alter the current and voltage at various points in the electric circuit but they do not need an additional source of energy to perform their functions. **Active components** require additional sources of energy to perform their functions and may include vacuum tubes, transistors, and integrated circuits. Active components are used primarily to amplify transmitted AC signals or as logic devices in digital systems and are the basis of electroacoustic (audio) circuits, which are described in Chapter 14.

Resistance and Resistors

Resistance (*R*) opposes the flow of electric current through matter and converts the passing current into heat that dissipates into the environment or that can be used in a number of practical applications, such as cooking and heating. It is one of the three parts of electric impedance in AC circuits and the only opposition to current flow in DC circuits. The unit of electric resistance is the **ohm (Ω)**, named after German physicist Georg Ohm (1789–1854), who discovered the relationship between electric voltage and electric current, which is known as **Ohm's Law** (described later in this chapter).

A **resistor** is a component of an electric circuit that has a known resistance and provides a specific opposition to a current passing through the circuit. In other words, it provides a specific resistance to the flow of energy through a circuit and inhibits the flow of current. The resistance of the resistor depends on its material, size, and construction (e.g., mass resistor, wire resistor). Resistors usually look like tiny cylinders with thin wires coming from both ends (the wires connect the resistor to the circuit). The value of the resistance provided by the resistor and its tolerance are indicated either numerically on its surface (e.g., 100 Ω, 2%) or are coded by four colored stripes circling the resistor. If you would like to know more about the color codes of resistors, consult the website. **Link 13-3**

Since the current flow through a resistor results in heat generation, the shape and size (volume) of the resistor and the material from which it is made (commonly carbon) determine the amount of power the resistor can handle before it overheats. The resistance in a circuit can be adjusted by including more than one resistor in the circuit. In addition, some resistors, called **potentiometers,** offer adjustable resistance that can be changed by rotating a dial or moving a slider attached to the resistor. Uses of potentiometers include the volume control on a hearing aid and the level control on an audiometer. A potentiometer can be imagined as a dividing network in which a moving element controls how much of the initial signal is passed further toward the output.

Ohm's Law

Recall from Chapter 4 that the relationship between force and velocity depends on the opposition (resistance) of an object to a change in its state. Similarly, in the domain of electricity the relationship between the voltage and current depends on the opposition (resistance) of the medium to a flow of electrons. The relationship between the voltage (*E*), resistance (*R*), and current (*I*) in DC circuits is known as Ohm's Law.

Box 13.1 Ohm's Law

The intensity of an electric current is directly proportional to the voltage producing the current and inversely proportional to the resistance through which the current flows.

Mathematically, Ohm's Law can be written as follows:

$$I = \frac{E}{R} \tag{13.2}$$

where *I* is the current in amperes (A), *E* is the voltage in volts (V), and *R* is the resistance in ohms (Ω). This equation is often manipulated and also written in the following ways, depending on the unknown part of the equation:

$$E = I \times R \tag{13.3}$$

$$R = \frac{E}{I} \tag{13.4}$$

However, keep in mind that in each case resistance controls the relationship between voltage and current and it is not a result of their existence.

Example 13.1

What is the resistance of an electric conductor in a DC system if a 12-V electromotive force causes the flow of a 100-A current?

First, use Equation 13.4, because we know the electromotive force (*E*) and the current (*I*) and we need to find the resistance (*R*):

$$R = \frac{E}{I}$$

Substitute known variables and solve.

$$R = \frac{12\ V}{100\ A}$$

$$R = 0.12\ \Omega$$

The classic form of Ohm's Law presented in Equations 13.2 to 13.4 applies to the *resistance* seen in both DC and AC systems and it can be extended to include the total electric impedance of AC systems (described later in this chapter).

If we reconsider Equation 13.1, which describes electric power as a product of voltage and current ($P = E \times I$), and substitute either the E or I with Equation 13.3 or 13.2, respectively, the following two equations can be derived as follows:

$$P = E \times I$$

$$P = (I \times R) \times I \quad \text{or} \quad P = E \times \left(\frac{E}{R}\right)$$

and the simplified to Equations 13.5a and 13.5b:

$$P = R \times I^2 \tag{13.5a}$$

$$P = \frac{E^2}{R} \tag{13.5b}$$

These two forms of the power equation are very useful for performing practical calculations.

Example 13.2

What is the power produced by a system in which the resistance is 8 Ω and the current is 10 A?

Select Equation 13.5a, substitute known variables, and solve.

$$P = R \times I^2$$

$$P = 8\ \Omega \times 10^2$$

$$800\ \text{W}$$

Answer: The power produced by the system is 800 W.

Example 13.3

What is the power produced by a system in which the resistance is 4 Ω and the voltage is 20 V?

Select Equation 13.5b, substitute known variables, and solve.

$$P = \frac{E^2}{R}$$

$$P = \frac{20^2}{4}$$

$$P = 100\ \text{W}$$

Answer: The power produced by the system is 100 W.

PRACTICE PROBLEMS: OHM'S LAW

1. If resistance (R) = 1000 Ω and voltage (E) = 500 V in a DC circuit, what is the resulting current intensity?
2. If voltage (E) = 50 V and current intensity (I) = 200 A in a DC circuit, what is the overall resistance of the circuit affecting the current?
3. If resistance (R) = 200 Ω and current intensity (I) = 50 A in a DC circuit, what is the voltage that caused that current?
4. What is the intensity of the current flow through an AC circuit if the voltage (E) = 250 volts and the total electric resistance of the circuit is R = 10 Ω?
5. What is the power produced by a system that has resistance (R) = 2 Ω and is passing the current (I) = 0.1 A?
6. What is the power produced by a system that has resistance (R) = 4 Ω and is passing the current (I) = 0.02 A?
7. What is the power produced by a system that has resistance (R) = 8 Ω when a voltage (E) = 65 V is applied to the system?
8. What is the power produced by a system that has resistance (R) = 16 Ω and is operating with voltage (E) = 500 V applied to it?

Answers (If you need help with these problems, consult the website.) **Link 13-4**

1. 0.5 A
2. 0.25 Ω
3. 10,000 V
4. 25 A
5. 0.0002 W
6. 0.0016 W
7. 528.13 W
8. 15,625 W

Capacitance and Capacitors

Capacitance (C) is the ability of matter to store electric charge and sustain the existing voltage by opposing the flow of direct current. Capacitance is defined as the ratio of stored electricity (electric charge) (Q) to the applied voltage (E):

$$C = \frac{Q}{E} \tag{13.6}$$

Capacitance is measured in units called farads, named after British physicist Michael Faraday (1791–1867), who is considered the father of electricity. One farad (F) is the capacitance that causes an accumulation of 1 coulomb (C) of electric charge when 1 volt of DC voltage is applied.

A **capacitor** is an electric component that is capable of storing electrostatic charge. A capacitor consists of two parallel metal plates (sheets) separated by a narrow layer of a dielectric (insulating) material such as air, paper, ceramic, or plastic. The surface areas of both plates are relatively large and have an excess of free electrons. In an uncharged state, the number of electrons on each plate of the capacitor is the same. An applied voltage creates an imbalance of electrons, which concentrate on one of the plates. This creates a polarity in which opposite charges (+ and −) are located on the two plates of the capacitor. These opposite charges attract each other across the gap between the plates of the capacitor, which creates an electric field inside the capacitor that is retained even after the source of voltage is disconnected from the capacitor. When the electric field is created, the capacitor is said to be charged, and it acts as a storing device for electric charge. The capacitance (*C*) of the capacitor depends on the area of the plates and the distance between them:

$$C = \frac{\varepsilon \times A}{d} \qquad (13.7)$$

where *A* is the surface area of a single plate, *d* is the distance between the plates, and ε is the permittivity of the dielectric placed between the plates. The permittivity of the material defines its ability to provide isolation between opposite charges. The higher the permittivity is, the lower the current that passes through the dielectric due to a given potential difference. Equation 13.7 is based on the assumption that the area of the plates is much larger than the distance between the plates (i.e., $A >> d$).

Once the capacitor is charged, it can be discharged using a switch to connect the capacitor to the circuit, causing a sudden power surge. For example, in a flash camera, pushing the button on the camera activates a switch that connects a charged capacitor to the circuit, which uses the stored charge to activate the flash. In a television set, a capacitor can be rated up to 5000 volts, so a fully charged capacitor can give a harmful electric shock, even after the power source is turned off. This is the reason that high-voltage electric devices that have charged capacitors have labels warning consumers not to open the device, even when the power is turned off.

We have just discussed the way a capacitor acts when it is connected to a DC power source or has been charged and left alone. Let's also take a look at what happens when a capacitor is connected to an AC power source. Recall that in DC circuits the current always flows one way. So one plate of a capacitor always receives electrons and can build up a charge. This is the reason that capacitors can be used to block the flow of DC through an electric circuit. In an AC circuit, powered by a sinusoidal voltage, the flow of electrons is in one direction for half of each cycle and in the other direction for the other half of each cycle, so the way the capacitor works is quite different. During the first part of the cycle, electrons are stored up on one plate of the capacitor, and during the second part of the cycle, when the current flows in the reverse direction, the stored up electrons "discharge," which means they flow through the circuit back the way they came. This happens on both sides of the capacitor; thus, there is an alternating current flow through the circuit on both sides of the capacitor, even though electrons do not flow through the capacitor. The amount of opposition to the flow of current depends on the capacitance of the capacitor (i.e., the time needed by the capacitor to discharge) and the frequency of the applied AC voltage. Therefore, the capacitance creates an opposition to current that is frequency dependent. This frequency-dependent opposition to current produced by capacitance is called **capacitive reactance (X_C)** and it is described as:

$$Xc = \frac{1}{2\pi fC} \qquad (13.8)$$

where *C* is the capacitance of the capacitor in farads (F) and *f* is the frequency of the AC voltage in Hz.

Inductance and Inductors

Inductance (*L*) is the ability of matter to store energy in a magnetic field and resist changes in *current* (unlike capacitance, which resists changes in *voltage*). The inductance is defined as the ratio of stored magnetism (magnetic flux, *Φ*) to the current (*I*) producing this flux as follows:

$$L = \frac{\Phi}{I} = \frac{B \times A}{I} \qquad (13.9)$$

where *I* is the electric current in amperes and *Φ* is magnetic flux in webers (Wb). As discussed earlier in this chapter, magnetic flux is the product of magnetic flux density (magnetic field strength, *B*) and the surface area (*A*) of the matter passing the flux. This relationship was inserted in the far right-hand part of Equation 13.9. The unit of inductance is the **henry** (H) named after American physicist Joseph Henry (1797–1878), known for his work on magnetism.

An **inductor** is an electric component that has a high inductance and prevents changes in the magnetic field produced by a passing current. An inductor is a thin coil of wire wrapped around an insulating core (the dielectric). The inductance of the inductor can be fixed or variable and it is determined by the number of turns of wire material and the wire diameter. When an electric current flows through the coil, it generates a magnetic field, which in turn generates its own current that opposes changes to the primary current. The dependence of inductance on the technical parameters of the inductor is given by Equation 13.10:

$$L = \frac{\mu n^2 A}{l} \qquad (13.10)$$

where *L* is inductance in henries, *A* is the cross section of the coil in m^2, *n* is the number of turns in the coil, *l* is the length of the coil in meters resulting from the number and the size of turns, and μ is the permeability of the coil core. Permeability is the property of a material that indicates its ability to respond to a magnetic field, that is, the degree of magnetization of the material that is caused by the presence of an external magnetic field. Ferromagnetic materials represent an example of materials with high permeability.

An inductor behaves quite differently from a capacitor. A capacitor does not allow DC to flow through the circuit, whereas an inductor does not oppose the DC at all. However, an inductor opposes AC, and the higher the frequency of the passing AC, the greater the opposition of the inductance to the current flow. This frequency-dependent opposition to current produced by inductance is called **inductive reactance** (X_L) and it is described as:

$$X_L = 2\pi fL \qquad \textbf{(13.11)}$$

Since induction coils easily attenuate high-frequency signals in AC circuits, they are commonly used as surge protectors, because surges in electricity are rapid, high-frequency changes in current. The tiny doughnut-looking coils attached to some computer cables are examples of such protectors. Induction coils are also used to create a magnetic field in the write/read heads of both analog and digital magnetic recorders.

A combination of capacitors and inductors are used in AC/DC converters to filter out the AC current component at the DC output of the converter. In addition, they can be used in filters and equalizers to separate or modify signals of specific frequencies passing through a circuit and as tuning devices in signal generators and radio receivers.

Electric Impedance

The concept of electric impedance (Z) is analogous to that of mechanic impedance (Chapter 4). Actually, the term *impedance* was originally coined by the English physicist and mathematician Oliver Heaviside (1850–1925) in 1886 in reference to the opposition to current produced by AC circuits. It was not until several years later that this term was adopted in mechanics and acoustics.

Recall from Chapter 4 that the elements of mechanic impedance are resistance (friction) and reactance (X), and reactance can be further broken down into stiffness reactance (X_s), which depends on compliance (C), and mass reactance (X_m), which depends on mass (m). Similarly, the elements of electric impedance are resistance (R) and reactance (X), with the latter one consisting of capacitive reactance (X_C), which depends on capacitance (C), and inductive reactance (X_L), which depends on inductance (L).* The above electric components have analogous properties to their mechanic counterparts; therefore, electric impedance can be expressed in the same form as mechanic impedance, that is, as:

$$Z = \sqrt{R^2 + X^2} \qquad \textbf{(13.12a)}$$

and

$$\theta = \tan^{-1}\left(\frac{X}{R}\right) \qquad \textbf{(13.12b)}$$

where Z, R, and X are the magnitudes of impedance, resistance, and reactance, respectively, of electric systems and θ is a phase difference between the reactance and resistance of the impedance. The vector (geometric) addition of R and X is needed to account for the phase difference between various components of impedance.

Equation 13.12a is the same equation you saw in Chapter 4 for mechanic impedance and the same equation is also used for acoustic impedance. Therefore, the calculation steps shown in Chapter 4 can be applied to solve electric impedance problems.

*Inductance is abbreviated with an L in honor of physicist Heinrich Lenz.

Example 13.4

What is the total magnitude of electric impedance of a system if the resistance is 500 Ω and the total reactance is 1000 Ω?

Select Equation 13.12a.

$$Z = \sqrt{R^2 + X^2}$$

Substitute known variables and solve.

$$Z = \sqrt{500^2 + 1000^2}$$

$$Z = \sqrt{250{,}000 + 1{,}000{,}000}$$

$$Z = \sqrt{1{,}250{,}000}$$

$$Z = 1118.03$$

Answer: The total impedance is 1118.03 Ω.

In addition to the vector addition of R and X, the electric reactance (X) is also the difference between capacitive reactance (X_C) and inductive reactance (X_L). This is the same formula used in Chapter 4 to determine the total reactance in mechanic systems. The mathematic form of this formula is:

$$X = X_L - X_C \qquad \textbf{(13.13)}$$

where $X_C = \frac{1}{2\pi fC}$ and $X_L = 2\pi fL$, as per Equations 13.8 and 13.11. Similar to acoustic and mechanic impedance, electric impedance is expressed in ohms (Ω).

Example 13.5

What is the total reactance of an electric system if the capacitive reactance of a circuit is 500 Ω and the inductive reactance is 550 Ω?

Select Equation 13.13.

$$X = X_L - X_C$$

Substitute known variables and solve.

$$X = 550 - 500$$

$$X = 50\ \Omega$$

Answer: The total reactance is 50 Ω.

Please note in Example 13.5 that we have only calculated the magnitude of the reactance and that the phase angle would also be required in order to specify the direction of the impedance vector (see Chapter 4).

PRACTICE PROBLEMS: ELECTRIC IMPEDANCE

1. What is the total impedance of an electric system that has a resistance of 1000 Ω and a total reactance of 750 Ω?

2. What is the total impedance of an electric system that has a total reactance of 350 Ω and a resistance of 250 Ω?
3. What is the total reactance of an electric system that consists of 543 Ω of capacitive reactance and 782 Ω of inductive reactance?
4. What is the total reactance in an electric system with a capacitive reactance of 820 Ω and inductive reactance of 840 Ω?
5. What is the resistance of an AC circuit having an electric impedance of 1000 Ω and an overall reactance of 200 Ω?

Answers (If you need help solving these problems, consult the website.) **Link 13-5**

1. 1250 Ω
2. 430.12 Ω
3. 239 Ω
4. 20 Ω
5. 979.8 Ω

As discussed previously in the chapters on mechanic vibration (Chapter 4) and sound waves (Chapter 5), an important concept related to impedance is impedance matching. When a system transfers its energy to another system, the effectiveness of this transfer depends on the relationship between the impedances of both systems. The most effective transfer takes place when both impedances "match" each other, in other words, when they are equal. The concept of impedance matching in a mechanic system was discussed in detail in Chapter 4 while considering the behavior of two balls colliding on a pool table. The same concept applies to electric systems, with one difference. In the case of a mechanic collision, the whole energy of the system was transferred during the short time of collision, after which the balls were disconnected from each other. This type of collision is called an elastic collision and it represents the transfer of energy. In electric systems, it is a much more common scenario that the source of energy provides a constant supply of power and the source and the load are physically connected during a continuous power transfer process. If you would like more information regarding impedance matching in an electric system, see the website. **Link 13-6**

The optimal transfer of power that occurs when the impedances are matched is desirable for providing power to light bulbs and electric tools and for feeding an audio signal into a loudspeaker. However, the optimal transmission of power is not always the primary concern for every transmission of electricity. In some cases, the purpose of an electrical circuit is to optimize the transfer of current or voltage. For example, a microphone signal is usually a very low voltage that needs to be amplified to a much higher voltage before any further signal processing can be done. In such a case it is more beneficial to have the load (input) impedance of the microphone amplifier much larger than the source (output) impedance of the microphone than to keep both impedances equal.

Electric Circuits and Kirchhoff's Laws

An electric circuit includes a source of electricity and a more or less complicated network of components and connections between the two terminals of this source. Individual components can be connected in series, forming one continuous loop, or in parallel, forming several branches connecting the same two points. A **series circuit** is so named because all of the components in the circuit are connected to each other in a series. In a series circuit the same current flows through all the components causing changes in voltage (voltage drops) along encountered elements. A circuit that forms several branches connecting the same two points is called a **parallel circuit**, because the signal is split up and processed by two or more loops carrying different currents. Examples of simple series and parallel circuits are shown in Figure 13.5. In complex electric circuits, series and parallel circuits are mixed together, with some components being connected in series while others are connected in parallel.

If two components are connected in parallel, a different current passes through each loop but the voltage drop across each of these two loops is the same. The relationships between voltages and currents in serial and parallel electric circuits are described by a pair of Kirchhoff's Laws (frequently misspelled as Kirchoff's Laws or Kirchiff's Laws):

1. The sum of all electromotive forces and voltage drops in any circuit loop must equal zero (First Kirchhoff's Law).
2. The sum of all the currents arriving at and leaving from any juncture point in a circuit must equal zero (Second Kirchhoff's Law).

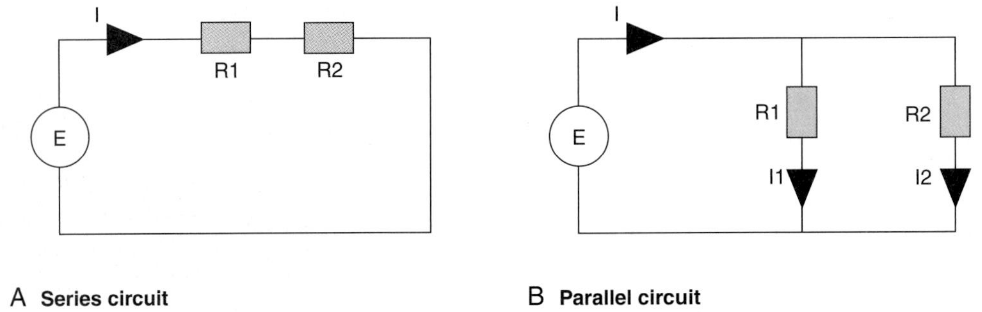

Figure 13.5. Examples of a series electric circuit **(A)** and a parallel electric circuit **(B)**.

To understand the First Kirchhoff's Law, consider walking in a large circle along hilly terrain. Sometimes you walk uphill and sometimes you walk downhill, but when you get back to the starting point, you have walked up as much as you have walked down (otherwise, you would not be back in the same place). In a circuit, there is a certain voltage as the electrical source leaves the battery terminal. The voltage will drop at various points in the circuit, and then will be increased by the battery. When it returns to the same point in the circuit, all the increases and decreases cancel each other and the total voltage change will equal zero. Similarly, for the Second Kirchhoff's Law, consider filling an empty container with water pouring from another container connected through a number of pipes of different diameters. If the diameter of the pipes differs, the streams of water in each pipe will be different. However, the time needed to fill the second container with a certain amount of water does not depend on the number and the cross sections of individual pipes as long as the overall cross section of all the pipes collectively stays the same.

For the series and parallel circuits shown in Figure 13.5, Kirchhoff's Laws can be written as $E + E_1 + E_2 = 0$ and $I + I_1 + I_2 = 0$, respectively. The above laws were named after German physicist Gustav Kirchhoff (1824−1887), who first formulated these laws. Note that Kirchhoff's Laws apply to both DC and AC circuits. If you would like more information about both laws and about electric components (impedances) in series and in parallel, see the website. **Link 13-7**

Switches and Transformers

Two other passive components commonly seen as part of electric circuits are electric switches and transformers. An **electric switch*** is a component used for opening (disconnecting) and closing (connecting) the pathway of an electric current. A simple switch has two pieces of metal called contacts. When the contacts touch one another, the pathway is closed. When they are separated, the pathway is open. There are many different types of switches, but their operations can always be described in terms of pole and throw. **Pole** indicates how many pathways are being opened or closed during each switch operation. **Throw** indicates how many positions a switch has. For example, if a switch operates two electric circuits simultaneously and you can set them in three different ways, this switch is called a "double-pole triple-throw switch." Some examples of simple switches are shown in Figure 13.6. Switches can also be differentiated on the basis of the type of **actuator,** that is, the moving part of the switch (toggle, rocker, push-button, etc.) or the type of contact made by the moving part (on–off switch, momentary switch, etc.).

An electric **transformer** is a component that matches the electric impedances of two AC circuits. It consists of a high-permeability metal core with two separate wire coils wound around the core as is shown in Figure 13.7. The two coils are

*In theoretical considerations such as mathematics and logic, a switch is called a gate.

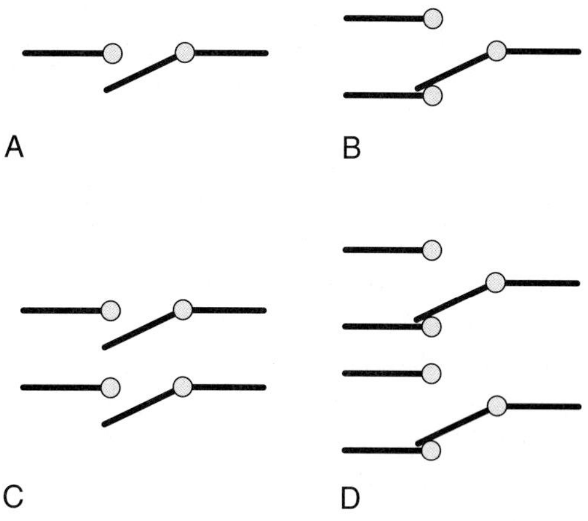

Figure 13.6. Examples of common switches: **(A)** single-pole single throw; **(B)** single-pole double throw; **(C)** double-pole single throw; and **(D)** double-pole double throw.

called the primary coil and the secondary coil and are connected to the source of the signal and the load, respectively.

The numbers of wire turns in the primary coil (N_p) and the secondary coil (N_s) define the **transformer ratio** (*r*).

$$r = \frac{N_s}{N_p} \qquad (13.14)$$

When no load is attached to the secondary coil, the primary coil behaves as a simple inductor. This is an open circuit transformer. However, when a load is connected to the secondary coil (closed circuit transformer), the magnetic field produced by the AC flowing in the primary coil induces a current in the secondary coil. The current in the secondary coil creates its own magnetic field, which opposes changes to the secondary current induced by the primary coil. The more wire turns the secondary coil of the transformer has, the larger its inductance and the stronger the magnetic field opposing the growth of current flowing in the secondary coil. However, at the same time, a large number of wire turns in the secondary coil results in a large voltage

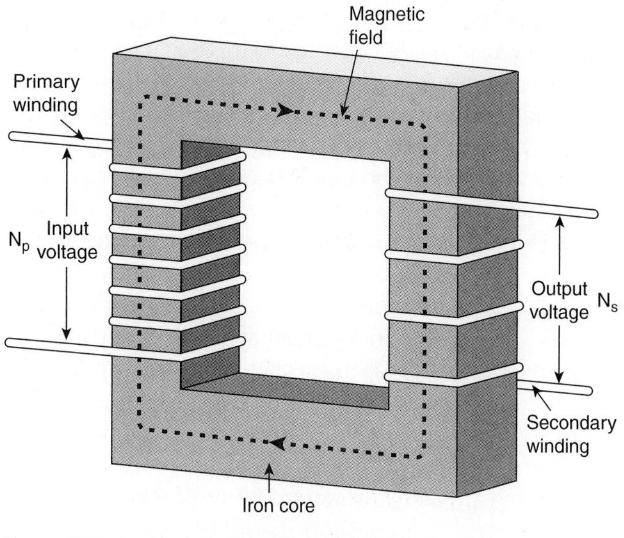

Figure 13.7. A schematic view of a transformer.

induced in the secondary circuit. As a result, the ratio of the voltage to the current in the secondary circuit is different than that in the primary circuit and the input and output of the transformer represent a conversion in electric impedance. If the transformer ratio (r) is properly selected, the transformer can match the impedance of the load connected to the secondary circuit (coil) to the impedance of the source of signal connected to the primary circuit (coil) and the other way around. The actual impedance change produced by a transformer is equal to r^2; that is:

$$Z_{out} = r^2 \times Z_{in} \tag{13.15}$$

where Z_{in} is the load impedance affecting the source and Z_{out} is the actual load impedance.

Although impedance transformation is one of the main applications of transformers, they are also equally important in providing electric isolation between the input and output of an electric circuit (when $r = 1$) and in converting asymmetric transmission lines to symmetric transmission lines or vice versa. The symmetry of the transmission lines will be discussed later in this chapter.

Active Components: Transistors and Integrated Circuits

All of the components of AC circuits that have been discussed thus far are passive components that can modify transmitted signals in various ways without using any supplementary source of energy. However, AC circuits also include active components, which use DC energy to operate, and they can modify a transmitted signal to a much greater degree and with much greater precision than passive components. They can also increase the power of a transmitted signal, a feat that passive components cannot accomplish because energy cannot be created or destroyed and it can only be converted from one form into another (Chapter 2). Active components can increase the power of a transmitted signal but at the cost of DC energy.

The heart of all electronic systems is an amplifier. An **amplifier** is a device that can boost (amplify) the power, voltage, or current of an electric signal by using energy from a supplementary DC source. The signal at the output of an ideal amplifier is identical in shape but proportionally larger than the input signal. Active devices utilize either electron (vacuum) tubes or semiconductor devices to process signals. Vacuum tubes are glass bulbs that can transmit current between two or more electrodes (anode, cathode, grids) located in their empty interior. Vacuum tubes with three (triode) or more (e.g., pentode, octode) electrodes can be used to amplify an AC signal, and they were the main parts of signal amplifiers until the development of semiconductor materials. A **semiconductor** is a material that conducts electricity under some conditions but not under others. This property makes semiconductors useful for building various electronic devices, such as semiconductor switches and amplifiers that can control the flow of an electric current. Since today's signal-processing technologies rely primarily on various forms of semiconductors, only semiconductor-based active components (transistors and integrated circuits) will be discussed in this book.

Semiconductor materials are typically silicon or germanium with some amount of impurities added to the base material. To understand the properties of semiconductor materials, it is important to realize that the valence shell of an atom has very specific properties and can only hold up to eight electrons (the first shell can hold only two electrons). When the valence shell is fully populated with these eight electrons, this atom is very stable and unlikely to take or give away electrons. Such atoms are called inert atoms or noble atoms. Atoms that have less than eight electrons in their valance shell try to merge together to create molecules so that their valence shell is fully populated. For example, an atom of silicon (Si) has only four electrons in its valence shell but it naturally forms Si_2 molecules (crystalline silicon) consisting of two atoms of Si. Crystalline silicon has no free electrons and is a very good insulator. Similarly, atoms of germanium have only four electrons in their valence shells but they create two-atom structures that are very stable and do not conduct any current. Thus, both silicon and germanium are very good insulators in their pure forms even though their atoms have only four valence electrons.

When specially selected impurities, that is, atoms that have more or less than four electrons on the valence shell, are added (doped) to silicon or germanium, they do not bond well with the base material. Such doped materials have some excess or deficit of electrons resulting in a limited flow of electrons across material, and this flow can be controlled. The typical impurities added to the silicon base of a semiconductor are boron or phosphorus. In the case of a germanium base, the typical impurities are indium or arsenic. When atoms of phosphorus, which have five electrons in the outer shell, are added to silicon, the phosphorus atoms use four of their valence electrons to bond with silicon atoms, leaving the fifth electron as a free electron that can drift within the material. This type of material, one that has some surplus of electrons, is called an N-type semiconductor. When atoms of boron, which have three electrons in their outer shell, are added to silicon, they create a P-type semiconductor. A P-type semiconductor has a deficit of electrons or, in other words, it has "holes" in the outer orbit of some of the atoms. Thus, in both of these cases, the added impurities increase the conductivity of the base material (silicon) because they either create a surplus of free electrons or create a condition in which atoms are trying to attract electrons from other atoms. If a DC voltage is applied to these materials, the free electrons (and holes) form a current passing through the material.

When P-type and N-type materials are connected together, they create a PN junction across which the free electrons in the N-type semiconductor want to move to the P-type semiconductor to fill existing "holes" and, similarly, the excess "holes" in the P-type semiconductor want to move to the N-type semiconductor. (Note: Since the "hole" is an empty space in a valence shell, the hole can easily accept an electron from another atom, thus passing the hole to the atom where it took an electron.) The process of creating electron—hole pairs is called recombination. However, only a limited number of electron—hole pairs can be recombined in a layer bordering the two materials because this action changes the initial electric neutrality of both the P-type and N-type materials. The N-type material becomes positively (+) charged at the PN border, preventing further movement of electrons toward the P-type material. Similarly, the P-type material becomes negatively (−) charged at the PN border, preventing further movement of "holes" traveling toward the N-type material. Thus, after the PN junction is made, a state of equilibrium develops in which a narrow insulating layer (called a depletion layer or depletion zone) between the materials is formed where the N material becomes positive and the P material becomes negative as a result of the recombined pairs in this layer. This state of equilibrium is shown in the left panel of Figure 13.8. The actual potential difference between the P and N charges that forms across the insulation layer is about 0.7 V for a silicon-based PN junction and about 0.4 V for a germanium-based PN junction.

Imagine now that an external DC voltage is applied to the silicon PN junction. If the "−" terminal of the battery is attached to the P-type element and the "+" terminal is attached to the N-type element, the battery will polarize the junction to an even higher degree, preventing any current from passing the junction. This type of polarized PN junction, illustrated in Figure 13.8B, is called a **reverse-biased** PN junction.

When the terminals of the battery are attached in reverse, the voltage of the battery works against the natural potential difference of the PN junction. This situation is shown in Figure 13.8C. When a battery voltage is larger than 0.7 V, it will result in a current flowing through the junction from the negative battery terminal through the PN junction to the positive terminal. This type of polarized PN junction is called a **forward-biased** PN junction.

In summary, a PN junction behaves as a conductor when polarized in one direction and as an insulator when polarized in the opposite direction. Thus, by changing the direction and amount of voltage polarizing the PN junction, the amount of current (flow of electrons) passing through the junction can be controlled.

The main forms of semiconductor components are diodes, transistors, and integrated circuits. A **diode** is a passive electronic component that passes electric current only in one direction. A semiconductor diode (e.g., Fig. 13.8) is a simple PN or NP junction that is not polarized. It has two terminals, called the collector (C) and the emitter (E). For a diode to pass the current, a positive voltage needs to be applied to the collector and a negative voltage to the emitter. The electrical symbol for a diode is shown at the bottom of the three panels in Figure 13.8. The left element of the symbol is the collector (▶) and the right element is the emitter (|). When the diode is polarized by an external voltage, it behaves as an insulator (Fig. 13.8B) or as a simple conductor (Fig. 13.8C). Diodes can be used as rectifiers (devices changing AC voltage into DC voltage), signal limiters, voltage regulators, switches, light receiving (photodiodes) and light emitting (LEDs) devices, and parts of more complex devices such as signal mixers, modulators, demodulators, and signal generators.

Transistors are built as two semiconductor junctions connected together in a PNP or NPN sandwich. The three parts (terminals) of the transistor are called the base (B; the middle layer of the sandwich), emitter (E), and collector (C). The polarization of the base in relationship to the emitter is

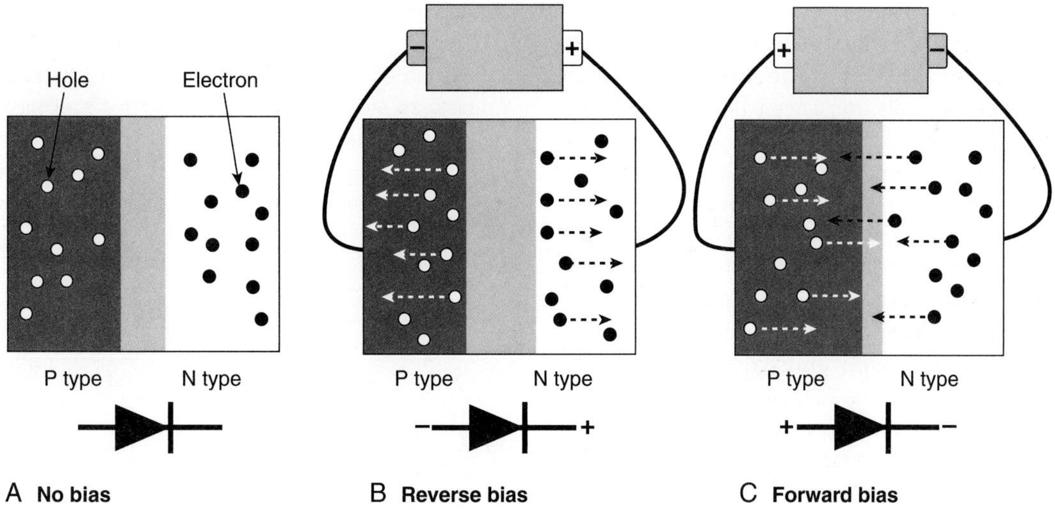

Figure 13.8. The PN junction consisting of P-type and N-type semiconductors connected together and left alone **(A),** reverse-biased **(B),** and forward-biased **(C).** The o symbols indicate extra holes, and the • symbols indicate free electrons. The symbol below each of the panels is an electrical symbol for a diode, which is a semiconductor component utilizing a single PN junction.

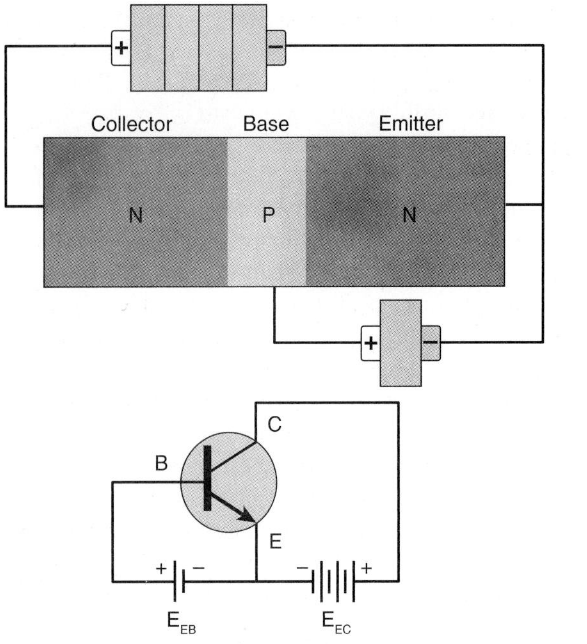

Figure 13.9. The basic operational schematic of an NPN transistor **(A)** and the electrical symbol for the NPN transistor **(B).**

called the bias. The basic diagram of an NPN transistor is shown in Figure 13.9.

Transistors have two main functions: to amplify a signal (analog systems) and to switch a signal on or off (digital systems). For the transistor to operate as an amplifier, both junctions need to be properly polarized. An easy way to remember the proper polarization of transistor junctions is to observe the NPN or PNP elements that make up the transistor. The letters of these elements indicate what polarity voltage, for example, positive (P) or negative (N), to use to set the correct barriers across both junctions. It is also important to note that in all transistors the base region is much narrower and much more lightly doped than the emitter and collector regions.

In the NPN transistor shown in Figure 13.9, the emitter–base junction is biased in the forward direction to facilitate the flow of electrons from the emitter to the electron-depleted base as an emitter current (I_E). The battery connected between collector and emitter has much higher voltage than the battery connected between emitter and the base, and this difference polarizes the base–collector PN junction in a reverse direction (the collector is much more positive than the base). The electrons of the I_E current entering the base recombine (fill) the holes in the base and they are lost as carriers of a current. However, the base region is very thin and lightly doped so that many of the electrons entering the base region cannot recombine with holes, so they either enter the positive terminal of the battery supplying the emitter–base junction or move toward the base–collector junction, where they come under the influence of a high collector–emitter potential difference. If the collector–base junction were not polarized, all the electrons leaving the emitter that did not recombine with the holes in the base region of the transistor would form a base current (I_B), which would enter the positive end of the battery polarizing the emitter–base junction. However, the collector–base junction is polarized in the reverse direction and to a much higher voltage than the emitter–base junction. Once the free electrons remaining in the base are attracted by the collector–emitter voltage, they move into the N-type collector and become a part of the collector current (I_C) that flows toward the positive terminal of the emitter–collector battery and returns to the emitter together with I_B. Since both I_C and I_B are parts of the emitter current (I_E), then, according to the Second Kirchhoff's Law:

$$I_E = I_B + I_C \quad \textbf{(13.16)}$$

Since the I_E depends on the emitter–base bias and because the collector current constitutes most of the emitter current, a small change in the emitter–base voltage (E_{EB}) has a large effect on the value of the I_C current. In other words, a relatively small change of the emitter–base voltage (E_{EB}) results in a large change in the thickness of the insulting layer separating the base from the emitter and thus in the resulting number of electrons entering the base and being accelerated into the collector. Therefore, if the input signal controls the emitter–base voltage, small changes of the input signal will result in large changes of the collector current that can be considered the output signal of the transistor. In sum, the amplification action of the transistor results from the fact that a large change in the output collector current (and resulting large voltage drop caused by the collector current flowing through a load) is caused by a small change in the input base–emitter voltage. Some practical types of amplifiers will be discussed in Chapter 14.

The transistor can also operate as a switch that opens and closes the current path. The base lead is the toggle. When there is no positive voltage applied to the base, the transistor is off, no current passes through the transistor, and the switch is open. Conversely, when forward-bias is applied to the base, the transistor is on, the current flows, and the switch is closed.

An integrated circuit (IC), or **chip**, consists of a large number of electric components, active and passive, etched in a semiconductor material creating a complete electric circuit. Depending on the number of components contained in an IC, integrated circuits can be divided into:

SSI (small-scale integration) ICs containing up to 100 components

MSI (medium-scale integration) ICs containing 100 to 3000 components

LSI (large-scale integration) ICs containing 3000 to 100,000 components

VLSI (very large-scale integration) ICs containing 100,000 to 1,000,000 components

ULSI (ultra large-scale integration) ICs containing more than 1,000,000 components

Integrated circuits can be both analog and digital, meaning that they may be used as the building blocks of both analog and digital systems. Basic information about the analog audio systems is provided in Chapter 14 and digital systems are discussed in Chapter 15.

ELECTRIC INSTALLATIONS

Electric components are the building blocks of larger devices and systems. When various electric devices and systems work together, they form structures called **networks.** Networks can be wired or wireless (e.g., a radio network). The collection of cables and auxiliary elements that connect a system via wires is called an **electric installation.** All devices included in a wired network need to be connected by pairs of wires to complete the circuit (keep the circuit as a closed loop) and to transmit voltage (potential difference) from one device to another. In addition, in low-voltage AC circuits, such as most audio systems, the installations need to be protected from various noise sources (electric noise) and from signals leaking from other systems **(crosstalk).** Electric noise consists of three main elements: **thermal noise** generated by the components involved in signal transmission, **transmitted noise** received with the original signal, and **interference noise** induced in the transmission wires by electromagnetic fields generated by power lines, various motors and engines, home appliances, radio and TV stations, medical equipment, and some natural phenomena. The first two types of noise are controlled by the selection of proper wires, components, and devices used for building transmission circuitry and by various noise reduction techniques that eliminate nonelectric and transmitted noise. The most dominant noise, and the one that is the most difficult to suppress, is interference noise. Every time an electric charge moves in a space or passes along a conductor, it generates an electromagnetic field. To protect audio signals against the adverse effects of various forms of electromagnetic interference (EMI), radio frequency interference (RFI), and interchannel crosstalk, the transmission lines carrying audio signals must be properly grounded, shielded, and balanced (made symmetric).

Ground and Grounding

Grounding is the act of connecting all electric circuits to one common point that has a very low resistance. This point is called a **ground.** The two types of grounds in electric systems are earth (power ground, safety ground) and chassis (signal ground, shield ground).

All typical installations delivering power from the power plant to buildings have outlets with three connecting wires. A pair of wires (hot wire, common wire) is used to deliver power from the power plant and the third wire is used as a power ground.

The main purpose of a power ground is to ensure the safety of people operating electric equipment. A power ground is provided by connecting an enclosure or the main metal mass of electric equipment to a ground electrode, which is a conductor buried in the ground (thus the origin of the name earth ground). For example, wall outlets providing electricity to houses have connections for three wires. Two of them deliver the required electric voltage and the third one is for the earth ground, established locally for a building, factory, or laboratory. The earth normally has a very low resistance and easily absorbs all unwanted electricity. Since electric current always attempts to find the path of least resistance, it will easily flow to the ground. If during an equipment failure or unskilled operation an electric potential appears on the surface of the equipment, it will be transferred immediately to the earth by the grounding conductor rather than affecting the user. If equipment is not grounded, the body of a person touching the equipment may constitute the pathway of least resistance and a person will absorb all the leaking electricity and experience an electric shock caused by the current passing through the body. The passing current may cause a small reaction, such as a mild tingling in the fingers, or a much larger one, such as intense muscle contractions (including the heart), severe burns at the contact points, and even death. To avoid potential contact with harmful electricity, all high-power, high-voltage, and high-current electric and electronic devices that use large amounts of electricity must be grounded.

The signal ground, also called the common or chassis ground, provides a common reference voltage point for all electric devices and their parts. This type of ground is needed to avoid the flow of unwanted, spurious, signal-related currents through a system. All wires and metal parts of electric equipment serve as conductors and may transmit unwanted currents, resulting in poor insulation between different current pathways in the circuit or in the creation of new unwanted currents induced by external electromagnetic fields. These currents may in turn produce their own electromagnetic field adding additional unwanted signals (noise and crosstalk). If two points in the system have different average potentials, they will always result in a current passing between these points. For example, some currents may carry small amounts of 60-Hz (50-Hz) signal from power lines, inducing an audible hum or buzz in other lines carrying the signals. They may also become carriers of spurious signals induced in their pathways by strong external electromagnetic fields created by power lines, thunderstorms, and other similar sources. To avoid or minimize such currents, all the devices and subsystems should be connected together in one place to make sure that there are no DC potential differences between the systems. This place is called a common point and it is usually the chassis of the device. In a system that has several separate devices, the common points of all individual devices should be connected together to one central common point forming a star-looking pattern of grounding wires.

Regardless of whether or not the safety ground wire (a "third" wire) connects a specific device to a local ground, the common ground wire in the power outlet is grounded at the power plant and it connects all energy receivers to the power plant ground. The main reason that one of the wires (terminals) in the power line is grounded is to prevent the accumulation of large static changes (mainly weather related) between two ungrounded wires. For example, grounding one of the wires provides an easy path to ground for lightening striking a power line. Without grounding, the huge charge transferred to a power line by lightening would travel directly to power receivers, potentially killing people and starting fires. All the chassis and shield grounds (signal grounds) should be connected to this ground regardless of the presence or absence of a safety ground. The five main things that need to be remembered in the grounding of various types of equipment are:

1. All the grounding wires should be as short as possible, solid (not a braided multiwire type), and thick to minimize their resistance.
2. All the grounding wires should directly connect individual devices to the common point of the system (common points of individual devices should not be connected in chain).
3. Grounding wires must not form any wire loops since such loops are the source of additional interference that completely defeats the purpose of grounding.
4. The central common point (central ground) should have a resistance as low as possible in reference to the earth ground.
5. The technical ground and the safety ground should be kept separate.

All audio devices should have separate common and power grounds. However, some low-current devices used in homes and offices have only a two-prong plug. This means that the maker of this equipment has determined that any malfunctions should not be harmful to the health of an operator. However, in such systems the hot and ground wires need to be clearly marked so they are not mixed up. This is the reason that most two-prong plugs are polarized via two different-sized prongs.

If you hear a low-frequency hum produced by audio or clinical equipment, it is most likely that the power plug is not properly polarized or that some form of ground loop was created by installation wires. A ground loop is created when there is more than one connection between the grounded equipment and the ground. The duplicate ground wires form a closed-loop receiving antenna that pick up interference noise. They also carry some current that generates its own electromagnetic field affecting transmitting circuitry. To avoid ground loops across power lines, it is strongly recommended that all devices that work together be connected to a single power outlet. When different devices are connected to different outlets, it is very likely that they will create ground loops in the power lines running in the walls of the building and induce hum and noise into the system.

It is also important to remember that if the original power wiring of an electric apparatus involves a three-wire system, it is prohibited by both common sense as well as electric code to connect only two basic power wires without the safety ground. Unfortunately, in many compromised practical situations, when users may not have all the matching plugs and sockets, the user may not connect the casing to a safety ground but instead may run a separate wire connecting the metal casing of the apparatus to the basic ground terminal of the power line. The ground impedance of such a line is likely too large to carry the fault current resulting from a malfunction of the apparatus, thus creating an unnecessary hazard of electric shock and fire (Fause, 1995).

Electromagnetic Shielding

Shielding is a method of reducing the amount of unwanted currents in the pathways of an electric device, caused by interfering electromagnetic fields. An electromagnetic shield is a partition separating electromagnetic fields existing in two regions of space. The purpose of the shield is to reduce the propagation of electromagnetic energy from one region of space to another (Fause, 1995). A good electromagnetic shield should be thick, conductive, continuous, and well grounded. It works by reflecting impinging electromagnetic waves due to an impedance mismatch and by absorbing and directing to ground the rest of the energy that was transmitted across the shield boundary.

A well-designed electromagnetic shield usually provides adequate protection against electric (electrostatic) and high-frequency electromagnetic fields; however, it does not offer much protection against static or low-frequency magnetic fields. An electric field is a high-impedance field since it is characterized by high voltage (potential difference) and low current leakage. A high potential difference in the external electric field rearranges the electric charges in the shield enclosing a wire or a piece of equipment. These charges create the opposite electric field inside the enclosure, which cancels out the effect of the outside field. The system also works the other way around, preventing leakage of an electric field from the inside of the enclosure to the outside. If electric equipment is surrounded by a conductive metal enclosure that is properly grounded (to drain any imbalance current to the ground), the static potential on the electromagnetic shield will always be zero, effectively protecting the device against external electrostatic fields.

Magnetic fields are low-impedance fields because they are produced by high currents and low-voltage leakage. Therefore, static and low-frequency magnetic fields can easily enter the shield (i.e., none of the field is reflected) and are only attenuated by absorption within the shield. For the shield to absorb a substantial amount of low-frequency magnetic energy, the shields should be relatively thick and less conductive than they need to be to protect against electric fields. However, high-frequency magnetic fields, such as radio-frequency fields and microwave fields, are well attenuated by conductive (low impedance) electromagnetic shields because at high frequencies even a highly conductive shield has a relatively high impedance (inductance), which creates some potential differences in the shield in response to impinging electromagnetic waves and results in a new magnetic field that opposes and cancels the effects of the original field. Thus, the electromagnetic shield prevents external electric and radio-frequency electromagnetic fields from entering shielded devices and it prevents the internal electric and radio-frequency electromagnetic fields generated inside the shield from propagating outside of the shielded region. When it is absolutely necessary to protect a given space against low-frequency magnetic fields, the space should be surrounded by separated electromagnetic and magnetic shields, although this solution is very costly and very heavy.

Electromagnetic shielding is typically made of a highly conductive material, such as copper, and has the form of metal plates surrounding pieces of equipment and wire mesh conduit surrounding the electric wires. This type of shield is frequently referred to as a Faraday cage or Faraday shield. Most audio and other communication equipment, together with connecting cables, have some form of Faraday shielding. Wires surrounded by such shields are called shielded wires or shielded cables* and are used for protecting low-voltage signals, such as microphone signals, against electromagnetic fields produced by stronger signals. Elevators and some concrete and steel building structures also work well as Faraday shielding, preventing telephone reception from mobile phones. High-security government and military offices are also enclosed in Faraday shields to prevent electromagnetic eavesdropping. An example of a Faraday shield preventing electromagnetic energy from spreading out is a shield surrounding the cooking chamber of a microwave oven. The main considerations in developing good electromagnetic shielding are (Fause, 1995):

1. The shield material must be a good electric conductor.
2. The number and size of openings in the shield must be minimized.
3. The shield must encompass as much of the system as possible.
4. The shield needs to be grounded or at least connected to a much larger mass of a conductive material to eliminate flow of spurious currents through the shield.
5. The shield should not carry any current other than the drain current induced by the external fields.

The last two requirements cannot be overemphasized since any conductive material exposed to an electromagnetic field behaves as an antenna radiating this field. Thus, any flow of energy in the shield is potentially dangerous to signals protected by the shield. If the magnitude of the transmitted signals is sufficiently large, such as the signals transmitted through loudspeaker cables, they do not need shielding since their voltage levels greatly exceed the levels of noise induced by external electromagnetic fields.

Balanced and Unbalanced Lines

Recall that a conductive electromagnetic shield does not offer much protection against static and low-frequency (50 to 60 Hz) magnetic fields. In other words, highly conductive materials offer no opposition to DC or low-frequency magnetic fields, which penetrate through the shield. However, as a magnetic field propagates through space, its intensity decreases with the distance from the field source and in proportion to the permeability of the material through which the field propagates. Thus, effective protection against a low-frequency magnetic field should include (Rich, 1982):

1. Good spatial separation between the signal circuitry and the source of the magnetic field
2. Thick and permeable magnetic screens (e.g., made of steel)
3. Perpendicular directions of signal lines and power lines (source of magnetic interference) running through equipment or space
4. Minimal distance between two wires in a pair of wires carrying the same signal to minimize the size of wire loops exposed to magnetic fields

The fourth item requires a more detailed analysis. Any pair of wires carrying a signal and connecting two pieces of equipment forms a loop. Recall that the larger the number of wire loops and the larger the size of the loops are, the larger the voltage magnitude induced in an inductor (coil). Thus, to minimize the effects of magnetic fields on a transmitted signal, the pairs of wires conducting the signal need to be arranged in such a way that they do not create large loops; that is, both wires in a pair should run tightly together. It is also beneficial to twist the wires around each other since such an arrangement further decreases the voltage induced in the wires by both electromagnetic and magnetic interferences. The twisted configuration changes the phase relationship between the direction of the field and direction of the wire so that the resulting currents induced in different pieces of both wires are out-of-phase and cancel each other out. The larger the number of twists per meter is, the greater the reduction in crosstalk between the pairs of wires and the lower the current inducted by external fields. Note, however, that for the twisted pair to reduce the effects of interfering fields, neither of the two wires can be grounded.

A typical pair of wires in which one wire is grounded is an example of an unbalanced (asymmetric) transmission line. The unbalanced nature of the line results from the fact that changes in the electric potential are different in each of the two wires; that is, they are not mirror images of each other.

*A cable is a group of wires running together in a plastic conduit. The wires in the cable may be shielded individually, the cable may be shielded as a whole, or it may not be shielded at all.

In a typical grounded circuit, one wire (the ground) always has a zero potential and all the AC changes are seen as variations in the electric potential of the hot wire. An example of an unbalanced shielded line is the coaxial cable used in TV installations in which one conductor is grounded and forms a shield around the hot conductor. The problem with such unbalanced lines is that grounding and shielding are not a sufficient means to protect small transmitted signals against electric noise induced by high-intensity magnetic and electromagnetic interferences. In addition, the wire used as a shield carries the signal in the form of a return current, making the shield less effective. However, further protection against interfering external fields, and especially magnetic fields, can be provided by making the transmission line symmetric (balanced). The interferences induced in each wire of a balanced line are in-phase and cancel each other out at the receiver (load), which responds to the difference in voltage between the wires. An ungrounded pair of wires and the twisted pair of wires discussed above are examples of balanced lines. However, such lines do not provide any of the benefits resulting from using shielding and grounding techniques. Thus, to maximize the protection of the signal circuitry against all interfering fields and crosstalk, the connecting lines should be balanced, shielded, and grounded. To create such a line, a line carrying audio or other signals needs to have three conductors (wires): two conductors for transmitting the signal and a reference ground conductor, which may also serve as a shield for the two other wires. A line that provides the advantages of all three protective techniques is a twisted (balanced) shielded pair of wires with the shield connected to the chassis ground at its driven end or both ends (Whitlock, 1994; Macatee, 1994). Such connecting lines are used in most scientific, clinical, and professional audio applications when the transmitted signals are very small. If balanced and unbalanced pieces of equipment need to be connected together, such matching can be accomplished using special balanced transformers that convert one type of signal transmission into the other one.

Summary

An external force, called the voltage (electromotive force, potential difference), is required for electric current to flow. The voltage can be stationary, resulting in a direct current, or the voltage can oscillate in time, resulting in an alternating current. An alternating current will result when an acoustic signal is converted into an electric signal or when power is generated by a power plant and sent along power transmission lines. Most electric devices, such as electric stoves, refrigerators, fans, and shavers, use AC power for their operation. However, devices that transmit and process information, such as computers, audiometers, and audio equipment, require DC power for their proper operation. An example of a DC power source is a battery.

An electromagnetic field is the interaction between the electric field generated by the presence of particles possessing an electric charge and the magnetic field generated by the relative movement of these particles in space.

Electric impedance is the opposition to the flow of electrons through matter. Matter that has low electric impedance and conducts electricity easily is called a conductor, matter that has high electric impedance and does not easily conduct electricity is called an insulator, and matter that can conduct electricity under some conditions but not under others is called a semiconductor.

An electric circuit is a pathway for the flow of electric current. In a series circuit, each electric component leads to only one other component in a long line from the beginning to the end of the circuit creating one continuous loop. In a parallel circuit, at one or more points the output from one component may be sent to two or more other components at the same time.

The main passive electric components that form DC circuits are resistors. The main passive components that form AC circuits are resistors, capacitors, and inductors. Auxiliary components that are used in either DC or AC circuits include switches, transformers, light devices, fuses, and diodes. Passive components can only modify AC signals but cannot increase their power. Active components can increase the power of AC signals by using supplementary DC power.

Electric systems include various electric components and devices that are connected together through wires and cables. Such systems are susceptible to electric hum and noise produced by poor wiring or by extraneous electromagnetic fields. The adverse effects of electric noise and hum can be reduced by proper grounding, shielding, and balancing of the equipment and connecting cables.

Key Points

- The magnitude of an electric current is measured in amperes. One ampere is equal to 1 coulomb of electrons (6.24×10^{18} electrons) passing through a point of observation in 1 second.
- The magnitude of a voltage depends on the difference in charge between two poles and it is measured in volts, where 1 V is the force needed to perform 1 J of work to move a charge of 1 C between the two poles.
- In the United States, public power is transmitted as an alternating current with a standard frequency of 60 Hz and voltage of 220 V (V_{rms}).
- The unit of electric power is the watt. The power consumption in DC systems is equal to the product of voltage (E) and electric current (I). To determine power consumption in AC systems, the RMS magnitude of the AC signal must be determined.
- Both electric and magnetic fields can be thought of as families of invisible lines of force connecting the two opposing poles of the source of the field and organizing particles of matter along these lines.
- Electric impedance is composed of resistance, capacitance, and inductance.
- Resistance, measured in ohms, opposes the flow of electricity through a circuit and converts the passing current into heat.
- An electric switch is an electric component used for opening and closing the pathway of an electric current.
- A transformer is an electric component that can change electric impedance, provide electric isolation between the input and the output of an electric circuit, and convert asymmetric transmission lines to symmetric transmission lines.
- A semiconductor is a material that conducts electricity under some conditions and works as an insulator under others. This property makes semiconductors useful for controlling the flow of electric current.
- Grounding is the process or act of connecting all electric circuits to one common point that has very low resistance to ensure the safety of people operating electric equipment.

CHAPTER 14

Audio Signals and Devices

Chapter Outline

Objectives

- To discuss the concepts of electroacoustic and electromechanic transduction
- To list and briefly describe different types of electroacoustic transducers including microphones, loudspeakers, and earphones
- To discuss the functions of audio devices such as amplifiers and filters
- To introduce the concepts of linear and nonlinear amplifiers
- To introduce and discuss the concept of linear and nonlinear signal distortions
- To discuss the harmonic and intermodulation distortion products that result from nonlinear signal processing
- To discuss the similarities and differences between limiters and compressors
- To introduce the concept of an audio system and related basic terminology

Key Terms

Amplifier
Audio signal
Automatic gain control (AGC)
Band-pass filter
Band-reject filter
Circumaural earphones
Closed earphone
Comb filter effect
Condenser microphone (electrostatic microphone)
Crossover network
Directional microphone
Directivity factor (*Q*)
Directivity index (DI)
Dynamic microphone
Dynamic range
Earphone
Electroacoustic chain (audio chain)
Electroacoustic transducer (audio transducer)
Electroacoustics
Electromechanic transducer
Equalizer
Filter
Free-field microphone
Frequency response
Gain
Graphic equalizer
Harmonic distortion
Headphone
Headset

High-pass filter
Input impedance
Input signal
Insert earphone
Intermodulation distortion
Line amplifier
Linear amplifier
Linear distortion
Loudspeaker
Loudspeaker system
Low-pass filter
Monophonic system
Nonlinear amplifier
Nonlinear distortions
Omnidirectional microphone
Open earphone
Output impedance
Output signal
Peak clipping
Piezoelectric microphone
Power amplifier
Preamplifier
Pressure microphone
Receiver
Saturation level
Signal compressor
Signal controller
Signal distortion
Signal limiter
Signal monitor
Signal processor
Signal transducer
Signal transformation
Stereophonic system
Supra-aural earphone
Transducer
Transfer function (input/output function)
Transmitter
Voltage amplifier

AUDIO SIGNALS

When an acoustic signal travels through the environment, it can be transmitted and modified by a variety of different absorbing and reflecting materials (Chapter 6) and by various resonating cavities (e.g., a Helmholtz resonator). All of these modifications are performed in real time when the sound wave is propagating. However, acoustic signals also need to be stored for use at different times and transmitted over distances much larger than the distance the original sound wave traveled. In many practical applications, transmitted signals also need to be amplified and processed (modified) in various complex ways, which are difficult or impossible to attain by acoustic means. Therefore, for the purposes of storing, transmitting over long distances, and reproducing sound, acoustic signals are converted into an electric form, processed in this form, and converted back into acoustic signals for final delivery. The electric representation of the acoustic signal is commonly referred to as an **audio signal,** from the Latin *audio* meaning "I hear." The concept of an audio signal was introduced at the beginning of Chapter 13. An audio signal is an electric waveform having frequencies within the acoustic range that is audible to humans. There are a number of different forms in which an audio signal can be stored. Some of these forms are electric (e.g., computer file), whereas some others are mechanic (e.g., vinyl record), magnetic (e.g., cassette tape), or optic (e.g., compact disc). However, a common feature of all audio signals is that they need electricity for storage and reproduction.

The devices that are used to convert an acoustic signal into an audio signal or vice versa are called audio transducers. A **transducer** is a device that converts one type of energy into another. A device that transfers acoustic energy into electric energy (or vice versa) is called an **audio transducer** or **electroacoustic transducer.** Similarly, a device that transfers mechanic energy into electric energy (or vice versa) is called an **electromechanic transducer.***

Audio science, traditionally called **electroacoustics,** is the science concerned with the conversion between acoustic energy and electric energy and the processing and transmission of audio signals. The source of audio signals is usually a microphone or mechanic sensor, whereas transmission and processing of these signals is performed by a variety of audio devices such as amplifiers, filters, equalizers, and compressors, in order to provide the desired technical and esthetic effects. In addition, audio signals can be synthesized (created) within an electric system for the purpose of converting it at a later point to an auditory stimulus. These signals include pure tones, synthesized noises, sound created by electronic musical instruments, and so forth. Audio signals are converted at their final destination into their acoustic form by loudspeakers or earphones. A signal pathway that consists of devices that convert sound waves into audio signals, transmit and process audio signals, and finally convert them back into sound is called an electroacoustic (audio) chain. An **electroacoustic chain** is a sequence of devices (or processing steps) that transforms an audio signal into its desired form. An electroacoustic chain can be as simple as a single audio device or it can contain many devices connected in series with various input and output options. More complex audio systems consist of two or more electroacoustic chains that are

*The terms electroacoustic transducer and electromechanic transducer are used regardless of whether energy is transformed to or from its electrical state. This is the commonly accepted usage and the process of transforming acoustic or mechanic energy into electric energy is never called acoustoelectric and mechanoelectric transduction, respectively.

called channels. Regardless of the complexity of the audio system, the system usually begins and ends with an audio transducer.

AUDIO TRANSDUCERS

As mentioned above, a transducer is a device that converts one form of energy into another. More specifically, electroacoustic and electromechanic transducers convert acoustic and mechanic energy into electric energy or vice versa. Depending on the direction of transduction, transducers can be divided into audio **receivers** and audio **transmitters.** Receivers convert input energy (acoustic or mechanic) into electric energy and transmitters convert electric energy into output energy (acoustic or mechanic). Unfortunately, the above common use of the term *transmitter* is reversed in the hearing aid literature, where transmitters are called hearing aid receivers. Students of hearing science should be prepared to encounter this opposite term when they begin to explore hearing aid technology. In addition, in the field of telecommunications, the terms *transmitter* and *receiver* are used to indicate devices that allow wired or wireless transmission of electric signals over large distances. In electroacoustics, however, the receiver means a device that *receives* sound (or vibration) and the transmitter indicates a device that *emits* sound (or vibration) and this is the meaning of these terms that we will use in this text. A microphone is an example of an electroacoustic receiver. A contact microphone and a gramophone pick-up (part of the obsolete record player) are examples of electromechanic receivers. Loudspeakers, earphones, and insert earphones are examples of electroacoustic transmitters and a bone vibrator is an example of an electromechanic transmitter.

Recall from previous chapters that sound is a mechanic vibration converted into an acoustic wave. Therefore, the technology that is used for electro*mechanic* and electro*acoustic* transduction can be considered the same technology except for one thing. Although both require the transduction of an electric signal to a mechanic signal, electroacoustic transduction also requires the mechanic signal to be transduced into an acoustic signal. This additional conversion is performed by a mechanoacoustic transducer; this principle of operation is shown in Figure 14.1.

The mechanoacoustic transducer is simply a mechanic arm (piston) driving a membrane that radiates acoustic energy when driven by a mechanic force. A **membrane,** also called a diaphragm, is a thin sheet-like material (in this case metal) that is fixed along its edges and has a certain amount of stiffness, which allows it to vibrate.

Figure 14.1 shows that when a force (F) at the input of a device acts on a membrane surface (S), a pressure (p) will result. The pressure will depend on the magnitude of the force and on the area of the surface as follows:

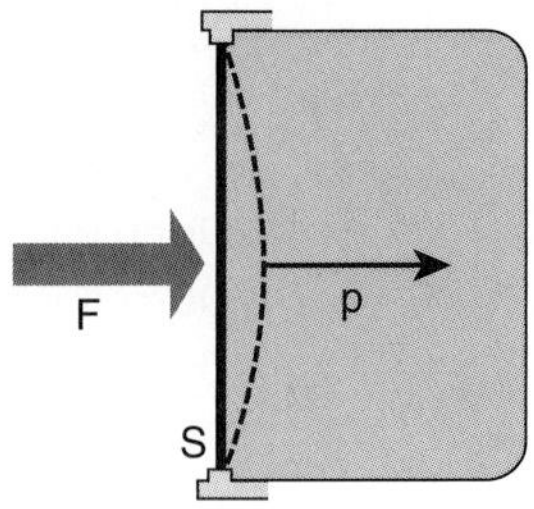

Figure 14.1. The principle of a mechanoacoustic conversion.

$$p = \frac{F}{S} \tag{14.1}$$

This equation should be familiar, because the relationship between pressure, force, and area was discussed, as it relates to acoustics, in Chapter 5. When acoustic energy is converted into mechanic energy, the transducer operates in the opposite direction, but in the same way as described in Equation 14.1, with acoustic pressure as the input and mechanic force as the output. Since both electroacoustic and electromechanic transducers use the same basic type of technology and they only differ in the form of input or output signal, they will both be referred to from this point on as audio transducers, without a separate discussion of the electroacoustic and electromechanic transducers.

Some transducers are capable of converting energy in just one direction (e.g., to act only as a receiver or only as a transmitter), whereas others can convert energy in both directions, acting as both a transmitter and a receiver. Transducers that can convert energy in both directions are called reciprocal transducers or reversible transducers. Transducers that only convert energy in one direction are called nonreciprocal transducers or nonreversible transducers. A classification of selected electroacoustic transducers based on their principle of operation is provided in Table 14.1.

Transducers involve the interaction between the physical characteristics of two different fields of physics. The process of converting one type of energy into another is based on a similarity between the principles governing mechanic, acoustic, and electric phenomena. In all three of these domains we have the same concepts of power (work, energy) and impedance. There are also similar functional relationships between the magnitudes associated with each domain. For example, in the mechanic domain force causes an object to move, in the acoustic domain pressure causes particles to move, and in the electric domain electromotive force causes current to flow. These functional similarities are called the electro-mechano-acoustic (EMA) analogies. The most common set of EMA analogies applicable to hearing science is shown in Table 14.2.

The main application of the EMA analogies is in the analysis of interactions between various physical systems.

Table 14.1. Audio Transducers Based on Their Principle of Operation

Type of Transducer	Principle of Operation
Reciprocal transducers	
Electromagnetic transducer	An electromagnetic transducer has a moving ferromagnetic element and a stationary coil. A ferromagnetic element (e.g., metal membrane) moves in response to acoustic waves in the magnetic field of an electromagnet and this movement creates changes in the current passing through the wiring of the electromagnet (receiver) or the reverse of this happens and a varying electric current passing through the wiring of the electromagnet creates a varying magnetic field that pulls or pushes the metal membrane located in this field (transmitter).
Electrodynamic (dynamic, magnetoelectric) transducer	An electrodynamic (dynamic, magnetoelectric) transducer has a stationary magnet and a membrane attached to a moving coil. The coil attached to the membrane moves in response to acoustic waves, which then induces a current in the coil (receiver), or the reverse of this happens and a flow of varying electric current through a suspended coil located in a magnetic field makes the coil and the attached membrane move (transmitter).
Electrostatic (condenser, electret*)	An electrostatic device is a capacitor (condenser) with one of its electrodes fixed and another one having the form of a membrane, each holding opposite charges. Movement of the movable electrode creates changes in the capacitance between the electrodes and these changes result in changes in a voltage between the electrodes (receiver) or the reverse of this happens and changes in the voltage applied to the electrodes affect the capacitance of the device and force the movable electrode to move (transmitter).
Piezoelectric (crystal) transducer	Piezoelectricity is a property of some crystals (e.g., quartz) in which the crystal changes dimensions in response to an applied voltage (transmitter) or the reverse of this happens and the piezoelectric crystal produces a voltage in response to an applied mechanic force acting on two opposing surfaces of the crystal (receiver).
Nonreciprocal transducers	
Carbon transducer	A carbon device has the form of a container loosely filled with carbon granules, which change their resistance to passing current in response to movements of the membrane enclosing the container. Carbon transducers can only operate as a receiver. Carbon microphones were used in all old telephones before the advent of dynamic and other newer microphones.
Laser transducer	A laser device has the form of a laser beam that is reflected from a vibrating surface responding to changes in the acoustic wave arriving at the surface. The small deflections of the vibrating surface (e.g., the vibrating glass from a window) are measured by comparing arriving and reflected laser beams and these differences are converted into an electric voltage to form the audio signal. Laser transducers described above can only operate as a receiver.
Gas plasma (plasma ion, corona) transducer	A gas plasma device is a chamber in which the electrical field electrically charges (ionizes) gas enclosed in a quartz tube connecting two electrodes. A sufficiently strong field frees so many free electrons that electricity begins to flow through a tube in the form of a visible light arc (such as an arc seen during metal welding) between both electrodes. The variable electric field affects the form and intensity of the arc, which heats the air surrounding the quartz tube and makes the air move back and forth in the form of acoustic pressure. A gas plasma loudspeaker (e.g., ionophone) has no moving parts and thus is a very effective loudspeaker at high frequencies.

**An electrostatic (condenser) microphone requires a polarized direct current voltage to work. An electret microphone has a layer of polarized dielectric (electret) placed between the plates of the microphone that eliminates the need for the voltage to be polarized.*

▶ **Table 14.2.** Basic Electro-Mechano-Acoustic Analogies

Mechanics	Acoustics	Electricity
Power	Power	Power
Force	Acoustic pressure	Voltage
Velocity	Particle velocity	Current
Displacement	Volume displacement*	Charge
Friction	Acoustic resistance	Resistance
Mass	Acoustic mass (inertance)	Inductance
Compliance (antonym: stiffness)	Acoustic compliance (antonym: elastance)	Capacitance

**Volume displacement is the amount of the medium that is temporarily displaced during wave propagation.*

For example, if an acoustic and a mechanic system interact, there exists a common translation between a characteristic that appears in an acoustic system and the similar characteristic in a mechanic system. In addition, EMA analogies make it easier to explain complex phenomena. For example, a concept that may be very difficult to grasp in electronics may have a counterpart in mechanics that is much easier to explain. Thus, understanding concepts related to the physical domain can help with the comprehension of a similar phenomenon observed in another domain.

Microphones

A microphone is an electroacoustic receiver that converts acoustic signals into audio (electric) signals. Microphones differ in their principle of operation and specific construction details, but all of them operate in the same basic way. Acoustic energy arriving at the membrane of the microphone is converted into mechanic energy, and this energy is subsequently converted into electric energy. The two basic classes of microphones are **pressure microphones** and **gradient (velocity) microphones.** A pressure microphone has a thin membrane that moves in response to changes in sound pressure at its front surface (Fig. 14.2A). The membrane is connected to some type of electric or magnetic element, depending on the specific transducer (Table 14.1), which converts the movement of the membrane into an electric signal. A pressure microphone is an **omnidirectional microphone,** that is, a microphone in which the response is the same regardless of the direction of the incoming signal. This holds true only for low and middle acoustic frequencies since at high frequencies all microphones are directional due to wave scattering and acoustic shadow effects.

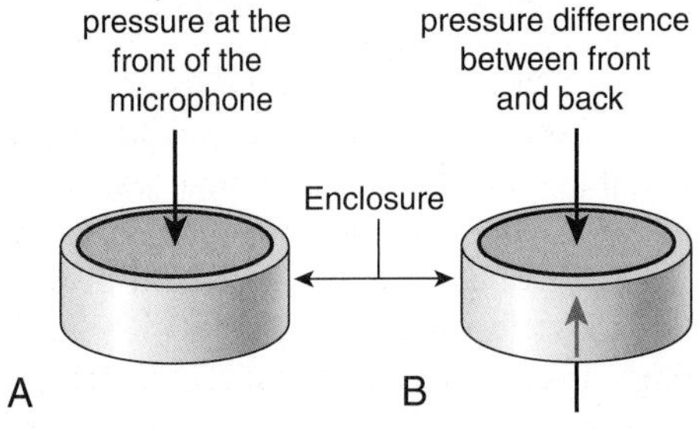

Figure 14.2. A pressure microphone **(A)** and a gradient microphone **(B).**

A **gradient microphone** (velocity microphone) responds to the difference in sound pressure (pressure gradient) between sound waves arriving at the front and the back of the microphone (Fig. 14.2B). The microphone response depends on the direction of sound waves; therefore, a gradient microphone is a **directional microphone.** If the sound is arriving from the side of the microphone (90° or 270°), then the signal will be identical at the front and back of the microphone and the microphone will not respond. From all other directions, the sound reaching the front and back of the microphone will differ, and the microphone will respond.

To examine how a specific microphone responds to sounds arriving from various directions, the directional characteristics of several basic types of microphones are shown in Figure 14.3. The graphs show a cross section (in the horizontal plane) of the three-dimensional characteristic of a microphone. The graphs have the form of a polar plot (Fig. 14.3A) in which the magnitude of the received sound is shown as a function of the azimuth (angle) of the sound source. The farther a response is plotted from the center of the polar plot, the greater the magnitude of the microphone response.

An omnidirectional microphone (Fig. 14.3B) responds equally well to sound from any direction, so the three-dimensional directional characteristic of this microphone is a sphere and the polar plot (cross section) is a circle. The small line located in the center of the figure shows the position of the microphone membrane and indicates that the membrane is facing 0° azimuth. The perfect circle surrounding the central point in Figure 14.2B shows that regardless of the azimuth (angle) of an approaching sound wave, the microphone response is the same (omnidirectional). An omnidirectional microphone is the optimal microphone to use if you want to record all of the sounds in an environment regardless of the location of various sound sources. For example, this type of microphone is used to pick up the voices of several simultaneous talkers or to measure background noise levels. One common application of an omnidirectional microphone is during a conference. An omnidirectional microphone is often positioned in the center of a conference table pointing straight up. This microphone will respond equally well regardless of the direction of the talker.

Gradient microphones have a much more directional three-dimensional characteristic than omnidirectional microphones. The polar pattern shown in Figure 14.3C represents a bidirectional (dipole, figure-of-eight) gradient microphone. The directivity pattern of the figure-of-eight

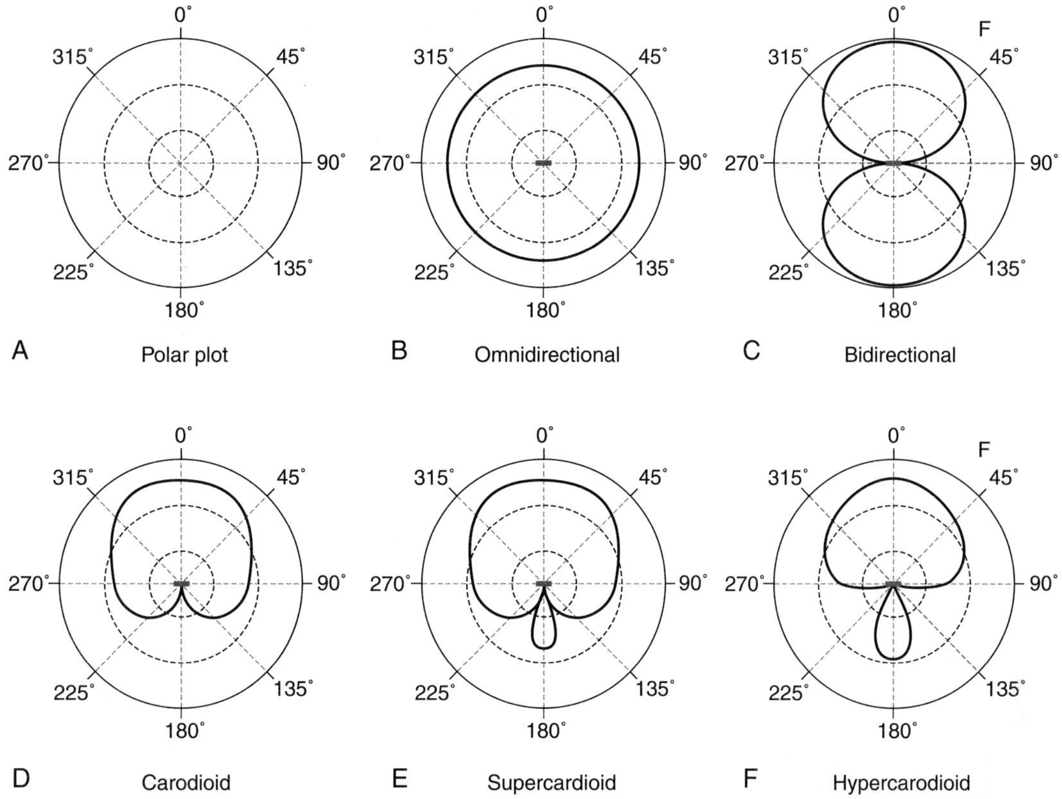

Figure 14.3. Illustration of a simple polar plot **(A).** The sound level created by a microphone located in the center and facing 0° is shown for an omnidirectional microphone **(B),** a bidirectional microphone **(C),** a cardioid microphone **(D),** a supercardioid microphone **(E),** and a hypercardioid microphone **(F).**

gradient microphone shows that the microphone responds most effectively to sounds originating from 0° and 180° (the front and back of the microphone) and the microphone does not respond when sounds originate on either side of the microphone. If the front or back of the gradient microphone is partially covered and/or the microphone has more than one membrane, the figure-of-eight directivity pattern can be made asymmetric and the microphone will emphasize only a single direction. A microphone that emphasizes only a single direction is called a unidirectional microphone. Most gradient microphones are unidirectional microphones.

The four basic types of unidirectional microphones are cardioid, supercardioid, hypercardioid, and shotgun microphone. The directional characteristic of a cardioid microphone is shown in Figure 14.3D. A cardioid microphone provides about 6 dB of attenuation (decrease) in sound intensity for sounds arriving from the sides of the microphone compared to sounds arriving from the front. Sounds arriving from the rear of the microphone are typically attenuated by about 15 dB to 25 dB. The supercardioid microphone (Fig. 14.3E) provides about 8.7 dB of attenuation at the sides and 11.4 dB at the rear and has two directions of maximum sound rejection at 125° and 235°. The hypercardioid microphone (Fig. 14.3F) provides about 12 dB of attenuation at the sides and 6 dB of attenuation at the rear and has two directions of maximum sound rejection (null points) at 110° and 250°. More complex directional patterns can be created by combining microphones with various directional characteristics together. The shotgun microphone (not shown) is a super-directional microphone in which the directional pattern resembles a very narrow supercardioid pattern. Shotgun microphones are the main microphones used in TV and film settings, as well as by wildlife naturalists to make realistic recordings of birds and animals.

Recall that the directivity patterns shown in Figure 14.3 are only valid at low and middle frequencies. At high frequencies all the microphones have very directional and complicated spatial characteristics. The frequency range in which the characteristics shown in Figure 14.3 can be considered accurate depends on the relationship between the sound wavelength and the dimensions of the microphone.

Based on the principle of operation (Table 14.1), the three most common types of microphones are (1) piezoelectric microphones, (2) dynamic microphones, and (3) condenser (electrostatic) microphones. The basic construction of each of these microphones is illustrated in Figure 14.4.

In a **piezoelectric microphone** (Fig. 14.4A), the input acoustic pressure acts on a membrane that is attached to one end of a piezoelectric bimorph (two piezoelectric plates bonded together through the surface perpendicular to their

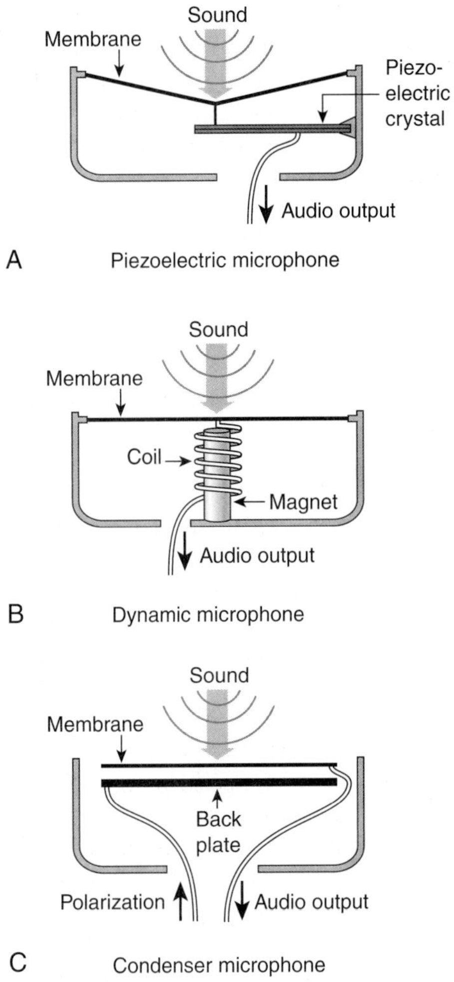

Figure 14.4. Principles of operation of piezoelectric **(A)**, dynamic **(B)**, and condenser **(C)** microphones.

polarization). Membrane vibrations result in a bending of the bimorph and the generation of varying charges on both sides of the bimorph. The end of the bimorph opposite to the end connected to the membrane is attached to two electrodes that convey the generated difference in electrical potential to the input of a microphone preamplifier (discussed later in this chapter). A **dynamic microphone** (Fig. 14.4B) uses electromagnetic induction. A coil is attached to the microphone membrane and the coil moves in a magnetic field. This induces a current in the coil. In a **condenser microphone** (Fig. 14.4C) the input acoustic pressure acts on a membrane that forms one plate of a large polarized (charged) capacitor (the capacitor is also referred to as a condenser in this application). The changes in the acoustic pressure move the membrane, which affects the distance between the plates of the condenser and subsequently affects its capacitance (Chapter 13). Since the plates of the condenser hold fixed charges, changes in the capacitance result in changes in the voltage across the plates that mimic the changes in acoustic pressure and result in the conversion of the acoustic signal into its electric form.

A number of technical parameters describe individual microphones and indicate the potential applications and limitations of specific microphones. The main technical parameters characterizing the operation of microphones are:

1. **Input sensitivity.** This is the ratio of the microphone output (in mV_{rms}) to its input (in Pa or dB SPL). For example, a microphone may have a sensitivity of 1 mV/Pa.
2. **Maximum (undistorted) input signal.** This is the highest sound pressure (in Pa or dB SPL) that the microphone is capable of converting into an electric signal without distortion. For example, the maximum (undistorted) input signal of a microphone may be 125 dB SPL.
3. **Frequency response.** This is the function (curve) showing the relationship between the magnitude of the microphone output and the signal frequency for the same magnitude of input signal. For example, if the frequency response is 50 Hz to 20,000 Hz (±3 dB), the microphone is converting the acoustic pressure in the frequency range from 50 Hz to 20,000 Hz into an electric signal with a tolerance (precision) of ±3 dB. The smaller the tolerance is, the flatter the frequency response is.
4. **Internal (self) noise.** Internal noise is the output of the microphone when there is no input. For example, if a microphone produces at its output a voltage corresponding to a 20-dB SPL signal at the input, even with no input signal, the internal noise can be said to be equivalent to 20 dB SPL.
5. **Dynamic range.** The dynamic range is the range between the noise level at the output with no signal at the input and the maximum undistorted signal at the output. An example of the dynamic range of a microphone is 80 dB.
6. **Output impedance.** This is the electric impedance (Chapter 13) measured at the output of a microphone. For example, a microphone may have an output impedance of 200 Ω.

One additional important technical parameter of microphones, which describes the overall selectivity of the microphone, is the **directivity factor (Q)**, which is related to the directivity pattern of the microphone. The directivity factor of a microphone indicates how much more sound energy would be captured by an omnidirectional microphone having the same on-axis sensitivity as a given directional microphone when the sound source is located on the axis of the microphone. The directivity factor expressed in dB is called the **directivity index (DI)** and is defined as:

$$DI = 10 \log Q \qquad \textbf{(14.2)}$$

The values of Q and DI depend on the sound frequency and are usually listed in the technical specifications of microphones for a 1000-Hz tone. Typical values of Q and DI for the most common polar plots shown in Figure 14.2 are

▶ **Table 14.3.** Directivity Factor and Directivity Index of the Most Common Directional Characteristics of Microphones

Polar Pattern	Mathematical Function	Directivity Factor (Q)	Directivity Index (DI) (dB)
Omnidirectional	$r = r_o = \text{const}$	1	0
Figure-of-eight (dipole)	$r = r_o \cos\theta$	3	4.8
Cardioid	$r = r_o(1 + \cos\theta)/2$	3	4.8
Supercardioid	$r = r_o(1 + 2\cos\theta)/3$	3.7	5.7
Hypercardioid	$r = r_o(1 + 3\cos\theta)/4$	4	6

given in Table 14.3. Even greater values of DI can be observed in the case of very directional microphones such as shotgun microphones (super-unidirectional microphone for commercial purposes) or parabolic microphones (microphone with an added parabolic dish, used outdoors for activities such as recording bird calls).

When you examine the technical specifications for measurement microphones, you will notice that they are described by another set of labels including free-field microphone, pressure microphone, and random incidence microphone. These labels are related to the frequency response of the microphone at high frequencies when the microphone is facing incoming sound waves, that is, when the microphone is pointed toward the sound source at a 0° angle of incidence. At low and middle frequencies, the frequency response of all three types of microphone is identical.

A **free-field microphone** is a microphone designed for measurements in a free field where sound travels with relatively few reflections, such as in open outdoor space (Chapter 6). This type of microphone responds to a single direction of sound arrival and its frequency response is corrected to compensate for the disturbance of the sound field caused by the presence of the microphone. Therefore, this microphone measures the sound pressure coming from a single direction that would exist at the microphone location if the microphone were not present.

A **pressure microphone** used for sound measurement is an omnidirectional microphone that responds uniformly to all directions of incoming sounds without any correction for the changes in the sound pressure level caused by the presence of the microphone in the sound field. Therefore, this microphone measures the sound pressure that actually exists in front of its membrane. Pressure microphones are mainly used with couplers and sound measurement devices, for the calibration of earphones where the measurement needs to account for the presence of the microphone.

A **random incidence microphone**, or diffuse-field microphone, is also an omnidirectional pressure microphone that responds uniformly to sound arriving simultaneously from all directions (similar to the pressure microphone), but its response is corrected to compensate for the presence of the microphone in the sound field. Thus, this microphone is used to measure sound pressure arriving from all directions that would exist at the microphone membrane if the microphone were not present. The output signals of a pressure microphone and random incidence microphone are usually very similar and in most practical cases these types of microphones can be used interchangeably.

In summary, a free-field microphone is used to measure sound pressure produced by a sound source in open space and free-field environments, a random incidence microphone is used to measure the sound pressure produced by a specific sound source in a specific environment, and the pressure microphone is used to measure the sound pressure that exists in a specific environment including the effects of the microphone present in this environment.*

Certain basic rules are important to know when using microphones for sound recording, transmission, or measurement. One of them is that the microphone has to be kept away from the human body and other large objects. This is because placing a microphone close to the human body (absorption) or to a large hard object (reflection) may affect the amount of energy acting on the microphone membrane. For that reason, a sound level meter (SLM, device used to measure sound pressure) needs to be held away from the body during sound level measurements.

If a talker's voice is recorded, the microphone should be kept away from the talker's lips and off-axis of the talker's mouth to record the speech as it is heard by other people. Some speech sounds, especially the plosives (e.g., "b" and "p"), are accompanied by a blast of air that may cause an audible "pop" sound and other sound distortions when they hit the membrane directly. The off-axis position of the microphone also improves the reception of sibilants (e.g., "s," "th," "sh") that produce a wind-like effect if the microphone is positioned straight in front of the lips.

Special hands-free microphones are designed to be clipped to clothes or hung at the chest via a loop around the neck. These microphones are called lavaliere microphones or lapel microphones. Due to the close proximity of these microphones to the clothing and somewhat distant location from the direct path of radiated speech, these microphones have a very poor high-frequency response (above 5 kHz). Therefore, they are designed with a special push-on grill that creates a resonance chamber that enhances sound pressure at the microphone membrane in the 5-kHz to 8-kHz frequency range. If these microphones are used as normal distant microphones, their recording will have an unnaturally enhanced high-frequency region.

In contrast to the high-frequency absorption seen when a microphone is placed near the body, setting a microphone close to a reflective surface can boost some frequencies more than others. Thus, special microphones called pressure zone

*Random incidence and pressure microphones can be used to measure the free-field–like sound pressure produced by a sound source if they are used in a relatively absorptive environment and the microphone membrane is held parallel to the direction of wave propagation.

microphones (PZMs) or boundary microphones (e.g., Crown PZM-30) are designed to work best when mounted on reflective surfaces. These microphones usually use a miniature electret microphone placed very close to a reflective surface (e.g., about 1 mm) and facing the reflective surface, to increase the sound pressure reaching the microphone. Thus, they similarly capture all the reflections in a wide frequency range. These types of microphones are often placed on conference tables or at the hard surface of a podium for conference presentations.

Low-frequency enhancement of the microphone output can also be created by the **proximity effect** when the talker holds a directional microphone very close to the mouth. When the directional microphone is held far away from a sound source, the distance from the source to both sides of the microphone is about the same. When the talker or vocalist holds the microphone at the lips, however, the difference in distance to both sides of the microphone can be as large as 5 to 10 times. This difference results in a large difference in sound pressure levels between the front and the back of the microphone; thus, this microphone responds only to the front wave. This in turn boosts the amount of low-frequency energy arriving at the microphone membrane that can be as large as 10 to 15 dB at frequencies below 200 Hz. This effect may be beneficial for a singer who wants to sound more deep and powerful, but it changes the natural spectral properties of the singer's or talker's voice. Note that the proximity effect does not apply to omnidirectional microphones since they only respond to the front wave, independent of their position in respect to the sound source.

Another important rule about the use of microphones is that the microphone needs to be protected from wind by a special windscreen. The windscreen is necessary to eliminate the high noise levels caused by air particles pushed onto the microphone membrane by natural wind pressure, air conditioning systems, air pressure from a singer's voice, and so forth. It is also important to remember that microphones are very susceptible to changes in atmospheric conditions and should be kept at a constant temperature and humidity. For example, condenser microphones are especially prone to damage from high humidity. If moisture condenses between the plates of the microphone, it may cause a new current pathway in the microphone that may burn the plates or destroy the preamplifier.

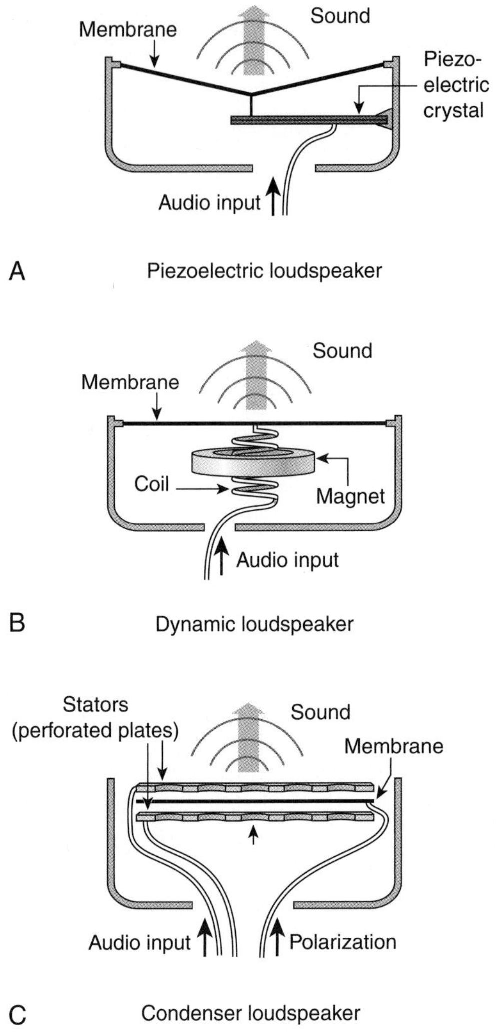

Figure 14.5. The basic parts of a piezoelectric loudspeaker **(A)**, a dynamic loudspeaker **(B)**, and a consider loudspeaker **(C)**.

Loudspeakers

A **loudspeaker** is an electroacoustic transmitter that converts audio signals into acoustic waves propagating through space. Loudspeakers perform the exact opposite sound conversion to microphones. A piezoelectric loudspeaker, shown in Figure 14.5A, works in exactly the opposite way as the piezoelectric microphone described earlier. A piezoelectric bimorph (two piezoelectric plates fused together and polarized in the direction of their common surface) is connected at one of its ends to two electrodes. The application of an audio signal to the electrodes forces one plate to expand and another plate to shrink. Since the plates are connected together, they cannot move independently and the whole bimorph bends back and forth in response to the varying audio signal. The far end of the bimorph is connected to the center of the membrane that oscillates in response to the bimorph movements. Some other types of piezoelectric loudspeakers use piezoelectric membranes that bend up and down in response to an applied voltage.

The most common type of loudspeaker is a dynamic (magnetoelectric, moving coil) loudspeaker, shown in Figure 14.5B. The audio signal supplied by a power amplifier is fed into a voice coil attached to the loudspeaker's membrane. The voice coil is located in a magnetic field produced by a permanent magnet. The magnetic field produced by a current passing through a coil interacts with the magnetic field from the magnet surrounding the coil, causing the coil to move in and out of the magnet's magnetic field (see the "right-hand rule" described in Chapter 13). Since the coil is attached to the membrane of the loudspeaker, the membrane moves with the coil, producing a sound that reflects the voltage changes of the audio signal.

A condenser loudspeaker (Fig. 14.5C) has a membrane that is placed between two fixed perforated plates (called stators). The audio signal is delivered between the two fixed places while the membrane is polarized and holds some charge. The membrane and hard plates act as a pair of capacitors, so when an audio signal is applied to the plates, one of the plates becomes more positive and the other one less positive. This results in a movement of the membrane away from one plate toward the other. The vibrations of the membrane push air through the holes in the plates, creating a sound wave that mirrors the shape of the audio signal.

Loudspeakers can be classified into several different types depending on the way the loudspeaker is built and how emits sound. Three common types of loudspeakers are planar, cone, and horn loudspeakers. A planar electrostatic loudspeaker is similar to a condenser microphone with a large flat membrane that vibrates in response to changes in electrical potential applied between the plates of the loudspeaker. A planar magnetic loudspeaker consists of a flat membrane stretched over a frame and a strong permanent magnet. The membrane can be made of aluminum or plastic (with an etched metal coil). Current passing through the membrane creates a magnetic field that interacts with the magnetic field of the permanent magnet, pushing or pulling the membrane in respect to the position of the permanent magnet. Planar magnetic loudspeakers are usually very thin and can be hung on a wall or used as free-standing units.

Cone loudspeakers have cone-shaped membranes that are either round or elliptic in shape; the cone-like design means a relatively large surface area can be used with a relatively small loudspeaker dimension. This design also improves the directivity of sound radiation, improves the power handling of the loudspeaker, and makes the loudspeakers more durable. While flat membrane loudspeakers operate as plane wave sources, cone loudspeakers operate more like point (spherical wave) sources.

A horn loudspeaker is a planar magnetic loudspeaker with an attached horn to improve the impedance matching with the surrounding air (cone loudspeakers also provide impedance matching, but to a lesser extent). Flat, high-frequency loudspeakers are generally small and light. They work well in low-intensity, high-frequency applications but they do not produce a lot of power. To improve their power output, they are coupled with long horns that effectively amplify the sound. The horn can be straight or it can be bent in a convoluted way to save some space. The most effective horns are exponential horns, in which the diameter of the horn increases in an exponential manner.

The most important technical parameters that are used to describe properties and limitations of various loudspeakers are:

1. **Efficiency or input sensitivity.** This is the ratio of the sound pressure level emitted by a loudspeaker measured at a distance (usually 1 m) from the loudspeaker membrane to the power of the audio signal applied to the loudspeaker. Loudspeaker efficiency is expressed in dB SPL per W or Pa/W and is usually defined for a 1-kHz signal, for example, 100 dB SPL per W or 200 Pa/W.
2. **Power handling capability (power rating).** This is the maximum continuous electrical power that the loudspeaker can handle without being damaged. An example of the power that a loudspeaker can handle is 300 W.
3. **Frequency response.** This is the function (curve) showing the relationship between the magnitude of the loudspeaker output and the signal frequency for the same magnitude of the input signal. For example, if the frequency response is 80 Hz to 14,000 Hz (±6 dB), the loudspeaker is producing acoustic pressure in the frequency range from 80 Hz to 14,000 Hz with a tolerance (precision) of ±6 dB.
4. **Input impedance.** This is the electric impedance (Chapter 13) measured at the input of the loudspeaker, for example, 4 Ω.
5. **Maximum continuous output signal.** This is the greatest sound pressure level that can be continuously produced by the loudspeaker, for example, 105 dB SPL.
6. **Directivity factor (Q).** The directivity factor of a loudspeaker is defined as the ratio of the sound intensity produced by a given loudspeaker at a point located at a predetermined distance on the main axis of the loudspeaker to the sound intensity produced at the same point by an omnidirectional loudspeaker supplied with the same power.

In analyzing a loudspeaker's behavior, it is important to note that the membrane of the loudspeaker emits sound in two opposite directions: toward the front and toward the back of the loudspeaker. So a loudspeaker is a natural dipole-type source of sound (Chapter 5). The sounds produced by the front and back of the loudspeaker's membrane arriving at the same point in space can interfere with one another, causing local peaks and dips of sound pressure depending on whether they are in-phase or out-of-phase at a specific frequency (Chapter 6). This phenomenon is called the **comb filter effect** since alternating peaks and dips in the frequency domain create a sound spectrum that looks like a comb. The peaks and dips of the comb can distort the original sound and should be avoided. The comb effect can be eliminated by mounting the loudspeaker in an infinite partition (baffle) that separates the front and the back of the loudspeaker, such as a wall or ceiling. Another solution is to mount a loudspeaker in a box that covers its sides and back. This box is called a closed enclosure to differentiate it from an open enclosure, which does not close the loudspeaker at its back and allows some reflections of sound from the surface behind the loudspeaker. If the loudspeaker is placed in a closed enclosure, the energy radiated by the back of the loudspeaker can be suppressed by lining the interior of the enclosure with an absorbing material or the energy can be reflected toward the front in the appropriate phase by a special construction called a reflex bass.

A full-range (wideband) loudspeaker must have a large membrane to push the large amount of air that needs to be moved for the loudspeaker to generate loud *low*-frequency sounds. However, a large membrane has a large mass, which is difficult to move at *high*-frequencies. Therefore, in many cases the wideband sound reproduction is created by two, three, or more loudspeakers of different sizes that reproduce different frequency ranges. These specialized loudspeakers are called subwoofer loudspeakers (very low-frequency loudspeakers), woofer loudspeakers (low-frequency loudspeakers), midrange loudspeakers (middle-frequency loudspeakers), and tweeter loudspeakers (high-frequency loudspeakers). Individual loudspeakers that are part of multiloudspeaker assemblies are called loudspeaker drivers or, simply, drivers. Drivers are connected to the audio source through a special filter called a **crossover network** that directs high-frequency energy to the high-frequency loudspeakers, low-frequency energy to the low-frequency loudspeakers, and so on. A single driver (loudspeaker) or several drivers (loudspeakers) with a crossover network and their enclosure are called a **loudspeaker system.** Loudspeaker systems can have different-sized and -shaped enclosures and different front panel arrangements. In addition, loudspeaker systems can include various types of loudspeakers and/or multiple loudspeakers of the same kind to improve the range of transmitted frequencies and power handling. The main considerations in the design of multiloudspeaker systems are the loudspeakers, an appropriate crossover network that provides a very smooth and flat overall frequency response, and a proper size of enclosure in which the sound radiation at low frequencies is not attenuated by the high stiffness of the enclosed air. Multiloudspeaker systems with two or more loudspeakers located at different places in the same enclosure create signals of different frequencies coming to the listener from different points in space, and this should be taken into consideration in some applications.

Earphones

An **earphone** is an electroacoustic transmitter that converts audio signals into acoustic pressure for delivery directly to the human ear. The purpose of the loudspeaker is to deliver sound into an open space to create the spatial impression of sound surrounding a listener or a group of listeners. The main purpose of earphones is to deliver a signal to the ears of a single listener while eliminating the listener from the acoustic effects of the environment. The main difference between the loudspeaker and the earphone is the difference in the air impedance loading the membrane of the transducer. In the case of the loudspeaker, the air impedance is about 40 Ω and is practically frequency independent in the audio range, whereas the impedance of the air in the closed ear canal is much larger and varies more with frequency.

The two basic categories of earphones are over the ear and in the ear. One or two earphones together with a system for holding them on the listener's head is called a **headphone system** or **headphones.** If a headphone system also incorporates a communication microphone, this system is called a **headset.** A system of an earphone and a microphone designed to be held in the hand during communication is called a **handset.**

Earphones can be inserted into the ear canal **(insert earphones)** or into the concha **(earbuds)** or placed over the ear. Earphones placed over the ear and resting on the antihelix/helix of the pinna are called **supra-aural earphones,** and those that rest over the head and surround the pinna are called **circumaural earphones.** Insert earphones are used with portable audio equipment and for hearing testing purposes. Earbuds are used mainly for entertainment purposes and are sold together with personal stereo systems (e.g., mp^3 players and portable CD players). They differ from insert earphones in that they do not close the ear canal (they are also usually of poorer quality than a medical-quality insert earphone). The main advantage of earbuds is that they are lightweight and small. Supra-aural earphones are larger and heavier than either of the two previous types. They are usually supported by a headband and have flat rubber or foam cushions resting against the pinnae. Circumaural earphones are the largest and generally the heaviest of all the earphone types. They surround the pinna and rest against the skull encapsulating the ear. They usually have a much better low-frequency response than supra-aural earphones due to the smaller air leakage and additional resonance space under the earphone earmuffs. They also provide better isolation from environmental noises compared with supra-aural earphones. Examples of insert earphone models are the line of the Etymotic Research ER earphones (e.g., ER-3A), Shure E-3, and Westone UM-2. Examples of earbuds are AKG-K14P, Beyer DTX-20, and Sony MDR EX-81. Examples of supra-aural earphone models are the Telephonics TDH-39, -49, and -50P; Bayer DT-48; and Sennheiser HD-414. Examples of circumaural earphones include the Beyer DT-990; Sony MDR-V6, AKG K-240, and K-270; and Sennheiser HDA-200 and HD-250.

Two important considerations in selecting earphones for various applications is the amount of closure around the back of the membrane of the earphone and the amount of attenuation (isolation) from the external world that the earphones provide. Both of these factors can be affected by the openings in the back of the earphone enclosure making an enclosure of either the open or closed type. A **closed earphone** has a solid back that creates an air-filled cavity between the enclosure and the membrane of the earphone. This solid back means the sound produced by the earphone cannot be heard easily at a distance from the listener's head. The closed earphone design also isolates a listener from external sounds. The most important effect of the closed enclosure, however, is its resonance character, which causes a significant boost in the reproduction of low frequencies by the earphone. An **open earphone** has openings in the back of the enclosure connecting the back side of the earphone membrane with the external world. This connection decreases the isolation of the listener from external noises and makes sounds reproduced by the earphone audible in the space close to the listener. The main effect of these openings, however, is a less resonant and flatter frequency response, which improves the overall sound balance of the earphone. The differentiation between open and closed earphones is most important in the case of circumaural earphones, but any type of earphone can be of either open or closed type. Examples of closed earphones are the Sennheiser HAD-200 and HD-250 (circumaural) and Sennheiser HD-25 (supra-aural). The main technical parameters that characterize earphones are:

1. **Input sensitivity.** This is the ratio of the sound pressure level emitted by the earphone measured in a special coupler simulating the human ear to the power of the audio signal applied to the earphone. Earphone efficiency is expressed in dB SPL per W or Pa/W and it is usually defined for a 1-kHz signal, for example, 110 dB/mW at 1 kHz.
2. **Frequency response.** This is the function showing the relationship between the magnitude of the earphone output and the signal frequency for the same magnitude of the input signal, for example, from 30 Hz to 18 kHz (± 6 dB).
3. **Input impedance.** This is the electric impedance measured at the input of the earphone, for example, 16 Ω.
4. **Power handling capacity (power rating).** This is the maximum power applied to the earphone that the earphone can sustain without being damaged, for example, 100 mW.
5. **Maximum continuous output signal.** This is the greatest sound pressure level that can be continuously produced by the earphone, for example, 115 dB SPL.

Earphone types are the same as the previously discussed loudspeaker types since the only difference between earphones and loudspeakers is the manner in which they match the load impedance. Therefore, popular earphones include dynamic (magnetoelectric) earphones, condenser (electrostatic) earphones, and piezoelectric earphones (see Fig. 14.5 for basic components).

AUDIO SIGNAL PROCESSING

Once the acoustic signal is converted into an audio signal, it is processed and transmitted by the electronic components connected in the electroacoustic chain. These components, together with audio transducers, are collectively called audio devices or electroacoustic devices. Audio devices can be classified in several ways. The main classification is based on the general function of the device. According to this classification, audio devices can be divided into:

1. **Signal transducers,** which convert one form of energy into another
2. **Signal controllers,** which adjust the signal intensity, mix the signals, and direct signals toward specific outputs
3. **Signal monitors,** which acquire and display information about signal properties such as level, spectral content, and so forth
4. **Signal processors,** which modify the signal properties according to certain processing rules

Transducers were already discussed in the previous section of this chapter. Four basic types of **signal controllers** used in the electroacoustic chain are mixers, splitters, attenuators, and amplifiers. Their role is to direct audio signals to the desired channel and set an appropriate signal level, but they are not intended to change the form of the signal. The role of mixers (signal adders) and splitters (signal separators) is to add audio signals together or to direct them toward more than one output. The role of attenuators (signal reducers) and amplifiers (signal boosters) is to provide the appropriate signal levels for processing by other electroacoustic devices. The amount of change in the signal level provided by attenuators or amplifiers can be fixed or variable. A variable attenuator is a device equipped with a variable resistor (e.g., a continuous potentiometer or step attenuator) that is used to make the adjustment.

Signal monitors include various types of signal measuring and monitoring devices such as voltmeters (e.g., peak program meters, volume unit [VU] meters, and sound level meters), ammeters, phase meters, power meters, and so forth. Their function is to measure some characteristic of sound (e.g., peak magnitude, RMS magnitude, phase, spectrum) and then provide a visual display of this information. Common types of video displays used by signal monitoring devices include analog meters (e.g., VU meter), digital numeric displays (e.g., digital sound level meter), signal traces (e.g., oscilloscope), and spectrum displays. For example, a VU meter indicates the relative signal strength reaching the meter. The display provides a needle deflection somewhere between about −20 and +3 units. Optimal sound transmission occurs when the VU meter indicates a value close to 0 units.

Signal processors (or audio processors) modify audio signals and eliminate noise and crosstalk that interfere with the transmission of desired signals. Signal processors include filters, equalizers, compressors, noise gates, limiters, expanders, companders, time compressors, time expanders, and reverberators. A list of the main audio processors used in electroacoustic chains with short descriptions of their function is included in Table 14.4.

Each of the devices listed in Table 14.4 has a number of classes, variants, and special applications that are discussed in books on electroacoustics and audio technologies. Similarly, there are a variety of signal controllers and signal displays. In this book only audio amplifiers and selected classes of audio processors—limiters, compressors, filters, and equalizers—will be described in greater detail. These are four devices commonly seen in hearing science applications.

Table 14.4. Basic Types of Signal Processors Used in Audio Systems

Audio Processor	Function
Filter	A device that passes signal components of certain frequencies while eliminating others
Equalizer	A device that changes the relative intensities of various frequency components of the signal spectrum
Limiter (clipper)	A device that prevents the signal from exceeding a certain predetermined magnitude
Compressor	A device that changes the dynamic range of the signal by decreasing the difference between the strongest and the weakest signal
Expander	A device that changes the dynamic range of the signal by increasing the difference between the strongest and the weakest signal
Compander	A combination of COMPressor and expANDER that decreases the dynamic range of the signal being transmitted through a noisy channel and restores the original dynamic range at the end of transmission to minimize the effect of noise on the transmitted signal
Noise gate	A device that eliminates background noise from a signal by passing only signals whose magnitudes exceed a certain threshold value and reducing to zero a signal that is lower than the threshold magnitude
Time compressor	A device that periodically discards small segments of the signal to make the whole signal shorter (based on a predetermined duration)
Time stretcher	A device that periodically replicates small segments of the signal to make the whole signal longer (based on a predetermined duration)
Time delay device	A device that delays one signal in respect to another signal so that both signals can arrive together or in a predetermined time order
Reverberator	A device that adds synthetic reflections to the original sound in order to improve the spatial properties of the signal; it makes the sound appear to be in an environment with some sound reflections

Amplifiers

An audio signal generated by a microphone is usually very small and needs to be increased in size to be used by other audio devices and transducers. This function is performed by an electronic (audio) amplifier. An **amplifier** is a device that increases the voltage (voltage amplifier), current (current amplifier), or both (power amplifier) of a transmitted signal. It does so by taking power from its direct current (DC) power supply and using it to replicate the input signal with a larger—usually much larger—magnitude at its output. The main difference between voltage, current, and power amplifiers is their input and output impedance. A typical **voltage amplifier** has high input impedance and low output impedance, a typical **current amplifier** has low input impedance and high output impedance, and a **power amplifier** has high input impedance and very low output impedance, matching the impedance of the load to maximize the power transfer (impedance matching). Thus, the decision of whether to use a voltage, current, or power amplifier in a specific application depends on the signal source impedance and amplifier load impedance.*

Three basic terms characterize amplifier operation: input signal, output signal, and gain. The **input signal** is the magnitude of the signal that enters the amplifier, the **output signal** is the magnitude of the signal that exits the amplifier, and the **gain** is the ratio (difference in dB) of the output signal to the input signal. In other words, the gain indicates how many times the input signal was amplified by the amplifier. For example, if the amplifier is fed with a 100-mV signal and produces 1 V at its output, its gain is 10 times or 20 dB. Similarly, if the input signal is 40 dB re: 1 mV and the output signal is 60 dB, the gain is 20 dB.

Voltage amplifiers are the most common amplifiers used in audio applications. They are usually divided into two main classes based on the voltage levels that they amplify: preamplifiers (low-voltage amplifiers) and line amplifiers (high-voltage amplifiers). **Preamplifiers** are small, low-noise amplifiers with very high input impedance that are designed to amplify low-level electric signals produced by various sensors (e.g., microphones, biologic electrodes, and so forth). They are usually connected directly (not through a cable) to a transducer or other low-signal device to minimize the effects of external noise and cable impedance on transmitted signals. The output signals of many microphones, and of electrodes used in medical testing, are often very small (e.g., 0.1 to 10 mV) and require a preamplifier. **Line amplifiers** are used when the signal source is relatively high or for subsequent stages of amplification after the initial signal has been amplified by a preamplifier. Line amplifiers are cheaper than preamplifiers and produce higher voltage levels at the output than preamplifiers, but they are also less sensitive and have lower input impedance, so they are generally used only when the input signal voltage is relatively high and reaches a nominal line level input voltage of 0.3152 V_{rms}, which is –10 dB re: 1 V_{rms}. The typical line voltage levels used in professional audio equipment is 0.775 V_{rms}.

*In some modular audio systems, where different components can be placed in different places, all components, including amplifiers, have the same input and output impedance (usually 600 Ω) so the signal levels at specific points of the system are always the same regardless of the combination of the modules being used.

Current amplifiers are used to amplify signals when the voltage source can only supply a very low current or to separate circuits with very different impedances (buffer amplifier). In this case, the amplifier should have low input impedance and provide an output current that is independent of the amplifier load.

Power amplifiers increase the power of audio signals and transfer this power to loudspeakers, earphones, or mechanic vibrators. Depending on their construction, power amplifiers may produce audio power ranging from as little as 0.1 to 1 W for earphones and bone vibrators to greater than 1 kW for high-power loudspeakers. If the power requirements are less than 0.1 W, no special power amplifier is usually needed and a line amplifier can handle the load.

The main technical parameters of audio amplifiers are:

1. **Input sensitivity.** This is the minimum magnitude of the input signal required to produce a predetermined magnitude of output signal or a specific signal-to-noise ratio at the output (e.g., 10 mV).
2. **Frequency response.** This is the function showing the relationship between the amplifier output and the signal frequency for the same magnitude of the input signal. An example of the frequency response of an amplifier is 5 Hz to 25 kHz (± 0.5 dB).
3. **Dynamic range** (signal-to-noise ratio). This is the range between the noise level at the output for short-circuited (no signal) input and the maximum undistorted signal at the output. An example of the dynamic range for an amplifier is 90 dB.
4. **Input impedance.** This is the electrical impedance measured at the input of the amplifier (e.g., 2 MΩ).
5. **Output impedance.** This is the electrical impedance measured at the output of an amplifier (e.g., 10 kΩ).
6. **Maximum (undistorted) output voltage.** This is the maximum output the amplifier can produce without distortion (e.g., 10 V).

The relationship between the magnitude of the output signal and the magnitude of the input signal of an amplifier or attenuator is called the **transfer function** or **input–output function** (I/O function). Most audio amplifiers are **linear amplifiers,** which means that their transfer function forms a straight line. In other words, it means that the magnitude of the output signal is linearly related to the magnitude of the input signal. Three examples of linear transfer functions are shown in Figure 14.6A. When both axes of the input–output graph are expressed in linear units (e.g., volts), the gain of the amplifier is equal to the slope of the transfer function, that is, the slope (*slope* $= \frac{\Delta y}{\Delta x}$) of the line.

If the ratio of the output signal to the input signal is 1:1, the signals have identical magnitudes and the amplifier does not provide any amplification. For the amplifier to amplify the input signal, the ratio of the input and output signals must be larger than 1 (e.g., Figure 14.6A, line a, where the slope = 3.5 because the ratio of the output to the input is 35/10). Conversely, if the ratio of the input and output signals is less than 1 (e.g., Fig. 14.6A, line c, where the slope is about 0.3 because the ratio of the output to the input is 20/70), it means that the "amplifier" is not actually amplifying the signal and is, in fact, acting as an attenuator, decreasing the input signal.

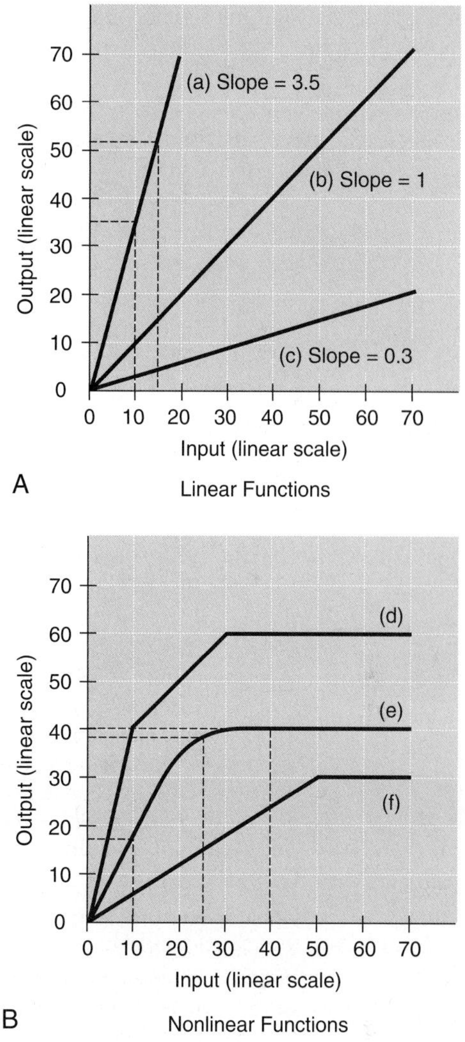

Figure 14.6. Examples of linear **(A)** and nonlinear **(B)** transfer functions.

In contrast to a linear amplifier, a **nonlinear amplifier** has a transfer function that is not a straight line. In the case where the transfer function is not linear, the amount of gain (amplification) provided by the amplifier varies as a function of the magnitude of the input signal. Figure 14.6B shows three nonlinear transfer functions. To illustrate the difference between linear and nonlinear amplifiers, let us analyze the linear transfer function shown by line a and the nonlinear transfer function shown by line e in Figure 14.6B. In the case of a linear transfer function, the gain of the amplifier is the same regardless of the input. When the input on the linear function a is 10, the output is 35 (35:10 = gain of 3.5), and when the input is 15, the output is 52.5 (52.5:15 = gain of 3.5). When the input on the nonlinear function e is 10, the output is 18 (18:10 = 1.8 gain); when the input is 25, the output is 37.5 (37.5/25 = 1.5 gain); and when the input is 40, the output is 40 (1:1 = no gain).

Nonlinearity of transmitting systems is a rule rather than an exception. Each linear system becomes nonlinear if the magnitude of the input signal exceeds a certain value. The main problem created by nonlinearity is signal distortion, called nonlinear distortion, which is signal level dependent and easily audible. Two types of nonlinear distortions, harmonic distortions and intermodulation distortions, are described in the next section of this chapter. A system's nonlinearity is not always an undesirable property, however, and many electric and audio system applications depend on nonlinear signal processing to achieve specific goals. Note, for example, that the nonlinear transfer function shown in Figure 14.6B, line f, is initially linear and becomes nonlinear after the signal input exceeds a value of 50. If such a system operates for input signals below this value, it would behave as a linear amplifier. When the input level exceeds this value, the amplifier produces some nonlinear distortions but it will also protect the output system against excessive signal levels. For example, a loudspeaker connected to the output of a properly designed and implemented (i.e., programmed) amplifier will never have a signal large enough to damage the loudspeaker, because the amplifier will become nonlinear beyond a certain critical input. Similarly, if a hearing aid is properly designed, hearing aid users will never get a signal that is too loud for the user.

Many power amplifiers are also nonlinear amplifiers because they are much more efficient than linear amplifiers. That means that they consume less DC power to deliver the same signal level at the output. The more nonlinear the amplifier is, however, the higher the level of nonlinear distortions, so a power advantage is associated with a decrease in signal quality. This tradeoff between power consumption and amplifier nonlinearity is, for example, of constant concern in hearing aid design. For example, a hearing aid should deliver clear speech, but if the batteries drain too quickly, then they have to be changed quite often, which makes the operation of the hearing aid expensive and inconvenient. If the battery life is maximized, however, the hearing aid may not provide sufficient amplification for the user.

There are several types of power amplifiers that differ in power consumption and signal quality. The main types are class A, B, AB, C, and D amplifiers. This classification is based on the duration of time during which the current flows through the amplifier during each wave period. A class A (linear) amplifier conducts current throughout the entire period of the waveform. That means that the whole peak-to-peak range of the input signal is processed by this amplifier. This type of amplifier produces no nonlinear distortions; however, it is very inefficient, with only as little as 20% of its energy used to amplify the signal and 80% of its energy wasted as heat. The class B amplifier processes only the positive or negative portions of the signal and two such amplifiers working in a push–pull mode can process the whole signal. Since each class B amplifier processes a two times smaller voltage signal than the class A amplifier, even two class B amplifiers waste less energy than one class A amplifier since power is proportional to voltage in the second power ($P \sim E^2$). However, push–pull class B amplifiers generate some unavoidable signal distortions as a result of the crossover needed to recombine both parts of the signal after amplification. This problem is minimized in class AB amplifiers that process a little bit more than half of the signal range to avoid the crossover distortions but are less efficient than the class B amplifier. Another class of power amplifiers are class D amplifiers, which use fast switching in the form of pulse modulation to considerably reduce the heat produced during signal transmission. If the frequency switching is much higher than the highest frequency of the transmitted signal, its nonlinear product can be easily filtered out and a class D amplifier can operate as a highly linear and efficient amplifier. Modern hearing aids and assistive devices use predominantly class D and class AB amplifiers.

Signal Transformations and Distortions

Many electroacoustic devices are designed not only to transmit audio signals, but also to change audio signals in predetermined ways to achieve a desired effect at the end of the transmission process. A modification of the original input signal leading to a desired change in the form of the output signal is called **signal transformation.** All of the devices listed in Table 14.4 perform signal transformations. If the change in the signal was not intended but was caused by limitations of the transmission channel, this change is called a **signal distortion.** The actual results of a transformation and a distortion can be identical; they both introduce signal deformation. The difference lies in whether the changes in the output signal were intentional or not.

Signal distortions can be divided into two main classes: linear distortions and nonlinear distortions. **Linear distortions** are frequency-dependent changes in gain that subsequently cause a change in the spectral components of the signal. These differences are independent of the magnitude of the input signal. Linear distortions result in changes in the temporal form of the transmitted signal, but since they are independent of the magnitude of the input signal, the waveform of the output signal is the same for small and large magnitudes of the input signal. This means that a linear distortion can be measured for any level of input signal.

The two different categories of linear distortion are frequency distortion and time delay (phase) distortion. Frequency distortions are caused by changes in the attenuation or gain of the signal as a function of frequency. The most frequent causes of frequency distortions are a limited bandwidth of a transmitting device and resonance properties of one of its elements. For example, a telephone has a limited bandwidth, and speech sounds above about 3400 Hz are removed from the signal. This is why speech on the telephone has such a distinct sound. Time delay (phase) distortions are caused by differences in the time needed for signals of different frequencies to be transmitted by a device. Recall that differences in time are directly related to differences in the phase of a sine wave (Chapter 3). Therefore, phase distortions, similar to frequency distortions, affect the shape of the output signal even though the transmitting system has a linear transfer function.

Nonlinear distortions are signal deformations that occur when the transfer function of the transmitting device is not linear and the shape of the output signal depends on the amplitude of the input signal. This type of transfer function was discussed in the previous section of this chapter. Nonlinear distortions result in the generation of new components in the output signal that were not present in the input signal but are correlated with the input signal. In contrast to linear distortions, the measured amount of nonlinear distortion depends on the magnitude of the input signal.

The two most common types of nonlinear distortions are harmonic distortion and intermodulation distortion. **Harmonic distortions** are harmonics of the signal (i.e., integer multiples of the signal) appearing at the output of a nonlinear device when the signal input includes sinusoidal components (e.g., a pure tone or pure tones). They appear at the output of nonlinear systems regardless of whether the signal is a pure tone or a complex signal. **Intermodulation distortions** are differential (one frequency minus another) and summation (one frequency plus another) tones that appear at the output of a nonlinear device when its input consists of two or more sine waves. The specific frequencies of the intermodulation distortions (f_d) for a signal consisting of two sine waves (f_1 and f_2) can be calculated as follows:

$$f_d = af_1 \pm bf_2 \qquad \textbf{(14.3)}$$

where f_1 and f_2 are the two frequencies of the input signal and a and b are small integers (1, 2, 3, and so forth). If either a or b is equal to zero, the calculated frequency is a harmonic of one of the two sine waves.

Example 14.1

If two sine waves with frequencies of 1000 Hz and 1200 Hz comprise the input signal to a nonlinear system, list two possible nonlinear distortion product frequencies.

First, select Equation 14.3.

$$f_d = af_1 \pm bf_2$$

Substitute known variables. We know that one frequency is 1000 Hz and the other is 1200 Hz, so include these.

$$f_d = a(1200) \pm b(1000)$$

Next, consider that the problem asked for two possible nonlinear distortions. From the text, we known that a and b are small integers, so let's select 1 for a and 2 for b and solve.

$$f_d = (1 \times 1200) \pm (2 \times 1000)$$

$$f_d = 1200 \pm 2000$$

$$f_d = 1200 + 2000 = 3200 \quad \text{and}$$

$$f_d = 1200 - 2000 = 800$$

Possible Answer: Two possible frequencies of the nonlinear distortion products are 3200 Hz and 800 Hz.

Another type of distortion appearing in audio systems is transient intermodulation (TIM) or slew-rate distortion. Transient intermodulation distortions are nonlinear distortions in electronic circuits that use negative feedback loops to improve their linearity. The larger the output signal of the system is, the less the system pushes the gain of the system, keeping signal transmission within the linear portion of the system's transfer function. When the input signal level changes rapidly (e.g., during the onset or offset of the signal), there is a time delay in the feedback loop controlling the gain of the system that causes additional time-specific nonlinear distortions.

Limiters and Compressors

Limiters and compressors are nonlinear devices that control the level of an audio signal and keep it under certain limits. The engineering challenge in designing limiting systems is to minimize the audibility of nonlinear distortions produced during signal processing. Examine again the transfer function shown in Figure 14.6B, line f. The transition from the linear part to the nonlinear part is instantaneous; that is, a straight linear slope becomes instantly a line parallel to the x axis. This type of nonlinear system is called a **hard signal limiter** and when the signal level exceeds the threshold of action, it becomes suddenly distorted to a great degree. A **signal limiter** is a device that passes low-level signals below a certain threshold value and clips off the peaks of the stronger signals. This type of operation is called **peak clipping.*** The maximum level that can be reached by the output signal of an amplifier is called the **saturation level.**

Signal limiting does not need to be hard and may be obtained by a gradual change in the input–output function slope. An example of a **soft signal limiter** is shown in Figure 14.6, line e. Soft signal limiting is less audible and more acceptable than hard signal limiting, although both systems may have the same clipping level. Still, both types of signal limiting provide an unacceptably high level of nonlinear distortion for many types of audio systems including hearing aids. For example, Harris at al. (1961), Jerger et al. (1966), and Olsen and Carhart (1967) reported that speech intelligibility decreases quite rapidly as the amount of nonlinear distortion in the speech signal increases. Therefore, modern signal level control is based on a more advanced signal processing technique called **automatic gain control** (AGC) and the devices using this technique are generally referred to as **signal compressors** or just compressors.

Signal compressors control the audio signal by changing the dynamic range of the signal, so that the difference between the strongest and weakest signal parts of the signal is made smaller (the waveform is "squeezed" so the amplitude is smaller but the waveform shape is reasonably well maintained compared to a peak clipper).

*Peak clipping is sometimes used as a desirable signal transformation to restore some harmonics to a signal when the original harmonics were filtered out due to the limited bandwidth of a transmission system. It is also used as a sound effect in music, especially in the processing of bass guitar sounds.

Examples of two transfer functions of signal compressing devices such as those used in hearing aids are shown in Figure 14.7 as curves a and b. Their shapes resemble the shapes of the transfer functions of the non-linear amplifiers shown in Figure 14.6 but they are not the same thing. Note that the transfer functions of the signal compressing devices in Figure 14.7 are expressed in logarithmic units (dB) unlike the transfer functions of non-linear amplifiers shown in Figure 14.6. With linear coordinates, a linear transfer function is represented with a straight line inclined at a 45° angle and the gain of the device is calculated as the output level minus the input level of the signal. Both devices, represented by a and b functions, are linear devices for input signals up to 40 dB; device a provides 30 dB of amplification and device b provides 10 dB of amplification. In the case of device a, an input signal of 30 dB results in an output signal of 60 dB. Above 40 dB, both of the devices become signal compressors with different degrees of AGC. In the case of device a, an input signal of 60 dB results in an output signal of 70 dB (10 dB amplification) and an input signal of 70 dB results in an output signal of 70 dB (0 dB amplification). In the case of device a, it compresses the output signal to 70 dB for all input signals larger than 40 dB. In the case of device b, it compresses the output signal gradually approaching 70 dB. Thus the gain of both systems varies depending on the input signal. It has to be stressed that although compression results in a nonlinear treatment of the input signal, its principle is different from signal limiting provided by classical non-linear amplifiers and the compression introduces only minimal nonlinear distortions. The difference between signal limiting and signal compression is shown in Figure 14.8.

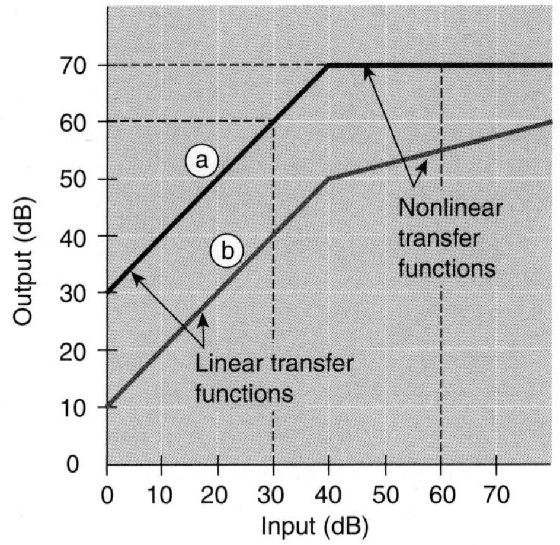

Figure 14.7. An input–output function with a logarithmic scale for the *x* and *y* axes.

A basic AGC system controls signal dynamics so that despite variations in the input level, the average output level of the device is constant and set at a predefined level. A compressor uses variable AGC to provide a smooth transition from linear signal processing (AGC turned off) to nonlinear signal processing at compression threshold (AGC turned on). Typical audio compressors are characterized by a short attack time (they act quickly to reduce the gain for very intense signals) and a long release time (they stop compressing the signal gradually) to minimize the signal distortion heard during compressor operation.

Two main operational principles of signal compression are input compression and output compression. Output

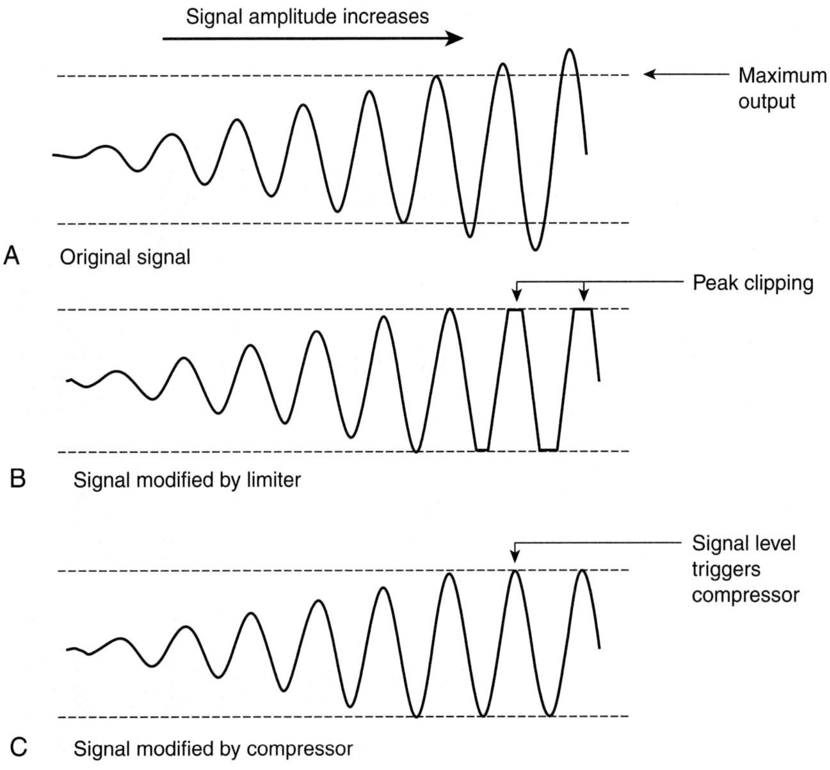

Figure 14.8. Comparison of peak clipping caused by a limiter and compression caused by a compressor.

compressors use a **negative feedback loop** to control the signal level, thus reducing nonlinear distortions. A negative feedback loop is a system in which the output signal is used to control the gain. The larger the output signal of the system is, the lower the system gain, thereby keeping an output signal below a certain output level. In contrast, input compressors vary the gain of the amplifier by monitoring the input signal level. Above a certain level, the gain is reduced.

Filters and Equalizers

Filters and equalizers are devices used to modify transmitted signals in the frequency domain. The purpose of both of these devices is to affect the spectral content of the signal and change the proportions between energies carried by the various frequency components.

A **filter** is a device that restricts the passage of energy to a specific frequency range called the filter band. Theoretical filters are "all-or-nothing" devices that either pass the signal of a specific frequency without any change or eliminate it completely. In reality, this never happens, and filters pass or stop "most" of the signal energy but not all of it. Consider, for example, a white noise signal appearing at the input of an acoustic filter. Depending on the filter characteristics, some of the components that make up the white noise will pass through the filter and some will be stopped (rejected) by the filter. Figure 14.9 shows the outputs of various types of filters passing a white noise signal. The filter types shown in Figure 14.9 are the four basic types of filters used in signal processing applications: low-pass filter, high-pass filter, band-pass filter, and band-reject (notch, stop-band) filter. A **low-pass (LP) filter,** as its name implies, passes the low-frequency energy and does not pass the high-frequency energy (notice the high-frequency energy is missing in the filter output). Such filters are used, for example, to remove ultrasonic ringing (high-frequency oscillations) or high-frequency noise from a sound. To understand the concept of a low-pass filter, consider a child playing on the beach and using a plastic sieve. The child puts all manner of sand, shells, rocks, and so forth into the sieve and shakes it. What comes out on the other side of the sieve is only sand and very small particles. Thus, the sieve acts as a filter, passing only the small materials and holding back the large materials. The low-pass filter passes only low frequencies and holds back high frequencies.

In contrast, a **high-pass (HP) filter** passes the high-frequency energy and blocks the low-frequency energy. Such filters are used, for example, to eliminate the 60-Hz hum produced by alternating current (AC) power. A **band-pass (BP) filter** passes a band of frequencies centered on a certain frequency and a **band-reject (BR) filter** (notch filter, stop-band filter) rejects a range of frequencies and passes frequencies that are lower or high than this band. These filters are used, for example, to eliminate the 60-Hz hum produced by an AC power supply.

Filter properties are characterized by a number of parameters. The main five filter parameters are (1) the upper cutoff frequency (f_U), (2) the lower cutoff frequency (f_L), (3) the center frequency (f_c), (4) the bandwidth (BW or Δf), and (5) the slope of the filter (Q). All of these characteristics apply to BP and BR filters but only the cutoff frequencies and slope apply to LP and HP filters. The characteristics of a BP filter and its bandwidth are shown Figure 14.10. The center frequency (f_c) of the filter is the frequency in the center of the band.* The upper cutoff frequency (f_U) is the frequency above the center frequency at which the signal intensity is 3 dB lower than the intensity at the center frequency. The lower cutoff frequency (f_L) is the frequency below the center frequency at which the

*The center frequency is usually the arithmetic mean of the upper and lower cutoff frequencies (i.e., $(\frac{f_L + f_U}{2})$); however, in some applications the center frequency is instead the geometric mean of the filter cutoff frequencies (i.e., $\sqrt{f_L + f_U}$).

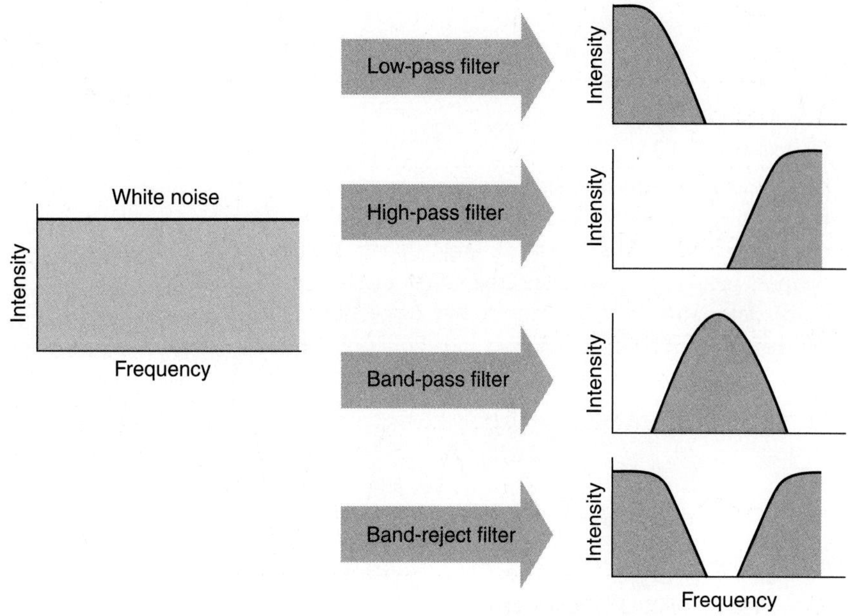

Figure 14.9. The concepts of four basic filters: low-pass (LP) filter, high-pass (HP) filter, band-pass (BP) filter, and band-reject (BR) filter.

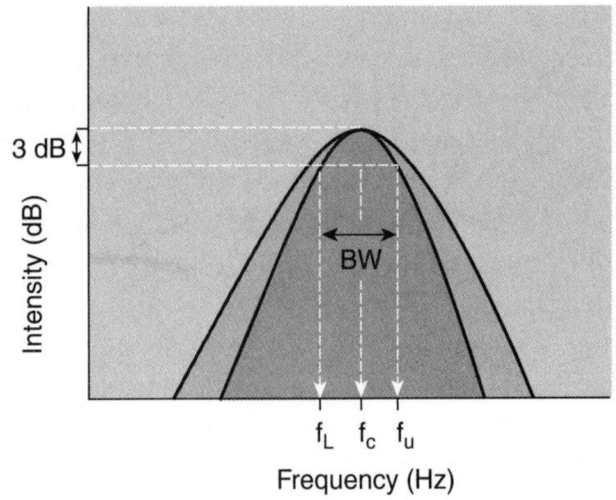

Figure 14.10. Characteristic parameters of a band-pass filter. The bandwidth, lower cutoff frequency (f_L), upper cutoff frequency (f_U), center frequency (f_c), and bandwidth are shown for the smaller dark gray band. The light gray band illustrates a band with a gentler slope compared to the dark gray band.

signal intensity is 3 dB lower than the intensity of the signal at the center frequency. The bandwidth (BW) is the width of the filter's operational band, that is, the width of the frequency band between the two 3-dB down points on either side of the band. The 3-dB decrease in signal level corresponds to a 50% drop in signal intensity and this decrease is the standardized value for determining a bandwidth of any device. The slope of the filter, also called roll-off rate, rejection rate, or skirt rate, is measured in decibels per octave (dB/octave) and may not be constant across the whole slope of the filter. Two different attenuation rates are illustrated in Figure 14.10. The dark gray band represents a filter with a steeper slope rate than the light gray band.

The selectivity of the filter (shown by the steepness of the filter slope) is characterized by the quality factor (Q). The higher the Q value is, the higher the selectivity of the filter. Q is defined as the ratio of the resonance (center) frequency (f_c) to the bandwidth (ΔB) of the curve.

$$Q = \frac{f_c}{\Delta B} \tag{14.4}$$

Example 14.2

Assume that an electroacoustic filter has two pass bands with center frequencies of 200 Hz and 1000 Hz and the respective bandwidths of 100 Hz and 200 Hz. Which of the pass bands has greater selectivity (Q value)?

To determine Q values insert the respective bandwidths and the center frequencies into Equation 14.4.

For the first band:

$$Q = \frac{f_c}{\Delta B}$$

$$Q = \frac{200}{100}$$

$$Q = 2$$

For the second band:

$$Q = \frac{f_c}{\Delta B}$$

$$Q = \frac{1000}{200}$$

$$Q = 5$$

Answer: The selectivity of the second band (Q = 5) is greater than that of the first one (Q = 2).

The above discussion applies to electric (audio) filters, but it can be extended to filters of any origin such as mechanic, acoustic, or biologic (neurologic) filters. For example, the concepts of mechanic resonance, critical band, and head-related transfer function are different forms of signal filtering.

As discussed previously, a filter is a device that either passes or stops all signal energy at a given frequency. In contrast, an **equalizer** is a device that attenuates to various degrees specific components of the signal spectrum to reshape the spectrum. In essence, an equalizer can be treated as a bank of filters operating side to side, each with different attenuation provided in the pass band. The frequency response of an equalizer may be fixed or adjustable. An example of an adjustable equalizer is a frequency response control in a hearing aid. An example of a fixed equalizer is the frequency response of a loudspeaker or an earphone.

Three basic types of equalizers are used in audio systems: shelf equalizers, graphic equalizers, and parametric equalizers. The most common type of equalizer is a **shelf equalizer,** which changes the proportion between low- and high-frequency energy in the sound spectrum. Examples of shelf filters are the treble and bass controls of an amplifier that change the proportion between the amounts of high- and low-frequency energy in the output signal.

A **graphic equalizer** is a set of adjacent band-pass filters equipped with a volume (gain) control for each channel in the form of a vertical slider. The shape of the sound spectrum is selected by adjusting the level controls of individual filters. The name *graphic* equalizer comes from the fact that the positions of individual sliders on the front panel of a filter resemble the contour of the equalizer's frequency response. Typical audio graphic equalizers are made by 4 to 30 relative bandwidth filters (e.g., one-third octave band filters). Graphic equalizers are commonly seen in home stereo systems. A digital form of this can be seen on computer screens, with virtual sliders controlled by a mouse.

A **parametric equalizer** is a small set of serial or parallel tunable filters with adjustable parameters such as bandwidth, center frequency, filter slope, and so forth that are tuned to compensate for some deficiencies of an audio system. This type of filter can be set, for example, as a notch filter to eliminate acoustic feedback caused by a hearing aid, or as a number of harmonically related notch filters set to eliminate 60-Hz hum and all of its harmonics during the restoration of old archival sound recordings. Parametric filters can also be used to enhance the spectral properties of specific phonemes when teaching foreign languages or to equalize music recordings in which some music instruments or vocalists are too strong or too weak.

AUDIO SYSTEMS

An audio system is a group of audio devices connected together for sound recording, transmission, or reproducing purposes. An audio system can be a single-channel device or a multichannel device in which several channels are used simultaneously to capture, process, and reproduce various sounds. An audio system that has a single transmission channel is called a single channel system or **monophonic** ("mono") **system.** In a monophonic system the sound can be captured by one microphone (or several microphones if their signals are combined together), transmitted though a single signal processing channel, and reproduced by a single loudspeaker (or several loudspeakers if they reproduce the same signal). An audio system with two channels that transmit correlated signals carrying spatial information about some real or imaginary space is called a **stereophonic** ("stereo") **system.** The purpose of a stereophonic system is to create or recreate the natural impression of sounds arriving from various directions. A critical property of a stereophonic system is that it transmits two correlated signals, called the left signal (LS) and right signal (RS), that are the bases for spatial sound reproduction. These two signals can be reproduced by a pair of loudspeakers or a pair of earphones. Classic two-channel loudspeaker systems, however, do not provide a full immersion of the listener in the sound field. In other words, they do not provide convincing and accurate reproduction of an acoustic environment. Much better spatial reproduction can be obtained by various surround sound (home theater) systems. The two basic types of surround sound system are discrete surround sound systems and matrix surround sound systems. Both types of systems provide several audio channels rather than two channels of classic stereophony, which is the simplest discrete system. Typical discrete surround sound systems provide four or more separate audio signals that are transmitted separately and delivered to separate loudspeakers. Discrete surround sound systems require several transmission channels, making these systems expensive and not compatible with typical two-channel systems. Examples of discrete surround sound systems are Dolby Digital and Dolby Digital plus. These systems provide high-quality surround sound.

Matrix surround sound is a two-channel or more sound where individual channels are carrying several coded signals that are later decoded and distributed among several loudspeakers. An example of a matrix system is the Dolby Pro-Logic System. The drawback of matrix surround sound is that the number of relatively independent audio signals and the width of their bandwidths are quite limited in order to be transmitted in two-channel format.

Most current commercial home theater systems deliver transmitted signals to several loudspeakers surrounding the listener and one or two low-frequency (woofer) channels (recall that low frequencies are not easily localizable so they do not need to be presented by the loudspeakers surrounding the listener). Such systems, depending on the number of channels, are denoted 4.1 (four surround channels and one low-frequency channel), 5.1, 6.1, 7.1, 10.2, and so forth.

Good reproduction of spatial sound is not limited to loudspeaker reproduction. Current systems of headphone reproduction can provide good immersion of the listener in an acoustic environment by using binaural head recordings or processing two-channel stereophonic signals with the head-related transfer function of the listener creating convincing out-of-the-head auditory spatial sound. Such systems are usually referred to as binaural audio or 3-D audio systems.

Summary

Acoustic signals are converted into electric audio signals for the purposes of storing, reproducing, and processing the signals. The conversion of a signal among acoustic, mechanic, and electric forms is conducted by a transducer. Transducers can be divided into receivers and transmitters. Receivers convert acoustic or mechanic energy into electric energy and transmitters convert electric energy into acoustic or mechanic energy. A microphone is an electroacoustic receiver that converts acoustic signals into audio signals. Loudspeakers and earphones are electroacoustic transmitters that convert audio signals into acoustic waves. Once the acoustic signal is converted into an audio signal, it is processed and delivered by signal controllers and audio processors.

Electroacoustic (audio) processing equipment includes transducers, audio controllers (e.g., amplifiers, mixers, and switches), signal processors (e.g., compressors and filters), and audio displays (e.g., VU meters and spectrum analyzers). If a signal change is intended, this change is called a signal transformation. If a signal change is not intended and is instead caused by the limitations of a transmission channel, it is called signal distortion. Distortions are generally divided into linear distortions, which are independent of the input signal amplitude, and nonlinear distortions, which occur when the shape of the output signal depends on the amplitude of the input signal. Nonlinear distortions result in the generation of new components in the output signal that were not present in the input signal including harmonic and intermodulation tones.

Key Points

- A transducer is a device that converts one type of energy into another. Electroacoustic and electromechanic transducers convert acoustic and mechanic energy into electric energy and vice versa.
- Reciprocal transducers can act as both a transmitter and a receiver, whereas nonreciprocal transducers can operate either as a transmitter or a receiver but not both.
- There are two basic classes of microphones based on the way they are designed: pressure microphones and gradient (velocity) microphones. Pressure microphones are omnidirectional microphones and gradient microphones are directional microphones.
- The three most common types of microphones based on their principle of operation are piezoelectric microphones, dynamic microphones, and condenser (electrostatic) microphones.
- One important parameter of microphones is the directivity factor, which indicates how selective a microphone is for sound coming from the front of the microphone.
- Two earphones together with a system for holding them over the ears are called headphones. If a headphone system also incorporates a communication microphone, this system is called a headset or a handset.
- An amplifier is a device that increases the magnitude of a signal.
- Filters and equalizers are devices that modify the spectral content of a signal. A filter is a device that restricts the passage of energy in a specific frequency range and an equalizer is a device that changes the spectral properties of the transmitted signal.
- The four basic types of filters are low-pass filter, high-pass filter, band-pass filter, and band-reject (notch, stop-band) filter.
- The five main parameters used to describe filters are the upper cutoff frequency, the lower cutoff frequency, the center frequency, the bandwidth, and the slope of the filter.
- Harmonic distortions are the harmonics of an input sine wave and intermodulation distortions are the differential and summation tones created by two or more sine waves.

Chapter Outline

CHAPTER 15

Digital Signal Processing

Objectives

- To explain the nature of a digital signal including how binary code can be used to represent numbers and signals
- To describe the basic processes behind converting an analog audio signal into a digital signal and vice versa including the concepts of quantization and sampling rate
- To review the common errors associated with conversion between analog and digital formats including aliasing, imaging, and quantization error
- To introduce the concept of digital storage and how a CD is imprinted with binary code

Key Terms

Aliasing error
Antialiasing filter
Anti-imaging filter (reconstruction filter)
Binary code
Bit
Byte
Central processing unit (CPU)
Computer (digital) word
Digital audio
Digital code
Digital signal
Digitization
Dither
Hybrid system
Imaging error (aperture error)
Nyquist frequency
Nyquist-Shannon sampling theorem
Oversampling
Processing algorithm
Quantization
Quantization error
Sampling
Sampling rate
Sigma-delta conversion
Word size (word length)

A **digital signal** is a stream of information that is presented as a sequence of numbers called a **digital code.** The word *digital* comes from the word *digit,* which means number. The digital code can be used to represent a signal (e.g., acoustic, video), to perform operations on a signal (e.g., multiplication, inversion, etc.), and to indicate the location of a signal or program in the computer memory (i.e., memory address). This means that digital code can be used by computers to store, process, and transmit information.

Every natural signal can be converted into a digital code, that is, converted into a sequence of numbers that indicate the magnitude of the signal at different moments in time. For example, a digital acoustic signal is a sequence of numbers that represents an analog acoustic signal in which samples of the magnitude of the signal have been taken at specific periodic moments in time and approximated.

The difference between an analog and a digital signal is similar to the difference between watching a continuous action and watching a sequence of photographs representing that action. If the photographs are taken in a very fast sequence, that is, if they are separated by very small time intervals, they can capture the details of the action so well it appears that the action is continuous. For example, when you watch a movie in a theater, you watch a picture-by-picture (digital) representation of an analog action performed by the actors and you do not notice anything missing. Another analogy between an analog and a digital signal is the comparison of an analog clock and a digital clock. A standard analog wall clock has a hand that sweeps all the way around the clock showing all time points. In contrast, a digital wall clock takes more of a "snapshot" of the time and then shifts from number to number in chunks. Thus, the analog clock gives the exact time and the digital clock approximates the correct time in chunks.

An analog signal is a continuous signal and a digital signal is an approximation of the analog signal by a sequence of numbers. The reason that analog signals are converted into digital signals is that digital signals are more immune to noise and distortion than analog signals. In addition, many operations on digital signals are much simpler than the same operations performed on analog signals because mathematical manipulation of a series of numbers is very easy. Operations on numbers that represent a natural signal are called digital signal processing (DSP) to differentiate them from analog signal processing (ASP), which was discussed in Chapter 14. In analog signal processing, alternating current (AC) electrical signals are directly modified by changing their temporal and spectral properties via the use of electronic components such as capacitors, inductors, and so forth. In contrast, DSP performs all modifications by completing mathematical operations (e.g., adding, subtracting, multiplying) on numbers.

DSP is at the heart of many types of modern technology including wireless phones, CD players, MP3 players, digital hearing aids, and so forth. The design of DSP circuitry requires some knowledge of high-level mathematics and computer science that are beyond the scope of this textbook. The basic concepts and rules of DSP are quite simple, however, and need to be known to understand and properly use digital equipment. The purpose of this chapter is to explain the nature of the digital signal, the basic processes behind converting an analog signal into a digital signal and vice versa, digital signal processing, and digital storage (recording).

DIGITAL SIGNALS

Digital signals are just numbers. To express a natural phenomenon as a digital signal, an analog signal is converted by an analog-to-digital converter (ADC or A/D converter) into a digital code that is manipulated by a dedicated DSP circuit on a microprocessor chip. This microprocessor chip is usually referred to in the computer literature as the **central processing unit (CPU).** If you want to know more about computers, see the website. **Link 15-1**

Once the digital signal has been processed by the digital circuitry, the digital code is translated back into an analog signal by a digital-to-analog converter (DAC or D/A converter). A schematic diagram of a basic DSP system is shown in Figure 15.1A. In actual audio DSP systems, some degree of analog processing usually takes place prior to and after the digital signal processing. This analog processing is indicated by the

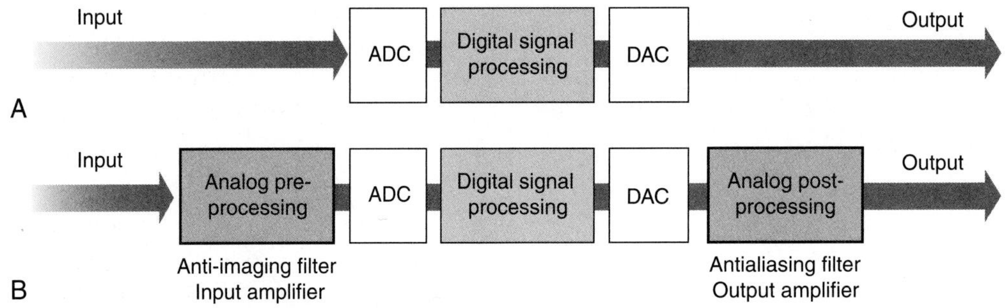

Figure 15.1. The digital **(A)** and analog plus digital **(B)** elements of signal processing circuitry.

darker gray boxes in Figure 15.1B. Systems that include both ASP and DSP are frequently called **hybrid systems.**

The main systems that process digital signals are computers. For computers to process information, the digital information must be in binary code. In **binary code,** all signals are represented numerically by two digits, 0 and 1. The binary code can represent any signal, from a single letter typed on a keyboard to the complex electrical signal created by speaking into a microphone. For example, pressing a single letter on a keyboard may send the computer a series of signals such as 01100001. For the purposes of this chapter, we will focus primarily on the use of binary code to indicate an acoustic signal, although we will introduce the reader to how numbers are represented in binary code.

The binary code indicates a stream of changes between two states of a given physical variable such as voltage or current. These two states are called *low* and *high* or *off* and *on,* where a code of 0 represents low or off and a code of 1 represents high or on. Each available space where a 0 or 1 must appear in the binary code is called a **bit,** which is short hand for the phrase binary digit of information. The term *bit* was first used in 1946 by American statistician John Tukey (1915–2000) for describing a digital signal. The bit is the smallest amount of information that can be processed by binary computers. The amount of information obtained in one bit is the same as the amount of information obtained by asking a yes-or-no question; that is, the answer is either "yes" or "no" or, in binary language, the answer is either "0" or "1." To represent more complex information such as numbers and letters, bits are combined into larger units called **bytes.** A byte is a contiguous sequence of eight bits that are combined together to represent a coded number, letter, or other symbol. For example, a byte may look like this: 10000001 or 11010010. The word *byte* was coined in 1956 by IBM engineer Werner Buchholz, who wanted to differentiate between a bit and a sequence of bits. To understand the byte coding used to represent a number, consider a number represented by the byte 10000001. The sequential steps needed to convert this byte into its decimal number are shown in Table 15.1. Each bit in a byte represents a sequential binary number (multiplication by 2) starting from the right. When the bit is "1," the number is present, and when the bit is "0," the number is absent. The byte represents a partial sum of 2^n numbers, where n = 0, 1, 2, 3, 4, 5, 6, or 7. Note that the bit numbers start from zero. Thus, a byte has eight bits labeled 0 to 7 from right to left.

The byte shown in Table 15.1 has two "1" bits in positions 0 and 7. This means that the numbers 2^7 and 2^0 are present in the coded number while all other 2^n numbers are not present. In other words, it means that the coded decimal number is $2^7 + 2^0 = 129$. As you can deduce from this example, the greatest number that can be expressed by a byte is $2^7 + 2^6 + 2^5 + 2^4 + 2^3 + 2^2 + 2^1 + 2^0 = 255$. If we want to represent both the numbers and the alphanumeric symbols (e.g., letters) by single bytes, we must use one of the bits in the byte to indicate whether the byte is a number (1) or a symbol (0), reducing the number of available positions for coding and thus limiting the range of numbers and symbols per byte to 127 each. If we want to use the digital code to represent numbers larger than 255 and more complex structures (like whole words or complex software commands), chains of signal codes composed of several bytes must be created. Such chains are called **computer (digital) words.** A computer word is a fixed-sized group of bytes that are handled together by a computer as a unit of information. Words vary in length based on individual computer CPUs and they can contain from one to several bytes. Since a byte is eight bits longs, words can be 8, 16, 32, 64, or 128 bits or even longer. The number of bits in a word is called the **word size** or **word length.** In some information compression schemes the concept of a half-byte word called a **nibble** is also used. This coding takes advantage of the fact that most letter codes in ASCII (American Standard Code for Information Exchange) share the same first four bits and the actual information is contained in the last four bits. Thus, if properly coded, one byte can carry information about two letters rather than one, halving the amount of transmitted data. If you would like to know more about binary numbers (i.e., operations performed on binary numbers), see the website. **Link 15-2**

▶ **Table 15.1.** Schematic Process of Representing Numbers in Byte Sequences

7	6	5	4	3	2	1	0	Bit number
2^7	2^6	2^5	2^4	2^3	2^2	2^1	2^0	Sequential powers of 2
1	0	0	0	0	0	0	1	An example of one byte of binary code
Yes	No	No	No	No	No	No	Yes	Is the bit turned on?
√							√	Which bits are added?
2^7							2^0	What are the binary numbers?
= 128							= 1	What do the binary numbers equal in decimal numbers?
			128 + 1 = 129					Add these two numbers

PRACTICE PROBLEMS: DIGITAL SIGNALS

1. How many bits are used in the following code: 110011?
2. How many bytes are used in the following code: 1001000101010100?
3. Assuming all eight bits are used to code for a number, what digital number is represented by the binary number 11110010?
4. Assuming all eight bits are used to code for a number, what digital number is represented by the binary number 00000011?

Answers (If you need help with these problems, consult the website.) **Link 15-3**

1. 6
2. 2
3. 242
4. 3

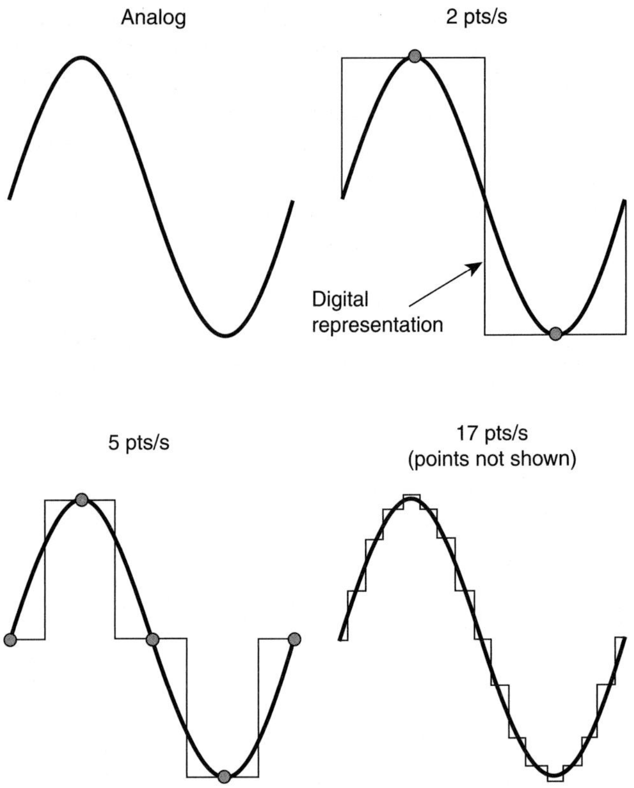

Figure 15.2. An original analog signal (thick line) and three analog output signals obtained after the analog-to-digital converter (ADC) and digital-to-analog converter (DAC) for sampling rates of 2, 5, and 17 Hz (samples per second). The sampled points are shown by round symbols on two of the output waveforms.

CONVERTING AN ACOUSTIC SIGNAL TO A DIGITAL CODE

Three basic steps are used in converting analog signals into digital signals. These three steps are sampling, quantization, and digitization. **Sampling** is the process of measuring the magnitude of a signal at specific moments in time. **Quantization** is the process of representing the instantaneous magnitude of a sound by one number from a limited set of predetermined normalized values called quantized levels. In other words, quantization involves the estimate of the magnitude of an analog signal at specific points in time using a limited set of numbers, which are determined based on the precision of the quantization system. The last step in converting an analog signal into a digital signal is digitization. **Digitization** is a process of converting the quantized values into binary form. In other words, it is the process of converting decimal (base 10) numbers into binary (base 2) numbers.

Sampling

To be converted into digital form, the waveform of an analog signal must be sampled, that is, measured at discrete time intervals. The value of each sample is equal to the value of the waveform at a sampling point. The term **sampling rate** specifies the number of times per second the magnitude of the signal is measured. For example, a sampling rate of 44.1 kHz indicates that the signal magnitude is measured 44,100 times per second. The higher the sampling rate, the more often the waveform is sampled (measured) in each second, creating a more accurate representation of the signal in the digital domain.

Three examples shown in Figure 15.2 illustrate what happens when an analog signal is converted into a digital signal using three different sampling rates. The upper left panel shows the original analog signal and the three other panels show the output analog signals as they would appear after being processed with a sampling rate of 2, 5, or 17 samples per second (Hz). Notice that after the conversion processes, the sine wave sampled two times per second (shown with two points on the waveform) now resembles a square wave rather than the original sine wave, and the greater the sampling rate, the closer the final waveform shape is to the original waveform.

An important rule involving sampling is the **Nyquist-Shannon sampling theorem** (Shannon, 1949), which states that for the sampled signal to represent no loss of information, the sampling rate must be at least twice the highest frequency in the spectrum of the original signal. It can be shown mathematically that if this condition is met, the reconstructed signal is practically identical to the original signal. The highest frequency in a sampled signal that can be reconstructed with no loss of information by a given converter is called the **Nyquist frequency**, after Harry Nyquist (1889–1976), a Swedish scientist who determined this relationship in 1928. Thus, the sampling rate should be at least twice as great as the Nyquist frequency to meet the Nyquist-Shannon theorem requirements. For example, if the Nyquist frequency is 22,050 Hz, the sampling rate should be 44,100 samples per second or higher to avoid distortions in the reconstructed signal. Looking at this from an equipment capabilities point of view, it means that the highest frequency properly processed by an ADC–DAC system that is sampling at 44,100 Hz is 20,050 Hz.

PRACTICE PROBLEMS: SAMPLING RATE

1. What is the highest signal frequency that can be processed without loss of information if the sampling frequency is 48,000 Hz?
2. What is the highest signal frequency that can be processed without loss of information if the sampling frequency is 50,200 Hz?
3. What sampling rate should be used by a DSP system if the highest signal frequency is 10,000 Hz?
4. What sampling rate should be used by a DSP system if the Nyquist frequency is 6000 Hz?
5. What is the minimum sampling rate of a DSP system processing signals in the 50-Hz to 20,000-Hz frequency range that is needed to avoid distortion of the reconstructed signal?

Answers (If you need help with these problems, consult the website.) **Link 15-4**

1. 24,000 Hz
2. 25,100 Hz
3. 20,000 Hz
4. 12,000 Hz
5. 40,000 Hz

Quantization and Digitization

Quantization is the process of representing a continuous (infinite) set of sampled values, such as real numbers, by a discrete (limited) set of values. Each signal sample is adjusted (rounded off) to the closest numerical value permitted by the quantization step of the converter. The quantized values are subsequently digitized, that is, converted into binary numbers expressed by a sequence of 0s and 1s. Depending on the precision of quantization (digital resolution), digitized signals may have groups of binary numbers extending from 1 (1-bit converter) to n (n-bit converter). To follow the process of converting analog samples into digital numbers, consider the sine wave shown in the left panel of Figure 15.3. The waveform magnitude extends from –10 V to 10 V and a point marked on the waveform has an instantaneous magnitude of 6.70 V. To translate this value into a digital code, 6.70 must be represented by a series of 0s and 1s (binary code). Conversion of 6.70 into a binary code requires a series of steps involving both quantization and digital representation of the sampled signal. In each of these steps a decision regarding a quantized value and its digital representation is made by choosing either 0 or 1 for signal representation. In making these decisions "1" is used to represent a "yes, it *is* higher than *x*" decision and "0" is used to represent a "no, it *is not* higher than *x*" decision regarding the value of the signal.

The right panel in Figure 15.3 shows the values of the transmitted signal resulting from 1-, 2-, 3-, and 4-bit processing. Let us assume that we want to use a 1-bit code to describe the signal. This means that the value 6.70 V can be represented by only one digit: 1 (high signal) or 0 (low signal). The value 6.70 V lies in the upper half of the voltage range from –10V to 10V and, therefore, would be assigned a code of 1 because we answer "yes" to the question of whether the value of the signal is larger than 0 V. Thus, a 1-bit conversion can only tell us whether the signal value lies

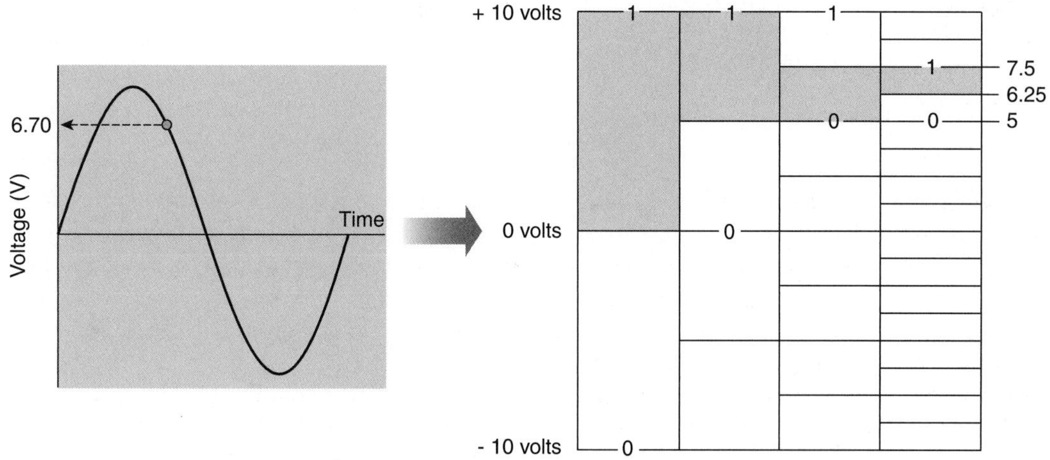

Figure 15.3. The process of signal quantization (*right panel*) of a sinusoidal signal (*left panel*). The values 0 and 1 in the right panel represent the digital code assigned to each quantized value.

above or below 0 V. Let us now consider a 2-bit conversion. The first bit will be the same as before, indicating that the signal value lies in the upper half of the original range, so this bit indicates that the signal magnitude is between 0 V and 10 V. The second bit provides information regarding whether the signal value lies in the upper (1) or lower (0) half of the new range defined by the first bit, that is, whether it is higher or lower than 5 V. Since 6.70 V is higher than 5 V, the second bit is again 1 and the 2-bit code is 11. This code means that the signal value is in the 5-V to 10-V range.

To increase the precision of the converted value, one needs to increase the number of bits even further. The 3-bit code of 6.70 V is 011, indicating that the number is between 5 V and 7.5 V (notice the code is arranged from *right to left*). Similarly, the 4-bit code is 1011, indicating that the number is between 6.25 and 7.5V. If this process was continued, and we used an 8-bit converter, the value of 6.70 V becomes the sequence 10101011.

In the example shown in Figure 15.3 the magnitude of the sine wave was converted into a digital signal using a 4-bit conversion. The original signal range was divided into 16 ($2^4 = 16$) subranges and the specific signal value was described as belonging to one of these specific subranges. Therefore, using the 4-bit conversion, there are 16 possible magnitude values that the input signal can be converted into and that the DSP unit can process (i.e., 0000, 0001, 0010, 0011, 0100, 0101, 0111, 0110, 1000, 1001, 1010, 1011, 1100, 1101, 1110, 1111). If we had added another bit, the number of divisions would double to 32, increasing by two times the accuracy of the approximation of the magnitude. The number of total divisions can be calculated using the formula $d = 2^n$ where d is the number of possible magnitude ranges and n is the number of bits. For example, to determine the number of divisions possible with a 12-bit processor, raise 2 to the 12th power: $d = 2^{12} = 4096$. Therefore, the number of divisions (subranges) for a 12-bit processor is 4096.

Current CD players and most other commercial digital audio equipment use a 16-bit processing scheme, which results in $2^{16} = 65{,}536$ possible quantized magnitude values. Recall from previous chapters that each doubling of signal level corresponds to a 6-dB change in the signal level. Thus, a 16-bit processor results in a signal dynamic range of 16×6 dB = 96 dB. This means that this processor can capture and convey changes in signal values that are as large as 96 dB. This dynamic range is sufficient for most audio applications because the signal that is transmitted with a 96-dB signal-to-noise ratio is, to most listeners, perceptually identical to the original analog signal. As 24-bit and 32-bit processors become more affordable, this bit rate may increase in future applications

To determine the speed required for high fidelity DSP of audio signals and to envision the resulting size of the digital signal stored as a file, consider a CD player with a 16-bit processor operating at a sampling rate of 44,100 Hz. In such a system the magnitude of the signal is measured and recorded 44,100 times per second using 16 bits of data for each sampled value. This means that the system must be able to transmit and process $44{,}100 \times 16 = 705{,}600$ bits per second. Looking at this number from the signal storage point of view, it means that each second of this signal requires about 705,600 bits/8 bits = 88,200 bytes (B) of storage. This is equal to 88.2 kilobytes (kB) of storage on a digital medium.

Recall that in the decimal system kilo stands for 1000. In the binary progression, the closest number to 1000 is 1024 (2^{10}), so kilo means 1024. This creates some confusion as both conventions are used in describing the size of digital files. According to decimal convention, which is recommended by the International System of Units (SI) and used by this textbook, 1 kB = 10^3 B; 1 megabyte (MB) = 10^6 B; and 1 gigabyte (GB) = 10^9 B. According to binary convention, which is used by most of the hardware and software manufacturers, 1 kB = 2^{10} = 1024 B; 1 MB = 2^{20} = 1,048,576 B; and 1 GB = 2^{30} = 1,073,741,824 B. Due to the common use of both of these conventions, a caution is needed when interpreting the size of digital storage. For example, a 3-minute-long piece of music processed with a 44,100-Hz sampling rate and 16-bit resolution (that is not compressed) will require 15.9 MB or 15.1 MB space depending on the convention that was used in calculating the size of the file.

PRACTICE PROBLEMS: QUANTIZATION

1. Using the same strategy employed in Figure 15.3, determine the coding if the voltage had been –6.70 V using a 6-bit processor.
2. Using the same strategy employed in Figure 15.3, determine the coding if the voltage had been 0.6 V using a 6-bit processor.
3. How many divisions are created in an 8-bit processor?
4. How many divisions are created in a 10-bit processor?
5. How many bits per second does a CD player with a 14-bit processor operating at a sampling rate of 44,100 Hz generate?
6. What is the sampling rate used by a 12-bit computer sound card that produces 264,600 bits per second?
7. How much hard disc space in MB is needed to store 6 minutes of music recorded at 352,800 bits per second?

Answers (If you need help with these problems, consult the website.) **Link 15-5**

1. 100100
2. 100001
3. 256
4. 1024
5. 617,400 bits per second
6. 20,050 Hz
7. Slightly less than 16 MB

ERRORS IN DIGITAL SYSTEMS

When an acoustic signal is converted from its analog form to a digital form and then back from its digital form to an analog form, the resulting signal is only an approximation of the original sound. With today's high-end technology (16-bit conversion with 44,100 Hz or higher sampling rate), we usually do not pay much attention to the difference between the original and digitally processed however, signals because the difference is perceptually small and not obtrusive. However, signal processing by the A/D and D/A converters introduces several types of errors, that, under some conditions, may result in audible distortions.

The main types of conversion errors observed in ADC and DAC converters include aliasing error, imaging error, and quantization error. All of these translation errors introduce distortion into the output signal. Aliasing and quantization introduce distortion into the ADC step and imaging introduces distortion into the DAC step. In a high-quality DSP system these distortions are barely if at all detectable, but in a low-quality or damaged DSP system the amount of distortion in the output may be large enough to substantially affect the sound quality.

Aliasing error is the distortion of the digital signal caused by a sampling rate that is too low in relationship to the highest frequency of the input signal. As a result, too few signal samples are taken to clearly describe the input signal. This situation is shown in Figure 15.4A. The input signal is sampled at the points indicated. Notice that the samples are taken so sparingly that they may actually represent a much lower frequency (bottom line in Fig. 15.4A) than the actual frequency of the input signal.

A visual analogy of aliasing error is commonly seen in TV car commercials. In some commercials the tires of a fast-moving car appear to move backward (i.e., the lines in a

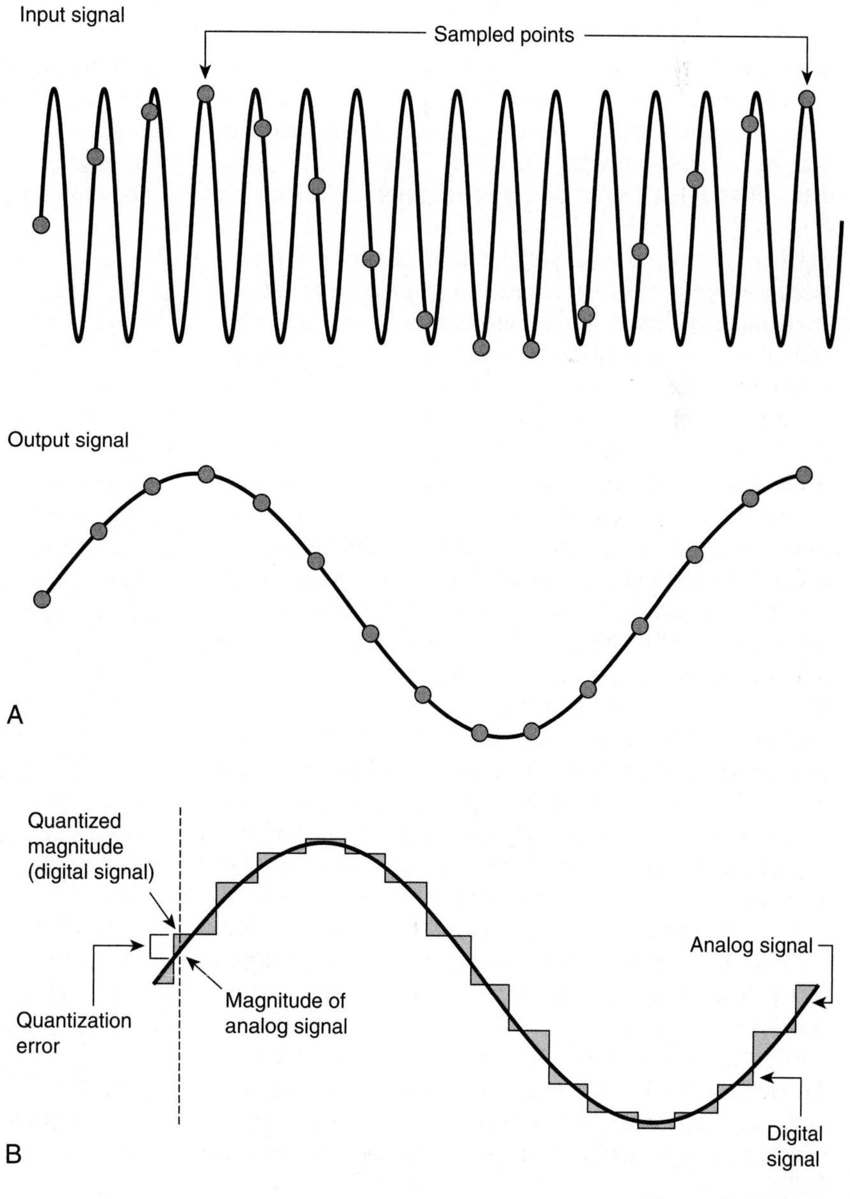

Figure 15.4. (A) Aliasing error caused by too few samples (•) taken during the processing of the input signal. The result is a new frequency at the output of the signal. **(B)** Quantization error shown as a difference between the actual magnitude of the signal and the quantized (digital) magnitude at a time point indicated with the dashed line.

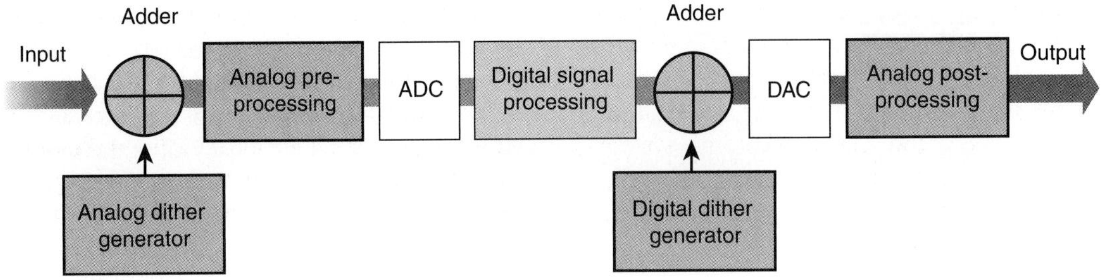

Figure 15.5. Basic block diagram of a digital signal processing (DSP) system with the location of analog and digital dither generators added.

hubcap appear to be moving backward). The wheel is obviously moving forward; it just looks like it is moving backward. This sensation is caused by the fact that the wheel is moving so fast that the sampling rate of the image (the "snapshots" of the moving image) is too low to capture the true motion of the wheel and, in fact, makes an error in the translation of the motion of the wheel onto the film. Thus, the spokes for the wheel appear to be going backward, because there are not enough pictures taken of the wheel to accurately represent the speed of the wheel. In a digital processing system, this error can be avoided by using a low-pass filter before the ADC, to remove frequencies higher than the Nyquist frequency. This type of filter is called an **antialiasing filter.**

Imaging error (aperture error) is the introduction of high-frequency distortion into the signal at the point where the signal is converted back from its digital form to an analog signal. This error is due to the instability (jitter) of the sampling clock in the DSP system. As a result, the samples of the original signal appear at slightly different times at the DAC than they were taken at the ADC, affecting the high-frequency content of the signal. When the signal is put back together, the pieces are put back into the wrong place, slightly, in time. This error is based on differences in the digital clocks between the ADC and DAC. In commercial systems the imaging error is very small and practically inaudible. If the clock frequency is not well controlled, however, it may create problems. To protect against imaging (aperture) errors, a low-pass **anti-imaging (reconstruction) filter** can be used at the output of the D/A converter.

The concept of signal quantization was described earlier in the chapter. When comparing an analog signal to a digital signal, any difference between the actual amplitude of the analog signal and the derived amplitude of the digital signal is called **quantization error.** The maximum quantization error is equal to one half of the spacing between two adjacent quantized levels permitted by the digital conversion process (one half of the least significant bit, i.e., the bit on the far right). The concept of quantization error is shown in Figure 15.4B.

Quantization error (rounding error) is the dominant type of error seen in DSP. The products of quantization error can be heard as noise when the signal is converted back to an acoustic signal. The greater the number of processing bits is, the smaller the quantization error and the better the digital resolution, however, the higher the cost of the D/A converter and the greater the power consumption. In addition, the more extensive the signal processing is, the greater the effect of rounding error on the form of the final signal. Thus, to prevent rounding errors (quantization noise) from being audible, many DSP systems use higher digital resolution than needed for the conversion process itself.

The main problem caused by quantization error is that the erroneous products created by the quantization process are correlated with the transmitted signal and therefore, if they are present, they have a characteristic quality and are easily heard in the output signal. This correlation makes the digital noise created by the quantization error much more unpleasant and easier to hear than the wideband random noise heard in analog systems. Unfortunately, large amounts of quantization error are generated by low-bit (less than 16-bit) processors. Thus, to make the quantization error less audible, a certain amount of random noise is frequently added to both the input and the output signals to mask the quantization error. This noise is called **dither** from the Middle English verb *didderen*, meaning "to tremble." The human ear is more forgiving of random noise compared to the same amount of correlated noise and the dither makes DSP errors more acceptable. As illustrated in Figure 15.5, dither generators are placed in a signal processing system at the input stage to the ADC (to eliminate the "digital quiet" when no signal is at the input and to eliminate nonlinear distortions) and at the output stage (to eliminate output distortions and mask audible correlated noise).

DIGITAL AUDIO APPLICATIONS

Once an analog signal is converted into its digital form, a variety of different processing techniques can be employed to modify the signal. The field of DSP that concerns auditory signals is called digital audio. **Digital audio** includes the processes of transmission, storage, amplification, filtering, summation, multiplication, equalization, compression, and so forth, of audio signals in digital format. Many of these processes can also be conducted using an analog signal via the electrical components discussed in Chapters 13 and 14, but in many cases DSP is a faster, cheaper, and more precise method to modify signals. In many cases DSP is the only feasible method of signal processing. Three examples of digital audio applications discussed in this chapter are digital filters, digital hearing aids, and digital recording systems. These three examples illustrate the most common DSP applications in the audio domain.

Digital Filters

Analog and digital filters have the same purpose, namely to change the signal as it passes through the filter, and usually both analog and digital filters are used as parts of DSP systems. Analog filters are used to limit and shape the bandwidth of the signal before it is digitized and to filter out distortion after the signal has been converted back to an analog signal. These two main types of analog filters used in DSP circuits are called antialiasing filters and anti-imaging filters and they were described previously in this chapter.

A digital filter is a mathematical algorithm that takes one sequence of numbers (the input signal) and produces a new sequence of numbers (the output signal). In other words, it is a mathematical formula (algorithm) for changing one digital signal into another. It can be utilized in the DSP system as a piece of software (computer program) stored in the computer memory or as hardware circuitry through a properly interconnected set of integrated circuit (IC) chips. Digital filters are a fundamental tool in digital audio systems and in any digital data acquisition and processing application. They are used, for example, in such operations as noise reduction, signal analysis, and automatic speech recognition.

A digital filter differs from an analog filter only in the way the filtering process is implemented. Analog filters consist of electronic circuits built from resistors, capacitors, and inductors that affect continuous signals and modify them in the time and frequency domains. A digital filter conducts the same operations in a mathematical form. Thus, it is important to realize that a digital filter can do anything that an analog filter can do and even more. In addition, some filter designs would be impractical to construct in an analog form, because of the complexity and expense of the filter. To find out more about digital filters, consult the website. **Link 15-6**

Digital Hearing Aids

A digital hearing aid is a hearing enhancing device that processes sound in a digital format. The DSP circuits also facilitate easy programming and allow switching between various modes of operation. A schematic block diagram of a digital hearing aid is identical to the diagram presented in Figure 15.1B. The input of the system is a microphone and the output is a miniature loudspeaker emitting acoustic signals directly to the ear canal of the user. The original acoustic signal is captured by the microphone and converted into an electric analog of the acoustic signal. A low-pass filter at the input of the hearing aid limits the upper frequency limit of the input signal to approximately 4000 to 6000 Hz. This bandwidth prevents the creation of aliasing errors while still allowing for high-fidelity (quality) speech output. The ADC converts the analog signal into a digital signal. The digital signal proceeds to the microprocessor, which is the IC chip that stores the processing algorithm. The **processing algorithm** is a computer program containing a set of instructions for the manipulation of the digital signal. Processing algorithms are loaded into and stored in the permanent read-only memory (ROM) of the microprocessor. Microprocessor algorithms are capable of controlling a variety of hearing aid features including the frequency response (the spectrum of the output signal), acoustic feedback control (the ability to control the "whistling" noise heard when an amplified sound from a loudspeaker leaks back into the microphone), noise suppression (the ability to decrease background noise), adaptive directional microphone response (the ability of the hearing aid to enhance the signal where the microphones are aimed), and compression schemes (e.g., the strategies the hearing aid uses to control soft and loud sounds). After manipulation, the digital signal is converted back into an analog signal with the use of a DAC, processed through a final stage of amplification, and then converted into an acoustic signal and delivered to the ear via the miniature loudspeaker. (Note: In some cases, rather than using a DAC, the digital signal is sent directly to a class D integrated receiver.)

The main quality issue for digital hearing aids is quantization error, which introduces audible and unpleasant noise. The more bits of processing power the hearing aid has, the smaller the quantization error, and the lower the amount of correlated noise appearing in the output signal. For hearing aid applications, however, the use of high-precision ADC and DAC is prohibitively expensive in terms of size and power consumption and is often limited to 14 or fewer bits.

The impact of quantization error on the quality of the output signal of a digital hearing aid can be reduced by adding dither to the transmitted signal or by using a special digital processing scheme called sigma-delta conversion. The concept of adding dither to a transmitted signal has already been discussed. **Sigma-delta conversion** is the process of quantizing the voltage difference between very small sampling steps with a low number of processing bits. Instead of numerically quantizing the absolute magnitude of the signal from baseline, quantization estimates the magnitude by comparing the difference between one point and the next in a signal (i.e., from one sampled voltage point to the next). Since the relative change in signal magnitude between adjacent points in time is much less than the difference in magnitude between each point and the baseline, the signal can be quantized with fewer bits to provide the same information about signal changes. The resulting amount of quantization noise can be further reduced by using a special sampling method called oversampling. **Oversampling** is a technique of sampling an analog signal at a sampling frequency much higher than twice the Nyquist frequency. Low-bit converters, such as 1- and 2- bit converters, produce large amounts of quantization noise but are very fast and allow high oversampling, such as 64 × the Nyquist frequency, that is, on the order of 3 MHz. Since the digitization noise created by quantization error is equally distributed across the transmitted frequency band, its amount in the output signal can be drastically reduced by applying a low-pass filter with a cutoff frequency equal to the Nyquist frequency. Thus, low-bit converters with high oversampling rates can result in sound quality similar to high-bit converters operating in the regular frequency band.

Digital Recording

Digital recording is a method of storing an audio (or video) signal in a digital format for further processing and reproduction. Audio signals can be stored on a variety of digital media such as magnetic tape, digital audio tape (DAT), and compact disc (CD).

A digital signal can be stored in two basic forms for future use: as the signal itself (audio file or raw binary file) or as a compressed data file. The first form, usually referred to as a pulse code modulation (PCM) signal, is used for audio or video CDs and magnetic tapes that can be played from dedicated players. The other form is used to store the data on a computer or on a data CD-ROM. These data files need to be converted into signal files before they can be played. The main advantage of the compressed data file for storage is that it takes up less space since it allows for additional signal coding and compression, which reduces the file size. Recall that a raw 3-minute-long binary audio file sampled at 44.1 kHz using a 16-bit converter takes about 15 MB of digital storage, whereas a corresponding data file can occupy only 3 MB or less. Examples of data audio files are WAV (an uncompressed digital file format derived from the analog source used by Windows), MP3, MPG, and AIFF files. Data files include a header that contains information about the signal sampling rate, bit resolution, compression scheme, and so forth. During playback, the header is read and the data file is converted into an appropriate signal file and played through the system. Typical sampling rates used for storing audio signals are 22,050, 44,100, and 48,000 Hz. Typical bit resolutions are 8, 12, 16, or 24 bits. A digital audio signal stored with a 24-bit/48 kHz sampling scheme is practically indistinguishable from its analog original form and is the highest quality digital signal needed for storing and processing.

Figure 15.6 illustrates the structure of digital data recorded on an audio CD. The disc is 1.2 mm thick and has a 120 mm diameter with a 15-mm-diameter hole in the center to allow the disc to be rotated by a motor. The disc typically holds 74 minutes of audio data recorded with a 16-bit/44.1 kHz sampling rate. The disc is made of pure polycarbonate vinyl (the same material that is used for motorcycle helmets and bulletproof "glass") with a thin layer of reflective pure aluminum protected by a layer of acrylic lacquer (to protect the aluminum from oxidation) attached to its surface. The disc label is attached at the top of the protective layer. During the recording process the stream of 0s and 1s is converted into a series of small indentations (called **pits**) and bumps (called **lands**) into the aluminum layer of the CD. The pits and lands represent the sequence of 0s and 1s in the binary data.

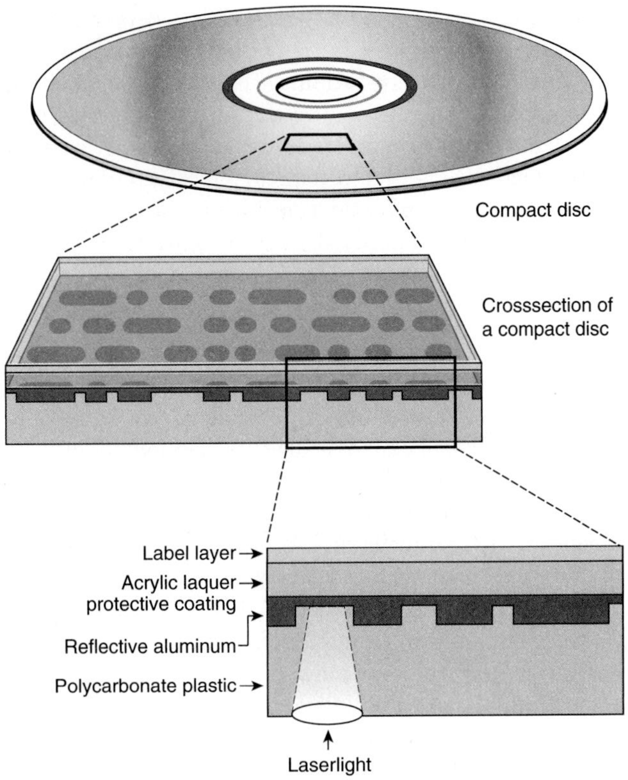

Figure 15.6. A cross section of a CD illustrating lands and pits.

The stream of pits is arranged as a single, tightly packed, continuous spiral track of data beginning at the center of the disc and progressing toward its outer ridge. The overall length of the track can be as long as 5 km. The direction of the recording is in the opposite direction compared to the direction used on vinyl audio records. Each pit is approximately 120 nm deep by 500 nm wide, and its depth is equal to one quarter of the wavelength of the laser beam. The minimum length of the pit is 0.83 μm. The pattern of pits and lands embedded in the disc matter is subsequently pressed into the top surface of the plastic layer of the CD and a layer of aluminum conforming to the surface of the disc is applied for reflectivity. This recording process is the pressing technique used in mass production of commercial CDs. A different recording technique is used in CD-R and CD-RW recorders. CD-R and CD-RW recorders use a burning technique in which a laser beam melts, to a different degree, the crystalline metal alloy covering the disc, creating regions (pits and lands) with various reflectivity on the disc's surface.

During the playback process, the laser beam of the optical read-head of a CD player scans the surface of the disc from beneath, through the polycarbonate plastic layer. The difference in thickness of the plastic layer between the pits and lands is about one quarter of the laser wavelength leading to a half-wavelength difference between light reflected from the aluminum layer covering the pits compared to the lands. The distractive interference of the light reflected from a pit reduces the intensity of the reflected light compared to the light intensity reflected from a land. The low- and high-intensity levels of reflected light are recorded through a photodiode and converted into a sequence of 0s and 1s in the reconstruction of the binary signal.

The main advantage of digital recording over analog recording is that the signals are recorded as sequences of only two states (0 and 1), which are very robust, are noise free, and do not deteriorate as much over time as analog recordings. When a digital signal is transferred between two digital devices, there is no loss of signal and no noise or distortions added. Since the manipulation of digital signals is also easier, more precise, faster, and inexpensive, one can expect the replacement of all analog audio recording systems with DSP systems.

Summary

A digital signal is created when an analog signal is converted into binary code by an analog-to-digital converter. A digital-to-analog converter is used to convert the digital signal back to its analog form after processing. The binary code is a series of 0s and 1s, which indicate the magnitude of the signal sampled a certain number of times per second. The highest frequency component in the signal should not exceed the Nyquist frequency, which is equal to one half of the sampling rate. In the ADC and DAC processes, several different types of errors can result in audible distortions. These errors include aliasing error, which occurs when there are frequencies in the input signal above the Nyquist frequency; imaging error, in which there is instability in the sampling clock; and quantization error, which is the difference between the actual amplitude of the analog signal and the derived amplitude of the digital signal.

Once an analog signal is converted into its digital form, a variety of different processing strategies can be employed to modify the signal including filtering, amplification, and storage. A digital filter is a mathematical formula used to modify the signal. A digital hearing aid is a hearing enhancing device that processes sound in a digital format, and a digital recording is a recorded signal that is stored in a digital format.

Key Points

- Every natural signal can be converted into a sequence of numbers that indicates the magnitude of the signal at different points in time.
- Operations on numbers that represent a natural signal are called digital signal processing to differentiate them from analog signal processing, where nondigital electrical signals (e.g., AC signals in a circuit) are directly modified by changing their temporal and spectral properties via the use of electronic components.
- In binary code, all signals are represented by a stream of 0s and 1s, which indicates changes between the on (low) and off (high) states of a signal.
- Each available space where a 0 or 1 must appear in the binary code is called a bit.
- A byte is a sequence of eight bits that are combined together to represent a coded number, letter, or other symbol. A word is a larger group of bits used to code longer numbers or more complex codes.
- Quantization is the process of representing the instantaneous magnitude of a sound by one number from a limited set of numbers, which are determined based on the precision of the quantization system.
- The sampling rate describes how many times per second the instantaneous magnitude of the signal is measured. The higher the sampling rate is, the more accurate the frequency representation of the signal.
- The highest frequency in the sampled signal that can be reconstructed with no loss of information is called the Nyquist frequency. The sampling rate should be at least two times the Nyquist frequency.
- Aliasing error is the introduction of low-frequency distortion into the signal due to the presence of

frequencies in the input signal that are above the Nyquist frequency.

- Imaging or reconstruction error is the introduction of high-frequency distortion into the signal due to instability (jitter) of the system clock that puts the samples of the signal back together in DAC at slightly different times than they were taken in ADC.
- Quantization error is a difference between the actual amplitude of the analog signal and the derived amplitude of the digital signal and it is dependent on the resolution of the ADC.
- The two main types of analog filters used in DSP circuits are antialiasing filters and anti-imaging filters. An antialiasing filter is a low-pass filter placed before the ADC and an anti-imaging filter is a low-pass filter placed after the DAC.
- A digital filter is a mathematical algorithm that takes one sequence of numbers (the input signal) and produces a new sequence of numbers (the output signal).
- One solution for minimizing quantization error in digital hearing aids is to use a special digital processing scheme called sigma-delta conversion, in which the quantization amplitude is obtained by comparing the difference between one point and the next in a signal (at an extremely rapid rate) rather than comparing each point with the baseline amplitude.
- A signal can be stored as a raw binary file or as a data file. Data file storage takes up less space because it allows for additional signal coding and compression, which reduces the file size. Examples of data audio files are WAV, MP3, MPG, and AIFF files.

Glossary

Abducens nerve the sixth cranial nerve (CN VI), which controls the movement of one extraocular muscle (muscles that move the eyeball): the lateral rectus muscle

Abscissa the horizontal axis of a two-dimensional graph

Absolute difference an amount by which one quantity is larger than another one

Absolute measurement measurements involving absolute differences (e.g., subtraction) between two quantities

Absolute threshold the minimum value of a stimulus that elicits a specific reaction a certain percentage of the time (usually 50%)

Absorbed sound wave the sound wave that has entered a boundary

Absorption see **sound absorption**

Absorption coefficient the measure of the effectiveness of a medium and its boundaries in absorbing sound wave energy

Acceleration (*a*) the rate of change in velocity, that is, $a = \frac{\Delta v}{\Delta t}$, where Δv and Δt are changes in velocity and time, respectively

Acoustic effect a phenomenon that affects sound waves traveling through a medium including absorption, refraction, reflection, interference, and diffraction

Acoustic energy the energy that is transferred from a vibrating object to a medium and propagated through the medium in the form of density changes

Acoustic impedance the opposition to the flow of sound energy through a medium

Acoustic nerve see **auditory nerve**

Acoustic power the power radiated by a sound source

Acoustic pressure the magnitude of change in the local atmospheric pressure caused by the vibration of a sound source

Acoustic reflex a bilateral middle ear muscle contraction in response to a loud sound in one or both ears

Acoustic resonance the state in which the frequency of an external force matches the resonance (natural) frequency of an acoustic system causing the system to absorb the maximum amount of external energy and to produce the strongest response to excitation

Acoustic shadow an area behind an obstacle that a direct sound wave does not enter or in which the sound intensity is greatly reduced

Acoustic system a small closed or semiclosed space in which the dimensions of the space are smaller or comparable to the wavelength of the propagating sound wave

Acoustician someone who studies the physical properties of sound

Acoustics the study of the physical properties of sound

Action potential stimulus-related potential (neuron firing) in an individual neuron in response to external stimulation, which is sufficient in intensity to cause an electrical impulse to be conducted down the axon of the neuron

Active component an electronic component that requires additional sources of energy to perform its functions; examples include vacuum tubes, transistors, and integrated circuits

Actuator the moving part of a switch or the type of contact made by the moving part of a switch

Aditus ad antrum a narrow bony passageway in the posterior bony wall of the middle ear that connects the tympanum to the antrum

Adjacent side (of a triangle) the side of a right triangle that forms the specific angle θ (theta) with the hypotenuse

Admittance the ease with which a system can vibrate due to an applied force; the inverse of impedance

Afferent neuron a neuron that carries sensory information (i.e., touch, taste, smell, hearing, and vision) from the peripheral nervous system to the central nervous system

Air conduction the process by which an acoustic signal travels through the structures of the outer and middle ear and arrives at the inner ear

Aliasing error the distortion of a digital signal caused by a sampling rate that is too low in relationship to the highest frequency of the input signal

Alternating current (AC) a current that periodically changes its direction; a current produced by an alternating voltage

Alternating voltage (AV) a difference in electric charge that periodically changes its magnitude and polarity

Ambient noise the background noise at a given place without any discernible components

Ampere (A) the current resulting from 1 coulomb of electricity passing through a point of observation in 1 second

Amplifier an active device that increases the voltage, current, or power of a transmitted signal

Amplitude the maximum (peak) magnitude of a periodic waveform

Amplitude density function the function that represents the relative percentage of time that a waveform magnitude has a given value

Amplitude distribution function the function that represents the relative percentage of time that a waveform magnitude is equal to or greater than a given value

Amplitude spectrum the distribution of the amplitudes of the sinusoidal components of a vector quantity as a function of frequency

Ampulla an enlargement at one end of each semicircular canal that houses a crista ampullaris

Anastomosis of Oort the place at which the olivocochlear neurons diverge from the vestibular nerve to enter the cochlea

Anatomy the study of a structure (e.g., the human body)

Anechoic chamber a specialized room with absorbing walls, ceiling, and floor that absorb all the arriving sound (each anechoic chamber has a lowest cutoff frequency below which it cannot be considered truly anechoic)

Angle (θ) the inclination of one line compared to another when the two lines intersect

Angle of incidence the angle at which a sound wave approaches a boundary

Angle of refraction the angle at which a sound wave proceeds through a material after passing through the surface of the material

Angular frequency (ω) a measure of how fast an object is rotating. The unit of angular frequency is radian per second (rad/s)

Angular gyrus parietal lobe gyrus that appears to integrate auditory information with other sensory information (e.g., visual, tactile)

Anions negatively charged ions

Annular ligament a ring-shaped ligament that holds the stapes footplate in the oval window

Annulus a ring-shaped ligament that holds the tympanic membrane in place along its lateral edges

Anterior toward the front

Anterior commissure a small fiber tract that connects the right and left temporal lobes and the right and left olfactory (smell) structures

Anterior ligament of the malleus a ligament that attaches the malleus to the anterior wall of the tympanic cavity

Anterior semicircular canal one of the three canals of the vestibular system; the canals contain the cristae ampullares, which function to detect angular acceleration of the body; the anterior semicircular canal is orthogonal to the posterior semicircular canal on the same side and parallel to the posterior semicircular canal on the opposite side

Anterior ventral cochlear nucleus (AVCN) one portion of the cochlear nucleus; receives auditory nerve projections and gives rise to the ventral acoustic stria (trapezoid body)

Antialiasing filter a low-pass filter inserted before the analog-to-digital (A/D) converter that is used to remove frequencies higher than the Nyquist frequency

Antihelix a cartilaginous ridge of the pinna that is medial to and generally parallel to the helix

Anti-imaging filter low-pass filter designed to prevent imaging error at the output of the digital-to-analog (D/A) converter

Antilog (antilogarithm) an operation that is the reverse of a logarithm; a number that is the object of the logarithm transformation

Antinodes the places in a vibrating mechanical system or in a sound field where the changes in a specific quantity are greatest

Antitragus a small cartilaginous projection of the pinna that is adjacent to the tragus (separated by the intertragal notch); superior to the ear lobe

Antrum a small chamber within the mastoid portion of the temporal bone that is posterior to the main middle ear cavity

Aperiodic vibration a vibration in which an object moves in an irregular and unpredictable manner around its point of equilibrium

Aperture error see **imaging error**

Apex (of the cochlea) the narrowest end of the spiral of the cochlea, where the scala tympani and scala vestibule join

Aqueduct of Sylvius see **cerebral aqueduct**

Arbor vitae fiber tracts projecting to and from the cortex of the cerebellum

Arcuate fasciculus a fiber tract that projects from Wernicke's area in the temporal lobe, around the back edge of the sylvian fissure, to Broca's area in the frontal lobe

Area (*A*) the amount of space occupied by a surface

Area triangularis see **Broca's area**

Atmospheric pressure a constant pressure exerted by the atmosphere on the surface of Earth

Atoms tiny building blocks with which all matter (solids, liquids, and gases) is composed; made up of three types of particles: protons, electrons, and neutrons

Attenuation a decrease in the magnitude of a signal

Audible sound a sound that can be heard

Audio chain a signal pathway that passes acoustic signals that have been converted into an electric (audio) form

Audio processor a device that is used to modify audio signals; audio processors include filters, equalizers, compressors, noise gates, limiters, expanders, companders, time compressors, time expanders, and reverberators

Audio receiver a transducer that converts acoustic or mechanic signals into electric (audio) signals

Audio signal an acoustic signal that has been converted into an electric form

Audio transducer device that transfers acoustic energy into electric energy or vice versa

Audio transmitter a transducer that converts electric (audio) signal energy into an acoustic or mechanic signal

Audition the act or process of listening

Auditory related to hearing or audition

Auditory association areas Cortical tissue (beyond Heschl's gyrus) that has been found to respond to auditory stimuli

Auditory distance estimation the process of determining how far one is from a sound source

Auditory nerve the portion of the vestibulocochlear nerve that relays auditory information from the cochlea to the central nervous system

Auditory response area the range of perceived intensities across frequency from the lowest intensity sound a human can perceive to the threshold of pain and from the lowest to highest frequency humans can hear

Auditory signal a signal that is intended to be heard

Auditory tube see **Eustachian tube**

Auricle see **pinna**

Auricular tubercle a bump of tissue along the edge of the helix, observed in some pinnae

Automatic gain control (AGC) a signal-processing device that automatically controls the output signal according to specific requirements

Average magnitude the average value of the magnitude of a waveform calculated across the whole period of the waveform

Average velocity (v_{avg}) the uniform velocity needed for an object to move across a certain distance (Δd) in a specific amount of time (Δt); that is, $v_{avg} = \frac{\Delta d}{\Delta t}$

Axons thin, thread-like extension of a neuron that carries nerve impulses and allows the nerve to communicate with other nerves via synaptic junctions

Azimuth the angle (θ) that represents the direction of a sound source in the horizontal plane

Azimuth estimation the process of determining the direction in the horizontal plane at which a sound is arriving at the listener

Background noise noise that is the sum of all sounds that interfere with a signal

Backward masking a masking paradigm in which a masking signal is presented slightly after an auditory signal of interest

Band-pass filter filter that passes a band of frequencies centered on a certain frequency

Band-reject filter filter that rejects a range of frequencies and passes frequencies that are lower or higher than this band

Bandwidth (Δf) the frequency range of a sound spectrum defined by a specific drop of sound energy at the lowest and highest frequency of the bandwidth

Bar a rigid, one-dimensional structure made of a material such as metal or wood that has a small cross section in comparison to its length; its shape is square or rectangular

Bark a unit of the bark scale, extending from 0 to 24

Bark scale a scale created by the range of audible frequencies considered as 24 side-by-side critical bands with end points and crossing points between the bands of 0, 100, 200, 300, 400, 510, 630, 770, 920, 1080, 1270, 1480, 1720, 2000, 2320, 2700, 3150, 3700, 4400, 5300, 6400, 7700, 9500, 12,000, and 15,500 Hz

Barometer an instrument that measures atmospheric pressure

Barometric pressure see **atmospheric pressure**

Base (of the cochlea) the widest coil of the spiral of the cochlea

Base number a number, such as 2 or 10, that defines the form (shape) of a logarithmic or exponential function

Basilar membrane the membrane that separates the scala media from the scala tympani; the organ of Corti is located on the scala media side of this membrane

Battery drain the current that is drawn from a battery

Beat frequency the number of times per second that the amplitude of a sound wave fluctuates

Beats slow periodic amplitude fluctuations caused when two sine waves that are very close in frequency interfere with one another

Bel (B) a logarithmic unit of power equal to the logarithm base 10 of the ratio of two powers such that the level in bels is equal to $log_{10}(\frac{P_2}{P_1})$, where P_2 and P_1 are respective powers

Bias a tendency to favor a particular type of response

Binary code code that represents all signals numerically using two digits, 0 and 1

Binaural related to two ears

Binaural advantage the improvement in auditory perception when a person is listening with two ears compared to one ear

Binaural localization cues localization cues created by differences in the acoustic characteristics of sounds as they arrive at the right ear and left ear

Binaural squelch a suppression of environmental sounds due to binaural listening, leading to improved speech intelligibility and signal identification; the brain is using binaural localization cues to separate sounds coming from different directions

Binaural summation an improvement in hearing sensitivity and sound loudness due to listening with two ears; if both ears have similar hearing thresholds, the binaural summation effect at the threshold is about 3 dB; binaural loudness is the sum of left and right ear monaural loudness

Bioelectric potentials the electric potentials (i.e., differences in electrical charge) existing between various areas within the human body

Bit binary digit of information; each available space where a 0 or 1 must appear in binary code

Boettcher cells support cells of the organ of Corti; found in the basal turn of the cochlea under the Claudius cells

Bone conduction the process by which an acoustic signal vibrates the bones of the skull to stimulate the cochlea; vibrations of the skull bones can result from either acoustic or mechanical stimulation of the skull

Bone conduction hearing aid a hearing aid that directly vibrates the bones of the skull for patients with outer and/or middle ear pathology; bone conduction hearing aids consist of a bone vibrator and supporting signal processing circuitry

Bone vibrator a device that is designed to vibrate the bones of the skull to transmit auditory signals

Bony labyrinth a cavity that contains the inner ear; located within the petrous portion of the temporal bone

Boundary a wall or other obstacle in a sound field that affects the way sound waves travel; a surface surrounding the space where sound waves propagate

Boundary microphone a microphone designed to receive reflections from reflective surfaces

Brachium of the inferior colliculus fiber projection from the inferior colliculus to the medial geniculate nucleus

Brain the portion of the central nervous system contained within the cranium and responsible for receiving and processing sensory information, transmitting motor commands to the body, and regulating body functions

Brainstem the lowest part of the brain that is structurally continuous with the spinal cord; contains the pons, medulla, and midbrain

Broadband noise a noise with acoustic energy distributed over a relatively wide frequency range

Broca's area the cortical tissue located in the inferior frontal gyrus of the language-dominant hemisphere (usually left) that is responsible for planning the motor actions for speech; lesions to this area result in an inability to express oneself by speech, also known as Broca's (or expressive) aphasia

Buckling effect see **catenary lever**

Bulk modulus of elasticity (K) a measure of stiffness in fluids and gases

Bushy cell a cell in the anterior ventral cochlear nucleus with multiple dendrites that resemble a bush

Byte a sequence of eight bits

Calculus a branch of mathematics concerning slopes and limits of functions as well as the area of the curve under a function

Capacitance (*C*) the ability of matter to store electric charge and sustain the existing voltage by opposing the flow of direct current; defined as the ratio of stored electricity (Q) to an applied voltage (*E*) such that $C = \frac{Q}{E}$

Capacitive reactance (X_c) frequency-dependent opposition to motion, such as electric current, produced by capacitance

Capacitor an electric component capable of storing electric change and providing a specified capacitance; a capacitor consists of two parallel metal plates separated by a narrow layer of insulating material such as air, paper, ceramic, or plastic

Cardioid microphone a directional microphone that provides about 6 dB of attenuation in sound intensity for sounds arriving from the sides of the microphone and about 15 to 25 dB of attenuation for signals arriving from the back of the microphone compared to sounds arriving from the front of the microphone

Cartesian coordinate system (rectangular coordinate system) a system for locating points on a plane or in three-dimensional space, referenced to orthogonal axes (e.g., *x*, *y*, *z*)

Cartilaginous portion of the ear canal the outer one third of the ear canal formed by a cartilaginous framework

Catenary lever the anatomic lever created because the umbo is displaced less than the rest of the tympanic membrane; as a result, the pressure at the umbo is about two times (6 dB) greater than the pressure across the entire membrane

Cavum concha the more inferior of the two parts of the concha; the portion of the concha closest to the external auditory meatus

Central auditory nervous system (CANS) a sound-processing network of afferent and efferent auditory fiber tracts and nuclei that connect the ear with the brain; a part of central nervous system (CNS)

Central nervous system the part of the nervous system consisting of the brain and spinal cord

Central processing unit (CPU) a microprocessor chip that controls a computer's operation

Central sulcus sulcus that separates the frontal and parietal lobes

Cerebellar cortex cell bodies located at the surface of the cerebellum

Cerebellopontine angle the angle created by the cerebellum and the pons

Cerebellum a structure posterior to the brainstem that receives information from the spinal cord and various sensory systems and coordinates the motion of the skeletal muscles in order to maintain equilibrium and posture

Cerebral aqueduct channel that connects the third to the fourth ventricle; part of the ventricular system

Cerebral cortex the cellular surface of each cerebral hemisphere

Cerebral hemispheres the right and left divisions of the brain

Cerebral peduncles two large fiber tracts connecting the brainstem with the brain; they look like pillars in an anterior view

Cerebrospinal fluid (CSF) a distillate of blood created by the choroid plexus; located in the ventricular system and in the subarachnoid space that surrounds the brain and spinal cord providing a protection function

Cerumen earwax

CGS System the original metric system proposed by the French Academy of Sciences that used the centimeter, the gram, and the second as the set of basic units

Characteristic frequency (CF) the frequency at which individual hair cells and nerve cells are tuned to respond most effectively

Chip an integrated circuit (IC)

Chladni figures figures that illustrate the distribution of the various nodes of vibration of a plate

Chladni patterns see **Chladni figures**

Chopper pattern a pattern of cell firing that is periodic, but the periodicity does not match the period of the stimulus; recorded from cells in the cochlear nucleus

Chorda tympani a branch of the facial nerve that crosses the epitympanum from the back of the tympanic cavity to the front just beneath the head of the malleus and incus; joins the lingual nerve to provide taste sensation to the anterior portion of the tongue

Choroid plexus vascular structure that produces cerebrospinal fluid (CSF)

Circular mode mode of vibration that runs in a circular manner in a plate or membrane

Circumaural earphones earphones that rest over the head and surround the pinna

Circumference a boundary line of an area or object (e.g., a circle); also the length of the line all the way around an area or object

Claudius cells support cells of the organ of Corti; adjacent to the Hensen cells

Clinical bone vibrator a bone vibrator used for hearing testing

Closed earphone earphone with a solid back that creates an air-filled cavity between the enclosure and the membrane of the earphone

Closed space indoor space; space enclosed in boundaries

Closed system a theoretical ideal system in which the only external force acting on the system is the activation force and once this force is taken away from the system, there are no additional external forces acting on it

Cochlea part of the inner ear that contains the sense organ of hearing (organ of Corti); the location in which mechanical motions generated by sound are coded into nerve impulses for transmission to the central nervous system

Cochlear amplifier an increase in the amplitude of an auditory signal at the level of the cochlea due to the motility function of the outer hair cells, which increase the magnitude of basilar membrane vibration

Cochlear duct see **scala media**

Cochlear microphonic an alternating current potential produced at the reticular lamina that mimics the vibration pattern of the basilar membrane; as the basilar membrane moves up and down, the cochlear microphonic alternates between positive and negative polarity, mimicking the shape of the input signal

Cochlear nerve see **auditory nerve**

Cochlear nucleus the most caudal auditory nucleus and the projection point for all auditory nerve fibers; located at the border of the medulla and the pons

Cochlear partition see **scala media**

Coefficient of damping (*a*) a measure describing the relationship between the coefficient of friction (*r*) and the mass (*m*) of a vibrating system, where $a = \frac{r}{2m}$

Coefficient of friction a unitless number that describes the resistance to sliding of two surfaces in contact with each other

Coincidence detectors nerve cells that only respond to concurrent signals from more than one neuron

Comb filter effect a signal interference in the form of multiple peaks and dips in sound pressure

Commissure of Probst see **dorsal commissure of the lemniscus**

Commissure of the inferior colliculus a fiber tract that connects the two inferior colliculi to allow information to cross between the two sides

Common factor a number by which all the numbers in a given set can be divided without a remainder

Communication bone vibrator a bone vibrator used for speech communication

Complex tone a sound that has more than one but a finite number of sinusoidal components

Complex vibration the combination of two or more sinusoidal vibrations that result in a nonsinusoidal vibration

Compliance (*C*) the inverse of stiffness (*K*); that is, $C = 1/K$

Component an individual element of a complex system (e.g., a sinusoidal component of a complex waveform or a component of an electric circuit)

Compound action potential (CAP) an alternating current potential generated by the simultaneous action potentials from many different neurons; the magnitude of the CAP depends on the number of activated neurons

Compression a bunching of particles causing an increased density in a medium; reduction of the signal dynamics

Compressional vibration a motion of a vibrating system in which different elements of the system vibrate in opposite directions

Computer word a chunk of binary code composed of one or more bytes that serves as the basic unit of information transfer in a given computer (digital system)

Concha a bowl-shaped depression that comprises the deepest groove in the pinna

Condenser microphone a microphone that uses variable capacitance to convert an acoustic signal into its electric form; acoustic pressure acts on a membrane that forms one plate of a large polarized capacitor; motion of the membrane causes a change in voltage between the plates

Conductance the ease with which energy travels through a frictional element in a system; the inverse of resistance

Conductor matter that has low electric impedance and allows free electrons to flow through it

Cone loudspeaker loudspeaker that uses a lightweight semirigid diaphragm (the cone) to emit sounds; a cone loudspeaker not enclosed in an enclosure acts as a dipole sound source

Cone of confusion an imaginary "cone" of space that defines the limits of human ability to detect the location of sound using binaural cues

Cone of light a light reflection off the tympanic membrane seen during otoscopic examination; observed on the anterior inferior quadrant in a normal ear

Constant a fixed number; a number that does not change

Constructive interference an increase in the amplitude of sound waves, when two or more sound waves travel through the same space and their compression and rarefaction phases occur together

Contact microphone a transducer that changes mechanical vibrations into an electric signal; a contact microphone can be used to convert the skull vibrations of a talker into an audio signal

Continuous noise a noise with relatively small fluctuations of level within a period of observation

Continuous spectrum a spectrum in which the energy is spread across a range of frequencies rather than at discrete sinusoidal components

Contralateral related to the opposite side

Coordinate system a set of numbers, such as distances or angles, that uniquely identify the position of specific points in space in reference to a central point called the origin

Corpora quadrigemina four round bumps on the dorsal surface of the midbrain, containing the superior colliculi of the visual system and the inferior colliculi of the auditory system

Corpus callosum a large C-shaped fiber tract that connects the right and left hemispheres and transfers information between them

Cortex a group of cell bodies located at the surface of the cortex (cerebral cortex) or cerebellum (cerebellar cortex)

Coulomb (*C*) the amount of electricity contained in 6.24×10^{18} (6.24 quintillion) electrons

Crista ampullaris sense organ of balance located within each of the three ampulla of the semicircular canals; responds to angular acceleration

Critical angle of incidence the smallest angle of incidence for which total internal reflection occurs

Critical band a range of frequencies that is integrated (summed together) by the neural system and affects the perception of various aspects of sound; the ear can be said to be a series of overlapping critical bands, each responding to a narrow range of frequencies

Critical band scale see **Bark scale**

Critical damping the amount of damping that causes an object to make only one vibration and then return to its natural (neutral) position

Critical distance the distance from the sound source at which the intensity of the direct and reflected sound fields are equal

Cross-links tiny fibers that connect individual hair cell stereocilia

Crossover network a multicircuit audio filter that directs high-frequency energy to the high-frequency loudspeakers, low-frequency energy to the low-frequency loudspeakers, and so on

Crosstalk audio signals that leak from one system into another

Crura of the antihelix the superior portion of the antihelix where it divides to form two folds separated by the triangular fossa

Crus of the helix the most medial aspect of the helix, which connects the helix to the side of the head and to the concha

Cupula a gelatinous mass that is part of the crista ampullaris; the stereocilia from the hair cells of the crista ampullaris project into the cupula and are sheared by the inertial lag of the cupula in relationship to the motion of the semicircular canal wall

Current a flow of electric charge through a conductor

Current amplifier an amplifier designed to amplify the input current

Cuticular plate a thickening at the top edge of the hair cell where the stereocilia are firmly anchored to the hair cell

Cycle one full repetition of a periodic motion

Cylindrical coordinates hybrid Cartesian-polar coordinates used to describe phenomena resulting from operations of line sources in three-dimensional space

Cymba concha the more superior of the two parts of the concha; the portion of the concha farthest from the external auditory meatus

Damped vibration the vibration of a system that involves some damping

Damping the effect of friction on a vibrating system

Darwin's tubercle see **auricular tubercle**

Decay time the time needed for a waveform to change from 90% to 10% of its peak value

Decibel (dB) a logarithmic unit of the ratio of two powers; one tenth of a bel, defined as $10 \times log(\frac{P_2}{P_1})$, where P_2 and P_1 are respective powers

Decussate to cross from one side to the other

Deiters cells support cells of the inner ear, which contain a cup-shaped depression that holds the bottom end of each outer hair cell and phalangeal processes that project to the reticular lamina

Dendrites neuron extensions that allow the nerve to communicate with other nerves at junctions called synapses; dendrites receive a signal and pass the signal to the cell body or axon

Density (ρ) the amount of matter in a given unit of volume

Depolarization a change in hair cell or nerve cell polarity (i.e., a change in electric potential) that occurs in response to a mechanical, electrical, or chemical stimulus

Destructive interference a decrease in the amplitude of at least one sound wave, when two waves travel through the same space and their compression and rarefaction phases occur together

Detection threshold the lowest intensity of a stimulus that can be detected a specific percentage of the time, usually 50%

Deterministic process an activity in which any future state of a process is a direct consequence of the previous states and can be predicted

Deterministic sound a sound in which the future behavior can be predicted mathematically or on the basis of previous observations

Diameter (*d*) a straight line connecting two points on the periphery (circumference, surface) of a figure (such as a circle or sphere) that passes through the center of the figure

Dielectric matter that has high electric impedance and allows very few electrons to flow through it; used to insulate, for example, two plates of a capacitor

Diencephalon the "in-between brain" located between two cerebral hemispheres at the inferior border; contains the thalamus and hypothalamus

Difference limen (DL) the smallest physical difference between two stimuli in which an observer can determine that the two stimuli are perceptually different; also known as just noticeable difference (jnd)

Difference threshold see **difference limen**

Diffraction see **sound diffraction**

Diffuse field microphone see **random incidence microphone**

Diffuse sound field an area filled with sound energy coming from all possible directions (with equal probability) and in which the sound pressure level is the same at all locations

Diffusion see **dispersion**

Digital audio the processes of transmission, storage, amplification, filtering, summation, multiplication, equalization, compression, and so forth, of audio signals in digital domain

Digital code a sequence of numbers

Digital signal stream of information that is presented as a sequence of numbers

Digitization the process of converting sampled quantized values into binary form

Diode an electronic device that passes electric current only in one direction

Dipole sound source a set of two identical monopole sound sources pulsating out-of-phase and separated by a small distance as compared to the wavelength produced by the source

Direct current (DC) a current produced by a unidirectional voltage

Direct sound field the sound field closest to a sound source where the sound energy is caused primarily by the sound source itself rather than reflections of the sound off barriers

Direct voltage (DV) a difference in electric charge that does not change its magnitude and polarity across time

Directional microphone microphone that preferentially responds to sounds arriving from a specific direction, usually to the front of the microphone

Directivity factor (Q) a measure of the directivity of a microphone

Directivity index (DI) the logarithmic measure of the directivity factor (Q) expressed in dB

Discrete spectrum see **line spectrum**

Discriminability index (d-prime, d') a statistic in signal detection theory that indicates the separation between noise (*N*) and signal plus noise (*S* + *N*) distributions

Dispersion a sound wave reflection pattern in which sound waves are reflected in many different directions due to a curved and/or rough wall surface

Displacement (*d*) a change in position in a given direction

Distance (*d*) the length of the line connecting two points

Distance estimation see **auditory distance estimation**

Distortional mechanism a bone conduction mechanism that results from alternating compressions and expansions of the bony labyrinth, which cause changes in the shape and size of the cochlear cavity and result in motion of the basilar membrane

Distributed property a property of an electric circuit that is distributed along the circuit

Dither random noise added to the input and/or output signals in a digital signal processing (DSP) system in order to mask correlated noise produced by quantization error

Doppler effect a shift in the frequency of a sound wave resulting from the movement of a sound source, the movement of a listener, changes in the medium, or a combination of these factors

Dorsal posterior (below the midbrain) or superior (above the midbrain)

Dorsal acoustic stria fiber tract originating in the dorsal cochlear nucleus and traveling primarily to the contralateral lateral lemniscus

Dorsal cochlear nucleus dorsal portion of the cochlear nucleus; receives auditory nerve projections and gives rise to the dorsal acoustic stria

Dorsal commissure of the lemniscus fiber projections from the dorsal nucleus of the lateral lemniscus to the opposite side of the brainstem

Driving frequency the frequency of an applied external force

Ductus reuniens a narrow channel of the inner ear membranous labyrinth that connects the cochlear duct to the saccule

Dynamic microphone a microphone that uses electromagnetic induction to convert sound into an electrical signal; motion of a microphone moves a magnet, which results in the induction of current in a coil of wire surrounding the microphone

Dynamic range the intensity range between the highest and the lowest value of a signal that can be transmitted by a specific channel or neuron; the highest value is determined by the saturation point (or the generation of distortions) and the lowest value is determined by intrinsic noise or the trigger level of the channel

Dynamics the study of energy

Ear the anatomic structure that contains the sense organs for hearing and balance

Earbuds earphones that are inserted into the concha

Ear canal see **external auditory canal**

Earphone an electroacoustic transmitter that converts audio signals into acoustic pressure delivered directly to the ear

Earth ground (power ground, safety ground) connection between an electronic device and the earth, so spurious current flows to the ground and not into a person

Echo the reflection of a sound wave that arrives so long after the original sound that it creates a repetition of the original sound

Efferent auditory pathway nerve pathway that travels from the cortex and various nuclei in the brainstem downward to modify the operating characteristics of lower level afferent neurons in the brainstem and the hair cells in the cochlea

Efferent neuron a neuron that carries information from the central nervous system to the peripheral nervous system

Efficiency the ratio of the sound pressure produced by a loudspeaker (or earphone) to its audio power at the input

Elastic medium matter that has the property of elasticity and is therefore capable of propagating sound waves

Elasticity the property of matter that allows matter to recover its form (size and shape) after it has been distorted (expanded or compressed)

Electric charge the amount of electricity

Electric circuit a closed loop connecting a source of electricity and the various elements conducting electric current

Electric component an electric element that has specified electric properties such as resistance, capacitance, and inductance

Electric current the flow of free electrons caused by the application of an applied voltage

Electric device a device that needs electricity to operate

Electric field the force field created by two opposite charges

Electric force see **electromotive force**

Electric impedance the total opposition of a matter to the flow of electric changes within the matter

Electric installation the collection of cables and auxiliary elements that connect the various pieces of an electric system

Electric load the final element of an electric circuit; the element that uses electricity for a specific work

Electric potential an electric charge measured in reference to a specific point

Electric potential difference difference in electric potential between two points

Electric source a natural phenomenon or device that generates an electric force

Electric switch a device used for opening and closing the pathway of an electric current

Electricity a form of energy resulting from the uneven distribution and directional flow of electrons

Electroacoustic chain see **audio chain**

Electroacoustic transducer see **audio transducer**

Electroacoustics the science concerned with the conversion between acoustic energy and electric energy and the processing and transmission of audio signals

Electromagnet the source of an electromagnetic field in which a current is passed through a coil of wire that is wrapped around a metal core

Electromagnetic field the interaction between the electric field generated by the presence of particles possessing an electric charge and the magnetic field generated by the relative movement of these particles in space

Electromagnetic wave a wave motion caused by an electric charge traveling through a system; does not require a medium and includes light and radio waves

Electromechanic transducer a device that transfers mechanic energy into electric energy or vice versa

Electromotility the ability of outer hair cells to change dimension in response to changes in the electrical potential of the cell

Electromotive force (EMF, *E*) an external force pushing free electrons to flow in an organized manner; measured in volts (V); the presence of opposing stationary charges that cause an electric current to flow

Electron one of three particles that make up an atom; carries a negative charge

Electrostatic microphone see **condenser microphone**

Elevation estimation the process of determining the angle between the horizontal plane passing through the ears of a listener and the direction in the vertical plane from which the sound is arriving

End correction an additional length that must be added to the mass of vibrating air to determine the resonance frequency of an acoustic system, which has the form of a tube (or other space) with an open end

Endocochlear potential the positive resting potential (approximately +80 mV) between the endolymph in the scala media and the perilymph in the scala vestibuli and scala tympani

Endolymph fluid located within the membranous labyrinth of the inner ear (e.g., in the scala media of the cochlea); this fluid is high in potassium and very low in sodium

Endolymphatic duct a narrow duct formed by the joining of the utricle and saccule; this duct projects from the membranous labyrinth of the inner ear to the endolymphatic sac

Endolymphatic sac a small membrane-covered cavity at the distal end of the endolymphatic duct; located in the dura mater (the outermost layer of the meninges)

Energy (*E*) the ability or capacity of an object to do work

Energy source a source of energy, such as a vibrating object, which can transfer energy to surrounding matter

Epithalamus a portion of the diencephalon concerned with emotion, behavior, and circadian rhythm (via the pineal gland, which synthesizes a hormone called melatonin in rhythm with the daily light cycle)

Epitympanum the superior portion of the tympanum

Equalizer a device that attenuates, to various degrees, specific components of a signal spectrum to reshape the spectrum

Equal-loudness contour see **equal-loudness curve**

Equal-loudness curve a line on a sound intensity versus frequency graph that connects points representing equally loud sounds

Equation a statement asserting the equality of two quantities

Equilibrium the rest or neutral position of a system, when it is not in a back-and-forth motion

Eustachian tube channel that begins on the anterior wall of the middle ear and connects the middle ear cavity with the nasopharyngeal cavity

Exocytosis fusion of the synaptic vesicles with the presynaptic membrane of a hair cell or nerve cell resulting in the release of neurotransmitter from the vesicles into the synaptic cleft

Exponent a number indicating the power to which a base number, such as 2 or 10, is raised (i.e., the number of times a base number is multiplied by itself)

Exponential notation see **scientific notation**

External absorption absorption of sound energy by a space boundary

External auditory canal the anatomic tube that begins at the external auditory meatus and extends medially to the tympanic membrane

External auditory meatus the external opening of the ear canal, located at the medial edge of the pinna

Facial nerve the seventh cranial nerve (CN VII), which provides sensory and motor innervation to the face; auditory system innervation includes sensory innervation to the outer ear and tympanic membrane and motor innervation to the stapedius muscle; a branch of the facial nerve called the chorda tympani travels through the middle ear

Fall time see **decay time**

Far sound field the sound field located some distance from a sound source in which the sound source is considered as a single entity and in which the sound pressure decreases uniformly as a function of distance

Fechner's Law the law stating that the magnitude of a sensation (R) increases proportionally with the logarithm of the stimulus intensity (I), such that $R = k \times \log_a(I)$

Fiber tract a group of nerve fibers

Filter a device that restricts the passage of energy to a specific frequency range, called the filter band

Final transient the motion of a system in response to a step-down function, that is, in response to the abrupt removal of the driving force

Fissures extremely deep sulci

Flux the quantity of electricity that can pass through a specific material in a specific period of time

Folia small folds seen on the surface of the cerebellum

Foramen magnum a large bony opening at the base of the skull through which the spinal cord enters the cranial cavity and is contiguous with the medulla

Force (*F*) the interaction between two objects or between an object and its environment, alternately defined as a push or pull

Force field an area in which a force such as gravity, electricity, or magnetism causes objects to be affected in certain ways (e.g., in an electric field, charged particles can attract or repel each other because of the electric force created by the charged particles)

Forward-biased junction a PN junction in which the orientation of a voltage works along the natural potential difference of the junction

Forced vibration a case in which a system is forced to vibrate in response to a continuous and periodic driving force

Forebrain the largest region of the brain; consists of the telencephalon and diencephalon

Fornix a curved bundle of nerve fibers connecting a structure called the hippocampus (associated with memory) with the diencephalon

Forward masking a masking paradigm in which a masking signal is presented slightly before an auditory signal of interest

Fourier Theorem a theorem stating that any complex oscillatory (vibratory) motion is the sum of various sinusoidal motions of varying amplitude, frequency, and phase

Free electron an electron that breaks away from its nucleus

Free-field microphone a microphone designed for measurements in a free field where sound travels with relatively few reflections, such as in open outdoor space

Free sound field a sound field in which sound wave propagation is not affected by space boundaries or objects; free-field sound pressure decreases 6 dB per doubling of distance from the sound source

Free vibration a case in which a system is left alone to vibrate at its resonance frequency after being activated by the short application of an external force

Frequency the number of repetitions (cycles) per second

Frequency domain representation of a phenomenon as a function of frequency

Frequency response the function showing the relationship between the magnitude of the output signal and the signal frequency for a constant magnitude of the input signal

Frequency spectrum see **amplitude spectrum**

Friction the force that opposes the relative motion or tendency to such motion of a body that is in contact with other bodies

Frontal lobe the most anterior of the lobes of the brain; responsible for voluntary skilled movements

Frontal/coronal a cut or slice that divides the body into front and back

Function the relationship between two sets of numbers

Fundamental frequency the lowest frequency of a vibrating system; the reciprocal of the fundamental period of a complex periodic wave

Fundamental period the amount of time it takes to complete one cycle of complex periodic vibration

Gain the ratio (difference in dB) of the output signal to the input signal

Ganglion a group of cell bodies in the peripheral nervous system

Gap junctions a series of channels through which potassium ions pass from the hair cells through the supporting cells and stria vascularis back to the endolymph of the inner ear

Gaussian distribution a common distribution of frequency of natural events such as height of a person; it is a probability density distribution function that looks like a bell-shaped curve centered at the most probable (mean) value of the distribution

Gradient microphone microphone that responds to the difference in sound pressure between sound waves arriving at the front and the back of the microphone

Graphic equalizer a set of adjacent band-pass filters equipped with a volume (gain) control for each channel in the form of vertical slider; the shape of the sound spectrum is selected by adjusting the level controls of individual filters

Gravity (*G* or *g*) the universal phenomenon that any two objects in the universe attract each other; a force (*G*) of attraction or acceleration (g) caused by this force

Gray matter see **cortex**

Greatest common factor (GCF) the largest common factor from a group of numbers; the greatest common factor from a set of harmonically related components is equal to the fundamental frequency

Ground the common point at which all electric circuits in a system are connected; the two types of grounds in electric systems are earth ground (power ground, safety ground) and chassis ground (signal ground, shield ground)

Ground wire the wire that connects an electric device to a common ground

Grounding the process or act of connecting all electric circuits to one common point that has a very low resistance, to protect the user from electric shock

Gyrus a bulge of cortex; the various gyri of the cortex are separated by the sulci

Habenula perforata tiny holes in the spiral lamina through which auditory nerve fibers pass

Hair cells sensory cells (auditory, vestibular) with tiny hairs called stereocilia projecting from one end; hair cells are responsible for changing mechanical motion into electrochemical impulses that can be transmitted by the nervous system

Handset a system consisting of an earphone and a microphone designed to be held in the hand during communication

Hard signal limiter a signal-limiting device that abruptly clips off signal values that exceed a certain threshold

Harmonic an integer multiple of the fundamental frequency

Harmonic distortion the nonlinear distortion of a sinusoidal signal resulting in the presence of signal harmonics at the output of the transmitting device

Harmonic motion a motion in which the acceleration of the object is directly proportional but opposite in direction to the displacement of the object from its equilibrium position

Harmonic relationship a relationship in which the components of a complex waveform are whole-number multiples of the fundamental frequency

Head-related transfer function (HRTF) a function relating the sound pressure at the entrance to the ear canal to the hypothetical sound pressure that would exist at the location corresponding to the center of the listener's head if the listener was not present

Headphone one or two earphones together with a system for holding them to the listener's head

Headset a headphone system that incorporates a communication microphone

Hearing the sense by which sound is perceived

Hearing area see **auditory response area**

Hearing level (HL) a logarithmic measure (expressed in dB HL) of the ratio of sound pressure in reference to the audiometric zero level

Hearing science the study of the physiologic, physical, psychological, and technical phenomena related to normal aspects of sound perception including the creation and transmission of auditory signals

Heavy damping the amount of damping that prevents an object from making even a single back-and-forth motion and results in a theoretically infinite time needed for an object to return to its equilibrium position

Helicotrema a narrow passage at the apex of the cochlea at which the scala tympani and scala vestibuli are connected

Helix the outer cartilaginous fold of the pinna that curves around the outside edge; it begins at the superior border of the lobule and ends at the crus of the helix

Helmholtz resonator an enclosed volume of air that creates a simple acoustic system with a single resonance frequency

Henry (H) a unit of inductance

Hensen cells inner ear support cells lateral to the outer hair cells

Heschl's gyrus the primary auditory cortex; receives projections from the medial geniculate body

High-pass filter a filter that passes high-frequency energy and blocks low-frequency energy

Hindbrain includes the pons, cerebellum, and medulla

Horizontal plane a cut or section that is parallel to the horizon; in reference to a standing person

Horizontal semicircular canal one of the three canals of the vestibular system that contain the cristae ampullares, which function to detect angular acceleration of the body; the horizontal canal is oriented at about 30° in relationship to the horizontal plane

Horn loudspeaker a loudspeaker with an attached horn to improve energy emission into the surrounding air; a horn improves the impedance matching between the loudspeaker and surrounding air

Hot wire the wire that supplies electric current and has some potential in reference to ground

Hybrid system system that includes both analog and digital signal processing

Hypotenuse the longest side of a right triangle

Hypothalamus part of the diencephalon; the chief autonomic center, responsible for the synthesis and release of hormones into the bloodstream (endocrine functions), controlling (together with the insular lobe) autonomic functions (e.g., respiration), and playing a role in growth, sexual and emotional behaviors, and eating and drinking behaviors

Hypotympanum the crescent-shaped inferior portion of the middle ear cavity located below the inferior border of the annulus and below the eustachian tube

Imaging error the introduction of high-frequency distortion into the signal at the point where the signal is converted back from its digital form to an analog signal; caused by instability (jitter) in the digital (DPS) sampling clock

Immittance a term developed for use with diagnostic testing of the middle ear to indicate either impedance or admittance; the use of impedance or admittance is preferable

Impedance the opposition to the flow of energy through a system

Impedance matching the practice of making the impedance of a load equal to the impedance of a source of power in order to transfer as much energy as possible from the source to the load

Impulse noise a single or occasionally repeated brief event caused by a sudden change in the motion of a sound source that causes a single oscillation in sound pressure, such as a gun shot

Incident wave a sound wave that arrives at a boundary

Incudostapedial joint the joint formed between the lenticular process of the incus and the head of the stapes

Incus one of the bones of the inner ear, attached at one end to the malleus and at the other end to the stapes; known as the anvil in nonprofessional terms

Indirect sound field see **reverberant sound field**

Inductance (*L*) the ability of matter to store energy in a magnetic field and resist changes in current; the ratio of stored magnetic flux (**Φ**) to the current (*I*) producing this magnetism, such that $L = \frac{\Phi}{I}$

Inductive reactance (X_L) frequency-dependent opposition to current produced by inductance

Inductor electric component that provides a specified inductance

Inertia the resistance of an object to a change in its state of motion (e.g., to be moved, to be redirected, or to be stopped)

Inertial middle ear mechanism a bone conduction mechanism that results from the inertial lag of the ossicular chain in comparison with the motion of the skull; this causes the stapes to move in and out of the oval window

Inertial vibration the motion of a vibrating system in which the entire vibrating object moves back and forth as a unit (e.g., at low frequencies the entire skull vibrates back and forth as a unit)

Inferior toward the bottom

Inferior colliculus part of the central auditory nervous system located on the dorsal aspect of the midbrain

Inferior semicircular canal see **posterior semicircular canal**

Initial transient the motion of a system in response to the sudden application of a driving force

Inner ear the portion of the ear that contains the vestibular and cochlear sense organs, which are responsible for generating neural impulses in response to mechanical motions; neural impulses generated here are later interpreted by the brain for sound perception and maintenance of balance

Inner ear mechanism bone conduction mechanisms that result in changes in the size and shape of the cochlea and cause an inertial lag between the walls of the bony labyrinth and the motion of the fluid and membranes within the bony labyrinth

Inner hair cells (IHCs) a single row of flask-shaped sensory cells in the organ of Corti of the inner ear; each inner ear contains approximately 3500 inner hair cells

Inner phalangeal cells support cells of the inner ear that provide structural support for the inner hair cells

Inner radial fibers type I afferent auditory nerve fibers that synapse with inner hair cells

Inner sulcus cells support cells of the inner ear that are medial to the inner hair cells and extend from the spiral limbus to the inside edge of the inner hair cells

In-phase the relationship between two waveforms that have the same frequency and the same initial phase

Input impedance the electric impedance measured at the input of the earphone or other electric device

Input sensitivity the ratio of the microphone output (in mV_{rms}) to its sound pressure input (in Pa or dB SPL)

Input signal the magnitude of the signal that enters the amplifier

Input-output function (I/O function) see **transfer function**

Insert earphone earphones that can be inserted into the ear canal

Instantaneous related to a specific moment in time

Instantaneous acceleration acceleration at a specific moment in time

Instantaneous magnitude the magnitude of a waveform at any given moment in time

Instantaneous velocity the velocity at a specific moment in time

Insula see **insular lobe**

Insular lobe a cortical structure located medial to the lateral fissure covered by the operculum (edges) of the frontal, temporal, and parietal lobes; responsible for autonomic processes such as regulating the internal environment of the human body

Insulator matter that has high electric impedance and prevents free electrons from flowing through it

Integer a positive or negative whole number or zero

Integrated circuit a complex, usually multifunctional, form of a semiconductor device

Interaural related to the difference between ears; "between ears"

Interaural intensity difference (IID) the difference in intensity of the sound wave arriving to the left ear and right ear

Interaural phase difference (IPD) the difference in phase of the sound wave arriving to the left ear and right ear

Interaural time difference (ITD) the difference in time of arrival of the sound wave arriving to the left ear and right ear

Interference see **sound interference**

Interference noise noise induced in transmission wires by electromagnetic fields generated by power lines, various motors and engines, home appliances, radio and TV stations, medical equipment, and some natural phenomena

Intermediate acoustic stria fiber tract originating in the posterior ventral cochlear nucleus and traveling primarily to the contralateral lateral lemniscus

Intermodulation distortion differential (one frequency minus another) and summation (one frequency plus another) tones that appear at the output of a nonlinear device when its input consists of two or more sine waves

Internal (self) noise the output of a microphone with no signal at its input

Internal absorption absorption of sound wave energy by the medium through which the sound wave is traveling

Internal auditory canal a bony canal in the petrous portion of the temporal bone through which the vestibulocochlear (VIII) and facial (VII) nerves travel

Internal capsule a large bundle of fibers that project through the diencephalon, connecting the cerebrum with the brainstem and cerebellum

Internal carotid artery paired artery that is one of two major conduits for blood to the brain; travels through a bony tunnel called the carotid canal, which is located anterior to the middle ear cavity

Internal jugular vein paired vein that is the major conduit for blood leaving the brain; travels through a bony tunnel called the jugular foramen, which is posterior to the middle ear cavity

International System of Units (SI) the system of standard international units for scientific measurement

Interneuron a neuron that provides communication between afferent and efferent neurons

Intertragal notch groove between the tragus and the antitragus

Inverse square law the law stating that in a free sound field the sound intensity is inversely proportional to the square of the distance from the sound source

Inverse thermal effect the bending of sound waves toward the ground when cold air is closer to the ground and warmer air is above it

Ion a charged particle; positive ions are called cations and negative ions are called anions

Ion channel a tiny opening in a cell membrane that allows ions to pass into and out of the cell

Ionized substance a substance containing a lot of charged particles

Ipsilateral related to the same side

Iso-loudness contour see **equal-loudness curve**

Isotope a variation of a chemical element in which the number of neutrons differs from that in its basic form

Isthmus (of the ear canal) a narrowing of the ear canal lateral to the tympanic membrane

Joule (J) the amount of work done when a 1-kg mass is moved 1 m

Judgment a human response to a test stimulus

Just noticeable difference (jnd) see **difference limen**

Kinematics the study of motion

Kinetic energy (E_k) the energy of motion that is carried by an object due to its velocity

Lateral toward the side

Lateral lemniscus the largest fiber tract in the auditory brainstem containing fiber projections from the cochlear nucleus and superior olivary complex, which then project to the inferior colliculus in the midbrain

Lateral olivocochlear bundle (LOCB) efferent neurons that project from the periolivary nuclei near the lateral superior olivary nucleus to the inner ear; these projections are primarily ipsilateral and synapse on the afferent nerve fibers below the inner hair cells

Lateral olivocochlear neurons see **lateral olivocochlear bundle**

Lateral semicircular canal see **horizontal semicircular canal**

Lateral sulcus sulcus that separates the frontal lobe (and part of the parietal lobe) from the temporal lobe

Lateral superior olivary (LSO) nucleus one of two relatively large nuclei (the lateralmost) located in the superior olivary complex

Lateralization the act of identifying the location of a phantom sound source within the head

Lavaliere microphone hands-free microphone that is clipped to clothes or hung at the chest via a loop around the neck

Law of Conservation of Energy a universal law stating that energy can change from one form to another but cannot be created or destroyed

Law of Universal Gravitation a universal law stating that the strength of gravity (a phenomenon in which any two objects attract each other) depends on the masses of both of the objects and the distance between them

Lenticular process of the incus the "L"-shaped bend at the end of the long process of the incus

Levator veli palatini muscle muscle located in the soft tissue lining the nasopharyngeal cavity; contraction of this muscle assists the tensor veli palatini in the opening of the eustachian tube

Level the logarithm of the ratio of two numbers

Light damping see **minimal damping**

Limbic lobe see **limbic system**

Limbic system telencephalon structures that anatomically border the telencephalon and the diencephalon and functionally border conscious and unconscious neurologic processing of drive-related (e.g., sex drive, eating and drinking behavior) and emotional behaviors

Line amplifier voltage amplifier used to increase a relatively large signal after the initial small signal has been amplified by a preamplifier

Line spectrum a spectrum that consists of one or more separate vertical lines

Linear amplifier an amplifier in which the magnitude of the output signal is linearly related to the magnitude of the input signal

Linear distortion frequency-dependent changes in signal gain that subsequently cause changes in the spectral composition of the output signal

Listener someone who is expecting to hear an auditory stimulus

Load a component attached to the output of the system; receiver of energy

Lobule earlobe; the most inferior portion of the pinna; the portion of the pinna that does not contain cartilage

Localization the process of determining the direction of incoming sound or the location of a sound source in space in terms of its azimuth and elevation

Localization cues the specific characteristics of received sounds that are used to determine the direction of incoming sound

Logarithm see **exponent**

Longitudinal fissure fissure that separates right and left hemispheres

Longitudinal waves waves in which the particles of the medium propagating the wave are displaced in the same direction as the wave propagation through the medium

Loudness the property of sound that allows sounds to be ordered on a scale extending from quiet (soft) to loud; loudness depends mainly on the intensity of sound

Loudness level the level of a sound that is judged to be equally loud compared to a reference sound; loudness level is measured in phons

Loudness scale a psychophysical scale in which the loudness of sound is quantified as a function of sound intensity; an example of the loudness scale is the sone scale

Loudspeaker an electroacoustic transmitter that converts audio signals into acoustic waves propagating through space

Loudspeaker system one or more loudspeakers working in the same enclosure

Low-pass filter filter that passes the low-frequency energy and does not pass the high-frequency energy

Lumped property a property of an electric circuit that is concentrated in one or several discrete locations

Mach number the ratio of the speed of an aircraft to the speed of sound

Macula the vestibular sense organ located within the utricle and saccule that responds to linear acceleration of the body or body position relative to gravity

Magnetic field force field created by moving electric charge

Magnetic force the push or pull exerted by a magnetic field

Magnetism the property of matter that results from the movement of charged particles, such as electrons, through the matter

Magnitude the quantity or extent of a property of an object

Malleus one of the bones of the inner ear, attached at one end to the tympanic membrane and at the other end to the incus; known as the hammer in nonprofessional terms

Manubrium of the malleus the most lateral aspect of the manubrium, which attaches to the tympanic membrane

Masking the ability of one sound (the masker) to completely block out or to decrease the audibility of another sound (the maskee)

Mass (*m*) the amount of matter that is present in a substance

Mass reactance (X_m) the ability of a mass to store energy and prevent its transmission through a system

Mass susceptance (B_m) the ease with which energy flows through a mass

Mastoid air cells air pockets that resemble a honeycomb within the mastoid portion of the temporal bone; surround the antrum

Maximum (undistorted) input signal the highest sound pressure (in Pa or dB SPL) that the microphone is capable of converting into an electric signal without nonlinear distortion

Maximum continuous output signal the greatest sound pressure level that can be continuously produced by a loudspeaker

Mean magnitude see **average magnitude**

Mechanic impedance impedance of a mechanic system; depends on the mass, stiffness, and friction coefficient of the system

Mechanic disturbance any event that causes a change in a medium at a specific location

Mechanic wave the transfer of mechanic energy from one molecule to another

Medial toward the middle

Medial geniculate body see **medial geniculate nucleus**

Medial geniculate nucleus nucleus in the thalamus that receives ascending auditory fiber projections from the inferior colliculus and from which fibers project to various parts of the cortex and cerebrum, most importantly to Heschl's gyrus (the primary auditory cortex)

Medial olivocochlear bundle (MOCB) efferent neurons that project from the periolivary nuclei near the medial superior olivary nucleus to the inner ear; these projections are primarily contralateral and synapse directly on the outer hair cells

Medial olivocochlear neurons see **medial olivocochlear bundle**

Medial superior olivary (MSO) nucleus one of two relatively large nuclei (the medialmost) located in the superior olivary complex

Medium a substance (matter) that occupies a space; a solid, fluid, or gas

Medulla see **medulla oblongata**

Medulla oblongata the most rostral portion of the spinal cord, contiguous with the spinal cord at the foramen magnum

Mel scale the scale relating frequency and pitch

Membrane a thin sheet-like material that is stretched and fixed along its edges to create stiffness

Membranous labyrinth an endolymph-filled structure enclosed by a membrane that is located within the bony labyrinth and that follows the curves and coils of the bony labyrinth; the membranous labyrinth contains the semicircular ducts, utricle, saccule, and cochlea, which are connected via various small communication channels

Mesencephalic aqueduct see **cerebral aqueduct**

Mesencephalon see **midbrain**

Mesotympanum the middle portion of the tympanic cavity

Metathetic continuum qualitative sensations for which a change in the stimulus elicits a change in the similarity (or dissimilarity) between two sensations rather than a change in the magnitude of sensation

Method of Adjustment a psychophysical method of threshold determination in which a listener manually adjusts test stimuli in a series of trials until the threshold has been determined

Method of Constant Stimuli a psychophysical method of threshold determination in which the value of the stimulus in individual trials is determined at random

Method of Limits a psychophysical method of threshold determination in which a stimulus is gradually increased and decreased by an examiner until the threshold has been obtained

Mho the traditional unit of admittance; mho is *ohm* spelled backwards, to indicate admittance is the inverse of impedance; the current term is *siemens*

Midbrain the most superior portion of the brainstem

Middle ear an air-filled cavity (about 2 cm^3 in volume) called the tympanic cavity or tympanum containing the ossicles

Middle ear mechanism see **inertial middle ear mechanism**

Midrange loudspeaker a loudspeaker that transmits midfrequency sounds

Minimal damping the amount of damping that allows a system to make several back-and-forth motions before retuning to its equilibrium position

Minimum audible angle (MAA) the smallest detectable difference in sound source location for stationary sound sources

Minimum audible movement angle (MAMA) the smallest detectable change in an angular location of a moving sound source

Missing fundamental when the greatest common factor of a group of harmonically related frequency components of a waveform is not present in the waveform, this waveform has a missing fundamental

MKS System (Metric System) the current international standard for physical measurement in which the meter, kilogram, and second are the basis for measurement

Mode the specific vibration pattern of a vibrating system associated with each resonance frequency of the system

Modiolus the central bony channel of the cochlea within which the spiral ganglia are located

Momentum (M) the product of mass (*m*) and velocity (*v*) of a moving object; that is, $M = m \times v$

Monaural related to one ear

Monaural localization cues localization cues that are created by the reflection and refraction of sound by the folds, cavities, and ridges of the outer ear

Monophonic system a single-channel audio system

Monopole sound source a pulsating sphere with a fixed center in space and a radius (*r*) that varies in a periodic pattern

Motility function see **electromotility**

Motor action see **electromotility**

N-Alternative Forced Choice (nAFC) a technique for determining threshold in which a listener is presented with a number (*n*) of observation intervals, one of which contains a signal, and the listener must select the interval that contained the signal

Narrowband noise a noise with acoustic energy concentrated in a relatively narrow band of frequencies

Nasopharyngeal cavity the upper part of the throat, behind the nasal cavity

Nasopharynx see **nasopharyngeal cavity**

Natural frequency see **resonance frequency**

Near sound field a sound field in which a large sound source acts as the sum of various small parts and the sound waves produced by different parts interfere with each other creating large and nonuniform local maxima and minima in acoustic pressure

Negative feedback loop a system in which the output signal is used to control the gain

Negative pole a pole that attracts positive energy

Nerve a collection of neurons that are bundled together, forming a communication pathway

Nerve fiber a thread-like extension that comes out of a cell body

Nerve impulse see **compound action potential**

Network a structure of various devices, circuits, and elements that are connected and operate together; a network can be wired or wireless

Neural potential see **action potential**

Neuron a cell that is capable of transmitting electrochemical information within the nervous system of the body

Neurotransmitter a chemical messenger that is released from the synaptic vesicles of a presynaptic membrane, travels across a synaptic cleft, and binds to specialized receptor cells on the postsynaptic membrane; this results in the transmission of information from one neuron to another, from a sense organ to a neuron, or from a neuron to a cell capable of a motor response

Neutron one of three particles that make up an atom; electrically neutral (it does not hold any charge)

Newton (N) the amount of force that causes a 1-kg mass to accelerate to 1 meter/s in 1 second

Newton's First Law of Motion an object at rest will remain at rest and an object in motion will remain in motion and move with uniform velocity unless acted upon by an external force

Newton's Second Law of Motion an object's acceleration is proportional to the force exerted on the object and inversely proportional to the mass of the object; that is, $F = M \times a$

Newton's Third Law of Motion for every action there is an equal and opposite reaction

Nibble half of a byte

Node a point or line in space or along a vibrating element at which the magnitude of displacement is zero for that mode of vibration

Noise an aperiodic vibration; a complex vibration that consists of energy spread across a range of frequencies rather than consisting of discrete frequency components that are harmonically related; unwanted sound

Nondirectional sound source a sound source that does not have any privileged direction of sound radiation; monopole sound source

Nonlinear device (amplifier) a device (amplifier) in which the shape of the output signal depends on the amplitude of the input signal

Nonlinear distortions signal deformations produced by nonlinear devices

Nonreciprocal transducer transducers that only convert energy in one direction

Nonreversible transducer see **nonreciprocal transducer**

Nonstationary noise a noise in which the spectrum and intensity change randomly over time and space and in which the average value cannot be reasonably predicted

Normal distribution see **Gaussian distribution**

Notch of Rivinus a tiny interruption in the tympanic sulcus

NP junction the junction between an N-type semiconductor and a P-type semiconductor; an N-type semiconductor has a surplus of electrons and a P-type semiconductor has a deficit of electrons

Nucleus a group of cell bodies in the central nervous system

Nucleus of the trapezoid body a collection of cell bodies located in the ventral acoustic stria (trapezoid body)

Nyquist frequency the highest frequency in a sampled signal that can be reconstructed with no loss of information by a given converter

Nyquist-Shannon sampling theorem the theorem stating that in order for a sampled signal to represent no loss of information, the sampling rate must be at least equal to twice the highest frequency in the spectrum of the original signal

Obturator foramen the hole between the crura of the stapes

Occipital lobe the most posterior of the lobes of the brain; responsible for visual perception and processing

Occlusion effect the increase in the intensity of bone-conducted sounds caused by the occlusion (covering) of the external ear

Octave a relative unit of frequency in which one octave represents a doubling in frequency

Octopus cell a cell primarily found in the posterior ventral cochlear nucleus, with tentacle-like dendrites

Oculomotor nerve the third cranial nerve (CN III), which controls the movement of four extraocular muscles (muscles that move the eyeball): the medial, superior, and inferior rectus muscles and the inferior oblique muscle

Offset time see **decay time**

Ogive curve a generic growth curve showing changes in a living organism's response due to changes in environmental conditions (e.g., a function representing changes in the percentage of correct responses as a function of the intensity of an auditory signal)

Ohm (Ω) the unit of impedance

Ohm's Law the law describing the relationship between the voltage (*E*), resistance (*R*), and current (*I*) in DC circuits

Olive a bulge located in the ventrolateral portion of the medulla caused by the underlying inferior olivary nucleus

Olivocochlear bundle efferent nerve fiber that projects from the periolivary nuclei of the superior olivary complex to the cochlea; composed of medial olivocochlear neurons and lateral olivocochlear neurons

Omnidirectional microphone a microphone in which the output is independent of the direction of the incoming sound

Omnidirectional sound source see **nondirectional sound source**

Onset pattern a pattern of cell firing in which cells fire only at the onset of a stimulus

Onset time see **rise time**

Open space outdoor sound field with no, or relatively few, boundaries

Open system a system in which various external forces (e.g., the force of friction) can act on the system during its operation

Opposite side (of a triangle) the side of a triangle that is not part of the specific angle θ (theta)

Order of operations the precise sequence of mathematical operations that are used to simplify the form of an equation; the order of operations is (1) operations within parentheses, (2) exponential operations including log and antilog operations, (3) multiplication and division, and (4) addition and subtraction

Ordinate the vertical axis of a two-dimensional graph

Organ of Corti the sense organ of hearing that runs along the entire length of the basilar membrane; located on the scala media side of the basilar membrane

Origin the central point of a coordinate system, such as (0, 0) in a two-dimensional or (0, 0, 0) in a three-dimensional Cartesian coordinate system

Orthogonal perpendicular; at right angles

Oscillation a back-and-forth movement between two states

Oscillator an object that can be set into oscillation

Osteotympanic mechanism see **outer ear mechanism**

Osseous portion of the ear canal the inner two thirds of the ear canal in which the underlining tissue is bone rather than cartilage

Ossicles the three bones of the middle ear: the malleus, incus, and stapes

Ossicular chain see **ossicles**

Ossicular lever the anatomic lever created due to a difference in the length of the malleus and the length of the incus; as a result, the force acting at the incus is about 1.15 times (about 1.2 dB) greater than the force acting at the malleus

Ossicular-inertial mechanism see **inertial middle ear mechanism**

Otoacoustic emissions very low-intensity sounds caused by the electromotility function of the outer hair cells; these sounds can be recorded in the ear canal via signal-averaging techniques

Otoconia tiny calcium carbonate crystals located within the otolithic membrane of the maculae in the utricle and saccule

Otolithic membrane a gelatinous membrane containing otoconia; the stereocilia of the hair cells of the maculae project into the otolithic membrane and are sheared when the otolithic membrane is pulled toward gravity or moved relative to the walls of the vestibule due to inertia

Otoscope an instrument that has a narrow tip, a light, and a magnifying lens; used for examination of the ear canal and tympanic membrane (otoscopic examination)

Outer ear the externally visible portion of the ear, which consists of the pinna and the external auditory canal

Outer ear mechanism a bone conduction mechanism in which vibrations of the skull cause vibrations of the ear canal and these vibrations generate acoustic waves; if the ear canal is unoccluded (not covered), most of sound energy exits the ear canal via the external auditory meatus; if the ear canal is occluded (covered), the sound energy is transmitted to the middle ear via tympanic membrane vibrations

Outer hair cells cylindrically shaped cells in the organ of Corti that are generally arranged in three rows along the length of the basilar membrane; there are approximately 12,000 outer hair cells per ear; these cells change in length in response to voltage changes across the cell membrane

Outer spiral fibers type II afferent auditory nerve fibers that project to the outer hair cells

Outer spiral sulcus cells inner hair cells support cells that begin at the Claudius cells and continue along the spiral ligament

Out-of-phase the relationship between two waveforms of the same frequency that have different initial phases

Output impedance the electric impedance measured at the output of a transmitting device

Output signal the magnitude of the signal that exits the amplifier

Overall sound power the amount of power in the frequency range (bandwidth) of a sound

Overdamping see **heavy damping**

Oversampling a technique of sampling an analog signal at a sampling frequency much higher than twice the Nyquist frequency

Overtone a harmonic other than the fundamental frequency

Paired comparison an n-alternative force choice (nAFC) technique with two intervals (i.e., 2AFC)

Parallel circuit a circuit that forms several branches connecting the same two points

Parametric equalizer an equalizer that consists of a small set of serial or parallel tunable filters with adjustable parameters such as bandwidth, center frequency, filter slope, and so forth

Parietal lobe the most superior of the lobes of the brain; responsible for tactile and proprioceptive (body position) perception, spatial orientation, conscious taste perception, and the integration of auditory information with other sensory information (e.g., visual, tactile)

Pars flaccida the superior portion of the tympanic membrane that is relatively loose (flaccid)

Pars tensa the portion of the tympanic membrane that is stretched taut; inferior to and larger than the pars flaccida

Partial a frequency component of a complex waveform

Particle velocity (v) the velocity of a molecule vibrating at the frequency of the sound wave as it passes that place in space

Passive component an electronic component that does not require additional sources of energy to perform its functions; examples include resistors, switches, lamps, and diodes

Pauser pattern a pattern of cell firing in which cells fire in response to the onset of a stimulus, stop firing for a brief time, and resume firing at a lower level

Peak clipping signal processing in which the magnitude peaks of stronger signals are clipped off by hard limiting

Pendulum a bob suspended from a fixed point on a thin arm that can swing freely back and forth when the pendulum is displaced from its rest position

Perception the act of recognition and interpretation of a stimulus based on previous experiences

Perilymph the fluid that fills the bony labyrinth (e.g., scala vestibuli and scala tympani of the inner ear); perilymph is high in sodium (Na) and low in potassium (K)

Perimeter see **circumference**

Period the time required for the completion of one cycle of a periodic motion

Periodic motion a motion that repeats itself in regular intervals

Periodic vibration a motion that repeats itself (e.g., a vibratory motion in which an object returns to the same point in space periodically during the motion)

Periodicity the concept that a periodic wave keeps repeating itself for an infinite amount of time

Periodicity pitch the pitch of the missing fundamental

Periolivary nuclei various small nuclei in the superior olivary complex that are the origin of the olivocochlear bundle

Peripheral nervous system one part of the nervous system (the other part is the CNS), which includes the nerves peripheral to the central nervous system, including the cranial nerves

Permanent magnet a magnet formed when the motions of electrons in neighboring atoms interact in such a way that the orbital motion of all the electrons of the group is aligned along the same axis; this can be natural (e.g., magnetite) or it can be created by an external process

Permeability (μ) the ability of a magnetic field to permit flux to enter the material

Permittivity (ε) the ability of an electric field to permit flux to enter the material

Phalangeal processes projections from the Dieters' cells that project around the outer hair cells and extend to the surface of the organ of Corti

Pharyngotympanic tube see **eustachian tube**

Phase a particular stage in the cycle of motion using the angles from a circle as the unit of measure

Phase angle (θ) the angle between the reference axis and the line connecting a point of interest with the origin

Phase locking a firing pattern of the inner hair cells in which the nerve firing is synchronized with the phase of the incoming auditory signal; thus, the nerve will only fire at certain phases of a periodic signal

Phase relationship the difference between the phases of two periodic waveforms as they cycle through time

Phase shift the relationship between the phase of one waveform and another where one is considered as the point of reference

Phase spectrum a spectrum display that indicates the initial ($t = 0$) phase angle of all the spectral components as a function of frequency

Phon a unit of loudness level

Phon curve see **iso-loudness curve**

Physiology the study of function and processes (e.g., processes taking place in living organisms)

Piezoelectric microphone a microphone that uses a piezoelectric effect to convert sound into electric signal; acoustic pressure acts on a membrane that is attached to one end of a piezoelectric crystal; the piezoelectric crystal creates a voltage in response to the applied pressure

Pink noise a noise that has spectrum density that is inversely proportional to frequency

Pinna the externally visible structure of the outer ear extending out from the side of the head at about a 30° angle around the external auditory meatus (opening) of the ear canal

Pitch the property of sound that allows sounds to be ordered on a scale extending from low to high; pitch depends mainly on the frequency of sound

Place code cochlear coding of auditory signals in which the place of maximal stimulation along the basilar membrane conveys the frequency of a sound wave

Place theory of hearing the theory attempting to explain the process of hearing based on place coding

Plane a two-dimensional surface

Plane wave a wave with a wavefront that has a straight surface

Planum temporale a cortical structure located medial to the lateral fissure (covered by the operculum [edges] of the frontal, temporal, and parietal lobes) and posterior to Heschl's gyrus; responds to auditory stimuli and is considered to be an auditory association area along with Wernicke's area

Plasticity the ability of the brain to reorganize itself in response to stimulation and learning

Plate a two-dimensional physical object in which the thickness of the object is much smaller than the length and width and it can vibrate without any structured support

PN junction see **NP junction**

Polar coordinate system a system for locating points in two-dimensional (plane) or in three-dimensional space including the distance of the line from the point in the space to the origin of the system and one (two-dimensional space) or two (three-dimensional space) angles created between the reference lines and the line connecting the point with the origin

Polarization the specific organization of invisible lines of force connecting the two opposing poles of the source of the field and organizing particles of matter along these lines; present in both electric and magnetic fields

Pole a contact that can be closed or opened in a switch; also a concentration of an electric charge

Pons the middle portion of the brainstem, between the medulla and the midbrain and ventral to the cerebellum; the fourth ventricle is located between the pons and cerebellum

Pontomedullary junction the junction between the pons and the medulla where the vestibulocochlear nerve enters the brainstem

Positive pole a pole that attracts negative energy

Postcentral gyrus parietal lobe gyrus located immediately posterior to the central sulcus; responsible for perception of sensation

Posterior toward the back

Posterior ligament of the incus a ligament that attaches the incus to the posterior wall of the tympanic cavity

Posterior semicircular canal one of the three canals of the vestibular system; the canals contain the cristae ampullares, which function to detect angular acceleration of the body; the posterior semicircular canal is orthogonal to the anterior semicircular canal on the same side and parallel to the anterior semicircular canal on the opposite side

Posterior ventral cochlear nucleus (PVCN) one portion of the cochlear nucleus; receives auditory nerve projections and gives rise to the intermediate acoustic stria

Potential difference see **electric potential difference**

Potential difference (*E*) see **electromotive force**

Potential energy (E_p) the energy of an object due to its position within a given physical system or environment

Potentiometer resistors that offer adjustable resistance that can be changed by rotating a dial or moving a slider attached to the resistor

Power (*P*) the rate at which a system gains or loses energy

Power amplifier an amplifier designed to maximize the power transfer to its electric load by matching the impedance of the load to its output impedance

Power ground see **earth ground**

Power handling capability the maximum continuous electrical power that the loudspeaker can handle without being damaged or producing nonlinear distortions

Power level the logarithm of the ratio of two powers

Power rating see **power handling capability**

Power spectrum a distribution of energy (power) as a function of frequency

Power spectrum density the average value of the power spectrum in a specific frequency band; that portion of the signal power contained in a 1-Hz wide bandwidth

Power spectrum density level a logarithmic measure of the power spectrum density expressed in dB in relation to some reference level (e.g., 10^{-12} W/m^2)

Power-of-10 notation see **scientific notation**

Preamplifier a low-noise, high-sensitivity amplifier that is used to amplify small input signals to the level acceptable for line amplifiers or power amplifiers

Precentral gyrus frontal lobe gyrus located immediately anterior to the central sulcus; responsible for coding of voluntary muscle movements

Pressure microphone an omnidirectional microphone that responds uniformly to all directions of incoming sounds without any correction for the changes in the sound pressure level caused by presence of the microphone in the sound field

Pressure transformer (of the middle ear) the pressure increase that results because of the size difference between the tympanic membrane and oval window; the tympanic membrane is 17 times larger than the oval window and this ratio results in about 17 times (about 25 dB) greater pressure at the oval window than the pressure at the tympanic membrane

Prestin a protein located in the outer hair cell wall that is associated with outer hair cell motility

Primary (afferent) ascending pathway the primary pathway containing ascending fibers from the peripheral auditory system to the cortex

Primary auditory area (A1) see **Heschl's gyrus**

Primary auditory cortex see **Heschl's gyrus**

Primary motor cortex see **precentral gyrus**

Primary somatosensory cortex see **postcentral gyrus**

Primary-like pattern a pattern of cell firing in which central auditory nervous system cells fire in a pattern that is similar to the signal in the auditory nerve

Probability (p) the likelihood that an event will occur under specific circumstances

Processing algorithm a computer program containing a set of instructions for the manipulation of a digital signal; processing algorithms are loaded into and stored in the permanent read-only memory (ROM) of a microprocessor

Propagation the process of conveying energy through space via a wave motion

Prothetic continuum quantitative sensations that vary in the quantity or magnitude of the sensation in response to a change in the stimulus

Proton one of three particles that make up an atom; carries a positive charge

Proximity effect increase in low-frequency emphasis of an auditory signal caused when a talker holds a directional microphone very close to the mouth

Psychoacoustician someone who studies human response to sound

Psychoacoustics the study of human response to sound; the study of the relationship between the acoustic stimuli and the sensation and perception of these stimuli

Psychometrics a branch of psychology that deals with measurement of psychological variables such as sensations, perceptions, aptitudes, and intelligence

Psychometry see **psychometrics**

Psychophysical measurement the measurement of sensation caused by a physical stimulus

Psychophysics the study of the relationship between the physical world and the perceptual world across all of the senses: hearing, taste, vision, smell, and touch

Pure tone a tone that has only one frequency component

Pyramidal eminence a bony projection of the posterior wall containing a tunnel from which the tendon of the stapedius muscle emerges

Pyramids prominent fiber bundles at the ventral surface of the medulla oblongata composed of descending motor fibers from the corticospinal tract

Pythagorean Theorem mathematical theorem stating that the sum of the squares of the two shorter sides of a right triangle are equal to the square of the hypotenuse

Quadrupole sound source a sound source consisting of two adjacent and out-of-phase dipole sound sources

Quality factor (Q) the ratio of the center frequency to the bandwidth of a resonance curve (response) curve of a system

Quantization the process of representing the instantaneous magnitude of a sound by one number from a limited set of predetermined normalized values called quantized levels

Quantization error any difference between the actual amplitude of an analog signal and the derived amplitude of the digital signal

Radial mode mode of vibration that runs across a plate or membrane

Radian a unit of the magnitude of an angle; 1 radian is the angle of a circle that is subtended by a segment of a circle equal in length to the radius of the circle

Radius (*r*) a line drawn from the central point of the circle or the sphere to any point on the circle or the sphere

Random incidence microphone an omnidirectional pressure microphone that responds uniformly to sound arriving simultaneously from all directions; response is corrected to compensate for the presence of the microphone in the sound field

Random process a process in which the outcome of an event is determined solely by chance

Random sound see **noise**

Rarefaction spreading of particles in a medium resulting in decreased density

Reactance the opposition of a system to a change in its state by the system's ability to store energy and prevent its transfer to or from another system

Reciprocal transducer transducers that can convert energy in both directions

Recognition threshold the lowest intensity of a stimulus at which the stimulus can be recognized a specific percentage of time, usually 50%

Reconstruction filter see **anti-imaging filter**

Reference level the value used as a reference magnitude in a ratio scale; the zero point of a relative scale

Receiver operating characteristic (ROC) the function showing the relationship between the hit rate and the false response rate; the function varies based on the value of d'

Reference point see **reference level**

Reflected sound wave sound wave that has "bounced" off a barrier back into the original medium in the opposite direction but at the same angle as an incidence wave

Reflection see **sound reflection**

Reflection coefficient the effectiveness of a boundary in reflecting sound waves; the ratio of the intensity of the reflected energy to the intensity of the incident wave

Refracted sound wave a sound wave that has bent around a boundary or has bent due to changes in the medium properties

Refraction see **sound refraction**

Reissner's membrane the membrane that separates the scala media from the scala vestibuli

Relative difference the ratio of two quantities

Relative measurement measurements involving relative differences (e.g., the ratio, a division) between two quantities

Resistance the opposition of a system to movement; resistance is the result of internal and external friction

Resistor electric component that provides a specified resistance

Resonance the state of a vibrating system in which no external force acts on the system and the system vibrates at its own frequency

Resonance curve a function showing the dependence of the amplitude of vibration of a vibrating system on the frequency of the driving force

Resonance frequency the frequency of the free back-and-forth motion (vibration, oscillation) of a system; the frequency at which a vibrating system moves back and forth when left alone

Response bias an internal criterion that dictates how a person will respond to a specific task under the condition of uncertainty

Response criterion (β) see **response bias**

Resting potentials a difference in electric charge between two areas in the human body (i.e., bioelectric potential) that exists in the natural state of an organism without the need for external stimulation

Reticular lamina the upper surface of the organ of Corti formed by the tops of the hair cells and supporting cells; the hair cell stereocilia project through this into the endolymph of the scala media

Reverberant sound field a sound field in which sound energy reflected from space boundaries dominates the sound energy propagating directly from the sound source

Reverberation multiple reflections of sound energy from the boundaries of an enclosed space

Reverberation chamber closed spaces with highly reflective surfaces that result in multiple strong reflections of sound energy from the space boundaries

Reverberation time the time needed for a sound pressure to decrease in intensity by 1000 times (60 dB) after the sound source has ceased its operation

Reverse-biased junction a PN junction in which the orientation of a voltage works against the natural potential difference of the junction

Reversible transducer see **reciprocal transducer**

Right ear advantage a slightly better speech recognition ability in listeners when sound is directed to the right ear compared to the left ear; attributed to the routing of a signal from the right ear to the left hemisphere, which is the language-dominant hemisphere in most people

Right triangle a triangle containing a right (90°) angle

Rise time the time needed for a waveform to change from 10% to 90% of its peak value

Rod a rigid one-dimensional structure made of a material, such as metal or wood, which has a small cross section in comparison to its length and is round

Rods (pillars) of Corti relatively rigid support cells in the organ of Corti that form a triangular tunnel between the inner and outer hair cells

Root mean square (RMS) value the quantity that characterizes the average power of a signal over a specific time period; if a signal *x* is broken down into a set of values corresponding to *n* consecutive moments in time (i.e., $x_1, x_2, \ldots, x_n$), the RMS magnitude (x_{rms}) is equal to x_i squared, averaged over a specific time period, and then the square root of this average value is determined

Rosenthal's canal channel in the center of the modiolus through which the auditory nerve fibers travel

Row-to-row cross-links fibers that connect adjacent stereocilia in different stereocilia rows on a hair cell

Saccule one of the two parts of the vestibule; contains a sense organ called a macula that responds to linear acceleration and head position relative to gravity

Safety ground see earth ground

Sagittal a cut that divides the body into right and left parts; if exactly on the midline, it is called a median sagittal cut; if to one side of midline, it is described as parallel to median sagittal or parasagittal

Sampling the process of measuring the magnitude of an analog signal at specific moments in time

Sampling rate the number of times per second the magnitude of an analog signal is measured

Saturation level a signal level beyond which further increases in the input signal do not affect the intensity of the output signal; see also **saturation point**

Saturation point the intensity level at which a hair cell or nerve cell is responding at its maximum level; intensity increases beyond this level will not increase the firing rate of the cell

Scala media the cochlear portion of the membranous labyrinth

Scala tympani one part of the cochlear portion of the bony labyrinth; the scala tympani extends along the length of the cochlea from the helicotrema to the round window

Scala vestibuli one part of the cochlear portion of the bony labyrinth; the scala vestibuli extends along the length of the cochlea from the vestibule to the helicotrema

Scalar a physical characteristic for which it is sufficient to provide a magnitude and a unit

Scale a graded measure of a specific sensation in which a faint sensation is located on one end of the scale and an increase in the degree of stimulation is associated with a point farther along the scale

Scaphoid fossa a groove underneath the curve of the helix

Scientific notation a way of representing very large or very small numbers in a condensed form, $a \times 10^n$, where a is a number equal to or greater than 1 but smaller than 10 and n is an exponent

Section a cut or slice in a specimen

Semicircular canals three canals of the vestibular system (anterior, posterior, and lateral), each of which contains a sense organ (crista ampullaris) that responds to angular acceleration of the body

Semiconductor a material that conducts electricity under some conditions but not under others

Semiconductor diode a simple semiconductor junction (PN or NP) that is not polarized

Sensation the awareness of an external stimulus or a change in the internal state of the body caused by an external stimulus

Sensation level (SL) a logarithmic measure, expressed in dB SL, of the ratio of the actual sound pressure to the threshold of hearing of the listener

Sensation magnitude the perceptual magnitude of a sensation caused by a physical stimulus

Series circuit a circuit in which all of the components are connected to each other in a series (i.e., in one loop)

Shearing motion the lateral motion of hair cell stereocilia that results in the opening and closing of mechanically gated ion channels in the membrane of the stereocilia

Shelf equalizers device that changes the proportion between low- and high-frequency energy in the sound spectrum

Shielding a method of reducing unwanted currents (caused by interfering electromagnetic fields) in an electric device by surrounding the circuit with a protective metal cover (shield)

Side-to-side cross-link a fiber that connects adjacent stereocilia in the same row of a hair cell

Siemens (S) a unit of admittance; the reciprocals of ohms

Sigma-delta conversion a special sampling scheme used in hearing aids; relies on oversampling

Signal compressor a device that decreases the dynamic range of the input signal in order to limit the output signal of the device

Signal controller device that adjusts the signal intensity, mixes signals, and directs signals toward specific outputs

Signal distortion a change in an audio signal that was not intended

Signal expander a device that expands the dynamic range of the input signal in order to improve the signal-to-noise ratio of the output signal

Signal limiter a device that limits the output signal by soft or hard clipping of its large values

Signal monitor a device that acquires and displays information about signal properties such as level, spectral content, and so forth

Signal processing the act of changing a signal according to some rules

Signal processing device see **signal processor**

Signal processor a device that modifies a signal

Signal transducer a device that converts energy from one form to another

Signal transformation a modification of an original input signal leading to a desired change in the output signal; an operation made by a signal-processing device

Signal-to-noise ratio the ratio of some measured aspect of a signal to some measured aspect of concurrent noise; usually expressed in a logarithmic form (i.e., x dB SNR)

Simple harmonic motion see **sinusoidal motion**

Simple vibration a vibration that has a sinusoidal form

Simplification the step-by-step process for making an equation progressively simpler

Simultaneous masking the masking resulting from the presence of two or more sounds presented at the same time

Sinusoidal motion the motion of an object in which changes in displacement, velocity, and acceleration are sinusoidal functions of time

Slope the incline (slant) of a line; expressed by the equation $slope = \frac{\Delta y}{\Delta x}$

Snell's Law the relationship between the speed of wave propagation and the angle of refraction

Soft signal limiter a signal-limiting device that gradually increases the amount of signal that is clipped off; soft limiting results in less noticeable signal distortion than hard limiting

Soma cell body

Sone a unit of loudness; 1 sone is defined as the loudness of a 1000-Hz tone with an intensity level of 40 dB SPL

Sone scale the most common loudness scale based on the sone

Sound a disturbance in an elastic medium that propagates through the medium as a longitudinal wave motion; a stimulus that causes an auditory sensation; an auditory sensation

Sound absorption a loss of sound energy as a sound wave is propagating through a medium, which results from absorption by the medium (internal absorption) and absorption by space barriers (external absorption)

Sound diffraction the bending of sound waves around barriers

Sound energy see **acoustic energy**

Sound field a space containing sound waves

Sound intensity the amount of sound power that travels through a specific area of the wavefront surface

Sound intensity level (IL) a logarithmic measure of the ratio of a specific sound intensity (I_2) to a reference sound intensity of 10^{-12} W/m^2 and expressed in decibels as

$$IL = 10 \times \log\left(\frac{I_2}{10^{-12}\frac{W}{m^2}}\right)$$

Sound interference the combination of two or more propagating sound waves; if overlapping waves of the same wavelength are in-phase, constructive interference occurs, and if the two waves are out-of-phase, destructive interference occurs

Sound level logarithm of the ratio of two sound intensities

Sound pressure see **acoustic pressure**

Sound pressure level (SPL) a logarithmic measure of the ratio of a specific sound pressure (p_2) and a reference sound pressure of 20 μPa and expressed in decibels as SPL $= 20 \times \log\left(\frac{p_2}{20\mu Pa}\right)$

Sound quality the property of sound that allows a human listener to scale sounds along emotional continua; sound quality can be measured on various quality scales such as pleasantness, clarity, annoyance, and so forth

Sound reflection the bouncing of sound waves off a boundary

Sound refraction the bending of sound waves due to a change in the speed of sound wave propagation; caused by sound waves entering a different medium or changes in temperature or wind

Sound source a mechanic disturbance that produces a sound

Sound wave a mechanic longitudinal wave propagating across a matter

Space of Nuel a perilymph-filled space surrounding the outer hair cells

Spatial orientation the act or process of determining the position of a sound source in space including its directional coordinates (azimuth and elevation) and the distance of the sound source from the listener

Spatial unmasking see **binaural squelch**

Specific acoustic impedance the opposition of a medium to the propagation of sound energy through the medium

Spectral analysis see **Fourier analysis**

Spectral envelope the overall outline of a spectrum as it changes across frequency

Spectrum a graphical representation of a complex waveform showing the distribution of waveform energy among its individual components; displayed as a function of frequency

Spectrum analysis see **Fourier analysis**

Spectrum component an individual sinusoidal element of a spectrum (displayed as a line in a line spectrum) with its length proportional to the amplitude of the element and located at a specific frequency

Spectrum envelope see **spectral envelope**

Spectrum level see **power spectrum density level**

Speech range the frequency range of speech sounds; 95% of speech energy is contained with the range from 80 to 12,000 Hz

Speed (*v*) the rate at which an object moves

Speed of sound (*c*) the rate at which sound energy propagates through a medium

Spherical wave a wave that propagates in all directions in space in the shape of an expanding sphere; the sound wave produced by a monopole sound source

Spinal cord the bundle of nerves extending from the base of the skull (where it is contiguous with the medulla of the brainstem) down the back; the point of origin for 31 pairs of spinal nerves that supply sensory and motor innervation to the body

Spiral ganglia the collection of cell bodies of the afferent auditory nerves; located in Rosenthal's canal within the modiolus of the cochlea

Spiral lamina a spiral, corkscrew-shaped bony shelf that projects from the side of the modiolus and partially divides the cochlear tunnel into smaller sections

Spiral ligament a ligament that connects the basilar membrane with the lateral wall of the body labyrinth

Spiral limbus the medial attachment point for Reissner's membrane

Standing wave a special case of wave interference in which sound bounces between two reflected parallel surfaces producing nodes and antinodes that are identical in nature to those observed in mechanical systems (e.g., strings)

Stapedius muscle a muscle located within the posterior wall of the tympanic cavity; the stapedius ligament attached to this muscle emerges from the wall of the middle ear and attaches to the neck of the stapes bone

Stapes the most medial and smallest of the middle ear bones; known as the stirrup in nonprofessional terms

Static electricity an electric charge that has accumulated at one specific location

Stationary noise a random sound that has average acoustic properties that do not vary over time or location in space

Steady-state time the time period during which a waveform has a relatively constant (steady) amplitude

Stem the base (foot, bottom) of a tuning fork that supports two emerging tines

Stereocilia tiny hair-like projections from one end of a hair cell that are responsible for changing mechanical motion into electrochemical impulses that can be transmitted by the nervous system

Stereocilia bundle a group of stereocilia on the top of each hair cell

Stereophonic system an audio system with several channels that transmit correlated signals carrying spatial information about some real or imaginary space

Stevens' Power Law the law stating that the magnitude of a sensation (*R*) increases based on the product of a constant (*k*) and the $\log_a$ of the stimulus magnitude, such that $R = k \times I^{\beta}$

Stiffness (*K*) a mechanic property of an elastic body that describes its opposition to a change in its dimensions by an external force; the inverse of compliance (*C*)

Stiffness reactance (X_c) the ability of the stiffness of a system to store energy and oppose its passage through a system

Stiffness susceptance (B_s) the ease at which energy travels through a spring element

Stimulus magnitude the strength of a physical stimulus (e.g., sound intensity)

Stimulus-related potential electrical potentials that are generated by stimulation

Stochastic process see **random process**

Stochastic sound see **noise**

Stria of Held see **intermediate acoustic stria**

Stria of Monaco see **dorsal acoustic stria**

Stria vascularis the vascular strip located on the lateral wall of the scala media

Striola the curved central line down the middle of each macula; on either side of the striola, hair cell kinocilium are oriented in opposite directions

Substitution the act of replacing something with something else (e.g., replacing a variable with a constant)

Subthalamus a small portion of the thalamus concerned with sensorimotor, association, and limbic functions

Subwoofer loudspeaker a loudspeaker that transmits very low-frequency sounds, usually in the 20-Hz to 150-Hz range

Sulcus a groove or valley in a cortex

Summating potential a direct current potential of the inner ear present during ear stimulation by a sound wave of sufficient intensity

Supercardioid microphone microphone that provides about 8.7 dB of attenuation for sounds arriving from the sides and about 11.4 dB at the rear; two directions of maximum sound rejection at 125° and 235°

Superior toward the top

Superior olivary complex a group of nuclei in the CANS located in the pons; the first location in the CANS that receives projections from both ears; this center plays a major role in coding for localization

Superior semicircular canal see **anterior semicircular canal**

Superior temporal gyrus the most superior of the three lateral temporal gyri; the posterior two thirds of the superior temporal gyrus, plus portions of the planum temporal, make up Wernicke's area

Supra aural earphone earphone placed over the ear and resting on the antihelix/helix of the pinna

Supramarginal gyrus parietal lobe gyrus located just above the posterior end of the lateral fissure; appears to integrate auditory information with other sensory information

Surface wave a mechanical wave motion observed on the surface of water; composed of both transverse and longitudinal vibration patterns

Susceptance (*B*) the ease with which energy travels through a mass or spring (stiffness) element in a system; the inverse (reciprocal) of reactance (*X*)

Sylvian fissure see **lateral fissure**

Symbol a conventional sign representing an object or an action

Synapse a junction between nerves through which neurotransmitter travels for communication

Synaptic cleft space between neurons

Synthesized signal a signal created by the combination of other signals

Tectorial membrane a membrane that extends from the spiral limbus out into the scala media over the entire organ of Corti, making contact with the tallest tips of the outer hair cell stereocilia

Tectum roof of the midbrain

Tegmen tympani the superior wall of the tympanum, a thin plate of bone separating the middle ear from the cranial cavity

Telencephalon the largest part of the brain; composed of large cerebral hemispheres that are divided into four large lobes-frontal, parietal, occipital, and temporal-and two smaller "lobes"-limbic and insular; the telencephalon undertakes the processing of conscious thoughts and intellectual functions, controls the initiation of body movement, and perceives sensations

Temperature gradient a change in temperature of the medium (e.g., with altitude)

Temporal code cochlear coding of auditory signals in which the rate of firing of hair cells and nerve fibers codes information about an auditory stimulus for transmission from the cochlea to the central nervous system

Temporal envelope the overall outline of a waveform as it changes over time

Temporal lobe the most lateral of the lobes of the brain; responsible for auditory processing, comprehension of language, higher order processing of visual information (e.g., recognizing faces or facial expression), and aspects of learning and memory (in combination with other brain centers including the hippocampus)

Temporal masking a masking paradigm in which two sounds arrive at a listener in a quick succession and the presence of one sound masks the other; includes forward masking and backward masking

Temporomandibular joint the jaw joint; anterior to the ear canal

Tensor tympani muscle a muscle located in the anterior wall of the middle ear; the tendon of the tensor tympani attaches to this muscle and emerges from the wall of the middle ear and attaches to the malleus

Tensor veli palatini muscle a muscle located in the soft tissue of the nasopharynx; attached to the cartilaginous portion of the eustachian tube; contraction of this muscle opens the cartilaginous portion of the eustachian tube during yawning and swallowing

Terminal threshold the threshold indicating the maximum value of a stimulus that elicits a given response (e.g., the terminal threshold for auditory sensation is the maximum intensity level at which a response is perceived as sound instead of pain)

Test stimulus a physical stimulus used in psychophysical studies

Thalamus the largest part of the diencephalon; responsible for directing all sensory information (except olfaction) to the proper area of the cerebrum; the medial geniculate nucleus of the CANS is part of the thalamus

Thermal effect the effect of bending sound waves away from the ground when warmer air is closer to the ground and colder air is above it

Thermal noise noise generated by the elements involved in signal transmission

Threshold the point at which the intensity level of a stimulus is just large enough to cause a change in the mental response of a person affected by the stimulus

Threshold of hearing the minimum value of an auditory stimulus that is detectable a specific percentage of the time (usually 50%)

Throw one of the positions of a switch during its operation

Timbre an attribute of auditory sensation by which a listener can judge that two sounds having the same loudness and pitch are different; the key factor permitting sound source recognition; varies with the spectral complexity of the sound

Time constant the time it takes for the amplitude of vibration to decrease by approximately 63%; a vibrating system is considered to cease its vibrations after the elapse of three time constants

Time domain representation of a phenomenon as a function of time

Time envelope see **temporal envelope**

Tip-to-side cross-link a fiber that connects adjacent stereocilia between the top (smaller cell) and the side (larger cell) of adjacent stereocilia across rows on a hair cell

Tissue a group of cells of unique structure and function

Tone a sound that has one (pure tone) or a finite (complex tone) number of distinct frequency components

Tonotopic organization the correspondence between stimulation frequency and place of stimulation along the cochlea

Tonotopicity see **tonotopic organization**

Total internal reflection a situation in which 100% of the sound energy reaching a boundary is reflected back into the original medium; total internal reflection occurs at the critical angle of incidence

Tragus a small cartilaginous projection of the pinna that is immediately anterior to the external auditory meatus

Trained listener a human listener who has been trained to listen to a specific stimulus and is, in general, more sensitive to specific changes in the stimulus than an untrained listener

Transducer a device that changes energy from one form to another

Transfer function the relationship between the magnitude of the output signal and the magnitude of the input signal

Transformer a device that matches the electric impedances of two AC circuits

Transformer ratio (*r*) the ratio of the numbers of wire turns in the secondary coil (N_s) and the primary coil (N_p) of a transformer such that $r = \frac{N_s}{N_p}$ of a transformer

Transient a short, aperiodic fragment at the beginning and the end of a periodic waveform; a state of motion that lasts only a very short time; it is normally seen after setting a system into vibration and after removing the driving force from a system

Transistor semiconductor active device that functions as an amplifier in analog systems and as a switch in digital systems

Transmitted noise noise in an audio signal that is received along with the signal of interest

Transverse cut that divides the body into top and bottom parts

Transverse fissure fissure that separates the cerebral hemispheres from the cerebellum

Transverse temporal gyrus see **Heschl's gyrus**

Transverse wave mechanical wave in which the particles of the medium are displaced in a direction that is perpendicular to the direction of the wave propagation through the medium

Trapezoid body the ventral acoustic stria; in cross section, this stria appears as a trapezoid in shape

Traveling wave see **transverse wave**

Triangular fossa a triangle-shaped indentation formed by the crura of the antihelix

Trigeminal nerve the fifth cranial nerve (CN V), which provides sensory and motor innervation to the front of the head via three branches: ophthalmic, maxillary, and mandibular; functions related to the auditory system include sensory innervation to the tympanic membrane and motor innervation to the tensor tympani and tensor veli palatini muscles

Trochlear nerve the fourth cranial nerve (CN IV), which provides motor innervation to one of the extraocular muscles (muscles that control eyeball movement): the superior oblique muscle

Tuning curve a curve representing changes in the threshold of a hair cell or auditory nerve cell response as a function of the stimulus frequency

Tunnel of Corti a triangular-shaped support structure created by the inner and outer rods (pillars) of Corti; located between the inner and outer hair cells

Tweeter loudspeaker a loudspeaker that transmits high-frequency sounds

Tympanic cavity an air-filled cavity of the middle ear containing the ossicles

Tympanic membrane a membrane located at the medial end of the external auditory canal and forming the lateral wall of the middle ear cavity; vibrations of this membrane change acoustic waves into the mechanic vibrations of the ossicles

Tympanic sulcus a ring-shaped groove in the temporal bone that is the insertion point for the edges of the tympanic membrane

Tympanosclerosis scarring of the eardrum that appears as white patches

Tympanum see **tympanic cavity**

Type I afferent neurons relatively large myelinated nerve fibers; type I afferent auditory nerve fibers project from the inner hair cells

Type II afferent neurons relatively thin nerve fibers that are not myelinated; type II afferent auditory nerve fibers project from the outer hair cells

Umbo the tip of the cone of the tympanic membrane

Underdamping see **minimal damping**

Unidirectional microphone a microphone that is designed to receive signals from a single direction

Unipolar (rectified) average magnitude the average absolute magnitude calculated over the whole period of the waveform, that is, the average magnitude calculated after inverting the negative half of the waveform

Unit a quantity accepted as a standard of measurement against which other measured quantities are compared

Upward spread of masking low-frequency maskers are better able to mask high-frequency signals than high-frequency maskers are to mask low-frequency signals; caused by the asymmetry of the excitation pattern along the basilar membrane

Utricle one of the two parts of the vestibule; contains a sense organ called a macula that responds to linear acceleration and head position relative to gravity

Vagus nerve the 10th cranial nerve (CN X); wanders all the way from the brainstem to the large intestines providing sensory and motor innervation to a number of structures; functions related to the auditory system include sensory innervation to the outer ear and tympanic membrane

Valence shell the outer shell of an atom

Valsalva maneuver a procedure that pushes air into the middle ear cavity via the eustachian tube; the procedure involves closing the mouth, pinching the nose, and blowing, which forces the eustachian tube to open and admit air

Variable a symbol representing an unknown number

Vector a physical characteristic that is described by a magnitude, a unit, and a direction

Velocity (*v*) the rate at which an object moves in a specific direction; the rate of change in the displacement of an object (i.e., $v = \frac{\Delta d}{\Delta t}$)

Velocity microphone see **gradient microphone**

Ventral anterior (below the midbrain) or inferior (above the midbrain)

Ventral acoustic stria fiber tract originating in the anterior ventral cochlear nucleus and traveling primarily to the contralateral superior olivary complex, with projections also directly to the lateral lemniscus; also known as the trapezoid body

Ventricle one of four fluid-filled cavities within the center of the brain containing cerebrospinal fluid

Vermis the wormlike center line that divides the two hemispheres of the cerebellum

Vestibular ganglion the collection of cell bodies of the afferent vestibular nerve; located in the internal auditory canal

Vestibular-ocular reflex (VOR) a reflex that allows the eyes to stay focused on an object even when the body is moving; due to a connection between the vestibular system and the oculomotor system, which controls eyeball movement

Vestibule the part of the bony labyrinth that contains the utricle and saccule

Vestibulocochlear anastomosis see **anastomosis of Oort**

Vestibulocochlear nerve the eighth cranial nerve (CN VIII), which conveys sensory information about hearing and balance to the central auditory nervous system

Vibration a back-and-forth motion that is mechanical, with elasticity acting as the restoring force

Vibrator an object that can be set into back-and-forth motion

Volt (V) unit of electromotive force (*E*)

Voltage (*E*) see **electromotive force**

Voltage amplifier an amplifier designed to amplify the voltage of a signal

Voltage drop the decrease in voltage caused by the flow of electric current through a specific component in an electric circuit

Volume (*V*) the amount of space occupied by a substance or an object; it is a three-dimensional measure commonly reported in cubic units of length, such as cubic centimeters (cc or cm^3) or cubic meters (m^3), or in units of fluid volume, such as liters

Watt (W) the unit of power that is defined as the ability of the system to do 1 joule of work in 1 second

Wave a change in energy concentration in a medium, which travels through the space

Wave motion see **wave**

Waveform a function representing changes of any physical quantity as a function of time

Waveform analysis see **Fourier analysis**

Waveform envelope see **temporal envelope**

Waveform synthesis the process of combining several individual sinusoidal motions into a complex waveform

Wavefront the imaginary line connecting leading points (or connecting any other in-phase points) of a wave propagating through a medium

Wavelength (λ) the shortest distance in space between two adjacent identical (same phase) points of a propagating wave

Wavelet a small spherical wave created when a wave travels through openings in a barrier

Weber's fraction the smallest perceived increment in a stimulus (ΔI) divided by the reference magnitude of the stimulus (I) is equal to a constant; that is, $\frac{\Delta I}{I} = K =$ constant; this constant is dependent on the type of stimulus

Weber's Law a general property of human perception that the smallest perceived change in stimulus intensity is proportional to the stimulus magnitude

Weight the force of gravity acting on an object

Wernicke's area a specialized area located in the temporal lobe of the language-dominant hemisphere (usually left); composed of the posterior two thirds of the superior temporal gyrus and some of the surrounding tissue including parts of the planum temporale; concerned with speech comprehension; lesions in this area result in an inability to comprehend spoken language, also known as Wernicke's aphasia or receptive aphasia

White matter myelinated fiber tracts, especially those of the cerebrum

White noise a noise that consists of an infinite number of sinusoidal components having the same amplitude, but random phase, that are spread evenly across a wide frequency range; a noise that has a spectrum density that is independent of frequency

Whole nerve action potential see **compound action potential**

Wind shear an increase in wind generally observed with increasing altitude

Woofer loudspeaker a loudspeaker that transmits low-frequency sounds

Work (W) the result of using energy; the effect of force (*F*) moving an object over a distance (*d*) (i.e., $W = \frac{F}{d}$)

YN (yes no) technique a threshold testing technique in which the listener is given a number of trials with some of them containing a signal and some of them not containing a signal and the listener is asked to respond "yes" or "no" at each trial

Young's modulus of elasticity (*K*) a measure of stiffness in solid matter

Zero level see **reference level**

References

Chapter 1

Cajori F. History of Mathematics. 2nd Ed. New York: McMillan, 1919:484.

O'Connor J, Robertson E. Roger Cotes, 2005. Available at: http://www-history.mcs.st-andrews.ac.uk/Biographies/Cotes.html. Accessed June 17, 2006.

Chapter 2

Mulligan JF. Introductory College Physics. 2nd Ed. New York: McGraw-Hill, Inc., 1991.

Chapter 3

International Standards Organization (ISO). Quantities and Units—Part 8: Acoustics, ISO 8000-8. Geneva, Switzerland: ISO, 2006.

Villchur E. Acoustics for Audiologists. San Diego, CA: Singular Publishing Group, 2000.

Chapter 4

Backus J. The Acoustical Foundations of Music. 2nd Ed. New York: W. W. Norton & Company, 1977.

Ellis A. On the history of musical pitch. *J Soc Arts* 1880;March 5. Reprinted in Studies in the History of Music Pitch. Amsterdam: Frits Knuf, 1968:44.

Lantz J, Petrak M, Prigge L. Using the 1000-Hz probe tone for immittance measurements in infants. *Hear J* 2004;57(10):34–42.

Rossing T. The Science of Sound. Reading, MA: Addison-Wesley, 1989.

Chapter 5

Bannon P. The molecular dynamics of air, 1996. Available at: http://www.ems.psu.edu/~bannon/moledyn.html. Accessed October 25, 2006.

Bohn D. Environmental effects on the speed of sound. *J Audio Eng Soc* 1988;36:223–231.

Corso JF. Bone-conduction thresholds for sonic and ultrasonic frequencies. *J Acoust Soc Am* 1963;35:1738–1743.

Fujimoto K, Nakagawa S, Tonoike M. Nonlinear explanation for bone-conducted ultrasonic hearing. *Hear Res* 2005;205:210–215.

Kleppe J. Engineering Applications of Acoustics. Norwood, MA: Artech House, 1989.

Lenhardt M, Skellett R, Wang P, et al. Human ultrasonic speech perception. *Science* 1991;253:82–85.

Russell DA, Titlow JP, Bemmen YJ. Acoustic monopoles, dipoles, and quadrupoles: an experiment revisited. *Am J Phys* 1999;67(8):660–664.

Chapter 6

Bate A. Note on the whispering gallery of St Paul's Cathedral, London. *Proc Phys Soc* 1938;50:293–297.

Beranek L. Music, Acoustics, and Architecture. New York: Wiley and Sons, 1962.

Brüel PV. Lydisolation og rumakustika. Åbo, Förlaget Bro, Sweden: Chalmers Technical University Press, 1946.

Harris C. Absorption of sound in air versus humidity and temperature. *J Acoust Soc Am* 1966;40:148–159.

Heimann D. Influence of metrological parameters on outdoor noise propagation. Paper ID: 113-IP/1-6. Proceedings of the Euronoise, 2003, Naples, Italy.

Hirschorn M. IAC Noise Control Reference Handbook. New York: Industrial Acoustics Company, 1989.

Lecklider T. The world of the near field. Evaluation Engineering, October 2005. Available at: http://www.evaluationengineering.com/archive/articles/1005/1005the_world.asp. Accessed October 19, 2006.

Porges G. Applied Acoustics. Los Altos, CA: Pennisula Publishing, 1977.

Lord Rayleigh (Strutt JW). The Theory of Sound. London, U.K.: Macmillan, 1877. Reprinted by Dover, 1979.

Spotts P. Battle of the whispers: Tourist attraction is research lab to solve mystery. *USA Today* (Science) 2006; June 4.

Tyndall J. Sound: A Course of Lectures Delivered at the Royal Institution of Great Britain. New York: D. Appleton and Company, 1867. (Cited by Calvert, 2000.)

Vitruvius Pollio (90–20 BC). De architectura libri decem. English edition: Vitruvius: Ten Books on Architecture. Transl, Ingrid D. Rowland. New York: Cambridge University Press, 1999.

Weston D. Ray acoustics for fluids. In: Crocker M, ed. Encyclopedia of Acoustics. New York: John Wiley and Sons, 1997:39–54.

Chapter 7

Martin W H. The transmission unit and telephone transmission reference systems. *Bell Syst Tech J* 1924;3:400–408.

Martin WH. Decibel—The name of the Transmission Unit. *Bell Syst Tech* J 1929;8:1–2.

Chapter 8

Alvord LS, Farmer BL. Anatomy and orientation of the human external ear. *J Am Acad Audiol* 1997;8:383–390.

Barr-Hamilton RM. The cupped hand as an aid to hearing. *Br J Audiol* 1983;17:27–30.

Battista RA, Equivel C. Middle Ear, Ossiculoplasty, Nov. 11, 2005. E-medicine from WebMD. Available at: http://www.emedicine.com/ent/topic219.htm. Accessed November 11, 2006.

Borg E. A quantitative study of the effect of the acoustic stapedius reflex on sound transmission through the middle ear of man. *Acta Otlarnygol* 1968;66:461–472.

Brask T. (1979). The noise protection effect of the stapedius reflex. *Acta Otolaryngol* 1979;360(Suppl.): 116–117.

Brenkman CJ, Grote JJ, Rutten WL. Acoustic transfer characteristics in human middle ears studied by SQUID magnetometer method. *J Acoust Soc Am* 1987;82:1646–1654.

Dallos P. The Auditory Periphery. New York: Academic Press, 1973.

Donaldson JA, Duckert LG. Anatomy of the ear. In: Paparella MM, Shumrick DA, Gluckman JL, et al. (eds.). Otolaryngology. Vol 1. Basic Sciences and Related Principles. 3rd Ed. Philadelphia: W.B. Saunders, 1991.

Fumagalli Z. Richerche morfologiche sull' apparato di transmissione del suono (Morphological research on the sound-transmission apparatus). *Arch Ital Otol Rinol Laringol* 1949;60(Suppl 1):ix, 323.

Gelfand SA. Hearing: An Introduction to Psychological and Physiological Acoustics. New York: Marcel Dekker, 1990.

Gelfand SA. Essentials of Audiology. 2nd Ed. New York: Thieme, 2001.

Glasscock ME, Shambaugh GE. Surgery of the Ear. 4th Ed. Philadelphia: W.B. Saunders, 1990.

Goode RL. The ideal middle ear prosthesis. In: Huttenbrink K-B (ed.). Middle Ear Mechanics in Research and Otosurgery. Dresden: Technical University of Dresden, 1997.

Gyo K, Goode RL, Miller C. Effect of middle ear modification on umbo vibration. Human temporal bone experiments with a new vibration measuring system. *Arch Otolaryngol Head Neck Surg* 1986;112:1253–1261.

Harris JD. Anatomy and Physiology of the Peripheral Auditory Mechanism. Austin, TX: Pro-Ed, 1986.

Helmholtz H. Die Mechanic der Gehorknöchelchen und des Trommelfells. Pflüg. *Arch Ges Physiol* 1868;1:1–60.

Helmholtz HL. On the Sensations of Tone as a Physiological Basis for the Theory of Music. New York: Dover Publishing Inc., 1954.

Ishijima K, Sando I, Balanan CD, et al. Functional anatomy of levator veli palatini muscle and tensor veli palatini muscle in association with Eustachian tube cartilage. *Ann Otol Rhinol Laryngol* 2002;111:530–536.

Killion M. Revised estimate of minimum audible pressure: where is the missing 6 dB? *J Acoust Soc Am* 1978;63: 1501–1508.

Kojo Y. Morphological studies of the human tympanic membrane. *J Oto-Rhino-Laryngol Soc Japan* 1954;57: 115–126 (in Japanese).

Lim DJ. Human tympanic membrane. An ultrastructural observation. *Acta Otolaryngol* 1970;70:176–186.

Liu T-C, Chen Y-S. Aging and external ear resonance. *Audiology* 2000;39:235–237.

Lucente FE. Anatomy, histology, and physiology. In: Lucente FE, Lawson W, Novick NL (eds.). The External Ear. Philadelphia: W.B. Saunders Company, 1995.

Lynch TJ, Nedzelnitsky V, Peake WT. Input impedance of the cochlea in cat. *J Acoust Soc Am* 1982;72: 108–130.

McElveen JT, Goode RL, Miller C, et al. Effect of mastoid cavity modification on middle ear sound transmission. *Ann Otol Rhinol Laryngol* 1982;91:526–532.

Møller AR. Hearing. Its Physiology and Pathophysiology. New York: Academic Press, 2000.

Pickles JO. An Introduction to the Physiology of Hearing, 2nd Ed. New York: Academic Press, 1982.

Puria S, Peake W, Rosowski J. Sound-pressure measurements in the cochlear vestibule of human-cadaver ears. *J Acoust Soc Am* 1997;101:2754–2770.

Rosowski J. Models of external- and middle-ear function. In: Hawkins H, McMullen T, Popper A, et al. (eds.). Auditory Computation. New York: Springer Verlag, 1996:16–61.

Spector GJ, Ge X. Development of the hypotympanum in the human fetus and neonate. *Ann Otol Rhinol Laryngol* 1981;90:1–20.

Teranishi R, Shaw EAG. External ear acoustic models with simple geometry. *J Acoust Soc Am* 1968;44:257–263.

Tonndorf J, Khanna SM. The role of the tympanic membrane in middle ear transmission. Ann Otolaryngol 1970;79:743–753.

Tonndorf J, Khanna SM. Tympanic membrane vibrations in human cadaver ears studied by time-averaged holography. *J Acoust Soc Am* 1972;52:1221–1233.

Von Békésy G. Experiments in Hearing. Transl., Ed., Wever E.G. New York: McGraw-Hill, 1960.

Wever EG, Lawrence M. Physiological Acoustics. Princeton, NJ: Princeton University Press, 1954.

Zemlin WR. Speech and Hearing Science: Anatomy and Physiology. 3rd Ed. Englewood Cliffs, NJ: Prentice-Hall, Inc., 1988.

Zwislocki J. (1975). The role of the external and middle ear in sound transmission. In: Tower DB (ed.), The Nervous System. Volume 3: Human Communication and Its Disorders. New York: Raven Press, 1975:45–55.

Chapter 9

Buckingham RA, Valvassori GE. Inner ear fluid volumes and the resolving power of magnetic resonance imaging: can it differentiate endolymphatic structures? *Ann Otol Rhinol Laryngol* 2001;110:113–117.

Brownell WE, Bader CR, Bertrand D, et al. Evoked mechanical responses of isolated cochlear outer hair cells. *Science* 1985;227:194–196.

Causse R. Développments récents dans le domaine de la physiologie de l'audition. *Rev Sci Paris* 1942;80: 371–383.

Cohen A, Furst M. Integration of outer hair cell activity in a one-dimensional cochlear model. *J Acoust Soc Am* 2004;115:2185–2192.

Dallos P, Billone MC, Durrant JD, et al. Cochlear inner and outer hair cells: functional differences. *Science* 1972;177:356–358.

Dallos P, Fakler B. Prestin, a new type of motor protein. *Nat Rev Mol Cell Biol* 2002;3:104–111.

Dimopoulos P, Muren C. Anatomic variations of the cochlea and relations to other temporal bone structures. *Acta Radiol* 1990;31:439–444.

Engel J, Knirsch M, Brandt N, et al. Persistence of CAV1.3 CA^{2+} channels in mature outer hair cells suggests afferent role of OHCs in hearing. *Acta Physiol* 2006;188(Suppl. 651):13200.

Furst M, Cohen A. Prediction of inner ear properties predicted by the dynamics of the cochlear amplifiers. *J Acoust Soc Am* 1994;95:3005–3006.

Gelfand SA. Hearing: An Introduction to Psychological and Physiological Acoustics. 3rd Ed. New York: Marcel Dekker, 1998.

Gold T. Hearing II. The physical basis of the action of the cochlea. *Proc Royal Soc Brit* 1948;135:492–498.

Kellaway PE. Cochlear microphonics: a critical review. *Arch Otolaryngol* 1944;39:203–210.

Kemp DT. Stimulated acoustic emissions from within the human auditory system. *J Acoust Soc Am* 1978;64: 1386–1391.

Kennedy HJ, Crawford AC, Fettiplace R. Force generation by mammalian hair bundles supports a role in cochlear amplification. *Nature* 2005;24:880–883.

Kiang NY, Watanabe T, Thomas EC, et al. Discharge patterns of single fibers in the cat's auditory nerve. Cambridge, MA: MIT Press, 1965.

Lieberman MC. Auditory nerve response from cats raised in a low-noise chamber. *J Acoust Soc Am* 1978;63:442–455.

Lim DJ. Functional structure of the organ of Corti: a review. *Hear Res* 1986;22:117–146.

Mann M. The nervous system in action. Chapter 8: Audition, 2002. Available at: http://www.unmc. edu/Physiology/ Mann/mann8.html. Accessed December 14, 2006.

Manoussaki D, Dimitriadis EK, Chadwick RS. Cochlea's graded curvature effect on low frequency waves. *Phys Rev Lett* (online) 2006;96(8):088701.

Nordang L, Oestreicher E, Arnold W, et al. Glutamate is the afferent neurotransmitter in the human cochlea. *Acta Laryngol* 2000;120:359–361.

Pickles JO, Comis SD, Osborne MP. Cross-links between stereocilia in the guinea pig organ of Corti and their possible relation to sensory transduction. *Hear Res* 1984;15:103–112.

Polyak SL, McHugh G, Judd DK. The Human Ear in Anatomical Transparencies. New York: Sonotone Corporation, 1948.

Rhode WS. Some observations on cochlear mechanics. *J Acoust Soc Am* 1978;64:158–176.

Ricci A. Active hair bundle movements and the cochlear amplifier. *J Am Acad Audiol* 2003;14:325–338.

Rose JE, Brugge JF, Anderson DJ, et al. (1967). Phase locked response to low-frequency tones in single auditory nerve fibers of the squirrel monkey. *J Neurophysiol* 1967;30:769–793.

Rutherford E. A new theory of hearing. *J Anat Physiol* 1886;21:166–168.

Santos-Sacchi J. Cochlear physiology. In: John AF, Santos-Sacchi J (eds.). Physiology of the Ear. 2nd Ed. San Diego, CA: Singular, 2001.

Seymour JC, Tappin JW. The effect of sympathetic stimulation upon the cochlear microphonic potentials. *Proc Roy Soc* 1951;44:755–759.

Spicer SS, Schulte BA. Differences along the place-frequency map in the structure of supporting cells in the gerbil cochlea. *Hear Res* 1994;79:161–177.

Steele KP. The benefits of recycling. *Science* 1999;285: 1363–1364.

Steele KP. The tectorial membrane of mammals. *Hear Res* 1983;9:327–359.

Tasaki I, Spyropoulos CS. Stria vasularis as source of endocochlear potential. *J Neurophysiol* 1959;22(2):149–155.

Ulfendahl M, Scarfone E, Flock Å, et al. Perilymphatic fluid compartments and intercellular spaces of the inner ear and the organ of Corti. *NeuroImage* 2000;12:307–313.

Von Békésy G. Experiments in Hearing. New York: McGraw-Hill, 1960.

Von Helmholtz H. (1862, 1877, 1885). Die Lehre von den Tonempfindungen als Physiologische Grundlage für die Theorie der Musik. English translation Ellis AJ, 1885, On the Sensations of Tone. Reprinted in 1954 by Dover, New York.

Wever EG. Theory of Hearing. New York: Wiley and Sons, 1949.

Wever EG, Bray CE. Action currents in the auditory nerve in response to acoustic stimulation. *Proc Natl Acad Sci* 1930;16:344–350.

Withnell RH, Shaffer LA, Lilly DJ. What drives mechanical amplification in the mammalian cochlea? *Ear Hear* 2002;23: 49–57.

Zheng J, Shen W, He DZ, et al. Prestin is the motor protein of cochlear outer hair cells. *Nature* 2000;405:149–155.

Chapter 10

Adams JC. Neuronal morphology in the human cochlear nucleus. *Arch Otolaryngol Head Neck Surg* 1986;112: 1253–1261.

Afifi A, Bergman R. Functional Neuroanatomy. Text and Atlas. New York: The McGraw-Hill Companies, Inc., 1998.

Aitkin LM. The Auditory Cortex. London: Chapman and Hall, 1990.

Arnesen AR, Osen KK. Fibre population of the vestibulocochlear anastomosis in the cat. *Acta Otolaryngol* 1984; 98:255–269.

Cant NB. Identification of cell types in the anteroventral cochlear nucleus that project to the inferior colliculus. *Neurosci Lett* 1982;32:241–246.

Chermack GD, Musiek FE. Central Auditory Processing Disorders: New Perspectives. San Diego, CA: Singular Publishing Group, 1997.

Ehret G. The auditory cortex. *J Comparat Physiol* 1997;181:547–557.

Ferragamo MJ, Oertel D. Octopus cells of the mammalian ventral cochlear nucleus sense the rate of depolarization. *J Neurophysiol* 2002;87:2262–2270.

Gannon PJ, Holloway L, Broadfield DC, et al. Asymmetry of chimpanzee planum temporale: humanlike pattern of Wernicke's brain language area homolog. *Science* 1998;279:220–222.

Giraud AL, Garnier S, Micheyl C, et al. Auditory efferents involved in speech-in-noise intelligibility. *Neuroreport* 1997;8:1779–1783.

Golding NL, Roberston D, Oertel D. Recordings from slices indicate that octopus cells of the cochlear nucleus detect coincident firing of auditory nerve fibers with temporal precision. *J Neurosci* 1995;15:3138–3153.

Joris PX, Carney LH, Smith PH, et al. Enhancement of neural synchronization in the anteroventral cochlear nucleus. I. Responses to tones at the characteristic frequency. *J Neurophysiol* 1994;71(3):1022–1036.

Joris PX, Smith PH, Yin CT. Enhancement of neural synchronization in the anterovental cochlear nucleus. II. Responses in the tuning curve tail. *J Neurophysiol* 1994;71(3):1037–1051.

Kiang NY-S, Watanabe T, Thomas EC, et al. Discharge Patterns of Single Fibers in the Cat's Auditory Nerve. Cambridge, MA: MIT Press, 1965.

Kopp-Scheinpflug C, Dehmel S, Dörrscheidt GJ, et al. Interaction of excitation and inhibition in anteroventral cochlear nucleus neurons that receive large endbulb synaptic endings. *J Neurosci* 2002;22(24):11004–11018.

Kumar UA, Vanaja CS. Functioning of the olivocochlear bundle and speech perception in noise. *Ear Hear* 2004; 25(2):142–146.

Levy KL, Kipke DR. Mechanisms of the cochlear nucleus octopus cell's onset response: synaptic effectiveness and threshold. *J Acoust Soc Am* 1998;103(4):1940–1950.

Louage DHG, van der Heijden M, Joris PX. Enhanced temporal response properties of anteroventral cochlear nucleus neurons to broadband noise. *J Neurosci* 2005;25(6):1560–1570.

Mannell RH. The brainstem auditory nuclei and centrifugal pathways, 2002. Available at: http://www.zainea.com/The%20Brainstem%20Auditory%20Nuclei.htm. Accessed April 10, 2007.

Masterton B, Jane JA, Diamond IT. Role of brainstem auditory structures in sound localization. I: trapezoid body, superior olive, and lateral lemniscus. *J Neurophysiol* 1967;30:341–359.

Masterton B, Thompson GC, Bechtold JK, et al. Neuroanatomical basis of binaural phase-difference analysis for sound localization: a comparative study. *J Compar Physiol Psychol* 1975;89(5):379–386.

Møller AR. Hearing. Its Physiology and Pathophysiology. New York: Academic Press, 2000.

Moore JK. The human auditory brain stem: a comparative view. *Hear Res* 1987;29:1–32.

Oertel D, Bal R, Gardner SM, et al. Detection of synchrony in the activity of auditory nerve fibers by octopus cells of the mammalian cochlear nucleus. *PNAS* 2000;97(22): 11773–11779.

Ostapoff EM, Feng JJ, Morest DK. A physiological and structural study of neuron types in the cochlear nucleus. II. Neuron types and their structural correlation with response properties. *J Compar Neurol* 1994;346:19–42.

Pfeiffer RR. Classification of response patterns of spike discharges for units in the cochlear nucleus: tone burst stimulation. *Exper Brain Res* 1966;1:220–235.

Rasmussen GL. An efferent cochlear bundle. *Anat Rec* 1942;82:441.

Rayes S. Auditory system: anatomic tour, 2006. Available at: http://serous.med.buffalo.edu/hearing/auditory_cortex.html. Accessed December 14, 2006.

Rhode WS, Smith PH. Encoding timing and intensity in the ventral cochlear nucleus of the cat. *J Neurophysiol* 1986;56(2):261–286.

Sahley TL, Nodar RH, Musiek FE. Efferent Auditory System: Structure and Function. San Diego, CA: Singular Publishing, 1997.

Seikel J, King D, Drumright D. Anatomy and Physiology for Speech, Language, and Hearing. San Diego, CA: Singular, 2000.

Spoendlin H, Schrott A. Analysis of the human auditory nerve. *Hear Res* 1989;43:25–38.

Chapter 11

Berger E, Kerivan J. Influence of physiological noise and the occlusion effect on the measurement of real ear attenuation at threshold. *J Acoust Soc Am* 1983;74:81–94.

Håkansson B, Brandt A, Carlsson P. Resonance frequencies of the human skull in vivo. *J Acoust Soc Am* 1994;95: 1474–1481.

Håkansson B, Carlsson P, Tjellström A. The mechanical point impedance of the human head, with and without skin penetration. *J Acoust Soc Am* 1986;80:1065–1075.

Killion M, Wilber L, Gudmundsen G. Zwislocki was right . . . a potential solution to the "hollow voice" problem of the amplified occlusion effect with deeply sealed earmolds. *Hear Instrum* 1988;39:14–18.

Stenfelt S. Hearing by bone conduction: physical and physiological aspects. Doctoral thesis, Chalmers University of Technology, Göteborg, Sweden, 1999.

Stenfelt S, Goode RL. Bone-conducted sound: physiological and clinical aspects. *Otol Neurol* 2005;26:1245–1261.

Stenfelt S, Hato N, Goode R. Factors contributing to bone conduction: the middle ear. *J Acoust Soc Am* 2002;111: 947–959.

Stenfelt S, Puria S, Hato N, et al. Basilar membrane and osseous spiral lamina motion in human cadavers with air and bone conduction stimuli. *Hear Res* 2003a;181:131–143.

Stenfelt S, Wild T, Hato N, et al. Factors contributing to bone conduction: the outer ear. *J Acoust Soc Am* 2003b;113: 902–913.

Stenfelt S, Håkansson B, Tjellström A. Vibration characteristics of bone conducted sound. *J Acoust Soc Am* 1999; 105(2):1084.

Tonndorf J, Jahn F. Velocity of propagation of bone-conducted sound in a human head. *J Acoust Soc Am* 1981;70:1294–1297.

Tonndorf J. Compressional bone conduction in cochlear models. *J Acoust Soc Am* 1962;34:1127–1131.

Tonndorf J. Bone conduction: studies in experimental animals: a collection of seven papers. *Acta Otolaryngol* 1966;213(Suppl):1–132.

Von Békésy G. Zur theorie des hörens bei der schallaufnahme durch knochenleitung. *Ann Phys* 1932;13:111–136.

Watson N, Gales R. Bone-conduction threshold measurements: effects of occlusion, enclosures, and masking devices. *J Acoust Soc Am* 1943;14:207–215.

Zwislocki J. Acoustic attenuation between the ears. *J Acoust Soc Am* 1953;25:752–759.

Chapter 12

American National Standards Institute (ANSI). Acoustical Terminology. ANSI S1.1-1994. New York: ANSI, 1994.

American Speech Language Hearing Association (ASHA). Guidelines for manual pure-tone threshold audiometry. *ASHA* 1978;20:297–301.

Chandler DW, Grantham DW. Minimum audible movement angle in the horizontal plane. *J Acoust Soc Am* 1992;91:1624–1636.

Cardozo, BL. Adjusting the method of adjustment: SD vs DL. *J Acoust Soc Am* 1965;37:786–792.

Elliott LL. Backward masking: monotic and dichotic conditions. *J Acoust Soc Am* 1962;34:1116–1117.

Fletch H. Auditory patterns. *Reviews of Modern Physics* 1940;12:47–65.

Glasberg BR, Moore BCJ. Derivation of auditory filter shapes from notched-noise data. *Hear Res* 1990;47:103–138.

Grantham DW. Auditory motion perception: snapshots revisited. In: Anderson TR, Gilkey RH (eds.). Binaural and

Spatial Hearing in Real and Virtual Environments. Mahwah, NJ: Lawrence Erlbaum, 1997.

Grantham DW. Detection and discrimination of simulated motion of auditory targets in the horizontal plane. *J Acoust Soc Am* 1986;79:1939–1949.

Gulick WL. Hearing: Physiology and Psychophysics. New York: Oxford University Press, 1971.

Hartman WM. Signals, Sound, and Sensation. Modern Acoustics and Signal Processing. Woodbury, NY: AIP Press, 1997.

Hawkins D, Prosek R, Walden B, et al. Binaural loudness summation in the hearing impaired. *J Speech Hear Res* 1987;30(1):37–43.

Hawley M, Litovsky R, Culling J. The effect of binaural hearing in the cocktail party: effect of location and the type of interferer. *J Acoust Soc Am* 2004;115:833–843.

Hughson W, Westlake HD. Manual for program outline for rehabilitation of aural casualties both military and civilian. *Trans Am Acad Ophthalmol Otolaryngol* 1944;48(Suppl.):1–15.

Middlebrook JC, Green DM. Sound localization by human listeners. *Ann Rev Psychol* 1991;42:135–159.

Mills AW. Auditory localization. In: Tobias JV (ed.). Foundations of Modern Auditory Theory. Vol. 2. New York: Academic Press, 1972:301–348.

Moore BCJ, Glasberg BR. Suggested formulae for calculating auditory-filter bandwidths and excitation patterns. *J Acoust Soc Am* 1983;74:750–753.

Moore BCJ, Peters RW, Glasberg BR. Auditory filter shapes at low center frequencies. *J Acoust Soc Am* 1990;88:132–140.

Pantev C, Hoke M, Lütkenhöner B, et al. Tonotopic organization of the auditory cortex: pitch versus frequency representation. *Science* 1989;246:468–488.

Scharf B. Critical bands. In: Tobias JV (ed.). Foundations of Modern Auditory Theory. Vol. 1. New York: Academic Press, 1970:157–202.

Shower EG, Biddulph R. Differential pitch sensitivity of the ear. *J Acoust Soc Am* 1931;3:275–287.

Stevens SS. The relation of pitch to intensity. *J Acoust Soc Am* 1935;6:150–154.

Stevens SS. On the theory of scales of measurement. *Science* 1946;103:677–680.

Stevens. SS. Mathematics, measurement and psychophysics. In: Stevens SS (ed.). Handbook of Experimental Psychology. New York: Wiley, 1951:1–49.

Stevens SS. Psychophysics. In: Steven G (ed.). Introduction to Its Perceptual, Neural, and Social Prospects. New York, NY: John Wiley & Sons, 1975.

Stevens SS, Volkman J. The relation of pitch to frequency: a revised scale. *Am J Psychology* 1940;53:329–353.

Stevens SS, Volkmann J, Newman EB. A scale for the measurement of the psychological magnitude pitch. *J Acoust Soc Am* 1937;8:185–190.

Wegel RL, Lane CE. The auditory masking of pure tone by another and its probable relation to the dynamics of the inner ear. *Physiol Rev* 1924;23:266–285.

Zwicker E, Fastl H. On the development of the critical band. *J Acoust Soc Am* 1972;52:699–702.

Zwicker E, Fastl H. Psychoacoustics. 2nd Ed. Heidelberg, Germany: Springer Verlag, 1999.

Zwicker E, Flottorp G, Stevens SS. Critical bandwidth in loudness summation. *J Acoust Soc Am* 1957;29:548–557.

Zwislocki J. Theory of temporal auditory summation. *J Acoust Soc Am* 1960;32:1046–1060.

Chapter 13

Fause KR. Fundamentals of grounding, shielding, and interconnection. *J Audio Eng Soc* 1995;43(6):498–516.

Gibilisco S. Electricity Demystified. New York: McGraw Hill, 2005.

Macatee S. Considerations in grounding and shielding audio devices. The 97th AES Convention (Preprint 3916), San Francisco, CA, November 10–13, 1994.

Rich A. Shielding and guarding. *Analog Dialogue* 1982: 16-3–16-19.

Whitlock B. Balanced lines in audio systems – facts, fiction, and transformers. The 97th AES Convention (Preprint 3917), San Francisco, CA, November 10–13, 1994.

Chapter 14

Harris JD, Haines H, Kelsey R, et al. The relation between speech intelligibility and the electroacoustic characteristics of low fidelity circuitry. *J Auditory Res* 1961;1:357–381.

Jerger J, Speaks J, Malmquist C. Hearing aid performance and hearing aid selection. *J Speech Hear Res* 1966;9:136–149.

Olsen WO, Carhart R. Development of test procedures for evaluation of binaural hearing aids. *Bull Prosthet Res* 1967;10:22–49.

Chapter 15

Shannon CE. The Mathematical Theory of Commumication. Urbana, IL: University of Illinois Press, 1949.

Additional Help in Basic Mathematics

Bleu BL. Forgotten Algebra: A Self-Teaching Refresher Course. 2nd Ed. Hauppauge, NY: Barrons Educational Series, Inc., 1994.

Dallos P, Billone MC, Durrant JD, et al. Cochlear inner and outer hair cells: functional differences. *Science* 1972;177:356–358.

Isaacs A. A Dictionary of Physics. New York: Oxford University Press, 1996.

Prout JH, Bienvenue GB. Acoustics for You. Malabar, FL: Krieger Publishing Company, 1991.

Ross DA. Master Math: Algebra. Franklin Lakes, NJ: Career Press, 1996.

Schwartz DA, Purve D. Pitch is determined by naturally occurring periodic sounds. *Hear Res* 2004;194:31–46.

Selby P, Slavin S. Practical Algebra: A Self-Teaching Guide. 2nd Ed. New York: John Wiley & Sons, Inc., 1991.

Slavin S. All the Math You'll Ever Need: A Self-Teaching Guide. 2nd Ed. New York: John Wiley & Sons, Inc., 1999.

Sperling A, Stuart M. Mathematics Made Simple. 5th Ed. Revised by Christine M. Peckaitis. New York: Broadway Books, 2001.

Townsend TH, Weiss MS. Understanding Decibels for Windows. Parrott Software, Inc.

Weidner R Sells R. Elementary Classical Physics. Vol. 1–3. 7th Ed. Boston, MA: Allyn & Bacon, 1971.

Index

Page numbers in *italics* denote figures; those followed by *t* denote tables; those followed by *b* indicate boxes.